a LANGE clinical manual

Poisoning & Drug Overdose

First Edition

**San Francisco Bay Area
Regional Poison Control Center**

Edited by
Kent R. Olson, MD
Medical Director
San Francisco Bay Area Regional Poison Control Center
San Francisco General Hospital
Adjunct Lecturer in Pharmacy
Assistant Clinical Professor of Medicine
University of California, San Francisco

Associate Editors

Charles E. Becker, MD
Chief, Division of Occupational Medicine & Toxicology
San Francisco General Hospital
Professor of Medicine

Neal L. Benowitz, MD
Chief, Division of Clinical Pharmacology
Professor of Medicine

James F. Buchanan, PharmD
Coordinator of Medical Information, Genentech, Inc.
Assistant Clinical Professor of Pharmacy

Frank J. Mycroft, PhD, MPH
Staff Toxicologist, HESIS
California State Department of Health Services
Assistant Clinical Professor of Environmental Health

John Osterloh, MD, MS
Director, Toxicology Laboratory
San Francisco Department of Public Health
Associate Professor of Clinical Laboratory Medicine

Olga F. Woo, PharmD
Poison Information Specialist
Assistant Clinical Professor of Pharmacy

APPLETON & LANGE
Norwalk, Connecticut/San Mateo, California

0-8385-1297-6

Notice: Our knowledge in clinical sciences is constantly changing. As new information becomes available, changes in treatment and in the use of drugs become necessary. The authors and the publisher of this volume have taken care to make certain that the doses of drugs and schedules of treatment are correct and compatible with the standards generally accepted at the time of publication. The reader is advised to consult carefully the instruction and information material included in the package insert of each drug or therapeutic agent before administration. This advice is especially important when using new or infrequently used drugs.

Copyright © 1990 by Appleton & Lange
A Publishing Division of Prentice-Hall

90 91 92 93 94 / 10 9 8 7 6 5 4 3 2 1

Prentice Hall International (UK) Limited, *London*
Prentice Hall of Australia Pty. Limited, *Sydney*
Prentice Hall Canada, Inc., *Toronto*
Prentice Hall Hispanoamericana, S.A., *Mexico*
Prentice Hall India Private Limited, *New Delhi*
Prentice Hall of Japan, Inc., *Tokyo*
Simon & Schuster Asia Pte. Ltd., *Singapore*
Editora Prentice Hall do Brasil Ltda., *Rio de Janeiro*
Prentice Hall, *Englewood Cliffs, New Jersey*

Senior Developmental Editor: Anne Marie Zwierzyna
Production Editor: Christine Langan
Designer: Steven M. Byrum

ISBN 0-8385-1297-6
ISSN 1048-8847

PRINTED IN THE UNITED STATES OF AMERICA

a LANGE clinical manual

Poisoning & Drug Overdose
First Edition

**San Francisco Bay Area
Regional Poison Control Center**

Edited by
Kent R. Olson, MD
Medical Director
San Francisco Bay Area Regional Poison Control Center
San Francisco General Hospital
Adjunct Lecturer in Pharmacy
Assistant Clinical Professor of Medicine
University of California, San Francisco

Associate Editors

Charles E. Becker, MD
Chief, Division of Occupational Medicine & Toxicology
San Francisco General Hospital
Professor of Medicine

Neal L. Benowitz, MD
Chief, Division of Clinical Pharmacology
Professor of Medicine

James F. Buchanan, PharmD
Coordinator of Medical Information, Genentech, Inc.
Assistant Clinical Professor of Pharmacy

Frank J. Mycroft, PhD, MPH
Staff Toxicologist, HESIS
California State Department of Health Services
Assistant Clinical Professor of Environmental Health

John Osterloh, MD, MS
Director, Toxicology Laboratory
San Francisco Department of Public Health
Associate Professor of Clinical Laboratory Medicine

Olga F. Woo, PharmD
Poison Information Specialist
Assistant Clinical Professor of Pharmacy

APPLETON & LANGE
Norwalk, Connecticut/San Mateo, California

0-8385-1297-6

Notice: Our knowledge in clinical sciences is constantly changing. As new
information becomes available, changes in treatment and in the use of drugs
become necessary. The authors and the publisher of this volume have taken
care to make certain that the doses of drugs and schedules of treatment are
correct and compatible with the standards generally accepted at the time of
publication. The reader is advised to consult carefully the instruction and
information material included in the package insert of each drug or
therapeutic agent before administration. This advice is especially important
when using new or infrequently used drugs.

Prentice Hall International (UK) Limited, *London*
Prentice Hall of Australia Pty. Limited, *Sydney*
Prentice Hall Canada, Inc., *Toronto*
Prentice Hall Hispanoamericana, S.A., *Mexico*
Prentice Hall India Private Limited, *New Delhi*
Prentice Hall of Japan, Inc., *Tokyo*
Simon & Schuster Asia Pte. Ltd., *Singapore*
Editora Prentice Hall do Brasil Ltda., *Rio de Janeiro*
Prentice Hall, *Englewood Cliffs, New Jersey*

Senior Developmental Editor: Anne Marie Zwierzyna
Production Editor: Christine Langan
Designer: Steven M. Byrum

ISBN 0-8385-1297-6
ISSN 1048-8847

PRINTED IN THE UNITED STATES OF AMERICA

Contents

Contents

Contributors

All contributing editors and authors were staff, faculty, or fellows affiliated
with the San Francisco Bay Area Regional Poison Control Center at the time
of their contributions.

Ilene B. Anderson, PharmD
Margaret Atterbury, MD
Georganne M. Backman
Charles E. Becker, MD
Neal L. Benowitz, MD
Bruce Bernard, MD
Paul D. Blanc, MD
Christopher R. Brown, MD
James F. Buchanan, PharmD
Chris Dutra, MD
Donna E. Foliart, MD
Gail M. Gullickson, MD
Patricia Hess Hiatt, BS
Jeffrey R. Jones, MPH, CIH
Kathryn H. Keller, PharmD
Michael T. Kelley, MD
Susan Kim, PharmD
Belle L. Lee, PharmD
Timothy McCarthy, PharmD
Howard E. McKinney, PharmD
Frank J. Mycroft, PhD, MPH
Kent R. Olson, MD
John D. Osterloh, MD, MS
Gary Pasternak
Mary Tweig, MD
Peter H. Wald, MD, MPH
Olga F. Woo, PharmD
Evan T. Wythe, MD
Peter Yip, MD

Preface

Poisoning & Drug Overdose provides practical advice for the management of poisoning and drug overdose and essential information about industrial chemicals and occupational illness. It will be useful to medical students, house officers, physicians, pharmacists, and nurses in the practice of emergency medicine, critical care, pediatrics, internal medicine, and occupational medicine. Industrial hygienists and professional toxicologists involved in government, research, and industry will also find it helpful.

This manual outlines a comprehensive approach to management, including essential advice on how to diagnose and treat poisoning and how to recognize and treat common complications. In addition, it brings together information not found elsewhere in toxicology texts: detailed information on the use, adverse effects, and availability of antidotes; pharmacokinetic data on drugs and poisons; a comprehensive table of industrial chemicals; and a table of known or suspected carcinogens.

The manual is divided into 4 sections and an index, each one identified by black tabs in the right margins. **Section I** guides the user through initial emergency steps to physical diagnosis, laboratory tests, and methods of decontamination. **Section II** provides information on diagnosis and treatment of approximately 150 common drugs and poisons. Icons at the beginning of each topic provide a quick reference on the availability of antidotes and the advisability of various decontamination methods. **Section III** describes the use and side effects of about 60 common antidotes and therapeutic drugs. **Section IV** describes the urgent medical evaluation and management of occupational illness and the medical management of industrial accidents. This section includes a table of common industrial chemicals and a table of known or suspected human carcinogens. The Index is comprehensive and extensively cross-referenced.

The manual allows the reader to move quickly from section to section to obtain needed information from each. For example, in managing a patient with theophylline intoxication, the reader will find specific information about theophylline toxicity in Section II, practical advice for management and complications such as seizures or hypotension in Section I, and detailed information about dosing and potential side effects of esmolol in Section III. In this way, a complete discussion of each complication, each toxin, and each antidote is provided in a consistent manner, but without repetition, in a conveniently sized manual.

Poisoning and Drug Overdose is not meant to replace or compete with works such as *Poisindex*. It does not list products by brand name or provide an ingredient index. We assume that if the product ingested has been identified, its ingredients are already known or *Poisindex* or a poison control center (see Table I—41, p 51) has been consulted for ingredient information.

Acknowledgements

This manual would not have been possible without the combined efforts of the staff, faculty and fellows at the San Francisco Bay Area Regional Poison Control Center, to whom I am deeply indebted. From its inception, this book has been a project by and for our poison center; therefore, we decided that all royalties from its sale will go directly to the poison center's operating fund and not to any individual.

On behalf of the authors and editors, my sincere thanks to Bill Banner, Bob Levin, Peter Wald, and Tom Kearney, who reviewed various portions of the manuscript and provided many excellent suggestions. I am also grateful for the expert advice and assistance we have received from the staff at Lange Medical Publications, including early guidance from Jane Townsend and very patient and dedicated ongoing help from Anne-Marie Zwierzyna.

Finally, I owe a special thanks to Donna, Bradley, Marlene, and Gregory, who patiently watched and waited while I labored over this book for the past three years.

Kent R. Olson, MD
San Francisco
January 1990

Section I. Comprehensive Evaluation and Treatment of Poisoning and Overdose

Kent R. Olson, MD

EMERGENCY EVALUATION AND TREATMENT

Even though they may not appear acutely ill, all poisoned patients should be treated as if they have a potentially life-threatening intoxication. Below is a checklist (Fig I–1) of emergency evaluation and treatment procedures. More detailed information on diagnosis and treatment for each emergency step is referenced by page and presented immediately following the checklist.

Quickly review the checklist to determine the scope of appropriate interventions and **begin needed life-saving treatment.** If further information is required for any step, turn to the cited pages for detailed discussion of each topic. Although the checklist is presented in a **sequential format,** many steps may be performed **simultaneously** (eg, airway management, naloxone and dextrose administration, gastric lavage).

AIRWAY

I. **Assessment.** The greatest contributor to death from drug overdose or poisoning is loss of airway protective reflexes with subsequent airway obstruction by the flaccid tongue, pulmonary aspiration of gastric contents, or respiratory arrest. All patients should be suspected of having a potentially compromised airway.
   A. **Patients who are awake** and talking are likely to have intact airway reflexes, but worsening intoxication can result in rapid loss of airway control.
   B. **In lethargic or obtunded patients,** the gag or cough reflex may give an indirect estimation of the patient's ability to protect the airway. If there is any doubt, it is best to perform endotracheal intubation (see below).
II. **Treatment.** Optimize airway position and perform endotracheal intubation, if necessary. Early use of naloxone, 0.4–2 mg IV (see pp 18 and 325), may awaken a patient intoxicated with opiates and obviate the need for endotracheal intubation.
   A. **Position the patient and clear the airway (see Fig 1–2)**
      1. **Optimize airway position** to force the flaccid tongue forward and to maximize the airway opening. The following techniques are useful.
         a. Place the neck and head in the **"sniffing" position,** with the neck flexed forward and the head extended (Fig I–2b). *Caution:* Do *not* use this position if there is any suspicion of neck injury.
         b. Apply the **"jaw thrust"** to create forward movement of the tongue without flexing or extending the neck. Pull the jaw forward by placing the fingers of each hand on the angle of the mandible just below the ears (Fig I–2c). (This motion also provides a painful stimulus to the angle of the jaw, the response to which gives an estimate of the patient's depth of coma.)
         c. Place the patient in a **head-down, left-sided position** that allows the tongue to fall forward and secretions or vomitus to drain out of the mouth (Fig I–2d).
      2. If the airway is still not patent, examine the oropharynx and **remove any obstruction or secretions** by suction, by a sweep with the finger, or with Magill forceps.
      3. The airway can also be maintained with **artificial oropharyngeal or nasopharyngeal airway devices.** These are placed in the mouth or

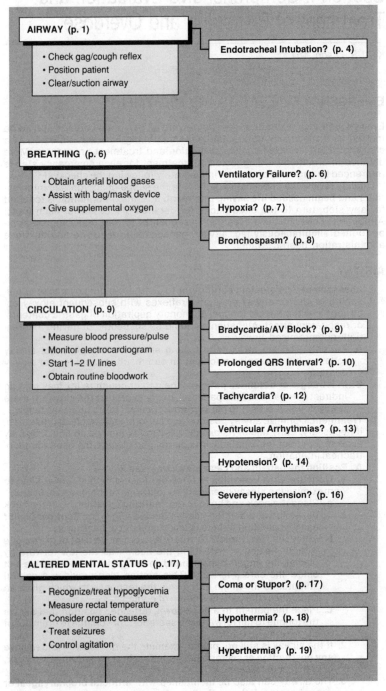

AIRWAY (p. 1)

- Check gag/cough reflex
- Position patient
- Clear/suction airway

Endotracheal Intubation? (p. 4)

BREATHING (p. 6)

- Obtain arterial blood gases
- Assist with bag/mask device
- Give supplemental oxygen

Ventilatory Failure? (p. 6)

Hypoxia? (p. 7)

Bronchospasm? (p. 8)

CIRCULATION (p. 9)

- Measure blood pressure/pulse
- Monitor electrocardiogram
- Start 1–2 IV lines
- Obtain routine bloodwork

Bradycardia/AV Block? (p. 9)

Prolonged QRS Interval? (p. 10)

Tachycardia? (p. 12)

Ventricular Arrhythmias? (p. 13)

Hypotension? (p. 14)

Severe Hypertension? (p. 16)

ALTERED MENTAL STATUS (p. 17)

- Recognize/treat hypoglycemia
- Measure rectal temperature
- Consider organic causes
- Treat seizures
- Control agitation

Coma or Stupor? (p. 17)

Hypothermia? (p. 18)

Hyperthermia? (p. 19)

Figure I–1. Checklist of emergency evaluation and treatment procedures. (Continued on p. 3.)

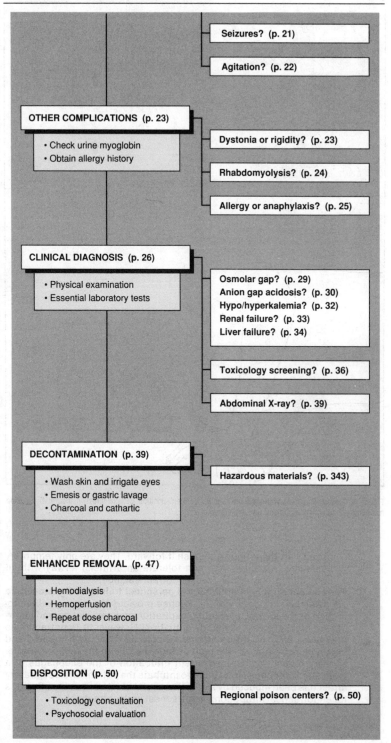

Seizures? (p. 21)

Agitation? (p. 22)

OTHER COMPLICATIONS (p. 23)
- Check urine myoglobin
- Obtain allergy history

Dystonia or rigidity? (p. 23)

Rhabdomyolysis? (p. 24)

Allergy or anaphylaxis? (p. 25)

CLINICAL DIAGNOSIS (p. 26)
- Physical examination
- Essential laboratory tests

Osmolar gap? (p. 29)
Anion gap acidosis? (p. 30)
Hypo/hyperkalemia? (p. 32)
Renal failure? (p. 33)
Liver failure? (p. 34)

Toxicology screening? (p. 36)

Abdominal X-ray? (p. 39)

DECONTAMINATION (p. 39)
- Wash skin and irrigate eyes
- Emesis or gastric lavage
- Charcoal and cathartic

Hazardous materials? (p. 343)

ENHANCED REMOVAL (p. 47)
- Hemodialysis
- Hemoperfusion
- Repeat dose charcoal

DISPOSITION (p. 50)
- Toxicology consultation
- Psychosocial evaluation

Regional poison centers? (p. 50)

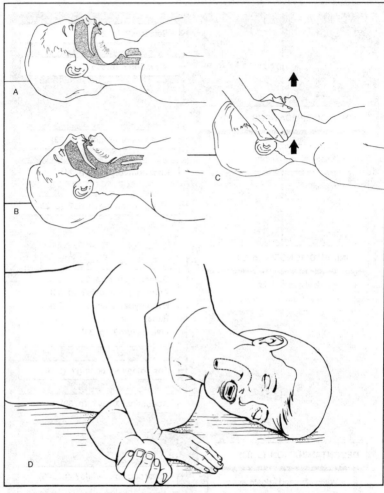

Figure I-2. Airway positioning. **A:** Normal position. **B:** "Sniffing" position. **C:** "Jaw thrust" maneuver. **D:** Left-side, head-down position, showing nasal and oral airway.

nose to lift the tongue and push it forward. They are only temporary measures. A patient who can tolerate an artificial airway without complaint probably needs an endotracheal tube.

B. Perform endotracheal intubation if personnel trained in the procedure are available. Intubation of the trachea provides the most reliable protection of the airway, preventing aspiration and obstruction and allowing for mechanically assisted ventilation. However, it is not a simple procedure and should be attempted only by those with training and experience. Complications include local trauma to the oropharynx, nasopharynx, and larynx; inadvertent intubation of the esophagus or a main stem bronchus; and failure to intubate the patient after respiratory arrest has been induced by a neuromuscular blocker. There are 2 routes for endotracheal intubation: nasotracheal and orotracheal.

1. Nasotracheal intubation. In nasotracheal intubation, a soft flexible tube is passed through the nose and into the trachea using a "blind" technique (Fig I–3a).
   a. Technique
   - **(1)** Instill local anesthetic and vasoconstrictor into the nose before the procedure to limit pain and bleeding. Use phenylephrine spray and 2% lidocaine jelly or 3–4 mL of a 5% cocaine solution.
   - **(2)** Pass the nasotracheal tube gently through the nose and into the nasopharynx. As the patient inspires, gently but firmly push the tube into the trachea. Success is usually marked by abrupt coughing.
   - **(3)** Check breath sounds to rule out accidental esophageal intubation or intubation of the right main stem bronchus.
   - **(4)** Secure the tube and fill the cuff balloon. (Tubes used for children do not have inflatable cuffs.)
   - **(5)** Obtain a chest x-ray to confirm appropriate tube placement.
   b. Advantages
   - **(1)** May be performed in a conscious patient without requiring neuromuscular paralysis.
   - **(2)** Once placed, it is better tolerated than orotracheal tube.
   c. Disadvantages
   - **(1)** Perforation of the nasal mucosa, with epistaxis.
   - **(2)** Stimulation of vomiting in an obtunded patient.
   - **(3)** Patient must be breathing spontaneously.
   - **(4)** Anatomically more difficult in infants because of anterior epiglottis.

2. Orotracheal intubation. In orotracheal intubation, the tube is passed through the mouth into the trachea under direct vision (Fig I–3b).
   a. Technique
   - **(1)** If the patient is not fully relaxed (eg, flaccid jaw and unrestricted neck mobility), induce neuromuscular paralysis with succinylcholine, 1–1.5 mg/kg IV (see p 326), or pancuronium, 0.1 mg/kg IV (see p 326). *Caution:* In children, succinylcholine may induce excessive vagal tone, resulting in bradycardia or asystole. Pretreat with atropine, 0.01 mg/kg IV, or use pancuronium for paralysis.
   - **(2)** Ventilate the patient manually with 100% oxygen while awaiting full paralysis (1–3 minutes).
   - **(3)** Using a lighted laryngoscope, visualize the larynx and pass the endotracheal tube into the trachea under direct vision.

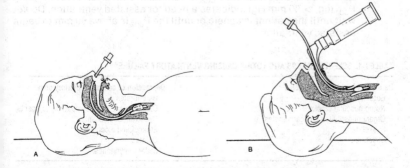

Figure I-3. Two routes for endotracheal intubation. **A:** Nasotracheal intubation. **B:** Orotracheal intubation.

          (4) Check breath sounds to rule out accidental esophageal intubation or intubation of the right main stem bronchus.

          (5) Secure the tube and inflate the cuff balloon. (Tubes used for children do not have inflatable cuffs.)

          (6) Obtain a chest x-ray to confirm appropriate tube position.

    b. Advantages

        (1) Performed under direct vision, making accidental esophageal intubation unlikely.

        (2) Insignificant risk of bleeding.

        (3) Patient need not be breathing spontaneously.

        (4) Higher success rate than that with nasotracheal route.

    c. Disadvantages

        (1) Frequently requires neuromuscular paralysis, creating risk of fatal respiratory arrest if intubation is unsuccessful.

        (2) Requires neck manipulation, which may cause spinal cord injury after neck trauma.

BREATHING

Along with airway problems, breathing difficulties are the major cause of morbidity and death in patients with poisoning or drug overdose. Patients may have one or more of the following complications: ventilatory failure, hypoxia, or bronchospasm.

  I. Ventilatory failure

    A. Assessment. Ventilatory failure has multiple causes, including failure of the ventilatory muscles, central depression of respiratory drive, and severe pneumonia or pulmonary edema. Examples of drugs and toxins that cause ventilatory failure and the causative mechanisms are listed in Table I–1.

    B. Complications. Ventilatory failure is the most common cause of death in poisoned patients.

      1. Hypoxia may result in brain damage, cardiac arrhythmias, and cardiac arrest.

      2. Hypercarbia results in acidosis, which may contribute to arrhythmias, especially in patients with cyclic antidepressant overdose.

    C. Differential diagnosis. Rule out:

      1. Bacterial or viral pneumonia.

      2. Viral encephalitis or myelitis (eg, polio).

      3. Traumatic or ischemic spinal cord or central nervous system injury.

      4. Tetanus, causing chest wall muscle rigidity.

    D. Treatment. Obtain arterial blood gases. The adequacy of ventilation is quickly estimated from the P_{CO2}; obtundation with an elevated or rising P_{CO2} (eg, > 60 mm Hg) indicates a need for assisted ventilation. Do **not** wait until the patient is apneic or until the P_{CO2} is above 60 mm to begin assisted ventilation.

TABLE I–1. SELECTED DRUGS AND TOXINS CAUSING VENTILATORY FAILURE[a]

Paralysis of ventilatory muscles	Depression of central respiratory drive
Botulin toxin	Barbiturates
Neuromuscular blockers	Clonidine and other sympatholytic agents
Organophosphates and carbamates	Cyclic antidepressants
Snakebite	Ethanol and alcohols
Strychnine	Opiates
	Sedative-hypnotics

[a] Adapted, with permission, from Olson KR, Pentel PR, Kelly MT: Physical assessment and differential diagnosis of the poisoned patient. *Med Toxicol* 1987;**2:**52.

1. **Assist breathing manually** with a bag-valve-mask device or bag-valve-endotracheal tube device until the mechanical ventilator is ready for use.
2. If not already accomplished, **perform endotracheal intubation.**
3. **Program the ventilator** for tidal volume (usually 15 mL/kg), rate (usually 12–15 breaths/min), and oxygen concentration (usually 30–35% to start). Frequently monitor the patient's response to ventilator settings by obtaining arterial blood gas values.
   a. If the patient has some spontaneous ventilations, the machine can be set to allow the patient to breathe spontaneously with only intermittent mandatory ventilation (usually 10–12 breaths/min).
   b. If the endotracheal tube was placed only for airway protection, the patient can be left to breathe entirely spontaneously with blow-by oxygen mist (T-piece).

II. **Hypoxia**
   A. **Assessment.** Examples of drugs or toxins causing hypoxia are listed in Table I–2. Hypoxia can be caused by the following conditions:
      1. **Insufficient oxygen** in ambient air (eg, displacement of oxygen by inert gases).
      2. **Disruption of oxygen absorption** by the lung (eg, due to pneumonia or pulmonary edema).
         a. **Pneumonia.** The most common cause of pneumonia in overdosed patients is pulmonary aspiration of gastric contents. Pneumonia may also be caused by intravenous injection of foreign material or bacteria, aspiration of petroleum distillates, or inhalation of irritant gases.
         b. **Pulmonary edema.** All the agents that can cause chemical pneumonia (eg, irritant gases, hydrocarbons) may also cause pulmonary edema. This usually involves alteration of pulmonary capillary permeability, resulting in **noncardiogenic** pulmonary edema (adult respiratory distress syndrome [ARDS]). In noncardiogenic pulmonary edema, the pulmonary capillary wedge pressure (reflecting left ventricular filling pressure) is usually normal or low. In contrast, **cardiogenic** pulmonary edema caused by cardiac-depressant drugs is characterized by low cardiac output with elevated pulmonary wedge pressure.
      3. **Cellular hypoxia,** which may be present despite a normal arterial blood gas value.
         a. Carbon monoxide poisoning (see p 109) and methemoglobinemia

TABLE I–2. SELECTED CAUSES OF HYPOXIA

Inert gases	**Pneumonia or noncardiogenic pulmonary edema**
Carbon dioxide	Aspiration of gastric contents
Methane and propane	Aspiration of hydrocarbons
Nitrogen	Chlorine and other irritant gases
Cardiogenic pulmonary edema	Cocaine
Beta blockers	Ethchlorvynol (IV and oral)
Cyclic antidepressants	Ethylene glycol
Quinidine, procainamide,	Metal fumes ("metal fumes fever")
and disopyramide	Mercury vapor
Verapamil	Nitogen dioxide
	Opiates
Cellular hypoxia	Paraquat
Carbon monoxide	Phosgene
Cyanide	Salicylates
Hydrogen sulfide	Sedative-hypnotic drugs
Methemoglobinemia	Smoke inhalation
Sulfhemoglobinemia	

(p 204) may severely limit oxygen binding to hemoglobin (and, therefore, oxygen-carrying capacity) without altering the P_{O_2}, because the routine blood gas determination measures dissolved oxygen in the plasma but does not measure actual oxygen content. In such cases, direct measurement of the oxygen saturation (with a co-oximeter but not a pulse oximeter) will reveal decreased oxyhemoglobin saturation.

    b. Cyanide poisoning (p 134) and hydrogen sulfide poisoning (p 169) interfere with cellular oxygen utilization, resulting in decreased oxygen uptake by the tissues, and may cause the venous oxygen saturation to be abnormally high.

B. Complications. Significant or sustained hypoxia may result in brain damage and cardiac arrhythmias.

C. Differential diagnosis
1. Erroneous sampling (eg, inadvertent venous blood gas).
2. Bacterial or viral pneumonia.
3. Pulmonary contusion caused by trauma.
4. Acute myocardial infarction with pump failure.

D. Treatment
1. **Correct hypoxia.** Administer supplemental oxygen as indicated based on arterial P_{O_2}. Intubation and assisted ventilation may be required.
     a. If carbon monoxide poisoning is suspected, give 100% oxygen (see p 109).
     b. See also treatment guides for cyanide (p 134), hydrogen sulfide (p 169), and methemoglobinemia (p 204).
2. **Treat pneumonia.** Obtain frequent sputum samples and initiate appropriate antibiotic therapy when there is evidence of infection.
     a. There is no basis for prophylactic antibiotic treatment of aspiration- or chemical-induced pneumonia.
     b. Although some physicians recommend corticosteroids for chemical-induced pneumonia, there is little evidence of their benefit.
3. **Treat pulmonary edema**
     a. Avoid excessive fluid administration. Pulmonary artery cannulation and wedge pressure measurements may be necessary to guide fluid therapy.
     b. Administer supplemental oxygen to maintain a P_{O_2} of at least 60–70 mm Hg. Endotracheal intubation and use of positive end-expiratory pressure (PEEP) ventilation may be necessary to maintain adequate oxygenation.

III. Bronchospasm

A. Assessment. Examples of drugs and toxins that cause bronchospasm are listed in Table I–3. Bronchospasm may result from the following:
1. **Direct irritant injury** from inhaled gases or pulmonary aspiration of petroleum distillates or stomach contents.
2. **Pharmacologic effects** of toxins, eg, organophosphate or carbamate insecticides or beta-adrenergic blockers.
3. **Hypersensitivity** or allergic reactions may also cause bronchospasm.

B. Complications. Severe bronchospasm may result in hypoxia and ventilatory failure.

TABLE I–3. SELECTED DRUGS AND TOXINS CAUSING BRONCHOSPASM

Beta blockers	Metal fumes ("metal fumes fever")
Chlorine and other irritant gases	Organophosphates and other anticholinesterases
Hydrocarbon aspiration	Smoke inhalation

C. **Differential diagnosis**
   1. Asthma or other preexisting bronchospastic disorder.
   2. Stridor caused by upper airway injury and edema (progressive airway edema may result in acute airway obstruction).
D. **Treatment**
   1. Administer supplemental oxygen.
   2. Remove the patient from the source of exposure to any irritant gas or other offending agent.
   3. Immediately discontinue any beta-blocker treatment.
   4. Administer bronchodilators:
      a. Aerosolized β_2 stimulant (eg, metaproterenol 0.6%, 2.5 mL in nebulizer [adult dose]).
      b. If this is not effective, and particularly for beta blocker-induced wheezing, give aminophylline, 6 mg/kg IV over 30 minutes.
   5. For patients with bronchospasm and bronchorrhea caused by organophosphate or other anticholinesterase poisoning, give atropine (see p 293).

CIRCULATION

I. **General assessment and initial treatment**
   A. **Check blood pressure and pulse rate and rhythm.** Perform cardiopulmonary resuscitation (CPR) if there is no pulse and advanced cardiac life support (ACLS) for arrhythmias and shock.
   B. **Begin continuous electrocardiographic (ECG) monitoring.** Arrhythmias may complicate a variety of drug overdoses, and all patients with potentially cardiotoxic drug poisoning should be monitored in the emergency department or an intensive care unit for at least 6 hours after the ingestion.
   C. **Secure venous access.** Antecubital or forearm veins are usually easy to cannulate. Alternative sites include femoral, subclavian, internal jugular, or other central veins. Central vein access is technically more difficult but allows measurement of central venous pressure and placement of pacemaker or pulmonary artery lines.
   D. **Draw blood** for routine studies (see p 28).
   E. **Begin intravenous infusion** of dextrose 5% in water (D5W); for children, use dextrose 5% in 0.25 normal saline. If the patient is hypotensive (see p 14), use normal saline, or other isotonic crystalloid solution.
   F. In seriously ill patients (eg, hypotensive, obtunded, convulsing, or comatose), **place a Foley catheter** in the bladder, obtain urine for routine and toxicologic testing, and measure hourly urine output.
II. **Bradycardia and atrioventricular (AV) block**
   A. **Assessment.** Examples of drugs and toxins causing bradycardia or AV block and their mechanisms are listed in Table I–4.
      1. Bradycardia and AV block are common features of intoxication with

TABLE I-4. SELECTED DRUGS AND TOXINS CAUSING BRADYCARDIA OR ATRIOVENTRICULAR BLOCK[a]

Cholinergic or vagotonic agents	**Sympatholytic agents**
Carbamate insecticides	Beta blockers
Digitalis glycosides	Clonidine
Organophosphates	Opiates
Physostigmine	**Other**
Membrane-depressant drugs	Phenylpropanolamine and other alpha-adrenergic agonists
Beta blockers	Calcium antagonists
Cyclic antidepressants	Lithium
Encainide and flecainide	Propoxyphene
Quinidine, procainamide, and disopyramide	

[a] Adapted, with permission, from Olson KR et al. *Med Toxicol* 1987;2:71.

calcium antagonists (see p 102) and drugs that depress sympathetic tone or increase parasympathetic tone. They may also result from severe intoxication with membrane-depressant drugs (eg, cyclic antidepressants, quinidine, other type Ia and type Ic antiarrhythmic agents).

2. Bradycardia or AV block may also be a reflex response (baroreceptor reflex) to hypertension induced by alpha-adrenergic agents such as phenylpropanolamine.
3. In children, bradycardia is commonly due to respiratory compromise and usually responds to ventilation and oxygenation.

B. **Complications**. Bradycardia and AV block frequently cause hypotension, which may progress to asystolic cardiac arrest.

C. **Differential diagnosis.** Rule out:
1. Hypothermia.
2. Myocardial ischemia or infarction.
3. Electrolyte abnormality (eg, hyperkalemia).
4. Metabolic disturbance (eg, hypothyroidism).
5. Intrinsic slow rate (common in athletes).
6. Cushing reflex (caused by severe intracranial hypertension).

D. **Treatment**. Do *not* treat bradycardia or AV block unless the patient is symptomatic (eg, syncope, hypotension). *Note:* Bradycardia may be a protective reflex to lower the blood pressure in a patient with life-threatening hypertension (see **VII**, below).
1. Maintain the airway and assist ventilation (see p 2) if necessary. Administer supplemental oxygen.
2. Rewarm hypothermic patients. A sinus bradycardia of 40–50/min is normal when the body temperature is 32–35 °C (90–95 °F).
3. Administer atropine, 0.01–0.03 mg/kg IV (p 293). If this is not successful, use isoproterenol 1–10 mcg/min IV (p 318), titrated to desired rate, or an emergency transcutaneous or transvenous pacemaker.
4. Use the following specific antidotes if appropriate:
   a. For beta-blocker overdose, give glucagon (p 314).
   b. For digitalis intoxication, use Fab fragments (p 304).
   c. For cyclic antidepressant or membrane-depressant drug overdose, administer sodium bicarbonate (p 296).
   d. For calcium antagonist overdose, give calcium (p 298).

III. **QRS interval prolongation**
A. **Assessment.** Examples of drugs and toxins causing QRS interval prolongation are listed in Table I–5.
1. QRS interval prolongation greater than 0.12 s in the limb leads (Fig I–4) is highly suggestive of serious poisoning by cyclic antidepressants (see p 136) or other membrane-depressant drugs (eg, propranolol). QRS interval prolongation in this setting reflects inhibition of sodium-dependent depolarization of cardiac tissue and is usually accompanied by QT interval prolongation, AV block, and depressed cardiac contractility. Normal QRS duration in patients with cyclic antidepressant overdose usually indicates a low risk for hypotension, arrhythmias, or seizures. A significant exception is the newer

TABLE I-5. SELECTED DRUGS AND TOXINS CAUSING QRS INTERVAL PROLONGATION[a]

Beta blockers (propranolol)	Hyperkalemia
Cyclic antidepressants	Phenothiazines (thioridazine)
Digitalis glycosides (complete heart block)	Propoxyphene
Diphenhydramine	Quinidine, procainamide, and disopyramide
Encainide and flecainide	

[a] Adapted, with permission, from Olson KR et al. *Med Toxicol* 1987;**2**:71.

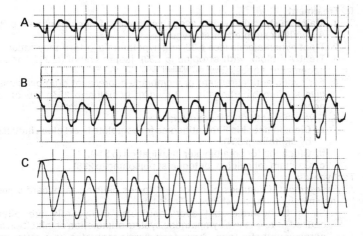

Figure I-4. Widened QRS interval caused by cyclic antidepressant overdose. **A:** Delayed intraventricular conduction results in prolonged QRS interval (0.18 s). **B** and **C:** Supraventricular tachycardia with progressive widening of QRS complexes mimics ventricular tachycardia. (Reproduced, with permission, from Benowitz NL, Goldschlager N: Cardiac disturbances in the toxicologic patient. Page 71 in: *Clinical Management of Poisoning and Drug Overdose.* Haddad LM, Winchester JF [editors]. Saunders, 1983.)

   antidepressant amoxapine, which causes serious central nervous system toxicity with normal QRS intervals.
   2. QRS interval prolongation may also be due to ventricular escape rhythm in a patient with complete heart block (eg, from digitalis or calcium antagonist poisoning).
B. **Complications.** QRS interval widening in cyclic antidepressant or membrane-depressant drug overdose is often accompanied by hypotension, AV block, and seizures.
C. **Differential diagnosis.** Rule out:
   1. Intrinsic conduction system disease (bundle branch block or complete heart block) due to coronary artery disease. Check an old ECG if available.
   2. Hyperkalemia with critical cardiac toxicity frequently appears as a sine wave pattern with markedly wide QRS complexes. These are usually preceded by peaked T waves (Fig I-7, p 33).
   3. Hypothermia with a core temperature of less than 32 °C (90 °F) often causes an extra terminal QRS deflection (J wave or Osborne wave), resulting in a widened QRS appearance (Fig I-5).

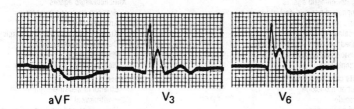

aVF   V₃   V₆

Figure I-5. Electrocardiogram of patient with hypothermia, showing prominent J waves. (Modified and reproduced, with permission, from Goldschlager N, Goldman MJ: Miscellaneous abnormal electrocardiogram patterns. Page 227 in: *Electrocardiography: Essentials of Interpretation.* Goldschlager N, Goldman MJ [editors]. Lange, 1984.)

D. Treatment

1. Maintain the airway and assist ventilation if necessary (see p 2). Administer supplemental oxygen.
2. Treat hyperkalemia (see p 32) and hypothermia (p 18) if they occur.
3. Treat AV block with atropine (p 293), isoproterenol (p 318), and a pacemaker if necessary.
4. For cyclic antidepressant or membrane-depressant drug overdose, give sodium bicarbonate, 1–2 meq/kg IV bolus (p 296); repeat as needed.
5. Give other antidotes if appropriate:
   a. Digoxin-specific Fab antibodies for complete heart block induced by digitalis (p 304).
   b. Glucagon for beta-blocker intoxication (p 314).
   c. Calcium for calcium antagonist poisoning (p 298).

IV. Tachycardia

A. Assessment. Examples of drugs and toxins causing tachycardia and their mechanisms are shown in Table I-6.

1. Sinus tachycardia and supraventricular tachycardia are often caused by excessive sympathetic system stimulation or inhibition of parasympathetic tone. Sinus tachycardia may also be a reflex response to hypotension or hypoxia.
2. Sinus tachycardia and supraventricular tachycardia accompanied by QRS interval prolongation (eg, with cyclic antidepressant overdose) may have the appearance of ventricular tachycardia (Fig I-4, p 11).

B. Complications. Simple sinus tachycardia (heart rate < 140/min) is rarely of hemodynamic consequence; children and healthy adults easily tolerate rates up to 160–180/min. However, sustained rapid rates may result in hypotension, chest pain, or syncope.

C. Differential diagnosis. Rule out:

1. Occult blood loss (eg, gastrointestinal bleeding, trauma).
2. Fluid loss (eg, gastritis, gastroenteritis).
3. Fever and infection.
4. Myocardial infarction.
5. Anxiety.
6. Intrinsic conduction system disease (eg, Wolff-Parkinson-White syndrome).

D. Treatment. If tachycardia is not associated with hypotension or chest pain, observation and sedation (especially for stimulant intoxication) are usually adequate.

1. For sympathomimetic-induced tachycardia, give propranolol, 0.01–0.03 mg/kg IV (p 338); or esmolol, 25–100 mcg/kg/min IV (p 311).

TABLE I-6. SELECTED DRUGS AND TOXINS CAUSING TACHYCARDIA[a]

Sympathomimetic agents	Anticholinergic agents
Amphetamines and derivatives	*Amanita muscaria* mushrooms
Caffeine	Antihistamines
Cocaine	Atropine and other anticholinergics
Ephedrine and pseudoephedrine	Cyclic antidepressants
Phencyclidine (PCP)	Phenothiazines
Theophylline	Plants (many)
Agents causing cellular hypoxia	**Other**
Carbon monoxide	Ethanol or sedative-hypnotic drug
Cyanide	withdrawal
Hydrogen sulfide	Hydralazine and other vasodilators
Oxidizing agents (methemoglobinemia)	Thyroid hormone

[a] Adapted, with permission, from Olson KR et al. *Med Toxicol* 1987;**2**:71.

TABLE I-7. SELECTED DRUGS AND TOXINS CAUSING VENTRICULAR ARRHYTHMIAS[a]

Ventricular tachycardia or fibrillation	QT prolongation or torsades de pointes
Amphetamines and other sympathomimetic agents	Amiodarone
Aromatic hydrocarbon solvents	Arsenic
Caffeine	Citrate
Chloral hydrate	Fluoride
Chlorinated or fluorinated hydrocarbon solvents	Organophosphate insecticides
Cocaine	Thallium
Cyclic antidepressants	
Digitalis glycosides	
Fluoride	
Phenothiazines	
Theophylline	

[a] Adapted, with permission, from Olson KR et al. *Med Toxicol* 1987;**2**:71.

    2. For anticholinergic-induced tachycardia, give physostigmine, 0.01–0.03 mg/kg IV (p 336); or neostigmine, 0.01–0.03 mg/kg IV. ***Caution:*** Do ***not*** use these drugs in patients with cyclic antidepressant overdose, because additive depression of conduction may result in asystole.

V. Ventricular arrhythmias
    A. Assessment. Examples of drugs and toxins causing ventricular arrhythmias are listed in Table I-7.
        1. Ventricular irritability is commonly associated with excessive sympathetic stimulation (eg, cocaine, amphetamines). Patients intoxicated by chlorinated, fluorinated, or aromatic hydrocarbons may have heightened myocardial sensitivity to the arrhythmogenic effects of catecholamines.
        2. Ventricular tachycardia may also be a manifestation of cyclic antidepressant or other membrane-depressant drug intoxication, although with these drugs true ventricular tachycardia may be difficult to distinguish from sinus or supraventricular tachycardia accompanied by QRS interval prolongation (Fig I-4, p 11).
        3. Agents that cause QT interval prolongation may produce "atypical" ventricular tachycardia (torsades de pointes). Torsades is characterized by polymorphous ventricular tachycardia that appears to rotate its axis continuously (Fig I-6). Torsades may also be caused by hypocalcemia or hypomagnesemia.
    B. Complications. Ventricular tachycardia with a pulse may be associated with hypotension or may deteriorate into pulseless ventricular tachycardia or ventricular fibrillation.
    C. Differential diagnosis. Rule out the following possible causes of ven-

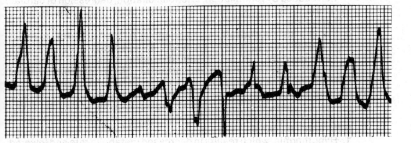

Figure I-6. Polymorphic ventricular tachycardia (torsades des pointes). (Modified and reproduced, with permission, from Goldschlager N, Goldman MJ: Effect of drugs and electrolytes on the electrocardiogram. Page 197 in: *Electrocardiography: Essentials of Interpretation.* Goldschlager N, Goldman MJ [editors]. Lange, 1984.)

tricular premature beats, ventricular tachycardia, or ventricular fibrillation.
1. Hypoxemia.
2. Hypokalemia.
3. Metabolic acidosis.
4. Myocardial ischemia or infarction.
5. Electrolyte disturbances (eg, hypocalcemia, hypomagnesemia) or congenital disorders that may cause QT prolongation and torsades.
D. **Treatment.** Administer CPR if necessary, and follow advanced cardiac life support (ACLS) guidelines for management of arrhythmias, with the exception that type Ia antiarrhythmic agents (eg, procainamide) should **not** be used, especially if cyclic antidepressant or membrane-depressant drug overdose is suspected.
1. Maintain the airway and assist ventilation if necessary (see p 2). Administer supplemental oxygen.
2. Correct acid-base and electrolyte disturbances.
3. **For ventricular fibrillation,** immediately apply direct current countershock at 3–5 J/kg. Repeat once if needed. Continue CPR if patient remains pulseless, and administer epinephrine, repeated countershocks, and lidocaine as recommended in ACLS guidelines.
4. **For ventricular tachycardia without a pulse,** immediately give a precordial thump or apply synchronized direct current countershock at 1–3 J/kg. If not successful, begin CPR and apply countershock at 3–5 J/kg; administer lidocaine and repeated countershocks as recommended in ACLS guidelines.
5. **For ventricular tachycardia with a pulse,** use lidocaine, 1–3 mg/kg IV (p 320); or phenytoin, 5–15 mg/kg IV (p 335). Do **not** use procainamide (Pronestyl) or other type Ia antiarrhythmic agents.
6. **For cyclic antidepressant or other membrane-depressant drug overdose,** administer sodium bicarbonate, 1–2 meq/kg IV (p 296), in repeated boluses until QRS interval narrows or serum pH exceeds 7.5.
7. **For "atypical" or polymorphic ventricular tachycardia (torsades):**
   a. Use overdrive pacing or isoproterenol, 1–10 mcg/min IV (p 318), to increase the heart rate (this makes repolarization more homogeneous and abolishes the arrhythmia).
   b. Alternately, administer magnesium sulfate, 1–2 g in adults, followed by infusion at 3–20 mg/min.
VI. **Hypotension**
A. **Assessment.** Examples of drugs and toxins causing hypotension and their mechanisms are listed in Table I–8.
1. Physiologic derangements resulting in hypotension include: volume loss due to vomiting, diarrhea, or blood loss; apparent volume depletion caused by venodilation; arteriolar dilation; depression of cardiac contractility; arrhythmias that interfere with cardiac output; and hypothermia.
2. Volume loss, venodilation, and arteriolar dilation are likely to result in hypotension with reflex tachycardia. In contrast, hypotension accompanied by bradycardia should suggest intoxication by sympatholytic agents, membrane-depressant drugs, calcium channel blockers, or cardiac glycosides or the presence of hypothermia.
B. **Complications.** Severe or prolonged hypotension can cause acute renal tubular necrosis, brain damage, and cardiac ischemia. Metabolic acidosis is a common finding.
C. **Differential diagnosis.** Rule out:
1. Hypothermia, which results in decreased metabolic rate and lowered blood pressure demands.

TABLE I-8. SELECTED DRUGS AND TOXINS CAUSING HYPOTENSION[a]

HYPOTENSION WITH RELATIVE BRADYCARDIA	HYPOTENSION WITH TACHYCARDIA
Sympatholytic agents	**Fluid loss or third spacing**
Beta blockers	Amatoxin-containing mushrooms
Bretylium	Arsenic
Clonidine, prazosin, and methyldopa	Colchicine
Hypothermia	Copper sulfate
Opiates	Hyperthermia
Reserpine	Iron
Tetrahydrozoline	Rattlesnake envenomation
	Sedative-hypnotic agents
Membrane-depressant drugs	
Beta blockers (mainly propranolol)	**Peripheral venous or arteriolar dilation**
Cyclic antidepressants	β_2-Stimulants (eg, metaproterenol, terbutaline)
Encainide and flecainide	Caffeine
Quinidine, procainamide, and disopyramide	Cyclic antidepressants
Propoxyphene	Hydralazine
	Hyperthermia
Others	Nitrites
Barbiturates	Sodium nitroprusside
Calcium antagonists	Phenothiazines
Cyanide	Theophylline
Fluoride	
Organophosphates and carbamates	
Sedative-hypnotic agents	

[a] Adapted, with permission, from Olson KR et al. *Med Toxicol* 1987;2:57.

    2. Hyperthermia, which causes arteriolar and venodilation and direct myocardial depression.

    3. Fluid loss caused by gastroenteritis.

    4. Blood loss (eg, from trauma or gastrointestinal bleeding).

    5. Myocardial infarction.

    6. Sepsis.

    7. Spinal cord injury.

D. Treatment. Fortunately, hypotension usually responds readily to empirical therapy with intravenous fluids and low doses of pressor drugs (eg, dopamine). When hypotension does not resolve after simple measures, a systematic approach should be followed to determine the cause of hypotension and to select the appropriate treatment.

    1. Maintain the airway and assist ventilation if necessary (see p 2). Administer supplemental oxygen.

    2. Treat cardiac arrhythmias that may contribute to hypotension (heart rate < 40–50/min or > 180–200/min [p 2]).

    3. Hypotension associated with hypothermia often will not improve with routine fluid therapy but will rapidly normalize upon rewarming of the patient. A systolic blood pressure of 80–90 mm Hg is expected when the body temperature is 32 °C (90 °F).

    4. Give a fluid challenge using normal saline, 10–20 mL/kg, or other crystalloid solution.

    5. Administer dopamine, 5–15 mcg/kg/min (p 307).

    6. Consider specific antidotes:

        a. Sodium bicarbonate (p 296) for cyclic antidepressant or membrane-depressant drug overdose.

        b. Glucagon (p 314) for beta-blocker overdose.

        c. Calcium (p 298) for calcium antagonist overdose.

        d. Propranolol (p 338) or esmolol (p 311) for theophylline, caffeine, or metaproterenol overdose.

    7. If the above measures are unsuccessful, insert a central venous pressure (CVP) monitor or pulmonary artery (PA) catheter to deter-

mine whether further fluids are needed and to measure the cardiac output (CO) and calculate the systemic vascular resistance (SVR = 80[MAP-CVP]/CO; normal SVR = 770–1500; MAP = mean arterial pressure). Select further therapy based on the results:

    a. If the central venous pressure or pulmonary artery wedge pressure remains low, give more intravenous fluids.

    b. If the cardiac output is low, give more dopamine (p 307) or dobutamine.

    c. If the systemic vascular resistance is low, administer norepinephrine (p 330).

VII. Hypertension

  A. Assessment. Hypertension is frequently overlooked in drug-intoxicated patients and often goes untreated. Many young persons have normal blood pressures in the range of 90/60 mm Hg to 100/70 mm Hg; in such a person an abrupt elevation to 170/100 is much more significant (and potentially catastrophic) than the same blood pressure elevation in an older person with chronic hypertension. Examples of drugs and toxins causing hypertension are listed in Table I–9. Hypertension may be caused by a variety of mechanisms:

    1. Amphetamines and other related drugs cause hypertension and tachycardia through generalized sympathetic stimulation.

    2. Selective alpha-adrenergic agents cause hypertension with reflex (baroreceptor-mediated) bradycardia or even AV block.

    3. Anticholinergic agents cause mild hypertension with tachycardia.

    4. Substances that stimulate nicotinic cholinergic receptors (eg, organophosphates) may initially cause tachycardia and hypertension, followed later by bradycardia and hypotension.

  B. Complications. Severe hypertension can result in intracranial hemorrhage, aortic dissection, myocardial infarction, and congestive heart failure.

  C. Differential diagnosis. Rule out:

    1. Idiopathic hypertension, which is common in the general population. However, without a prior history of hypertension it should not be initially assumed to be the cause of the elevated blood pressure.

    2. Increased intracranial pressure due to spontaneous hemorrhage, trauma, or other causes. This may result in hypertension with reflex bradycardia (Cushing reflex).

TABLE I–9. SELECTED DRUGS AND TOXINS CAUSING HYPERTENSION[a]

HYPERTENSION WITH TACHYCARDIA

Generalized sympathomimetic agents	Anticholinergic agents
Amphetamines and derivatives	Atropine and other anticholinergics
Cocaine	Antihistamines
Ephedrine	Cyclic antidepressants
Epinephrine	Phenothiazines
Levodopa	**Other**
LSD (lysergic acid diethylamide)	Ethanol and sedative-hypnotic drug withdrawal
Monoamine oxidase inhibitors	Nicotine (early stage)
Marihuana	Organophosphates (early stage)
Phencyclidine	

HYPERTENSION WITH BRADYCARDIA OR ATRIOVENTRICULAR BLOCK

Clonidine	Norepinephrine
Ergot derivatives	Phenylephrine
Methoxamine	Phenylpropanolamine

[a] Adapted, with permission, from Olson KR et al. *Med Toxicol* 1987;**2**:56.

D. Treatment. Rapid lowering of the blood pressure is desirable as long as it does not result in hypotension, which can potentially cause an ischemic cerebral infarction in older patients with cerebrovascular disease. For a patient with chronic hypertension, lowering the diastolic pressure to 100–110 mm Hg is acceptable. On the other hand, for a young person whose normal diastolic blood pressure is 60 mm Hg, the diastolic pressure should be lowered to 90–100 mm Hg.

1. **If hypertension is accompanied by a focally abnormal neurologic examination** (eg, hemiparesis), perform a computed tomography (CT) scan as quickly as possible. In a patient with a cerebrovascular accident, hypertension should not be treated unless specific complications of the elevated pressure (eg, heart failure, cardiac ischemia) are present. Consult a neurologist.

2. **For hypertension with little or no tachycardia,** use phentolamine, 0.02–0.1 mg/kg IV (see p 335); nifedipine, 0.1–0.2 mg/kg chewable capsule or liquid form (p 328); or nitroprusside, 2–10 mcg/kg/min IV (p 330).

3. **For hypertension with tachycardia,** add to the above treatment (see **2,** above) propranolol, 0.02–0.1 mg/kg IV (p 338); esmolol, 25–100 mcg/kg/min IV (p 311); or labetalol, 0.2–0.3 mg/kg IV (p 319). *Caution:* Do **not** use propranolol or esmolol alone to treat hypertensive crisis; beta blockers may paradoxically worsen hypertension if it is due primarily to alpha stimulation.

ALTERED MENTAL STATUS

I. Coma and stupor
A. Assessment.
Decreased level of consciousness is the most common serious complication of drug overdose or poisoning. Examples of drugs and toxins causing coma are listed in Table I–10.

1. Coma is most often a result of global depression of the brain's reticular activating system, caused by anticholinergic agents, sympatholytic drugs, generalized CNS depressants, or toxins that result in cellular hypoxia.
2. Coma sometimes represents a postictal phenomenon after a drug- or toxin-induced seizure.
3. Coma may also be caused by brain injury associated with infarction or intracranial bleeding. Brain injury is suggested by the presence of focal neurologic deficits and is confirmed by CT scanning.

TABLE I-10. SELECTED DRUGS AND TOXINS CAUSING COMA OR STUPOR[a]

General CNS depressants	**Cellular hypoxia**
Anticholinergics	Carbon monoxide
Antihistamines	Cyanide
Barbiturates	Hydrogen sulfide
Cyclic antidepressants	Methemoglobinemia
Ethanol and other alcohols	**Other or unknown mechanisms**
Phenothiazines	Bromide
Sedative-hypnotic agents	Diquat
Sympatholytic agents	Disulfiram
Clonidine	Hypoglycemic agents
Methyldopa	Lithium
Opiates	Phencyclidine
Tetrahydrozoline	Phenylbutazone and enolic acid derivatives
	Salicylates

[a] Adapted, with permission, from Olson KR et al. *Med Toxicol* 1987;**2**:61.

B. Complications. Coma is frequently accompanied by respiratory depression, which is a major cause of death. Other conditions that may accompany or complicate coma include hypotension (see p 14), hypothermia (p 18), hyperthermia (p 19), and rhabdomyolysis (p 24).

C. Differential diagnosis. Rule out:
1. Head trauma or other causes of intracranial bleeding.
2. Abnormal levels of blood glucose, sodium, or other electrolytes.
3. Hypoxia.
4. Hypothyroidism.
5. Liver or renal failure.
6. Environmental hyperthermia or hypothermia.
7. Serious infections such as encephalitis or meningitis.

D. Treatment
1. Maintain the airway and assist ventilation if necessary (see p 2). Administer supplemental oxygen.
2. Give dextrose, thiamine, and naloxone.
   a. Dextrose. All patients with depressed consciousness should receive concentrated dextrose unless hypoglycemia is ruled out with an immediate spot determination (eg, Dextrostix). Use a secure vein and avoid extravasation; concentrated dextrose is highly irritating to tissues.
      (1) Adults: Give 50% dextrose, 50 mL (25 g) IV.
      (2) Children: Give 25% dextrose, 2 mL/kg IV.
   b. Thiamine. Thiamine is given to prevent abrupt precipitation of Wernicke's syndrome due to thiamine deficiency in alcoholic patients and others with suspected vitamin deficiencies. It is *not* given routinely to children. Give thiamine, 100 mg, in the IV bottle or intramuscularly (p 340).
   c. Naloxone. All patients with respiratory depression should receive naloxone (p 325); if the patient is already intubated and being artificially ventilated, then naloxone is not immediately necessary and can be considered diagnostic rather than therapeutic. *Caution:* Although naloxone has no depressant activity of its own and can normally be given safely in large doses, it may precipitate abrupt opiate withdrawal. If amphetamines or cocaine has been injected along with heroin, reversal of the opiate-induced sedation may unmask stimulant-mediated hypertension, tachycardia, or psychosis. In addition, acute pulmonary edema is sometimes temporally associated with naloxone reversal of opiate intoxication.
      (1) Give naloxone, 0.4 mg IV (may also be given IM).
      (2) If there is no response within 1–2 minutes, give naloxone, 2 mg IV.
      (3) If there is still no response and opiate overdose is highly suspected by history or clinical presentation (pinpoint pupils, apnea, hypotension), give naloxone, 10–20 mg IV.
3. Normalize the body temperature (see hypothermia, p 18, or hyperthermia, p 19).
4. If there is any possibility of central nervous system trauma or cerebrovascular accident, perform a CT scan.
5. If meningitis or encephalitis is suspected, do a lumbar puncture and treat with appropriate antibiotics.

II. Hypothermia
A. Assessment. Hypothermia may mimic or complicate drug overdose and should be suspected in every comatose patient. Examples of drugs and toxins causing hypothermia are listed in Table I–11.
1. Hypothermia is usually caused by exposure to low ambient temperatures in a patient with blunted thermoregulatory response mecha-

TABLE I-11. SELECTED DRUGS AND TOXINS ASSOCIATED WITH HYPOTHERMIA[a]

Barbiturates	Opiates
Cyclic antidepressants	Phenothiazines
Ethanol and other alcohols	Sedative-hypnotic agents
Hypoglycemic agents	

[a] Adapted, with permission, from Olson KR et al. *Med Toxicol* 1987;2:60.

nisms. Drugs and toxins may induce hypothermia by causing vasodilation, inhibiting the shivering response, decreasing metabolic activity, or causing the person to lose consciousness in a cold environment.

2. The patient with a temperature lower than 32 °C (90 °F) may appear to be dead, with barely detectable pulse or blood pressure and with absent reflexes. The ECG may reveal an abnormal terminal deflection (J wave or Osborne wave, Fig I-5, p 11).

B. **Complications.** Because there is a generalized reduction of metabolic activity and less demand for blood flow, hypothermia is commonly accompanied by hypotension and bradycardia.

1. Mild hypotension (systolic blood pressure of 70–90 mm Hg) in a patient with hypothermia should *not* be aggressively treated; excessive intravenous fluids may cause fluid overload and further lowering of the temperature.

2. Severe hypothermia (temperature < 28–30 °C) may cause intractable ventricular fibrillation and cardiac arrest. This may occur abruptly, such as when the patient is moved or rewarmed too quickly or if CPR is performed.

C. **Differential diagnosis.** Rule out:

1. Sepsis.

2. Hypoglycemia.

3. Hypothyroidism.

4. Environmental hypothermia, caused by exposure to a cold environment.

D. **Treatment**

1. Maintain the airway and assist ventilation if necessary (see p 2). Administer supplemental oxygen.

2. Because the pulse rate may be profoundly slow (10/min) and weak, perform careful cardiac evaluation before assuming that the patient is in cardiac arrest. Do *not* treat bradycardia; it will resolve with rewarming.

3. Unless the patient is in cardiac arrest (asystole or ventricular fibrillation), rewarm slowly (using blankets, warm intravenous fluids, and warmed mist inhalation) to prevent rewarming arrhythmias.

4. For patients in cardiac arrest, usual antiarrhythmic agents and direct current countershock are frequently ineffective until the core temperature is above 32–35 °C (90–95 °F). Provide gastric or peritoneal lavage with warmed fluids and perform CPR. For ventricular fibrillation, bretylium, 5–10 mg/kg IV (see p 297), may be effective.

5. Open cardiac massage with direct warm irrigation of the ventricle, or partial cardiopulmonary bypass, may be necessary in hypothermic patients in cardiac arrest who are unresponsive to the above treatment.

III. **Hyperthermia**

A. **Assessment.** Hyperthermia (temperature > 40 °C or 104 °F) may be a catastrophic complication of intoxication by a variety of drugs and toxins (Table I-12).

1. Hyperthermia may be caused by excessive heat generation because

TABLE I-12. SELECTED DRUGS AND TOXINS ASSOCIATED WITH HYPERTHERMIA[a]

Excessive muscular hyperactivity, rigidity, or seizures	Impaired heat dissipation or disrupted thermoregulation
Amoxapine	Amoxapine
Amphetamines and derivatives	Anticholinergic agents
Cocaine	Antihistamines
Cyclic antidepressants	Cyclic antidepressants
Lithium	Phenothiazines and other antipsychotic agents
LSD (lysergic acid diethylamide)	**Other**
Maprotiline	Exertional heatstroke
Monoamine oxidase inhibitors	Malignant hyperthermia
Phencyclidine	Metal fumes fever
Increased metabolic rate	Neuroleptic malignant syndrome
Dinitrophenol and pentachlorophenol	Withdrawal from ethanol or sedative-hypnotic drugs
Salicylates	
Thyroid hormone	

[a] Adapted, with permission, from Olson KR et al. *Med Toxicol* 1987;**2**:59.

of sustained seizures, rigidity, or other muscular hyperactivity; increased metabolic rate; impaired dissipation of heat secondary to absent sweating (eg, anticholinergic agents); or hypothalamic disorders.

2. **Neuroleptic malignant syndrome (NMS)** is a hyperthermic disorder seen in patients chronically using antipsychotic agents and is characterized by hyperthermia, muscle rigidity (often "lead-pipe"), metabolic acidosis, and confusion.

3. **Malignant hyperthermia** is an inherited disorder that causes severe hyperthermia, metabolic acidosis, and rigidity after use of certain anesthetic agents.

B. **Complications.** Untreated hyperthermia is likely to result in hypotension, rhabdomyolysis, coagulopathy, cardiac and renal failure, brain injury, and death. Survivors often have permanent neurologic sequelae.

C. **Differential diagnosis.** Rule out:
   1. Sedative-hypnotic drug or ethanol withdrawal (delirium tremens).
   2. Exertional or environmental heat stroke.
   3. Thyrotoxicosis.
   4. Meningitis or encephalitis.
   5. Other serious infections.

D. **Treatment. Immediate rapid cooling** is essential to prevent death or serious brain damage.
   1. Maintain the airway and assist ventilation if necessary (see p 2). Administer supplemental oxygen.
   2. Administer glucose-containing intravenous fluids, and give concentrated dextrose bolus (p 315) if the patient is hypoglycemic.
   3. Rapidly gain control of seizures (p 21), agitation (p 22), or muscular rigidity (p 23).
   4. Begin external cooling with tepid (lukewarm) sponging and fanning. This evaporative method is the most efficient way of cooling. Other methods include iced gastric or colonic lavage or even ice-water immersion.
   5. Shivering often occurs with rapid external cooling, and shivering may generate yet more heat. Some physicians recommend chlorpromazine to abolish shivering, but this agent can lower the seizure threshold and may cause hypotension. It is preferable to use diazepam, 0.1–0.2 mg/kg IV (p 302); midazolam, 0.05–0.1 mg/kg IV (p 323); or neuromuscular paralysis (see below).
   6. The most rapidly effective and reliable means of lowering the tem-

perature is by neuromuscular paralysis. Administer pancuronium, 0.1 mg/kg IV (p 326); or vecuronium, 0.1 mg/kg IV. *Caution:* The patient will stop breathing; be prepared to ventilate and intubate endotracheally.

7. If muscle rigidity persists despite administration of neuromuscular blockers, a defect at the muscle cell level (ie, malignant hyperthermia) should be suspected. Give dantrolene, 1–10 mg/kg IV (p 300).

IV. Seizures

A. Assessment. Seizures are a major cause of morbidity and mortality from drug overdose or poisoning. Seizures may be single and brief or multiple and sustained and may result from a variety of mechanisms (Table I–13).

1. Generalized seizures usually result in loss of consciousness, often accompanied by tongue biting and fecal and urinary incontinence.
2. Other causes of muscular hyperactivity or rigidity (see p 23) may be mistaken for seizures, especially if the patient is also unconscious.

B. Complications

1. Any seizure can cause airway compromise, resulting in apnea or pulmonary aspiration.
2. Multiple or prolonged seizures may cause severe metabolic acidosis, hyperthermia, rhabdomyolysis, and brain damage.

C. Differential diagnosis. Rule out:

1. Serious metabolic disturbance (hypoglycemia, hyponatremia, hypocalcemia, hypoxia).
2. Head trauma with intracranial injury.
3. Idiopathic epilepsy.
4. Alcohol or sedative-hypnotic drug withdrawal.
5. Exertional or environmental hyperthermia.
6. Central nervous system infection such as meningitis or encephalitis.

D. Treatment

1. Maintain the airway and assist ventilation if necessary (see p 2). Administer supplemental oxygen.

TABLE I–13. SELECTED DRUGS AND TOXINS CAUSING SEIZURES[a]

Adrenergic-sympathomimetic agents	**Antidepressants and antipsychotics**
Amphetamines and derivatives	Amoxapine
Caffeine	Cyclic antidepressants
Cocaine	Haloperidol and butyrophenones
Phencyclidine	Loxapine
Phenylpropanolamine	Phenothiazines
Theophylline	
Others	
Antihistamines (diphenhydramine, hydroxyzine)	Fluoride
Beta blockers (primarily propranolol; not	Isoniazid
reported for atenolol, metoprolol, pindolol,	Lead and other heavy metals
or practolol)	Lidocaine and other local anesthetics
Boric acid	Lithium
Camphor	Mefenamic acid
Carbamazepine	Meperidine
Cellular hypoxia (eg, carbon monoxide, cyanide,	Metaldehyde
hydrogen sulfide)	Methanol
Chlorinated hydrocarbon solvents and insecticides	Phenols
Cholinergic agents (carbamates, nicotine,	Phenylbutazone
organophosphates)	Piroxicam
Cicutoxin and other plant toxins	Salicylates
Citrate	Strychnine (opisthotonus and rigidity)
DET (insect repellant)	Withdrawal from ethanol or sedative-
Ethylene glycol	hypnotic drugs

[a] Adapted, with permission, from Olson KR et al. *Med Toxicol* 1987;2:63.

2. Administer naloxone (p 18) if seizures are thought to be due to hypoxia caused by narcotic-associated respiratory depression.
3. Check for hypoglycemia and administer dextrose and thiamine as for coma (p 18).
4. Use one or more of the following anticonvulsants: **Caution:** Anticonvulsants can cause hypotension, cardiac arrest, or respiratory arrest if administered rapidly.
   a. Diazepam, 0.1–0.2 mg/kg IV (p 302).
   b. Midazolam, 0.1–0.2 mg/kg IM (useful when intravenous access is difficult; p 323).
   c. Phenobarbital, 10–15 mg/kg IV, slow infusion over 15–20 minutes (p 334).
   d. Phenytoin, 15–20 mg/kg IV, slow infusion over 25–30 minutes (p 335).
   e. Pentobarbital, 5–6 mg/kg IV, slow infusion over 8–10 minutes, then continuous infusion at 0.5–3 mg/kg/h titrated to effect (p 333).
5. Immediately check the rectal or tympanic temperature and cool the patient rapidly (p 19) if the temperature is above 40 °C (104 °F). The most rapid and reliably effective method of temperature control is neuromuscular paralysis with pancuronium, 0.1 mg/kg IV (p 326). **Caution:** If paralysis is used, the patient must be intubated and ventilated; in addition, monitor the electroencephalogram (EEG) for continued brain seizure activity because peripheral muscular hyperactivity is no longer visible.
6. Use specific antidotes if available:
   a. Pyridoxine for isoniazid (INH; p 339).
   b. Pralidoxime (2-PAM) or atropine, or both, for organophosphate or carbamate insecticides (p 337).

V. Agitation, delirium, or psychosis

A. **Assessment.** Agitation, delirium, or psychosis may be caused by a variety of drugs and toxins (Table I–14). In addition, such symptoms may be due to a functional thought disorder or metabolic encephalopathy resulting from medical illness.
1. Functional psychosis or stimulant-induced agitation and psychosis are usually associated with an intact sensorium, and hallucinations are predominantly auditory.
2. With metabolic encephalopathy or drug-induced delirium, there is usually alteration of sensorium (confusion, disorientation). Hallucinations, when they occur, are predominantly visual.

B. **Complications.** Agitation, especially if accompanied by hyperkinetic behavior and struggling, may result in hyperthermia (see p 19) and rhabdomyolysis (see p 24).

TABLE I-14. SELECTED DRUGS AND TOXINS CAUSING AGITATION, DELIRIUM, OR CONFUSION[a]

Predominant confusion or delirium	Predominant agitation or psychosis
Amantadine	Amphetamines and derivatives
Anticholinergic agents	Caffeine
Antihistamines	Cocaine
Carbon monoxide	LSD (lysergic acid diethylamide)
Cimetidine	Marihuana
Disulfiram	Phencyclidine (PCP)
Lead and other heavy metals	Phenylpropanolamine
Levodopa	Procaine
Lidocaine and other local anesthetics	Theophylline
Lithium	
Salicylates	
Withdrawal from ethanol or sedative-hypnotics	

[a] Adapted, with permission, from Olson KR et al. *Med Toxicol* 1987;2:62.

   C. Differential diagnosis. Rule out:
      1. Serious metabolic disturbance (hypoxia, hypoglycemia, hyponatremia).
      2. Alcohol or sedative-hypnotic drug withdrawal.
      3. Thyrotoxicosis.
      4. Central nervous system infection such as meningitis or encephalitis.
      5. Exertional or environmental hyperthermia.
   D. Treatment. Sometimes the patient can be calmed with reassuring words and by eliminating excessive noise, light, and physical stimulation. If this is not quickly effective, rapidly gain control of the patient in order to determine the rectal or tympanic temperature and to begin rapid cooling and other treatment if needed.
      1. Maintain the airway and assist ventilation if necessary (see p 2). Administer supplemental oxygen.
      2. Treat hypoglycemia (p 31), hypoxia (p 7), or other metabolic disturbances.
      3. Administer one of the following sedatives:
         a. Midazolam, 0.05–0.1 mg/kg IV over 1 minute (p 323), or 0.1–0.2 mg/kg IM (p 323).
         b. Diazepam, 0.1–0.2 mg/kg IV over 1 minute (p 302).
         c. Haloperidol, 0.1–0.2 mg/kg IM, or IV over 1 minute (p 315). *Note:* Do not give decanoate salt IV.
      4. If hyperthermia occurs as a result of excessive muscular hyperactivity, then skeletal muscle paralysis is indicated: Use pancuronium, 0.1 mg/kg IV (see p 326). *Caution:* Be prepared to ventilate and endotracheally intubate the patient after muscle paralysis.

OTHER COMPLICATIONS

  I. Dystonia, dyskinesia, and rigidity
    A. Assessment. Examples of drugs and toxins causing abnormal movements or rigidity are listed in Table I–15.
      1. **Dystonic reactions** are common with therapeutic or toxic doses of many antipsychotic agents and with some antiemetics. The mechanism is thought to be related to central dopamine blockade. Dystonias usually consist of forced, involuntary, and often painful neck rotation (torticollis); tongue protrusion, jaw extension, or trismus. Other extrapyramidal or parkinsonian movement disorders (eg, pill rolling, bradykinesia, masked facies) may also be seen with these agents.

TABLE I–15. SELECTED DRUGS AND TOXINS CAUSING DYSTONIAS, DYSKINESIAS, AND RIGIDITY[a]

Dystonia	Dyskinesias
Haloperidol and butyrophenones	Amphetamines
Metoclopramide	Anticholinergic agents
Phenothiazines	Antihistamines
Rigidity	Caffeine
Black widow spider bite	Cocaine
Lithium	Cyclic antidepressants
Malignant hyperthermia	Ketamine
Methaqualone	Levodopa
Monoamine oxidase inhibitors	Lithium
Neuroleptic malignant syndrome	Phencyclidine (PCP)
Phencyclidine (PCP)	
Strychnine	

[a] Adapted, with permission, from Olson KR et al. *Med Toxicol* 1987;**2**:64.

2. In contrast, **dyskinesias** are usually rapid, repetitive body movements that may involve small localized muscle groups (eg, tongue darting, focal myoclonus) or may consist of generalized hyperkinetic activity. The cause is not dopamine blockade but, more commonly, increased dopamine effect or blockade of central cholinergic effect.

3. **Rigidity** may also be seen with a number of toxins and may be due to central nervous system effects or spinal cord stimulation. Neuroleptic malignant syndrome (see p 20) is characterized by rigidity, hyperthermia, metabolic acidosis, and altered mental status. Rigidity seen with malignant hyperthermia (see p 20) is caused by a defect at the muscle cell level and may not reverse with neuromuscular blockade.

B. **Complications.** Sustained muscular rigidity or hyperactivity may result in rhabdomyolysis (see p 24), hyperthermia (p 19), ventilatory failure (p 6), or metabolic acidosis (p 30).

C. **Differential diagnosis.** Rule out:
   1. Catatonic rigidity caused by functional thought disorder.
   2. Tetanus.
   3. Cerebrovascular accident.
   4. Postanoxic encephalopathy.
   5. Idiopathic parkinsonism.

D. **Treatment**
   1. Maintain the airway and assist ventilation if necessary (see p 2). Administer supplemental oxygen.
   2. Check the rectal or tympanic temperature, and treat hyperthermia (p 19) rapidly if the temperature is above 39 °C (102.2 °F).
   3. **Dystonia.** Administer an anticholinergic agent such as diphenhydramine (Benadryl; p 305), 0.5–1 mg/kg IM or IV; or benztropine (Cogentin; p 295), 1–4 mg IM in adults. Follow with oral therapy for 2–3 days.
   4. **Dyskinesia.** Do **not** treat with anticholinergic agents. Instead, administer a sedative such as diazepam, 0.1–0.2 mg/kg IV (p 302); or midazolam, 0.05–0.1 mg/kg IV or 0.1–0.2 mg/kg IM (p 323).
   5. **Rigidity.** Do **not** treat with anticholinergic agents. Instead, administer a sedative (see **4**, above) or provide specific pharmacologic therapy:
      a. Intravenous calcium for black widow spider bite (p 298).
      b. Dantrolene (p 300) for malignant hyperthermia.

II. **Rhabdomyolysis**
   A. **Assessment.** Muscle cell necrosis is a common complication of poisoning. Examples of drugs and toxins causing rhabdomyolysis are listed in Table I–16.
      1. Mechanisms of rhabdomyolysis include prolonged immobilization on a hard surface, excessive seizures or muscular hyperactivity,

TABLE I-16. SELECTED DRUGS AND TOXINS ASSOCIATED WITH RHABDOMYOLYSIS

Excessive muscular hyperactivity, rigidity, or seizures	Direct cellular toxicity
Amphetamines and derivatives	Amatoxin-containing mushrooms
Cocaine	Carbon monoxide
Cyclic antidepressants	Colchicine
Lithium	Ethylene glycol
Monoamine oxidase inhibitors	**Other or unknown mechanisms**
Phencyclidine (PCP)	Barbiturates (prolonged immobility)
Seizures caused by a variety of agents	Ethanol
Strychnine	Hyperthermia caused by a variety of agents
Tetanus	Sedative-hypnotic agents (prolonged immobility)
	Trauma

hyperthermia, or direct cytotoxic effects of the drug or toxin (eg, carbon monoxide, colchicine, *Amanita phalloides* mushrooms).
  2. The diagnosis is made by finding hematest-positive urine with few or no intact red blood cells or an elevated serum creatine phosphokinase (CPK) level.
  B. Complications. Myoglobin released into the circulation may precipitate in the kidneys, causing acute tubular necrosis and renal failure. This usually occurs only when the serum CPK level exceeds 10,000 units. With severe rhabdomyolysis, hyperkalemia, hyperphosphatemia, and hypocalcemia may also occur.
  C. Differential diagnosis. Hemolysis with hemoglobinuria may also produce hematest-positive urine with no intact red blood cells.
  D. Treatment
  1. Establish a steady urine flow rate (2–3 mL/kg/h) with intravenous fluids. For massive rhabdomyolysis accompanied by oliguria, administer mannitol, 0.5 g/kg IV.
  2. Alkalinize the urine by adding 100 meq of sodium bicarbonate to each L of 5% dextrose. Acidic urine promotes deposition of myoglobin in the tubules.
  3. Provide intensive supportive care, including hemodialysis, for acute renal failure. Kidney function is usually regained in 2–3 weeks.
III. Anaphylactic and anaphylactoid reactions
  A. Assessment. Examples of drugs and toxins causing anaphylactic or anaphylactoid reactions are listed in Table I–17. These reactions are characterized by bronchospasm and increased vascular permeability that may lead to laryngeal edema, skin rash, and hypotension.
  1. **Anaphylaxis** occurs when a patient with antigen-specific immunoglobulin E (IgE) bound to the surface of mast cells and basophils is exposed to the antigen, triggering the release of histamine and various other vasoactive compounds.
  2. **Anaphylactoid reactions** are also caused by release of active compounds from mast cells but do not involve prior sensitization or mediation through IgE.
  B. Complications. Severe anaphylactic or anaphylactoid reactions can result in laryngeal obstruction, respiratory arrest, hypotension, and death.
  C. Differential diagnosis. Eliminate the following conditions.
  1. Anxiety, with vasodepressor syncope or hyperventilation.
  2. Pharmacologic effects of the drug or toxin (eg, procaine reaction with procaine penicillin).
  3. Bronchospasm or laryngeal edema from irritant gas exposure.
  D. Treatment
  1. Maintain the airway and assist ventilation if necessary (see p 2). Endotracheal intubation may be needed if laryngeal swelling is severe. Administer supplemental oxygen.

TABLE I-17. EXAMPLES OF DRUGS AND TOXINS CAUSING ANAPHYLACTIC OR ANAPHYLACTOID REACTIONS

Anaphylactic reactions (IgE-mediated)	Anaphylactoid reactions (not IgE-mediated)
Antisera (antivenins)	Acetylcysteine
Foods (nuts, fish, shellfish)	Blood products
Hymenoptera and other insect stings	Iodinated contrast media
Immunotherapy allergen extracts	Opiates
Penicillins and other antibiotics	Scombroid
Vaccines	Tubocurarine
Other or unclassified	
Exercise	
Sulfites	

2. Treat hypotension with intravenous crystalloid fluids (eg, normal saline) and place patient in supine position.
3. Administer epinephrine (p 309):
   a. Mild to moderate reactions: 0.3–0.5 mg SC (children, 0.01 mg/kg; maximum 0.5 mg).
   b. Severe reactions: 0.05–0.1 mg IV bolus every 5 minutes, or an infusion of 1–4 mcg/min.
4. Administer diphenhydramine (Benadryl; p 305), 0.5–1 mg/kg IV over 1 minute. Follow with oral therapy for 2–3 days.
5. Administer corticosteroid such as hydrocortisone, 200–300 mg IV; or methylprednisolone, 40–80 mg IV.

DIAGNOSIS OF POISONING

Diagnosis and treatment of poisoning often must proceed rapidly without the results of extensive toxicologic screening. Fortunately, in most cases the correct diagnosis can be made by using carefully collected data from the history, a directed physical examination, and commonly available laboratory tests.

I. **History.** Although frequently unreliable or incomplete, the history of ingestion may be very useful if carefully obtained.
   A. Ask the patient about all drugs taken, including nonprescription drugs or vitamins.
   B. Ask family members, friends, and paramedical personnel about any prescriptions or over-the-counter medications known to be used by the patient or others in the house.
   C. Obtain any available drugs or drug paraphernalia for later testing, but handle them very carefully to avoid poisoning by skin contact or inadvertent needle stick with potential for HIV transmission.
   D. Check with the pharmacy on the label of any medications found with the patient to determine if other prescription drugs have been obtained there.

II. **Physical examination**
   A. **General findings.** Perform a carefully directed examination emphasizing key physical findings that may uncover one of the common **autonomic syndromes;** this may suggest a certain class of drugs or toxins and specific empirical treatment. Important variables in the autonomic physical examination include blood pressure, pulse rate, pupil size, sweating, and peristaltic activity. The autonomic syndromes are summarized in Table I–18.
      1. **Alpha-adrenergic syndrome.** Hypertension with reflex bradycardia is characteristic. The pupils are usually dilated. (Examples: phenylpropanolamine, phenylephrine, methoxamine.)
      2. **Beta-adrenergic syndrome.** β_2-mediated vasodilation may cause hypotension. Tachycardia is common. (Examples: terbutaline, metaproterenol, theophylline, caffeine.)
      3. **Mixed alpha- and beta-adrenergic syndrome.** Hypertension is accompanied by tachycardia. The pupils are dilated. The skin is sweaty, although mucous membranes are dry. (Examples: cocaine, amphetamines, phencyclidine.)
      4. **Sympatholytic syndrome.** Blood pressure and pulse rate are both decreased (peripheral alpha blockers such as hydralazine may cause hypotension with reflex tachycardia). The pupils are small, often pinpoint. Peristalsis is often decreased. (Examples: agents that decrease central nervous system sympathetic output, such as centrally acting α_2 agonists [clonidine, methyldopa], opiates, phenothiazines.)
      5. **Nicotinic cholinergic syndrome.** Stimulation of nicotinic receptors at autonomic ganglia activates both parasympathetic and sympathetic systems, with unpredictable results. Excessive stimulation fre-

TABLE I-18. AUTONOMIC SYNDROMES[a,b]

	Blood Pressure	Pulse Rate	Pupil Size	Sweating	Peristalsis
Alpha-adrenergic	+ +	−	+ +	+	−
Beta-adrenergic	±	+ +	±	±	±
Mixed adrenergic	+ +	+ +	+ +	+ +	−
Sympatholytic	−	−	− −	−	
Nicotinic	+	+	±	+ +	+ +
Muscarinic	−	− −	− −	+ +	+ +
Mixed cholinergic	±	±	− −	+ +	+ +
Anticholinergic	+	+ +	+ +	− −	− −

[a] Key to symbols: + = increased; + + = markedly increased; − = decreased; − − = markedly decreased; ± = mixed effect, no effect, or unpredictable.
[b] Adapted, with permission, from Olson KR et al. Med Toxicol 1987;2:54.

quently causes depolarization blockade. Thus, initial tachycardia may be followed by bradycardia and muscle fasciculations may be followed by paralysis. (Examples: nicotine; in addition, the depolarizing neuromuscular blocker succinylcholine which acts on nicotinic receptors in skeletal muscle.)

6. **Muscarinic cholinergic syndrome.** Muscarinic receptors are located at effector organs of the parasympathetic system. Stimulation causes bradycardia, miosis, sweating, hyperperistalsis, bronchorrhea, wheezing, excessive salivation, and urinary incontinence. (Examples: There are no pure muscarinic drugs.)

7. **Mixed cholinergic syndrome.** Because both nicotinic and muscarinic receptors are stimulated, mixed effects may be seen. The pupils are usually miotic (pinpoint in size). The skin is sweaty, and peristaltic activity is increased. Fasciculations are a manifestation of nicotinic stimulation and may progress to muscle weakness or paralysis. (Examples: organophosphate and carbamate insecticides, physostigmine.)

8. **Anticholinergic syndrome.** Tachycardia with mild hypertension is common. The pupils are widely dilated. The skin is flushed, hot, and dry. Peristalsis is decreased, and urinary retention is common. Patients may have myoclonic jerking or choreoathetoid movements. Agitated delirium is common, and hyperthermia may occur. (Examples: atropine, scopolamine, benztropine, antihistamines, antidepressants; all these drugs are primarily antimuscarinic).

B. **Eye findings**
   1. **Pupil size** is affected by a number of drugs acting on the autonomic nervous system. Table I-19 lists common causes of miosis and mydriasis.
   2. **Horizontal gaze nystagmus** is common with a variety of drugs and toxins, including barbiturates, ethanol, carbamazepine, phenytoin, and scorpion envenomation. Phencyclidine (PCP) may cause horizontal, vertical, and even rotatory nystagmus.

C. **Abdominal findings.** Peristaltic activity is commonly affected by drugs and toxins; see Table I-18 on autonomic syndromes.
   1. Ileus may also be due to **mechanical factors** such as injury to the

gastrointestinal tract with perforation and peritonitis, or mechanical obstruction by a swallowed foreign body.
2. Abdominal distension and ileus may also be a manifestation of acute **bowel infarction,** a rare but catastrophic complication caused by prolonged hypotension or mesenteric artery vasospasm (caused, for example, by ergot or amphetamines). Radiographs or CT scan may reveal air in the intestinal wall, biliary tree, or hepatic vein.

D. **Skin findings**
1. **Sweating** or absence of sweating may provide a clue to one of the autonomic syndromes (Table I–18).
2. **Flushed red skin** may be caused by carbon monoxide poisoning, boric acid intoxication, chemical burns from corrosives or hydrocarbons, or anticholinergic agents. It may also be due to vasodilation (eg, phenothiazines or disulfiram-ethanol interaction).
3. **Pale coloration** with diaphoresis is frequently caused by sympathomimetic agents. Severe pallor should suggest possible arterial vasospasm, such as that caused by ergot (see p 146) or amphetamines (p 62).
4. **Cyanosis** may indicate hypoxia, sulfhemoglobinemia, or methemoglobinemia (p 204).

E. **Odors.** A number of toxins may have characteristic odors (Table I–20). However, the odor may be subtle and may be obscured by the smell of emesis or other ambient odors. In addition, the ability to smell an odor may vary; for example, only about 50% of the general population can smell the "bitter almond" odor of cyanide. Thus, the absence of an odor does not guarantee the absence of the toxin.

III. **Essential clinical laboratory tests.** Simple, readily available clinical laboratory tests may provide important clues to the diagnosis of poisoning and may guide the investigation toward specific toxicology testing.

A. **Routine tests.** The following tests are recommended for routine screening of the overdose patient:
1. Serum osmolality and osmolar gap.
2. Electrolytes for determination of sodium, potassium, and anion gap.

TABLE I–19. SELECTED CAUSES OF PUPIL SIZE CHANGES[a]

CONSTRICTED PUPILS	DILATED PUPILS
Sympatholytic agents	**Sympathomimetic agents**
Clonidine	Amphetamines and derivatives
Opiates	Cocaine
Phenothiazines	Dopamine
Tetrahydrozoline	LSD (lysergic acid diethylamide)
Cholinergic agents	Monoamine oxidase inhibitors
Carbamate insecticides	Nicotine
Nicotine	**Anticholinergic agents**
Organophosphates	Atropine and other anticholinergics
Physostigmine	Antihistamines
Pilocarpine	Cyclic antidepressants
Others	Glutethimide
Barbiturates	
Ethanol	
Heatstroke	
Isopropyl alcohol	
Phencyclidine (PCP)	
Pontine hemorrhage	
Sedative-hypnotic agents	
Subarachnoid hemorrhage	

[a] Adapted, with permission, from Olson KR et al. *Med Toxicol* 1987;2:66.

TABLE I-20. SOME COMMON ODORS CAUSED BY TOXINS AND DRUGS[a]

Odor	Drug or Toxin
Acetone	Chloroform, isopropyl alcohol
Acrid or pearlike	Chloral hydrate, paraldehyde
Bitter almonds	Cyanide
Carrots	Cicutoxin (water hemlock)
Garlic	Arsenic, organophosphates, thallium
Mothballs	Naphthalene, paradichlorobenzene
Pungent aromatic	Ethchlorvynol
Wintergreen	Methyl salicylate

[a] Adapted, with permission, from Olson KR et al. *Med Toxicol* 1987;2:67.

    3. Serum glucose.
    4. Blood urea nitrogen (BUN) and creatinine for evaluation of renal function.
    5. Hepatic transaminases and hepatic function tests.
    6. Urinalysis to check for crystalluria, hemoglobinuria, or myoglobinuria.
    7. Electrocardiogram (ECG).
    8. Stat serum acetaminophen level and serum ethanol level.
  B. Serum osmolality and osmolar gap. Serum osmolality may be measured in the laboratory with the freezing point depression osmometer or the heat of vaporization osmometer. Under normal circumstances the measured serum osmolality is approximately 290 mosm/L, and can be calculated from the sodium, glucose, and BUN. The difference between the calculated osmolality and the osmolality measured in the laboratory is known as the osmolar gap (Table I-21).
    1. Causes of elevated osmolar gap. (Table I-21.)
      a. The osmolar gap may be increased in the presence of low-molecular-weight substances such as ethanol, other alcohols, and glycols that contribute to the measured but not the calculated gap. Table I-22 describes how to estimate alcohol and glycol levels from the osmolar gap.
      b. Osmolar gap accompanied by anion gap acidosis should immediately suggest poisoning by methanol or ethylene glycol.
    Note: A falsely normal osmolar gap despite the presence of alcohols may result from using a heat of vaporization method for measuring osmolality, because the alcohols will boil off before the serum boiling point is reached.

TABLE I-21. CAUSES OF ELEVATED OSMOLAR GAP[a,b]

Acetone	Mannitol
Ethanol	Methanol
Ethyl ether	Propylene glycol
Ethylene glycol	Renal failure without dialysis
Isopropyl alcohol	

[a] Osmolar gap = measured - calculated osmolality.

Calculated osmolality = $2[Na] + \frac{[glucose]}{18} + \frac{[BUN]}{2.8} = 290$ mosm/L.

Na (serum sodium) in meq/L; glucose and BUN (urea nitrogen) in mg/dL.

Note: The osmolality may be measured as falsely normal if a vaporization point osmometer is used instead of the freezing point device, because volatile alcohols will be boiled off.
[b] Adapted, with permission, from Olson KR et al. *Med Toxicol* 1987;2:74.

TABLE I–22. ESTIMATION OF ALCOHOL AND GLYCOL LEVELS FROM THE OSMOLAR GAP[a]

Alcohol or Glycol	Molecular Weight (mg/mmol)	Conversion Factor
Acetone	58	5.8
Ethanol	46	4.6
Ethylene glycol	58	5.8
Isopropyl alcohol	60	6
Methanol	32	3.2
Propylene glycol	72	7.2

To obtain estimated serum level (in mg/dL), multiply osmolar gap by conversion factor.

[a] Adapted, with permission, from *Current Emergency Diagnosis & Treatment,* 3rd ed. Ho MT, Saunders CE (editors). Appleton & Lange, 1990.

   2. **Differential diagnosis**
      a. Patients with chronic renal failure who are not undergoing hemodialysis may also have an elevated osmolar gap owing to accumulation of low-molecular-weight solutes.
      b. False elevation of the osmolar gap may be caused by the use of an inappropriate sample tube (lavender top, EDTA; grey top, fluoride-oxalate; blue top, citrate); see Table I–31.
      c. Falsely elevated gap may also occur in patients with severe hyperlipidemia.
   3. **Treatment** depends on the cause. If ethylene glycol (p 151) or methanol (p 202) poisoning is suspected, based upon elevated osmolar gap not accounted for by ethanol or other alcohols and the presence of metabolic acidosis, then ethanol infusion therapy and hemodialysis may be indicated.
C. **Anion gap metabolic acidosis.** The normal anion gap of 8–12 meq/L accounts for unmeasured anions (eg, phosphate, sulfate) in the plasma. Metabolic acidosis is usually associated with an elevated anion gap.
   1. **Causes of elevated anion gap.** (Table I–23.)
      a. An elevated anion gap acidosis is usually due to accumulation of lactic acid or other unmeasured acid anions such as formate or oxalate.
      b. In any patient with an elevated anion gap, also check the osmolar gap; combined anion and osmolar gap suggests poisoning by methanol or ethylene glycol.
      c. A narrow anion gap may occur with overdose by lithium or bromide, both of which will increase the measured serum chloride level.
   2. **Treatment**
      a. Treat the underlying cause of the acidosis:

TABLE I–23. SELECTED DRUGS AND TOXINS CAUSING ELEVATED ANION GAP ACIDOSIS[a,b]

Benzyl alcohol	Hydrogen sulfide
Beta-adrenergic drugs	Ibuprofen
Caffeine	Iron
Carbon monoxide	Isoniazid
Cyanide	Methanol
Ethanol (ketoacidosis)	Phenformin
Ethylene glycol	Salicylates
Exogenous organic and mineral acids	Seizures
Formaldehyde	Theophylline

[a] Anion gap = [Na] · [Cl] · [HCO$_3$] = 8–12 meq/L.
[b] Adapted, with permission, from Olson KR et al. *Med Toxicol* 1987;**2**:73.

(1) Treat seizures (see p 21) with anticonvulsants or neuromuscular paralysis.

(2) Treat hypoxia (p 7) and hypotension (p 14) if they occur.

(3) Treat methanol (p 202) or ethylene glycol (p 151) poisoning with ethanol and hemodialysis.

(4) Treat salicylate intoxication (p 261) with alkaline diuresis and hemodialysis.

b. Treatment of the acidemia itself is not generally necessary, unless the pH is less than 7.0–7.1. In fact, mild acidosis may be beneficial by promoting oxygen release to tissues. However, acidemia may be harmful in poisoning by salicylates or cyclic antidepressants.

(1) In salicylate intoxication (p 261), acidemia enhances salicylate entry into the brain and must be prevented. Alkalinization of the urine promotes salicylate elimination.

(2) In cyclic antidepressant overdose (p 136), acidemia enhances cardiotoxicity. Maintain the serum pH at 7.45–7.5 with boluses of sodium bicarbonate.

D. Hyperglycemia and hypoglycemia. A variety of drugs and disease states can cause alterations in the serum glucose level (Table I–24). Blood glucose is determined by nutritional state, endogenous insulin levels, endocrine function, and the presence of various drugs or toxins.

1. Hyperglycemia, especially if severe (> 500 mg/dL) or sustained, may result in dehydration and electrolyte imbalance caused by the osmotic effect of excess glucose in the urine; shift of water from the brain into plasma may result in hyperosmolar coma. More commonly, hyperglycemia in the setting of poisoning or drug overdose is mild and transient.

Significant or sustained hyperglycemia should be treated if it is not resolving spontaneously or if the patient is symptomatic.

a. If the patient has altered mental status, maintain the airway, assist ventilation if necessary, and administer supplemental oxygen.

b. Replace fluid deficits with intravenous normal saline or other isotonic crystalloid solution.

c. Correct acid-base and electrolyte disturbances.

d. Administer regular insulin, 5–10 units IV initially, followed by infusion of 5–10 units/h, monitoring effects on serum glucose level (children: administer 0.1 unit/kg initially and 0.1 unit/kg/h).

2. Hypoglycemia, if severe (serum glucose < 40 mg/dL) and sustained, can rapidly cause permanent brain injury. For this reason, whenever hypoglycemia is suspected as a cause of seizures, coma, or altered

TABLE I–24. SELECTED CAUSES OF ALTERATIONS IN SERUM GLUCOSE

Hypoglycemia	Hyperglycemia
Akee fruit	β_2-adrenergic drugs
Endocrine disorders (hypopituitarism, Addison's disease, myxedema)	Corticosteroids
	Dextrose administration
Ethanol intoxication	Caffeine intoxication
Fasting	Diabetes mellitus
Hepatic failure	Diazoxide
Insulin	Excessive circulating epinephrine
Oral hypoglycemic agents	Glucagon
Propranolol intoxication	Theophylline intoxication
Renal failure	Thiazide diuretics
Reactive hypoglycemia	Vacor
Salicylate intoxication	

mental status, immediate empirical treatment with dextrose is indicated.

  a. If the patient has altered mental status, maintain the airway, assist ventilation if necessary, and administer supplemental oxygen.

  b. If available, perform rapid bedside blood glucose testing (now possible in most emergency departments).

  c. If the blood glucose is low (< 70 mg/dL) or if bedside testing is not available, administer concentrated dextrose 50%, 50 mL IV (25 g). In children, give 25% dextrose, 2 mL/kg (see p 315).

  d. In malnourished or alcoholic patients, also give thiamine, 100 mg IM or IV, to prevent acute Wernicke's syndrome.

E. Hyperkalemia and hypokalemia. A variety of drugs and toxins can cause serious alterations in the serum potassium level (Table I–25). Potassium levels are dependent upon potassium intake and release (eg, from muscles), diuretic use, proper functioning of the ATPase pump, serum pH, and beta-adrenergic activity. Changes in serum potassium do not always reflect overall body gain or loss but may instead be due to intracellular shifts (eg, acidosis drives potassium out of cells; beta-adrenergic stimulation drives it into cells).

  1. Hyperkalemia (serum K^+ > 5 meq/L) produces muscle weakness and interferes with normal cardiac conduction. Peaked T waves and prolonged PR intervals are the earliest sign of cardiotoxicity. Critical hyperkalemia produces QRS interval widening, AV block, ventricular fibrillation, and cardiac arrest (see Fig I–7).

  a. Hyperkalemia caused by **fluoride intoxication** (see p 154) is usually accompanied by hypocalcemia.

  b. **Digitalis intoxication** associated with hyperkalemia is an indication for administration of digoxin-specific Fab antibodies (p 304).

  2. Treatment of hyperkalemia. A potassium level higher than 6 meq/L is a medical emergency; greater than 7 meq/L is critical.

  a. Monitor the ECG. QRS prolongation indicates critical cardiac poisoning.

  b. Administer calcium chloride, 10–20 mg/kg IV (p 298), if there are signs of critical cardiac toxicity. *Caution:* Do *not* use calcium in patients with digitalis glycoside poisoning; intractable ventricular fibrillation may result.

  c. Sodium bicarbonate, 1–2 meq/kg IV (p 296), rapidly drives potassium intracellularly.

  d. Glucose plus insulin also promotes intracellular movement of potassium. Give 50% dextrose, 50 mL (25% dextrose, 2 mL/kg in children), plus regular insulin, 0.1 unit/kg IV.

  e. Kayexalate (sodium polystyrene sulfonate), 0.3–0.6 g/kg orally in 2 mL/kg sorbitol 70% is effective but takes several hours.

  f. Hemodialysis will rapidly lower serum potassium levels.

TABLE I-25. SELECTED DRUGS AND TOXINS AND OTHER CAUSES OF ALTERED SERUM POTASSIUM[a]

Hyperkalemia	Hypokalemia
Alpha-adrenergic agents	Barium
Angiotensin converting enzyme inhibitors	Beta-adrenergic drugs
Beta blockers	Caffeine
Digitalis glycosides	Diuretics (chronic)
Fluoride	Epinephrine
Lithium	Theophylline
Potassium	Toluene (chronic)
Renal failure	
Rhabdomyolysis	

[a] Adapted, with permission, from Olson KR et al. *Med Toxicol* 1987;2:73.

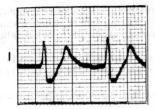
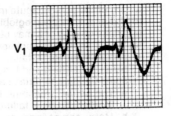

Figure I-7. Electrocardiogram of patient with hyperkalemia. (Modified and reproduced, with permission, from Gold-schlager N, Goldman MJ: Effect of drugs and electrolytes on the electrocardiogram. Page 199 in: *Electrocardiography: Essentials of Interpretation.* Goldschlager N, Goldman MJ [editors]. Lange, 1984.)

3. **Hypokalemia** (serum K^+ < 3.5 meq/L) may cause muscle weakness, hyporeflexia, and ileus. Rhabdomyolysis may occur. The ECG shows flattened T waves and prominent U waves. With severe hypokalemia, AV block, ventricular arrhythmias, and cardiac arrest may occur.
   a. **With theophylline, caffeine, or ß2-agonist intoxication,** intracellular shift of potassium may produce a very low serum K^+ level with normal total body stores. Patients usually do not have serious symptoms or ECG signs of hypokalemia, and aggressive potassium therapy is not required.
   b. **With barium poisoning** (p 87), profound hypokalemia may lead to respiratory muscle weakness and cardiac and respiratory arrest, and therefore intensive potassium therapy is necessary. Up to 420 meq has been given in 24 hours.
   c. **Hypokalemia resulting from diuretic therapy** may contribute to ventricular arrhythmias, especially those associated with chronic digitalis glycoside poisoning.
4. **Treatment of hypokalemia.** Mild hypokalemia (K^+ = 3–3.5 meq/L) is usually not associated with serious symptoms.
   a. Administer potassium chloride orally or intravenously. Do *not* give more than 10–15 meq/h IV (0.25–0.5 meq/kg/h in children).
   b. Monitor serum potassium and the ECG for signs of hyperkalemia from excessive potassium therapy.
   c. If hypokalemia is due to diuretic therapy or gastrointestinal fluid losses, measure and replace other ions such as magnesium, sodium, and chloride.
F. **Renal failure.** Examples of drugs and toxins causing renal failure are listed in Table I–26. Renal failure may be caused by a direct nephrotoxic

TABLE I-26. EXAMPLES OF DRUGS AND TOXINS AND OTHER CAUSES OF RENAL FAILURE

Direct nephrotoxic effect	**Rhabdomyolysis (see also Table I-16)**
Acetaminophen	Amphetamines and derivatives
Amanita phalloides mushrooms	Coma with prolonged immobility
Antibiotics (eg, aminoglycosides)	Carbon monoxide
Analgesics (eg, phenacetin)	Hyperthermia
Chlorinated hydrocarbons	Phencyclidine (PCP)
Ethylene glycol (oxalate)	Status epilepticus
Heavy metals (eg, mercury)	Strychnine
Hemolysis	
Arsine	
Methemoglobinemia	
Naphthalene	
Oxidizing agents (eg, chlorates)	

action of the poison; acute massive tubular precipitation of myoglobin (rhabdomyolysis), hemoglobin (hemolysis), or calcium oxalate crystals (ethylene glycol); or it may be secondary to shock due to blood or fluid loss or cardiovascular collapse.

1. **Assessment.** Renal failure is characterized by progressive rise in the serum creatinine and blood urea nitrogen (BUN) levels, usually accompanied by oliguria or anuria.

   a. The serum creatinine level usually rises about 1 mg/dL/d after total anuric renal failure.

   b. More abrupt rise should suggest rapid muscle breakdown (rhabdomyolysis), which increases the creatinine load and also results in elevated creatine phosphokinase (CPK) levels that may interfere with the serum creatinine determination.

   c. Oliguria may be seen before renal failure occurs, especially with hypovolemia. In this case, the BUN level is usually elevated out of proportion to the serum creatinine level.

2. **Complications.** The earliest complication of acute renal failure is hyperkalemia (see p 32); this may be more pronounced if the cause of the renal failure is rhabdomyolysis or hemolysis, both of which release large amounts of intracellular potassium into the circulation. Later complications include metabolic acidosis, delirium, and coma.

3. **Treatment**

   a. Prevent renal failure, if possible, by administering specific treatment (eg, acetylcysteine for acetaminophen overdose, BAL [dimercaprol] chelation for mercury poisoning, intravenous fluids for rhabdomyolysis or shock).

   b. Monitor the serum potassium frequently and treat hyperkalemia (see p 32) if it occurs.

   c. Do **not** give supplemental potassium, and avoid cathartics or other medications containing magnesium, phosphate, or sodium.

   d. Perform hemodialysis as needed.

G. **Hepatic failure.** A variety of drugs and toxins may cause hepatic failure (Table I-27). Mechanisms of toxicity include direct hepatocellular damage (eg, *A phalloides*), metabolic creation of a hepatotoxic intermediate (eg, acetaminophen, carbon tetrachloride), or hepatic vein thrombosis (eg, pyrrolizidine alkaloids).

1. **Assessment.** Laboratory and clinical evidence of hepatitis usually does not become apparent until at least 24–36 hours after exposure to the poison. Then transaminase levels rise sharply and may fall to normal over the next 3–5 days. If hepatic damage is severe, measures of hepatic function (eg, bilirubin, prothrombin time) will continue to worsen after 2–3 days, even as transaminase levels are returning to normal.

2. **Complications**

   a. Abnormal hepatic function may result in excessive bleeding owing to insufficient production of vitamin K-dependent coagulation factors.

TABLE I-27. EXAMPLES OF DRUGS AND TOXINS CAUSING HEPATIC DAMAGE

Acetaminophen	Halothane
Amanita phalloides mushrooms	Insecticides (chlorinated)
Aromatic hydrocarbons	Iron
Arsenic	Polychlorinated biphenyls (PCBs)
Carbon tetrachloride and other chlorinated hydrocarbons	Phosphorus
Copper	Pyrrolizidine alkaloids
Ethanol (chronic)	Thallium

TABLE I-28. DRUGS COMMONLY INCLUDED IN URINE OR GASTRIC SCREEN[a]

Alcohols Acetone Ethanol Isopropyl alcohol Methanol	**Phenothiazines** Chlorpromazine Prochlorperazine Promethazine Thioridazine Trifluoperazine
Anticonvulsants Carbamazepine Phenobarbital Phenytoin Primidone	**Sedative-hypnotics** Barbiturates Benzodiazepines Carisoprodol Chloral hydrate Ethchlorvynol
Analgesics Acetaminophen Salicylates	Glutethimide Meprobamate Methaqualone
Antihistamines Benztropine Chlorpheniramine Diphenhydramine Pyrilamine Trihexylphenidyl	**Stimulants** Amphetamines Cocaine and benzoylecgonine Phencyclidine (PCP) Strychnine
Opiates Codeine Dextromethorphan Hydrocodone Meperidine Methadone Morphine Oxycodone Pentazocine Propoxyphene	**Tricyclic antidepressants** Amitriptyline Desipramine Doxepin Imipramine Nortriptyline Protriptyline **Other drugs** Lidocaine Propranolol Quinidine and quinine

[a] Newer drugs in any category may not be included in screening.

   b. Hepatic encephalopathy may lead to coma and death, usually within 5–7 days of massive hepatic failure.
3. **Treatment**
   a. Prevent hepatic injury if possible by administering specific treatment (eg, acetylcysteine for acetaminophen overdose).
   b. Obtain baseline and daily transaminase, bilirubin, and glucose levels and prothrombin time.
   c. Provide intensive supportive care for hepatic failure and encepha-

TABLE I-29. DRUGS COMMONLY SCREENED FOR IN THE BLOOD

Alcohols Acetone Ethanol Isopropyl alcohol Methanol	**Sedative-hypnotics** Barbiturates Carisoprodol Chlordiazepoxide Diazepam Ethchlorvynol Glutethimide
Anticonvulsants Ethosuximide Carbamazepine Phenobarbital Phenytoin	Meprobamate Methaqualone **Analgesics** Acetaminophen Salicylates

TABLE I-30.   DRUGS AND TOXINS NOT COMMONLY INCLUDED IN TOXICOLOGY SCREENING[a]

Anesthetic gases	Ethylene glycol
Antiarrhythmic agents	Fentanyl and other opiate derivatives
Antibiotics	Fluoride
Antihypertensives	Formate
Benzodiazepines (newer generation)	Hypoglycemic agents
Beta blockers other than propranolol	Isoniazid
Bromide	Lithium
Borate	LSD (lysergic acid diethylamide)
Caffeine	Marihuana
Calcium antagonists	Noxious gases
Colchicine	Plant toxins
Cyanide	Pressors (eg, dopamine)
Digitalis glycosides	Solvents and hydrocarbons
Diuretics	Theophylline
Ergots	Vasodilators

[a] Many of these are available as separate specific tests.

lopathy (eg, glucose for hypoglycemia, fresh-frozen plasma for coagulopathy, lactulose for encephalopathy).

   d. Liver transplant may be the only effective treatment once massive hepatic necrosis has resulted in severe encephalopathy.

IV. Toxicology screening.* To maximize the utility of the toxicology laboratory, it is necessary to understand what the laboratory can and cannot do and how knowledge of the results will affect the patient. The routine "tox screen" is of minimal value in the initial care of the poisoned patient. On the other hand, specific toxicologic analyses and quantitative levels of certain drugs may be extremely helpful. Before ordering any tests, always ask these 2 questions: (1) How will the result of the test alter the approach to treatment? and (2) Can the result of the test be returned in a timely manner to affect therapy positively?

   A. Limitations of toxicology screens. Owing to long turnaround time, lack of availability, reliability factors, and the low risk of serious morbidity with supportive clinical management, toxicology screening is estimated to affect management in less than 15% of all cases of poisoning or drug overdose.

   1. Toxicology screens or panels may look specifically for only 40–50 drugs out of more than 10,000 possible drugs or toxins (or 6 million chemicals). However, these 40–50 drugs (Tables I–28 and I–29) account for more than 80% of overdoses.

   2. To detect many different drugs, screens utilize methods with broad specificity, and sensitivity may be poor for some drugs (analytic false-negatives). On the other hand, some drugs present in therapeutic amounts may be detected on the screen even though they are causing no clinical symptoms (clinical false-positives).

   3. Because many agents are not sought or detected (Table I–30), a negative toxicology screen does not always rule out poisoning; the negative predictive value of the screen is only about 70%. In contrast, ruling in a drug etiology with a positive screen is better, with a positive predictive value of about 90%.

   4. The specificity (reliability) of toxicologic tests is dependent on the method and the laboratory. The presence of other drugs, drug metabolites, disease states, or incorrect sampling may cause erroneous results (Table I–31).

*By John Osterloh, MD.

B. **Uses for toxicology screens**
   1. Broad (urine and blood) screening is essential whenever the diagnosis of brain death is being considered, to rule out common depressant drugs that might result in temporary loss of brain activity and mimic brain death.
   2. Toxicology screens may be used to confirm clinical impressions during hospitalization and can be inserted in the permanent medicolegal record.

C. **Approach to toxicology testing**
   1. Communicate clinical suspicions to the laboratory.
   2. Obtain gastric, blood, and urine specimens on admission and have the laboratory store them temporarily. If the patient rapidly recovers, they can be discarded.
   3. Urine and gastric specimens are the best samples for broad qualitative screening. Blood samples should be saved for possible quantitative testing, but blood is not a good specimen for screening for many common drugs, including psychotropic agents, opiates, and stimulants.

TABLE I-31. INTERFERENCES IN TOXICOLOGIC BLOOD TESTS.

Drug or Toxin	Method[a]	Causes of Falsely Increased Blood Level
Acetaminophen	SC	Salicylate, salicylamide, methyl salicylate (each will increase acetaminophen level by 10% of their level in mg/L); bilirubin; phenols; renal failure (each 1 mg/dL increase in creatinine = 30 mg/L acetaminophen).
	GC	Phenacetin.
	HPLC	Cephalosporins; sulfonamides.
	IA	Phenacetin.
Amphetamines	GC[b]	Other volatile stimulant amines (misidentified).
	IA[b]	Phenylpropanolamine, ephedrine, phenteramine, phenmetrazine, labetalol, others.
	TLC[b]	MDA (and several similar amines); labetalol.
Chloride	SC	Bromide (0.8 meq Cl = 1 meq Br).
Creatinine	SC	Ketoacidosis (may increase Cr up to 2–3 mg/dL); cephalosoporins; creatine (eg, with rhabdomyolysis).
Digoxin	IA	Endogenous digoxinlike natriuretic substances in newborns and in patients with renal failure (up to 1 ng/mL); oleander ingestion (other cardiac glycosides identified as digoxin); after digoxin antibody (Fab) administration.
Ethanol	SC[c]	Other alcohols, ketones (by oxidation methods); isopropyl alcohol (by enzymatic methods).
Ethylene glycol	SC	Other glycols; elevated triglycerides.
Isopropanol	GC	Skin disinfectant containing isopropyl alcohol used before venipuncture (highly variable, usually trivial, but up to 40 mg/dL).
Lithium	SC	Green-top Vacutainer specimen tube (contains lithium heparin) may cause marked elevation (up to 6–8 meq/L).

continued

TABLE I-31.   INTERFERENCES IN TOXICOLOGIC BLOOD TESTS (Continued)

Drug or Toxin	Method[a]	Causes of Falsely Increased Blood Level
Methemoglobin	SC	Sulfhemoglobin (cross-positive ~ 10% by co-oximeter); methylene blue (2 mg/kg dose gives transient false-positive 15% methemoglobin level); hyperlipidemia (triglyceride, 6000 mg/dL, may give false methemoglobin of 28.6%).
		Falsely decreased level with in vitro spontaneous reduction to hemoglobin in Vacutainer tube (~ 10%/h). Analyze within 1 hour.
Osmolality	Osm	Lavender-top (EDTA) Vacutainer specimen tube (15 mosm/L); gray-top (fluoride-oxalate) tube (150 mosm/L); blue top (citrate) tube (10 mosm/L).
		Falsely normal if vapor pressure method used (alcohols are volatilized).
Salicylate	SC	Phenothiazines,[b] acetaminophen; ketosis;[b] salicylamide; accumulated salicylate metabolites in patients with renal failure (~ 10% increase).
		Decreased or altered salicylate level: bilirubin; phenylketones.
	GC[c]	Methysalicylate; eucalyptol; theophylline.
	HPLC	Theophylline; antibiotics.
Theophylline	SC[c]	Diazepam; caffeine; accumulated theophylline metabolites in renal failure.
	HPLC	Acetazolamide; cephalosporins; endogenous xanthines and accumulated theophylline metabolites in renal failure (minor effect).
	GC	Phenobarbital (rare).
	IA	Caffeine; accumulated theophylline metabolites in renal failure.

[a]GC = gas chromatography (interferences primarily with older methods); HPLC = high-pressure liquid chromatography; IA = immunoassay; SC = spectrochemical; TLC = thin-layer chromatography.
[b]More common with urine test.
[c]Uncommon methodology.

4. Decide if a specific quantitative blood level may assist in management decisions (eg, use of an antidote or dialysis; Table I-32). Quantitative levels are helpful only if there is a predictable correlation between the serum level and clinical effect.

5. A regional poison control center (see Table I-41) or toxicology consultant may provide assistance in considering certain drug etiologies and in selection of specific tests.

TABLE I-32.   SPECIFIC QUANTITATIVE LEVELS AND POTENTIAL INTERVENTIONS[a]

Drug or Toxin	Potential Intervention
Acetaminophen	Acetylcysteine
Carboxyhemoglobin	100% Oxygen
Digitalis	Digitalis antibodies
Ethanol	Low level indicates search for other toxins
Ethylene glycol	Ethanol therapy, hemodialysis
Iron	Deferoxamine chelation
Lithium	Hemodialysis
Methanol	Ethanol therapy, hemodialysis
Methemoglobin	Methylene blue
Salicylate	Alkalinization, hemodialysis
Theophylline	Repeat-dose charcoal, hemoperfusion

[a]Adapted from Olson KR: Toxicology screens and asymptomatic poisoning. In: *Current Therapy in Emergency Medicine.* Callaham M (editor). Mosby, 1986.

TABLE I–33. RADIOPAQUE TABLETS[a,b]

Weakly visible	Moderate
Acetazolamide	Multivitamins with iron
Brompheniramine with phenylephrine and phenylpropanolamine	**Strongly visible**
Busulfan	Calcium carbonate
Chloral hydrate	Ferrous sulfate
Ferrous gluconate	Potassium chloride
Liothyronine	
Meclizine	
Perphenazine with amitriptyline	
Phosphorus	
Prochlorperazine	
Pseudoephedrine with dexbrompheniramine	
Sodium chloride	
Thiamine	
Tranylcypromine	
Trifluoperazine	
Trimeprazine	
Zinc sulfate	

[a] Sustained-release and enteric-coated drugs were *highly variable.*
[b] Adapted from Savitt DL, Hawkins HH, Roberts JR: The radiopacity of ingested medications. *Ann Emerg Med* 1987;**16**:331.

   V. Abdominal x-rays. Abdominal x-rays may reveal radiopaque tablets, drug-filled condoms, or other toxic material.
   A. The radiograph is useful only if positive; recent studies suggest that few types of tablets are predictably visible (Table I–33).
   B. Do **not** attempt to determine radiopacity of a tablet by placing it directly on the x-ray plate. This often produces a false-positive result because of an air-contrast effect.

DECONTAMINATION

   I. Surface decontamination
   A. Skin. Corrosive agents rapidly injure the skin and must be removed immediately. In addition, many toxins are readily absorbed through the skin and systemic absorption can only be prevented by rapid action. Table I–34 lists several corrosive chemical agents that also have systemic toxicity if absorbed through the skin.

TABLE I–34. EXAMPLES OF CORROSIVE CHEMICALS WITH SYSTEMIC TOXICITY[a]

Chemical Agent	Systemic Effects
Freons	CNS depression, arrhythmias
n-Hexane	Peripheral neuropathy
Hydrofluoric acid	Hypocalcemia, hyperkalemia
Methylene chloride	CNS depression, metabolism to carbon monoxide
Methyl butyl ketone	Peripheral neuropathy
Oxalic acid	Hypocalcemia, kidney injury
Paraquat	Pulmonary edema, fibrosis
Phenol	CNS depression; liver, kidney injury
Phosphorus (white)	Liver, kidney injury
Picric acid	Kidney injury
Potassium permanganate	Methemoglobinemia
Silver nitrate	Methemoglobinemia
Tannic acid	Liver injury

[a] From Edelman PA: Chemical and electrical burns. Pages 183–202 in: *Management of the Burned Patient.* Achauer BM (editor). Appleton & Lange, 1987.

1. Be careful not to expose yourself or other care providers to potentially contaminating substances. Wear protective gear (gloves,
   gown, goggles) and wash off exposed areas promptly. Contact a
   regional poison center for information about the hazards of the
   chemicals involved; in the majority of cases, health care providers
   are not at significant personal risk for secondary contamination, and
   simple measures such as emergency department gowns and plain
   latex gloves are sufficient protection. For radiation and other hazardous materials incidents, see also section IV, p 343.

2. Remove contaminated clothing and flush exposed areas with copious quantities of tepid (lukewarm) water or saline. Wash carefully
   behind ears, under nails, and in skin folds. Use soap and shampoo
   for oily substances.

3. There is rarely a need for chemical neutralization of a substance
   spilled on the skin. In fact, the heat generated by chemical neutralization can potentially create worse injury. Some of the few exceptions to this rule are listed in Table I–35.

B. **Eyes.** The cornea is especially sensitive to corrosive agents and hydrocarbon solvents that may rapidly damage the corneal surface and lead
to permanent scarring.

1. Act quickly to prevent serious damage. Flush exposed eyes with
   copious quantities of tepid tap water or saline. If available, instill
   local anesthetic drops in the eye first to facilitate irrigation.

2. Place the victim in a supine position under a tap or use intravenous
   tubing to direct a stream of water across the nasal bridge into the
   medial aspect of the eye (Fig I–8). Use at least 1 L to irrigate each eye.

3. If the offending substance is an acid or a base, check the pH of the
   tears after irrigation and continue irrigation if the pH remains abnormal.

4. Do **not** instill any neutralizing solution; there is no evidence that such
   treatment works, and it may further damage the eye.

5. After irrigation is complete, check the conjunctival and corneal sur-
   faces carefully for evidence of full-thickness injury. Perform a fluorescein examination of the eye using fluorescein dye and a Wood's
   lamp to reveal corneal injury.

6. Patients with serious conjunctival or corneal injury should be referred to an ophthalmologist immediately.

C. **Inhalation.** Agents that injure the pulmonary system may be acutely
irritating gases or fumes and may have good or poor warning properties
(see p 163).

1. Be careful not to expose yourself or other care providers to toxic
   gases or fumes without adequate respiratory protection (see p 348).

2. Remove the victim from exposure and give supplemental humidified
   oxygen, if available. Assist ventilation if necessary (see p 6).

3. Observe closely for evidence of upper respiratory tract edema, which
   is heralded by hoarse voice and stridor and may progress rapidly to

TABLE I–35. SOME TOPICAL AGENTS FOR CHEMICAL EXPOSURES TO THE SKIN[a]

Chemical Corrosive Agent	Topical Treatment
Hydrofluoric acid	Magnesium sulfate (Epsom salts) or calcium gluconate soaks
Oxalic acid	Calcium gluconate soaks
Phenol	Mineral oil or other oil
Phosphorus (white)	Copper sulfate 1% (colors embedded granules blue, facilitates removal)

[a] From Edelman PA: Chemical and electrical burns. Pages 183–202 in: *Management of the Burned Patient.* Achauer BM (editor). Appleton & Lange, 1987.

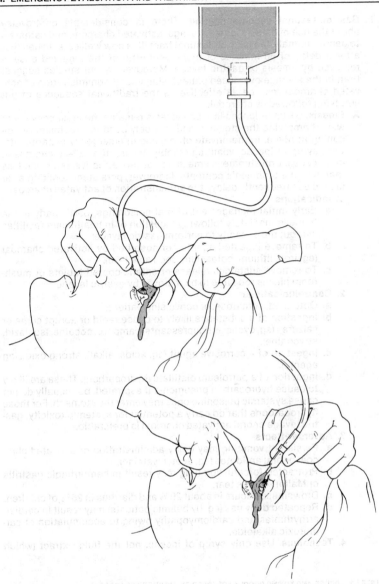

Figure I-8. Irrigation of the eyes after chemical injury, showing technique for irrigating both upper and lower eyelids.

complete airway obstruction. Endotracheally intubate patients with evidence of progressive airway compromise.

4. Also observe for late-onset noncardiogenic pulmonary edema resulting from slower-acting toxins, which may take several hours to appear. Early signs and symptoms include dyspnea, hypoxemia, and tachypnea (see p 163).

II. **Gastrointestinal decontamination**. There is considerable controversy about the use of emesis, gastric lavage, activated charcoal, and catharsis to decontaminate the gastrointestinal tract. It is now well established that after a delay of 60 minutes or more, very little of the ingested dose is removed by emesis or gastric lavage. Moreover, recent studies suggest that, in the average overdosed patient, simple oral administration of activated charcoal may be as effective as the traditional sequence of gut emptying followed by charcoal.

A. **Emesis.** Syrup of ipecac-induced emesis remains the most convenient way of emptying the stomach and is widely used for treatment of poisoning at home, in the private office, and in emergency departments. With syrup of ipecac, vomiting reliably occurs after 20–30 minutes in most cases. Unfortunately, emesis is not very effective, removing less than half the stomach's contents. Moreover, persistent vomiting after ipecac use frequently delays the administration of activated charcoal.

   1. **Indications**
      a. Early initial management of oral poisonings, particularly in the home immediately following ingestion or in health care facilities without the capacity to perform gastric lavage.
      b. To remove ingested agents not adsorbed by activated charcoal (eg, iron, lithium, potassium; see Table I–36).
      c. To remove sustained-release or enteric-coated tablets or mushroom pieces too large to be removed by gastric lavage.

   2. **Contraindications**
      a. Obtunded, comatose, or convulsing patient.
      b. Ingestion of a substance likely to cause rapid or abrupt coma or seizures (eg, cyclic antidepressants, camphor, cocaine, isoniazid, strychnine).
      c. Ingestion of a corrosive agent (eg, acids, alkali, strong oxidizing agents).
      d. Ingestion of a petroleum distillate (hydrocarbon). These are likely to cause hydrocarbon pneumonia if aspirated, but usually do not cause systemic poisoning once they enter the stomach. For those hydrocarbons that do carry a potential for systemic toxicity, gastric lavage or oral activated charcoal is preferable.

   3. **Adverse effects**
      a. Persistent vomiting may delay administration of activated charcoal or oral antidotes (eg, acetylcysteine).
      b. Protracted forceful vomiting may result in hemorrhagic gastritis or Mallory-Weiss tear.
      c. Drowsiness occurs in about 20% and diarrhea in 25% of children.
      d. Repeated daily use (eg, by bulimic patients) may result in cardiac arrhythmias and cardiomyopathy owing to accumulation of cardiotoxic alkaloids.

   4. **Technique.** Use only syrup of ipecac, not the fluid extract (which

TABLE I–36. DRUGS AND TOXINS POORLY ADSORBED BY ACTIVATED CHARCOAL[a]

Alkali	Iron
Cyanide[b]	Lithium
Ethanol and other alcohols	Mineral acids
Ethylene glycol	Potassium
Fluoride	

[a] Few studies have been performed to determine in vivo adsorption of these and other toxins to activated charcoal. Adsorption may also depend on the specific type and concentration of charcoal.

[b] Charcoal should still be given because usual doses of charcoal (60–100 g) will adsorb usual lethal ingested doses of cyanide (200–300 mg).

contains much higher concentrations of emetic and cardiotoxic alkaloids).

  a. Administer 30 mL of syrup of ipecac orally (15 mL for children under age 5 years; 10 mL for children under age 1 year; not recommended for children under age 9 months). After 10–15 minutes, give 2–3 glasses of water (there is no consensus on the quantity of water or the timing of administration).

  b. If emesis has not occurred after 20 minutes, give a second dose of ipecac. Repeat the fluid administration. Have the patient sit up or move around, as this sometimes stimulates vomiting.

  c. If the second dose of ipecac does not induce vomiting, then gastric lavage (see **II.B**, below) should be performed if gastric emptying is still desired. However, it is not necessary to empty the stomach to remove the ipecac.

  d. If ipecac is not available and a pharmacy or emergency department is not within a 20- to 30-minute drive, then soapy water solution may be used as an alternate emetic. Use only standard dishwashing liquid or lotion soap, 2 tablespoons in a glass of water. Do *not* use powdered laundry or dishwasher detergent or liquid dishwashing concentrate; these products are corrosive. There is no other accepted safe alternative to syrup of ipecac. Manual digital stimulation, copper sulfate, salt water, mustard water, apomorphine, and other emetics are unsafe and should not be used.

  e. It is not yet established whether coadministration of activated charcoal with ipecac will result in adequate emesis, although it has been shown that emesis will occur.

B. Gastric lavage. Gastric lavage is more invasive than ipecac-induced emesis, but it is a common procedure in most emergency departments and is safe if carefully performed. It is probably slightly more effective than ipecac, especially for recently ingested liquid substances. However, it does not reliably remove undissolved pills or pill fragments (especially sustained-release or enteric-coated products).

  1. Indications

    a. To remove ingested liquid and solid drugs and poisons.

    b. To administer activated charcoal and cathartics to patients unwilling or unable to swallow them orally.

    c. To dilute and remove corrosive liquids from the stomach and to empty the stomach in preparation for endoscopy.

  2. Contraindications

    a. Obtunded, comatose, or convulsing patients. Because it disturbs the normal physiology of the esophagus and airway protective mechanisms, gastric lavage must be used with caution in obtunded patients whose airway reflexes are dulled. In such cases, endotracheal intubation must be performed first to protect the airway.

    b. Ingestion of sustained-release or enteric-coated tablets. Lavage is unlikely to return intact tablets, even through a 40F orogastric hose. In such cases emesis followed by lavage, or whole bowel irrigation (see p 46), may be preferable to remove as many intact pills as possible.

    c. Ingestion of a corrosive substance. This is controversial; many gastroenterologists recommend that immediate lavage be performed after liquid caustic ingestion to remove corrosive material from the stomach and to prepare for endoscopy.

  3. Adverse effects

    a. Perforation of the esophagus or stomach.

    b. Nosebleed from nasal trauma during passage of the tube.

    c. Inadvertent tracheal intubation.

d. Vomiting and pulmonary aspiration in an obtunded patient without airway protection.

4. Technique

a. If the patient is obtunded, protect the airway by intubating the trachea with a cuffed endotracheal tube or, if only mildly depressed, by positioning the patient in the left lateral decubitus position (see Fig I-9).

b. Insert the largest possible gastric tube through the mouth or nose and into the stomach (36–40F in adults). Check tube position with air insufflation while listening over the stomach.

c. Immediately withdraw as much of the stomach contents as possible, and save the aspirate for possible toxicology screening.

d. Administer activated charcoal, 60–100 g (1 g/kg; see **II.C,** below)

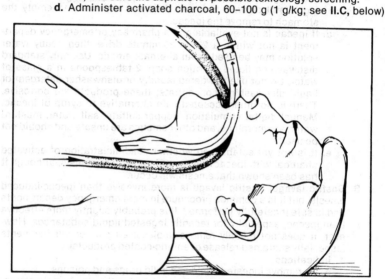

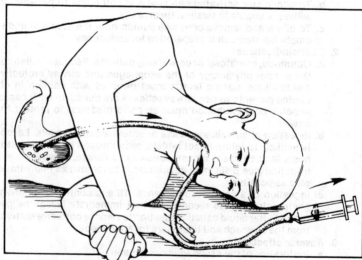

Figure I-9. Gastric lavage.

down the tube before starting lavage to begin adsorption of material that may enter the intestine during the lavage procedure.

e. Instill tepid (lukewarm) water or saline, 200–300 mL aliquots, and remove by gravity or active suction. Use repeated aliquots for a total of 2 L or until return is free of pills or toxic material. *Caution:* Excessive volume lavage can result in electrolyte imbalance or hypothermia in infants and small children.

C. **Activated charcoal.** Activated charcoal is a highly adsorbent yet harmless material made from distillation of wood pulp. Owing to its very large surface area, it is highly effective in adsorbing most toxins. Only a few toxins are poorly adsorbed to charcoal (Table I–36). Recent studies suggest that only activated charcoal has proved worthwhile in management of mild ingestions and that administration of activated charcoal alone should replace emesis and lavage procedures.

1. **Indications**
    a. Used after virtually any toxic ingestion to limit drug absorption from the gastrointestinal tract, even if the substance is not known to be well adsorbed to charcoal.
    b. Repeated oral doses of activated charcoal may enhance elimination of some drugs from the bloodstream (see p 49).

2. **Contraindications**
    a. Ileus or intestinal obstruction.
    b. Corrosive agent ingestion, unless other drugs or toxins have also been ingested (charcoal obscures endoscopic view).

3. **Adverse effects**
    a. Constipation or intestinal bezoar (can be prevented by coadministration of a cathartic).
    b. Distension of the stomach with potential risk of pulmonary aspiration.
    c. Many commercial products now available contain charcoal and the cathartic sorbitol in a premixed suspension. Although this is a convenient formulation, repeated doses may cause excessive diarrhea, dehydration, and hypernatremia, especially in young children and elderly persons.
    d. May bind coadministered ipecac or acetylcysteine (probably not clinically significant).

4. **Technique**
    a. Give activated charcoal, 60–100 g (1 g/kg) orally or by gastric tube. If the quantity of ingested substance is known, give at least 10 times the ingested dose of toxin by weight to prevent desorption of the toxin in the lower gastrointestinal tract.
    b. One or 2 repeat doses of activated charcoal may be given at 1- or 2-hour intervals to insure adequate gut decontamination.

D. **Cathartics.** Controversy remains over the use of cathartics to hasten elimination of toxins from the gastrointestinal tract. Most toxicologists use cathartics but also recognize that little data exist to support their efficacy.

1. **Indications**
    a. To enhance gastrointestinal transit of charcoal-toxin complex, decreasing likelihood of desorption of toxin or development of charcoal bezoar.
    b. To hasten passage of iron tablets and other ingestions not adsorbed by charcoal.

2. **Contraindications**
    a. Ileus or intestinal obstruction.
    b. Sodium- and magnesium-containing cathartics should *not* be used in patients with fluid overload or renal insufficiency.
    c. There is no role for oil-based cathartics (previously recommended for hydrocarbon poisoning).

3. Adverse effects

a. Severe fluid loss, hypernatremia, and hyperosmolarity may result from overuse or repeated doses of cathartics.

b. Hypermagnesemia may occur in patients with renal insufficiency who are given magnesium-based cathartics.

c. Abdominal cramping and vomiting may occur, especially with sorbitol.

4. Technique

a. Administer cathartic of choice (magnesium citrate 10%, 3–4 mL/kg; or sorbitol 70%, 1–2 mL/kg) along with activated charcoal or mixed together as a slurry.

b. Repeat one-half the original dose if there is no charcoal stool after 4–6 hours.

E. Whole bowel irrigation. Whole bowel irrigation has recently become a popular technique for elimination of toxins from the gut. The technique uses surgical bowel-cleansing polyethylene glycol electrolyte solutions that are formulated to pass through the intestinal tract without being absorbed. These are given in large quantity to force intestinal contents out by sheer volume. However, the effectiveness of this treatment has not yet been fully studied, and its role remains unclear.

1. Indications

a. Large ingestions of iron, lithium, or other drugs poorly adsorbed to activated charcoal.

b. Large ingestions of sustained-release or enteric-coated tablets (eg, Theo-dur, Ecotrin) known to be poorly removed by gastric tube.

c. Ingestion of foreign bodies or drug-filled packets or condoms.

2. Contraindications

a. Ileus or intestinal obstruction.

b. Obtunded, comatose, or convulsing patient unless airway is protected.

3. Adverse effects

a. Nausea and bloating.

b. Regurgitation and pulmonary aspiration.

c. Activated charcoal may not be as effective when given with whole bowel irrigation.

4. Technique

a. Give bowel preparation solution (CoLyte or GoLYTELY), 2 L/h by gastric tube (children, 500 mL/h), until rectal effluent is clear.

b. Be prepared for large volume stool within 1–2 hours. Pass a rectal tube or have the patient sit on a commode.

F. Other oral binding agents. Other binding agents may be given in certain circumstances to trap toxins in the gut, although activated charcoal is the most widely used effective adsorbent. Table I–37 lists some alternative binding agents and the toxin(s) for which they may be useful.

TABLE I-37. SELECTED ORAL BINDING AGENTS

Drug or Toxin	Binding Agent(s)
Calcium	Cellulose sodium phosphate
Chlorinated hydrocarbons	Cholestyramine resin
Digitoxin[a]	Cholestyramine resin
Heavy metals (As, Hg)	Demulcents (egg white, milk)
Iron	Sodium bicarbonate
Paraquat[a]	Fuller's earth, Bentonite
Potassium	Sodium polystyrene sulfonate (Kayexalate)

[a]ted charcoal is also very effective.

G. Surgical removal. Occasionally, drug-filled packets or condoms, intact tablets, or tablet concretions persist despite aggressive gastric lavage or whole gut lavage, and surgical removal may be necessary. Consult a regional poison control center (Table I–41) or a medical toxicologist for advice.

ENHANCED ELIMINATION

Measures to enhance elimination of drugs and toxins have been over-emphasized in the past. Although a desirable goal, rapid elimination of most drugs and toxins is frequently not practical and may be unsafe. A logical understanding of pharmacokinetics as they apply to toxicology (toxicokinetics) is necessary for the appropriate use of enhanced removal procedures.

I. **Assessment.** Three critical questions must be answered.
   A. **Does the patient need enhanced removal?** Ask the following questions: How is the patient doing? Will supportive care enable the patient to recover fully? Is there an antidote or other specific drug that might be used? Important indications for enhanced drug removal include:
      1. Obvious severe or critical intoxication with deteriorating condition despite maximal supportive care (eg, phenobarbital overdose with intractable hypotension).
      2. The normal or usual route of elimination is impaired (eg, lithium overdose in a patient with renal failure).
      3. The patient has ingested a known lethal dose or has a lethal blood level (eg, theophylline, methanol, paraquat).
      4. The patient has underlying medical problems that could increase the hazards of prolonged coma or other complications (eg, severe chronic obstructive pulmonary disease, congestive heart failure).
   B. **Is the drug or toxin accessible to the removal procedure?** For a drug to be accessible to removal by extracorporeal procedures, it should be located primarily within the bloodstream or in the extracellular fluid. If it is extensively distributed to tissues, it is not likely to be easily removed.
      1. **The volume of distribution (Vd)** is a numerical concept that provides an indication of the accessibility of the drug:

      Vd = apparent volume into which the drug is distributed
         = (amount of drug in the body)/(plasma concentration)
         = (mg/kg)/(mg/L) = L/kg

      A drug with a very large Vd has a very low plasma concentration. In contrast, a drug with a small volume of distribution is potentially quite accessible by extracorporeal removal procedures. Table I–38 lists some common volumes of distribution.
      2. **Protein binding** may affect accessibility; highly protein-bound drugs

TABLE I-38. VOLUME OF DISTRIBUTION OF SOME DRUGS AND TOXINS

Large Vd (> 5–10 L/kg)	Small Vd (< 1 L/kg)
Antidepressants	Theophylline
Phenothiazines	Phenobarbital
Lindane	Lithium
Phencyclidine (PCP)	Carbamazepine
Opiates	Alcohols
Digoxin	Salicylate

have low free drug concentrations and are difficult to remove by dialysis.

C. Will the method work? Does the removal procedure efficiently extract the toxin from the blood?

1. **The clearance (Cl)** is the rate at which a given volume of fluid can be "cleared" of the substance. Clearance may be calculated from the extraction ratio across the dialysis machine or hemoperfusion column, multiplied by the blood flow rate through the system:

$$\text{Clearance} = \text{extraction ratio} \times \text{blood flow rate}$$

   Note: The units of clearance are milliliters per minute. Clearance is not the same as elimination rate (milligrams per minute). If the blood concentration is small, the actual amount of drug removed is also small.

2. **Total clearance** is the sum of all sources of clearance (eg, renal excretion plus hepatic metabolism plus respiratory and skin excretion plus dialysis). If the contribution of dialysis is small compared with the total clearance rate, then the procedure will contribute little to overall elimination rate (Table I–39).

II. Methods available for enhanced elimination

A. Urinary manipulation. These methods require that the renal route be a significant contributor to total clearance.

1. Forced diuresis may increase glomerular filtration rate, and ion trapping by urinary pH manipulation may enhance elimination of polar drugs.

2. Alkalinization is commonly used for salicylate overdose, but "forced" diuresis (producing urine volumes of up to 1 L/h) is generally not used because of the risk of fluid overload.

B. Hemodialysis. Blood is taken from a large vein (usually femoral vein) using a double-lumen catheter and is pumped through the hemodialysis system. The patient must be anticoagulated to prevent clotting of blood in the dialyzer. Drugs and toxins flow passively across the semipermeable membrane down a concentration gradient into a dialysate (electrolyte and buffer) solution. Fluid and electrolyte abnormalities can be corrected concurrently.

1. Flow rates of up to 300–500 mL/min can be achieved, and clearance rates may reach 200–300 mL/min.

2. Characteristics of the drug or toxin that enhance its extractability include small size (molecular weight < 500 daltons), water solubility, and low protein binding.

C. Hemoperfusion. Using equipment and vascular access similar to that for hemodialysis, the blood is pumped directly through a column containing an adsorbent material (either charcoal or Amberlite resin). Systemic anticoagulation is required, often in higher doses than for hemodialysis, and thrombocytopenia is a common complication.

1. Because the drug or toxin is in direct contact with the adsorbent material, drug size, water solubility, and protein binding are not important limiting factors.

2. For most drugs, hemoperfusion can achieve greater clearance rates than hemodialysis. For example, the hemodialysis clearance for phenobarbital is 60–80 mL/min, whereas the hemoperfusion clearance is 200–300 mL/min.

D. Peritoneal dialysis. Dialysate fluid is poured into the peritoneal cavity through a transcutaneous catheter and drained off, and the procedure is repeated with fresh dialysate. The gut wall and peritoneal lining serve as the semipermeable membrane.

1. Peritoneal dialysis is easier to perform than hemodialysis or

TABLE I-39. ELIMINATION OF SELECTED DRUGS AND TOXINS[a]

Drug or Toxin	Volume of Distribution (L/kg)	Usual Body Clearance (mL/min)	Reported Clearance by:	
			Dialysis (mL/min)	Hemoperfusion[b] (mL/min)
Acetaminophen	0.8–1	400	150	190–300
Amitriptyline	6–10	500–800	NHD[c]	240[d]
Bromide	0.7	5	100	NA[e]
Digitoxin	0.6	4	10–26	NA
Digoxin	7–12	150–200	NHD	90–140
Ethanol	0.7	100–300	100–200	NHP[f]
Ethchlorvynol	2–4	120–140	20–80	150–300[d]
Ethylene glycol	0.6	200	100–200	NHP
Glutethimide	2.7	200	70	300[d]
Isopropyl alcohol	0.7	30	100–200	NHP
Lithium	0.6–1	25–30	50–100	NHP
Methanol	0.7	40–60	100–200	NHP
Methaqualone	5.8	130–175	23	150–270
Methotrexate	0.5–1	50–100	NA	54
Nortriptyline	20–40	500–1000	24–34	216[d]
Paraquat	2.8	200	10	50–155
Pentobarbital	0.8–1	27	40–55	200–300
Phenobarbital	0.8	2–15	60–75	100–300
Phenytoin	0.6	15–30	NHD	76–189
Salicylate	0.15	30	35–80	57–116
Theophylline	0.3–0.6	80–120	30–50	60–225

[a] Adapted from Pond SM: Diuresis, dialysis, and hemoperfusion: Indications and benefits. *Emerg Med Clin North Am* 1984;2:29.
[b] Hemoperfusion data are mainly for charcoal hemoperfusion.
[c] NHD, not hemodialyzable.
[d] Data are for XAD-4 resin hemoperfusion.
[e] NA, not available.
[f] NHP, not hemoperfusable.

    hemoperfusion and it does not require anticoagulation, but it is only about 10–15% as effective owing to poor extraction ratios and slower flow rates (clearance rates, 10–15 mL/min).

  2. However, peritoneal dialysis can be performed continuously, 24 hours a day: a 24-hour peritoneal dialysis with dialysate exchange every 1–2 hours is approximately equal to 4 hours of hemodialysis.

  E. Repeat-dose activated charcoal. Repeated doses of activated charcoal (20–30 g or 0.5–1 g/kg every 2–3 hours) are given orally or via gastric

TABLE I-40. DRUGS KNOWN TO BE REMOVED BY REPEAT-DOSE ACTIVATED CHARCOAL

Carbamazepine	Phenobarbital
Chlordecone	Phenylbutazone
Dapsone	Phenytoin
Digitoxin	Salicylate
Nadolol	Theophylline

tube. A constant slurry of activated charcoal in the intestinal lumen extracts drug or toxin from the gut wall in a kind of "gut dialysis" quite distinct from simple adsorption of ingested unabsorbed tablets. This technique is easy and noninvasive and has been shown to shorten the half-life of phenobarbital, theophylline, and several other drugs (Table I–40). *Caution:* Repeat-dose charcoal may cause serious fluid and electrolyte disturbance secondary to large-volume diarrhea, especially if premixed charcoal-sorbitol suspensions are used. Also, it should not be used in patients with ileus or obstruction.

DISPOSITION OF THE PATIENT

I. **Emergency department discharge or intensive care unit admission?**
   A. All patients with potentially serious overdose should be observed for at least 6 hours before transfer to a nonmedical (eg, psychiatric) facility or discharge. If signs or symptoms of intoxication develop during this time, admission for further observation and treatment is required.
   B. Beware of delayed complications from slow absorption of medications (eg, from a tablet concretion or bezoar, or sustained-release or enteric-coated preparations). If specific drug levels are determined, obtain repeated serum levels to be certain that they are decreasing as expected.
   C. Most patients admitted for poisoning or drug overdose will need observation in an intensive care unit, although this depends on the potential for serious cardiorespiratory complications. Any patient with suicidal intent must be kept under close observation.
II. **Regional poison control center consultation.** Consult with a regional poison control center to determine the need for further observation or admission, administration of antidotes or therapeutic drugs, selection of appropriate laboratory tests, or decisions about extracorporeal removal. An experienced clinical toxicologist is usually available for immediate consultation. See Table I–41 for a list of regional poison control centers (certified by the American Association of Poison Control Centers).
III. **Psychosocial evaluation**
   A. **Psychiatric consultation for suicide risk.** All patients with intentional poisoning or drug overdose should have psychiatric evaluation for suicidal intent.
      1. It is not appropriate to discharge a potentially suicidal patient from the emergency department without a careful psychiatric evaluation. Most states have provisions for the physician to place an emergency psychiatric hold, forcing involuntary patients to remain under psychiatric observation for up to 72 hours.
      2. Patients calling from home after an intentional ingestion should always be referred to an emergency department for medical and psychiatric evaluation.
   B. **Child abuse or sexual abuse**
      1. Children should be evaluated for the possibility that the ingestion was not accidental. Sometimes parents or other adults intentionally give children sedatives or tranquilizers to control their behavior.
      2. Accidental poisonings may also warrant social services referral. Occasionally children get into stimulants or other abused drugs that

TABLE I-41. AAPCC-CERTIFIED[a] REGIONAL POISON CONTROL CENTERS IN THE USA[b]

State	Poison Center	Phone Number
Alabama	Alabama Poison Center, Tuscaloosa	(800) 462-0800 (AL only) (205) 345-0600
	Children's Hospital of Alabama, Birmingham	(800) 292-6678 (205) 939-9201
Arizona	Arizona Poison and Drug Information Center, Tucson	(800) 362-0101 (AZ only) (602) 626-6016
	Samaritan Regional Poison Center, Phoenix	(602) 253-3334
California	Fresno Regional Poison Control Center, Fresno	(800) 346-5922 (209) 445-1222
	Los Angeles County Medical Association Regional Poison Control Center, Los Angeles	(213) 484-5151 (213) 664-2121 (for physicians) (800) 825-2722 (for physicians)
	San Diego Regional Poison Center, University of California, San Diego	(800) 876-4766 (CA only) (619) 543-6000
	San Francisco Bay Area Regional Poison Center, San Francisco	(800) 523-2222 (CA only) (415) 476-6600
	UC Davis Medical Center Regional Poison Center, Sacramento	(800) 342-9293 (CA only) (916) 453-3692
Colorado (also Montana, Wyoming)	Rocky Mountain Poison Center, Denver	(800) 332-3073 (CO only) (303) 629-1123 (800) 525-5042 (MT only) (800) 442-2702 (WY only)
Florida	Florida Poison Information Center, Tampa	(800) 282-3171 (FL only) (813) 253-4444
Georgia	Georgia Poison Control Center, Atlanta	(800) 282-5846 (GA only) (404) 589-4400
Kentucky	Kentucky Regional Poison Center, Louisville	(800) 722-5725 (KY only) (502) 589-8222
Maryland	Maryland Poison Center, Baltimore	(800) 492-2414 (MD only) (301) 528-7701
Massachusetts	Massachusetts Poison Control System, Boston	(800) 682-9211 (MA only) (617) 232-2120
Michigan	Blodgett Regional Poison Center, Grand Rapids	(800) 632-2727 (MI only) (616) 774-7851
	Poison Control Center, Children's Hospital Detroit	(800) 462-6642 (MI only) (313) 745-5711
Minnesota	Hennepin Regional Poison Center, Minneapolis	(612) 347-3141
	Minnesota Regional Poison Center, St Paul	(800) 222-1222 (MN only) (612) 221-2113

continued

TABLE I-41. AAPCC-CERTIFIED[a] REGIONAL POISON CONTROL CENTERS IN THE USA[b] (Continued)

State	Poison Center	Phone Number
Missouri	Cardinal Glennon Children's Hospital Regional Poison Center, St Louis	(800) 392-9111 (MO only) (800) 366-8888 (314) 772-5200
Montana	*See* Colorado	
Nebraska	Mid-Plains Poison Center, Omaha	(800) 642-9999 (NE only) (402) 390-5400 (800) 228-9515 (other states)
New Jersey	New Jersey Poison Information and Education System, Newark	(800) 962-1253 (NJ only) (201) 923-0764
New Mexico	New Mexico Poison and Drug Information Center, Albuquerque	(800) 432-6866 (NM only) (505) 843-2551
New York	Long Island Regional Poison Control Center, East Meadow	(516) 542-2323
	New York City Poison Center, New York City	(212) 340-4494 (212) 764-7667
Ohio	Central Ohio Poison Center, Columbus	(800) 682-7625 (OH only) (614) 228-1323
	Regional Poison Control System and Drug and Poison Information Center, Cincinnati	(800) 872-5111 (513) 558-5111
Oregon	Oregon Poison Center, Portland	(800) 452-7165 (OR only) (503) 279-8968
Pennsylvania	Pittsburgh Poison Center, Pittsburgh	(412) 681-6669
	Delaware Valley Regional Poison Center, Philadelphia	(215) 386-2100
Rhode Island	Rhode Island Poison Center, Providence	(401) 277-5727
Texas	North Texas Poison Center, Dallas	(800) 441-0040 (TX only) (214) 590-5000
	Texas State Poison Center, Galveston Houston Austin	(800) 392-8548 (TX only) (409) 765-9728 (713) 654-1701 (512) 478-4490
Utah	Intermountain Regional Poison Center, Salt Lake City	(800) 456-7707 (UT only) (801) 581-2151
Washington, DC	National Capitol Poison Center, Washington, DC	(202) 625-3333
West Virginia	West Virginia Poison Center, Charleston	(800) 642-3625 (WV only) (304) 348-4211
Wyoming	*See* Colorado	

[a] AAPCC, American Association of Poison Control Centers.
[b] AAPCC, Regional Certification Committee, January, 1990.

TABLE I-42. HUMAN TERATOGENS[a]

Alcohol (ethanol)
Alklyating agents (busulfan, chlorambucil, cyclophosphamide, mustine/mechlorethamine)
Antimetabolic agents (aminopterine, azauridine, cytarabine, fluorouracil, 6-mercaptopurine, methotrexate)
Carbon monoxide
Coumadins
Diethylstilbestrol (DES)
Disulfiram
Heparin
Lithium carbonate
Methyl mercury
Mercuric sulfide
Polychlorinated biphenyls (PCBs)
Phenytoin
Tretinoin (retinoic acid)
Trimethadione
Thalidomide
Tetracycline
Valproic acid

[a] From Bologa-Campeanu M et al: Prenatal adverse effects of various drugs and chemicals: A review of substances of frequent concern to mothers in the community. *Med Toxicol Adverse Drug Exp* 1988;**3**:307.

are left around the home. Repeated ingestions suggest overly casual or negligent parental behavior.

    3. Intentional overdose in a child or adolescent should raise the possibility of physical or sexual abuse. Teenage girls may have overdosed because of unwanted pregnancy.

IV. Overdose in the pregnant patient

    A. In general, it is prudent to check for pregnancy in any young woman with drug overdose or poisoning. Unwanted pregnancy may be a cause for intentional overdose, or special concerns may be raised about treatment of the pregnant patient.

    B. Inducing emesis with syrup of ipecac is probably safe in early pregnancy, but protracted vomiting is unwelcome, especially in the third trimester. Gastric lavage or oral activated charcoal is preferable in all trimesters.

    C. Some toxins are known to be teratogenic or mutagenic (Table I–42).

REFERENCES

Airway, Breathing, and Circulation

Benowitz NL, Goldschlager N: Cardiac disturbances in the toxicologic patient. In: *Clinical Management of Poisoning and Drug Overdose.* Haddad LM, Winchester JF (editors). Saunders, 1983.

Boehnert MT, Lovejoy FH Jr: Value of the QRS duration versus the serum drug level in predicting seizures and ventricular arrhythmias after an acute overdose of tricyclic antidepressants. *N Engl J Med* 1985;**313**:474.

Dronen SC et al: A comparison of blind nasotracheal and succinylcholine-assisted intubation in the poisoned patient. *Ann Emerg Med* 1987;**16**:650.

Ferguson RK, Vlasses PH: Hypertensive emergencies and urgencies. *JAMA* 1986;**255**:1607.

Pentel P, Peterson CD: Asystole complicating physostigmine treatment of tricyclic antidepressant overdose. *Ann Emerg Med* 1980;**9**:588.

Pentel PR, Benowitz NL: Tricyclic antidepressant poisoning: Management of arrhythmias. *Med Toxicol* 1986;**1**:101.

Shannon M, Lovejoy FH Jr: Pulmonary consequences of severe tricyclic antidepressant ingestion. *Clin Toxicol* 1987;**25**:443.

Sheppard D: Pharmacotherapy of asthma. *West J Med* 1985;**142**:700.

Woo OF et al: Atrioventricular conduction block caused by phenylpropanolamine. (Letter.) *JAMA* 1985;**253**:2646.

Coma and Altered Mental Status

Schwart JA, Koenigsberg MD: Naloxone-induced pulmonary edema. *Ann Emerg Med* 1987;**16**:1294.

Hypothermia

Brunett DD et al: Comparison of gastric lavage and thoracic cavity lavage in the treatment of severe hypothermia in dogs. *Ann Emerg Med* 1987;**16**:1222.

Hyperthermia

Rosenberg J et al: Hyperthermia associated with drug intoxication. *Crit Care Med* 1986;**14**:964.

Rhabdomyolysis

Patel R et al: Myoglobinuric acute renal failure in phencyclidine overdose: Report of observations in 8 cases. *Ann Emerg Med* 1980;**9**:549.

Anaphylactic Reactions

Barach EM et al: Epinephrine for treatment of anaphylactic shock. *JAMA* 1984;**251**:2118.

Seizures

York RC, Coleridge ST: Cardiopulmonary arrest following intravenous phenytoin loading. *Am J Emerg Med* 1988;**6**:255.

Agitation, Delirium, or Psychosis

Clinton JE et al: Haloperidol for sedation of disruptive emergency patients. *Ann Emerg Med* 1987;**16**:319.

Dystonia, Dyskinesia, and Rigidity

Corre KA, Niemann JT, Bessen HA: Extended therapy for acute dystonic reactions. *Ann Emerg Med* 1984;**13**:194.

Decontamination

Curtis RA, Barone J, Giacona N: Efficacy of ipecac and activated charcoal/cathartic: Prevention of salicylate absorption in a simulated overdose. *Arch Intern Med* 1984;**144**:48.
Edelman PA: Chemical and electrical burns. In: *Management of the Burned Patient*. Achauer BM (editor). Appleton & Lange, 1987.
Freedman GE, Pasternak S, Krenzelok EP: A clinical trial using syrup of ipecac and activated charcoal concurrently. *Ann Emerg Med* 1987;**16**:164.
Jones J et al: Cathartic-induced magnesium toxicity during overdose management. *Ann Emerg Med* 1986;**15**:1214.
Kulig K et al: Management of acutely poisoned patients without gastric emptying. *Ann Emerg Med* 1985;**14**:562.
Rosenberg PG, Livingstone DJ, McLellan BA: Effect of whole-bowel irrigation on the antidotal efficacy of oral activated charcoal. *Ann Emerg Med* 1988;**17**:681.
Tennenbein M, Cohen S, Sitar DS: Efficacy of ipecac-induced emesis, orogastric lavage, and activated charcoal for acute drug overdose. *Ann Emerg Med* 1987;**16**:838.

Diagnostic Workup

Olson KR, Pentel PR, Kelley MT: Physical assessment and differential diagnosis of the poisoned patient. *Med Toxicol* 1987;**2**:52.
Rygnestad T, Berg KJ: Evaluation of benefits of drug analysis in the routine clinical management of acute self-poisoning. *J Toxicol Clin Toxicol* 1984;**22**:51.
Savitt DL, Hawkins HH, Roberts JR: The radiopacity of ingested medications. *Ann Emerg Med* 1987;**16**:331.

Management of Complications Detected in Diagnostic Workup

Amitai Y, Lovejoy FH Jr: Hypokalemia in acute theophylline poisoning. *Am J Emerg Med* 1988;**6**:214.

Emmett M, Narins RG: Clinical use of the anion gap. *Medicine* 1977;**56**:38.

Gennari FJ: Serum osmolality: Uses and limitations. *N Engl J Med* 1984;**310**:102.

Lombard J, Wong B, Young JH: Acute renal failure due to rhabdomyolysis associated with cocaine toxicity. *West J Med* 1988;**148**:466.

Woodle ES et al: Orthotopic liver transplantation in a patient with *Amanita* poisoning. *JAMA* 1985;**253**:69.

Enhanced Elimination

Pond SM: Diuresis, dialysis and hemoperfusion: Indications and benefits. *Emerg Med Clin North Am* 1984;**2**:29.

Pond SM: Role of repeated oral doses of activated charcoal in clinical toxicology. *Med Toxicol* 1986;**1**:3.

Section II. Specific Poisons and Drugs: Diagnosis and Treatment

ACETAMINOPHEN
Kent R. Olson, MD

ANTIDOTE   IPECAC   LAVAGE   CHARCOAL

Acetaminophen is a widely used drug found in many over-the-counter and prescription analgesics and cold remedies. When it is combined with another drug such as codeine or propoxyphene, the more dramatic acute symptoms caused by the other toxin may mask the mild and nonspecific symptoms of early acetaminophen toxicity, resulting in delayed recognition and antidotal treatment.

I. **Mechanism of toxicity.** One of the products of normal metabolism of acetaminophen by the cytochrome P-450 mixed oxidase system is hepatotoxic. Normally, this reactive metabolite is rapidly detoxified by glutathione in the liver; however, in overdose, production of the toxic metabolite exceeds glutathione capacity and the metabolite reacts directly with hepatic macromolecules, causing liver injury. Renal damage may occur by the same mechanism owing to renal metabolism.

II. **Toxic dose**
   A. **Acute ingestion** of more than 140 mg/kg in children or 6 g in adults is potentially hepatotoxic.
      1. Children younger than 10–12 years of age appear to be less susceptible to hepatotoxicity because of the smaller contribution of cytochrome P-450 to acetaminophen metabolism.
      2. On the other hand, the margin of safety is lower in chronic alcoholics and other patients with induced cytochrome P-450 microsomal enzymes, because more of the toxic metabolite may be produced in these patients.
   B. **Chronic toxicity** has been reported after daily consumption of high therapeutic doses (5–6 g) by alcoholics.

III. **Clinical presentation.** Clinical manifestations depend upon the time after ingestion.
   A. **Early** after acute acetaminophen overdose, there are no symptoms other than anorexia, nausea, or vomiting.
   B. **After 24–48 hours,** when elevated prothrombin time (PT) and transaminase levels appear, hepatic necrosis becomes evident. If acute hepatic failure occurs, encephalopathy and death may ensue. Acute renal failure occasionally occurs.

IV. **Diagnosis.** Diagnosis is possible only if the ingestion is suspected early and a serum acetaminophen level is obtained. Therefore, many clinicians routinely order stat acetaminophen levels in all overdose patients, regardless of the history of substance ingested.
   A. **Specific levels.** Obtain a 4-hour postingestion acetaminophen level and use the nomogram (Fig II–1) to predict the range of severity. Falsely elevated acetaminophen levels may occur in the presence of high levels of salicylate (see Section I, Table I–31, p 37).
   B. **Other useful laboratory studies.** CBC, electrolytes, glucose, BUN, creatinine, liver and renal function tests, prothrombin time.

V. **Treatment**
   A. **Emergency and supportive measures**

LEGEND

Not Available or Not Indicated   See Text Before Administering   ANTIDOTE   IPECAC   LAVAGE   CHARCOAL

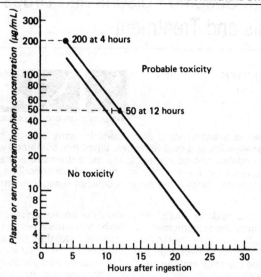

Figure II-1. Nomogram for prediction of acetaminophen hepatoxicity following acute overdosage. The upper line defines serum acetaminophen concentrations known to be associated with hepatotoxicity; the lower line defines serum levels 25% below those expected to cause hepatotoxicity. To give a margin for error, the lower line should be used as a guide to treatment. (Modified and reproduced, with permission, from Rumack BM, Matthew M: Acetaminophen poisoning and toxicity. *Pediatrics* 1975;**55**:871.)

1. **Treat vomiting,** which may delay the administration of antidote and charcoal (see below), with metoclopramide, 10–20 mg IV (children, 0.1 mg/kg [see p 322].
2. **Provide general supportive care for hepatic or renal failure** if it occurs. **Liver transplant** may be necessary for massive hepatic failure.
B. **Specific drugs and antidotes.** If the serum level falls above the possible toxicity line on the nomogram or if stat serum levels are not immediately available, start antidotal therapy with **acetylcysteine** (NAC, Mucomyst, p 289), 140 mg/kg orally. The effectiveness of this therapy depends on **early treatment,** before the metabolite accumulates; it is of minimal benefit if started after 12–16 hours. If vomiting interferes with oral acetylcysteine administration, give it by gastric tube.
C. **Decontamination**
1. Induce emesis or perform gastric lavage (see p 42).
2. Administer activated charcoal and a cathartic. Activated charcoal may interfere with absorption of the antidote acetylcysteine, and the use of charcoal therefore remains controversial. Charcoal may be removed by lavage before acetylcysteine is given, or the dose of acetylcysteine may be increased (see p 289).
3. Gut emptying is probably not necessary following small ingestions if activated charcoal is given promptly.
D. **Enhanced elimination.** Hemoperfusion effectively removes acetaminophen from the blood but is not generally indicated because antidotal therapy is so effective.

Reference

Smilkstein MJ et al: Efficacy of oral *n*-acetylcysteine in the treatment of acetaminophen overdose: Analysis of the national multicenter study (1976 to 1985). *N Engl J Med* 1988;**319**:1557.

AMANTADINE
Christopher R. Brown, MD

ANTIDOTE   IPECAC   LAVAGE   CHARCOAL

Amantadine is an antiviral agent that is also effective in the treatment of Parkinson's disease and for prophylaxis against the parkinsonian side effects of neuroleptic agents. It has also been advocated for use in therapy of cocaine addiction. Although there is limited information about its effects in acute overdose, it has been associated with seizures, arrhythmias, neuroleptic malignant syndrome, and death.

I. **Mechanism of toxicity.** Amantadine is thought to both enhance the release of dopamine and prevent dopamine reuptake in the peripheral and central nervous systems. In addition, it has anticholinergic properties, especially in overdose.

II. **Toxic dose.** The toxic dose has not been determined. Because the elimination of amantadine depends entirely on kidney function, elderly patients with renal insufficiency may develop intoxication with therapeutic doses.

III. **Clinical presentation**
   A. **Amantadine intoxication** causes agitation, visual hallucinations, nightmares, disorientation, delirium, slurred speech, ataxia, myoclonus, tremor, and sometimes seizures. Anticholinergic manifestations include dry mouth, urinary retention, and mydriasis. Rarely, ventricular arrhythmias including torsade de pointes (see p 13) and multifocal premature ventricular contractions may occur. Amantadine has also been reported to cause heart failure.
   B. **Amantadine withdrawal,** either after standard therapeutic use or in the days following an acute overdose, may result in hyperthermia and rigidity (possibly a form of neuroleptic malignant syndrome; see p 20).

IV. **Diagnosis.** The diagnosis is based on a history of acute ingestion or by noting the above-mentioned constellation of symptoms and signs in a patient taking amantadine.
   A. **Specific levels.** Serum levels are not readily available. Serum levels above 1.5 mg/L have been associated with toxicity.
   B. **Other useful laboratory studies.** CBC, glucose, electrolytes, BUN, creatinine, ECG.

V. **Treatment**
   A. **Emergency and supportive measures**
      1. Maintain the airway and assist ventilation if necessary (see p 2).
      2. Treat coma (p 17), seizures (p 21), arrhythmias (p 13), and hyperthermia (p 19) if they occur.
      3. Monitor the asymptomatic patient for at least 8–12 hours after acute ingestion.
   B. **Specific drugs and antidotes.** There is no known antidote. Although some of the manifestations of toxicity are due to anticholinergic effects of amantadine, physostigmine should not be used.
      1. Treat **tachyarrhythmias** with beta blockers such as propranolol (see p 338) or esmolol (p 311).
      2. **Neuroleptic malignant syndrome (NMS)** requires urgent cooling measures (p 19) and may respond to specific pharmacologic therapy with dantrolene (p 300). When NMS occurs in the setting of amantadine withdrawal, some have advocated using amantadine as therapy.
   C. **Decontamination**
      1. Induce emesis or perform gastric lavage (see p 42).
      2. Administer activated charcoal and a cathartic (see p 45).

3. Gut emptying is probably not necessary following small ingestions if activated charcoal is given promptly.

D. **Enhanced elimination.** Amantadine is not efficiently removed by dialysis, because the volume of distribution is very large (5 L/kg). The serum elimination half-life ranges from 12 hours to 34 days, depending on renal function. In a patient with no renal function, **dialysis** or **hemoperfusion** may be the only way to remove the drug.

Reference

Horadam VW et al: Pharmacokinetics of amantadine hydrochloride in subjects with normal and impaired renal function. *Ann Intern Med* 1981;**94**:454.

AMMONIA
Kent R. Olson, MD

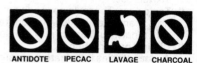

ANTIDOTE   IPECAC   LAVAGE   CHARCOAL

Ammonia is widely used as a refrigerant, a fertilizer, and a household and commercial cleaning agent. Anhydrous ammonia (NH_3) is a highly irritating gas that is very water-soluble. Aqueous solutions of ammonia may be strongly alkaline, depending on the concentration. Solutions for household use are usually 5–10% ammonia, but commercial solutions may be 25–30% or more. Addition of ammonia to chlorine or hypochlorite solutions will produce chloramine gas, an irritant gas with similar properties.

I. **Mechanism of toxicity.** Ammonia gas is highly water-soluble and rapidly produces an alkaline corrosive effect on contact with moist tissues such as the eyes and upper respiratory tract. Exposure to aqueous solutions causes corrosive alkaline injury to the eyes, skin, or gastrointestinal tract (see Caustic and Corrosive Agents, p 114).

II. **Toxic dose**
   A. **Ammonia gas.** The odor of ammonia is detectable at 50 ppm, and eye irritation is common at 100 ppm. The OSHA permissible exposure limit (PEL) for anhydrous ammonia gas is 50 ppm as an 8-hour time-weighted average (the ACGIH recommended TLV is 25 ppm). The level considered immediately dangerous to life or health (IDLH) is 500 ppm.
   B. **Aqueous solutions.** Dilute aqueous solutions of ammonia (eg, < 5%) rarely cause serious burns but are moderately irritating. More concentrated industrial cleaners (eg, 25–30%) are much more likely to cause serious corrosive injury.

III. **Clinical presentation.** Clinical manifestations depend on physical state and route of exposure.
   A. **Inhalation of ammonia gas.** Symptoms are rapid in onset owing to the high water-solubility of ammonia and include immediate burning of the eyes, nose, and throat, accompanied by coughing. With serious exposure, upper airway swelling may rapidly cause airway obstruction, preceded by croupy cough, hoarseness, and stridor. Bronchospasm with wheezing may occur. With very large exposure, noncardiogenic pulmonary edema may also occur.
   B. **Ingestion of aqueous solutions.** Immediate burning in the mouth and throat is common. With more concentrated solutions, serious esopha-

geal and gastric burns are common, and victims have dysphagia, drooling, and severe throat, chest, and abdominal pain. Hematemesis and perforation of the esophagus or stomach may occur. The absence of oral burns does not rule out significant esophageal or gastric injury.
  C. **Skin or eye contact with gas or solution.** Serious alkaline corrosive burns may occur.
IV. **Diagnosis.** Diagnosis is based on a history of exposure and description of the typical ammonia smell, accompanied by typical irritative or corrosive effects on the eyes, skin, and upper respiratory or gastrointestinal tract.
  A. **Specific levels.** There are no specific blood levels.
  B. **Other useful laboratory studies.** CBC, electrolytes, arterial blood gases, chest x-ray.
V. **Treatment**
  A. **Emergency and supportive measures.** Treatment depends on the physical state and the route of exposure.
    1. **Inhalation of ammonia gas**
      a. Observe carefully for signs of progressive upper airway obstruction, and intubate early if necessary (see p 4).
      b. Administer humidified supplemental oxygen and bronchodilators for wheezing (p 8). Treat noncardiogenic pulmonary edema (p 7) if it occurs.
      c. Asymptomatic or mildly symptomatic patients may be sent home after brief (1–2 hours) observation.
    2. **Ingestion of aqueous solution.** If a solution of 10% or greater has been ingested or if there are any symptoms of corrosive injury (dysphagia, drooling, pain), perform flexible endoscopy as soon as possible to evaluate for serious esophageal or gastric injury. Obtain a chest x-ray to look for mediastinal air, which suggests esophageal perforation.
    3. **Eye exposure.** After eye irrigation, perform fluorescein examination and refer to an ophthalmologist if there is evidence of corneal injury.
  B. **Specific drugs and antidotes.** There is no proved specific antidote for these or other common caustic burns. Although administration of corticosteroids is favored by many toxicologists in hopes of limiting esophageal scarring, this treatment is unproved and may be harmful in patients with perforation or serious infection.
  C. **Decontamination**
    1. **Inhalation.** Remove immediately from exposure, and give supplemental oxygen if available.
    2. **Ingestion**
      a. Immediately give **water** or **milk** by mouth to dilute the ammonia.
      b. Do **not** induce emesis.
      c. **Gastric lavage** is recommended in order to remove any liquid caustic in the stomach and to prepare for endoscopy; use a small, flexible tube to avoid injury to damaged mucosa.
      d. Do **not** use activated charcoal; it may obscure the endoscopist's view.
    3. **Skin and eyes.** Remove contaminated clothing and wash exposed skin with water. Irrigate exposed eyes with copious amounts of tepid water or saline (see p 40).
  D. **Enhanced elimination.** There is no role for dialysis or other enhanced elimination procedures.

Reference

Klein J, Olson KR, McKinney HE: Caustic injury from household ammonia. *Am J Emerg Med* 1985;3:320.

AMPHETAMINES
Neal L. Benowitz, MD

ANTIDOTE   IPECAC   LAVAGE   CHARCOAL

Dextroamphetamine and methylphenidate (Ritalin) are used for the treatment of narcolepsy and for attention-deficit disorders in children. Several amphetaminelike drugs (benzphetamine, diethylpropion, phendimetrazine, phenmetrazine, and phenteramine) are marketed as prescription anorectic medications for use in weight reduction (Table II–1). Methamphetamine and several other amphetamine derivatives (see also Lysergic Acid Diethylamide [LSD] and Other Hallucinogens, p 191), as well as a number of prescription drugs, are used orally and intravenously as illicit stimulants. "Ice" is a smokable form of methamphetamine.

Phenylpropanolamine, ephedrine, and other over-the-counter decongestants are discussed on p 238.

I. **Mechanism of toxicity.** Amphetaminelike drugs act primarily by activating the sympathetic nervous system via central nervous system stimulation, peripheral release of catecholamines, inhibition of neuronal reuptake of catecholamines, or inhibition of monoamine oxidase. The various drugs have different profiles of action resulting from different levels of central nervous system and peripheral stimulation.

All these drugs are well absorbed orally and are generally extensively metabolized by the liver. Excretion of most amphetamines is highly dependent on urine pH, with amphetamines being more rapidly eliminated in acid urine.

II. **Toxic dose.** These drugs have a low therapeutic index, with toxicity at

TABLE II-1. COMMON AMPHETAMINELIKE DRUGS

Drugs	Clinical Indications	Typical Adult Dose (mg)
Benzphetamine	Anorectant	25–50
Dextroamphetamine	Narcolepsy, hyperactivity (children)	5–15
Diethylpropion	Anorectant	25, 75 (SR)
Fenfluramine	Anorectant	20–40
Mazinol	Anorectant	1–2
Methamphetamine	Narcolepsy, hyperactivity (children)	5–15
Methylphenidate	Hyperactivity (children)	5–20
Phendimetrazine	Anorectant	35, 105 (SR)
Phenmetrazine	Anorectant	25, 75 (SR)
Phentermine	Anorectant	8, 30 (SR)
Pemoline	Narcolepsy, hyperactivity (children)	18.7–75

SR = Sustained-release.

levels only slightly above usual doses. However, a high degree of tolerance can develop after repeated use. Acute ingestion of more than 1 mg/kg of dextroamphetamine (or an equivalent dose of other drugs; see Table II–1) should be considered potentially life-threatening.

III. **Clinical presentation**
  A. **Acute central nervous system effects** of intoxication include euphoria, talkativeness, anxiety, restlessness, agitation, seizures, and coma. Intracranial hemorrhage may occur owing to hypertension or cerebral vasculitis.
  B. **Acute peripheral manifestations** include sweating, tremor, muscle fasciculations and rigidity, tachycardia, hypertension, acute myocardial ischemia, and infarction (even with normal coronary arteries). Inadvertent intra-arterial injection may cause vasospasm resulting in gangrene; this has also occurred with oral use of DOB (2,5- Dimethoxy-4-bromo-amphetamine; see Lysergic Acid Diethylamide [LSD] and Other Hallucinogens, p 191).
  C. **Death** may be caused by ventricular arrhythmia, status epilepticus, intracranial hemorrhage, or hyperthermia. Hyperthermia frequently results from seizures and muscular hyperactivity and may cause brain damage, rhabdomyolysis, and myoglobinuric renal failure (see p 19).
  D. **Chronic effects** of amphetamine abuse include weight loss, cardiomyopathy, stereotypic behavior (such as picking at the skin), paranoia, and paranoid psychosis. Psychiatric disturbances may persist for days or weeks. Following cessation of habitual use, patients may suffer fatigue, hypersomnia, hyperphagia, and depression lasting several days.

IV. **Diagnosis.** Diagnosis is usually based on a history of amphetamine use and clinical features of sympathomimetic drug intoxication.
  A. **Specific levels.** Amphetamine and many related drugs can be measured in **urine and gastric samples**, providing confirmation of exposure. However, serum levels do not correlate well with severity of clinical effects.
  B. **Other useful laboratory studies.** CBC, electrolytes, glucose, BUN and creatinine, CPK, urinalysis, urine myoglobin, ECG and electrocardiographic monitoring, CT scan of the head (if hemorrhage suspected).

V. **Treatment**
  A. **Emergency and supportive measures**
    1. Maintain the airway and assist ventilation if necessary (see p 2).
    2. Treat agitation (p 22), seizures (p 21), coma (p 17), and hyperthermia (p 19) if they occur.
    3. Continuously monitor the temperature, other vital signs, and the ECG for a minimum of 6 hours.
  B. **Specific drugs and antidotes.** There is no specific antidote.
    1. **Hypertension** (see p 16) is best treated with a parenteral vasodilator such as phentolamine (p 335) or nitroprusside (p 330).
    2. Treat **tachyarrhythmias** (pp 12–13) with propranolol (see p 338) or esmolol (p 311).
    3. Treat **arterial vasospasm** as described for ergots (p 146).
  C. **Decontamination**
    1. Do *not* induce emesis because of the risk of abrupt onset of seizures. Perform gastric lavage (see p 43).
    2. Administer activated charcoal and a cathartic (see p 45).
    3. Gut emptying is probably not necessary following small ingestions if activated charcoal is given promptly.
  D. **Enhanced elimination.** Dialysis and hemoperfusion are not effective. Repeat dose charcoal has not been studied. Renal elimination of dextroamphetamine may be enhanced by acidification of the urine, but this is not recommended because of the risk of aggravating the nephrotoxicity of myoglobinuria.

Reference

Kendrick WC, Hull AR, Knochel JP: Rhabdomyolysis and shock after intravenous amphetamine administration. *Ann Intern Med* 1977;86:381.

ANESTHETICS, LOCAL
Michael T. Kelley, MD, and
Neal L. Benowitz, MD

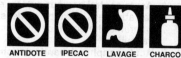

ANTIDOTE   IPECAC   LAVAGE   CHARCOAL

Local anesthetics are widely used to provide anesthesia via local subcutaneous injection; topical application to skin and mucous membranes; and epidural, spinal, and regional nerve blocks. In addition, lidocaine (see p 320) is used intravenously as an antiarrhythmic agent and cocaine (see p 127) is a popular drug of abuse. Commonly used agents are divided into 2 chemical groups: ester-linked and amide-linked (Table II-2).

TABLE II-2. COMMON LOCAL ANESTHETICS[a]

Anesthetic	Maximum Adult Single Dose[a] (mg)
Ester-linked	
Benzocaine[b]	N/A
Butacaine[b]	N/A
Chlorprocaine	800
Cocaine[b]	N/A
Cyclomethylcaine[b]	N/A
Hexylcaine[b]	N/A
Procaine	600
Proparacaine[b]	N/A
Propoxycaine	75
Tetracaine	15
Amide-linked	
Bupivacaine	400
Dibucaine	10
Etidocaine	400
Lidocaine	300
Lidocaine with epinephrine	500
Mepivacaine	400
Prilocaine	600

[a]Maximum single dose for subcutaneous infiltration.
[b]Used only for topical anesthesia.

I. **Mechanism of toxicity.** Local anesthetics bind to sodium channels in nerve fibers, blocking the sodium current responsible for nerve conduction and thereby increasing the threshold for conduction and reversibly slowing or blocking impulse generation. In therapeutic concentrations, this results in local anesthesia. In high concentrations, such actions may result in central nervous system and cardiovascular toxicity. In addition, some local anesthetics (eg, benzocaine) have been reported to cause methemoglobinemia (see p 204).

II. **Toxic dose.** Systemic toxicity occurs when brain levels exceed a certain threshold. Toxic levels can be achieved with a single large subcutaneous injection, with rapid intravenous injection of a smaller dose, or by accumulation of drug with repeated doses. The recommended maximum single subcutaneous doses of the common agents are listed in Table II–2.

    A. With local subcutaneous injection, peak blood levels are reached in 10–60 minutes, depending on the vascularity of the tissue and whether a vasoconstrictor such as epinephrine has been added.

    B. Ester-type drugs are rapidly hydrolyzed by plasma cholinesterase and have short half-lives. Amide-type drugs are metabolized by the liver, have longer duration of effect, and may accumulate after repeated doses in patients with hepatic insufficiency.

III. **Clinical presentation**

    A. Toxicity due to **local anesthetic effects** includes prolonged anesthesia and, rarely, permanent sensory or motor deficits. Spinal anesthesia may block nerves to the muscles of respiration, causing respiratory arrest, or may cause sympathetic blockade, resulting in hypotension.

    B. Toxicity resulting from **systemic absorption** of local anesthetics affects primarily the central nervous system, with headache, confusion, perioral paresthesias, slurred speech, muscle twitching, convulsions, coma, and cardiorespiratory arrest. Cardiotoxic effects include sinus arrest, atrioventricular block, asystole, and hypotension.

    C. **Methemoglobinemia** (see also p 204) may occur after exposure to benzocaine.

    D. **Allergic reactions** (bronchospasm, hives, and shock) are uncommon and occur almost exclusively with ester-linked local anesthetics. Methylparaben, used as a preservative in some multidose vials, may be the cause of some reported hypersensitivity reactions.

    E. Features of toxicity caused by **cocaine** are discussed on p 127.

IV. **Diagnosis.** Diagnosis is based on a history of local anesthetic use and typical clinical features. Abrupt onset of confusion, slurred speech, or convulsions in a patient receiving lidocaine infusion for arrhythmias should suggest lidocaine toxicity.

    A. **Specific levels.** Serum levels may confirm the role of local anesthetics in producing suspected toxic effects, but these must be obtained promptly because the levels rapidly fall. Serum concentrations of lidocaine greater than 6–10 mg/L are considered toxic.

    B. **Other useful laboratory studies.** CBC, electrolytes, glucose, BUN and creatinine, creatine phosphokinase (CPK), ECG and electrocardiographic monitoring, arterial blood gases, methemoglobin level.

V. **Treatment**

    A. **Emergency and supportive measures**

        1. Maintain the airway and assist ventilation if necessary (see p 2).

        2. Treat coma (p 17), seizures (p 21), hypotension (p 14), arrhythmias (pp 9–13), and anaphylaxis (p 25) if they occur.

        3. Monitor vital signs and ECG for at least 6 hours.

    B. **Specific drugs and antidotes.** There is no specific antidote.

    C. **Decontamination**

        1. **Parenteral exposure.** Decontamination is not feasible.

        2. **Ingestion**

    a. Do **not** induce emesis because of the risk of abrupt onset of seizures. Perform gastric lavage (see p 43).

    b. Administer activated charcoal and a cathartic (see p 45).

    c. Gut emptying is probably not necessary following small ingestions if activated charcoal is given promptly.

D. Enhanced elimination. There is no effective method for enhanced removal of local anesthetics.

Reference

Reynolds F: Adverse effects of local anaesthetics. *Br J Anaesth* 1987;**59**:78.

ANTIARRHYTHMIC DRUGS (NEWER)
Neal L. Benowitz, MD

ANTIDOTE   IPECAC   LAVAGE   CHARCOAL

Because of their actions on the heart, antiarrhythmic drugs are extremely toxic and overdoses are often life-threatening. Several classes of antiarrhythmic drugs are discussed elsewhere in Section II: type Ia drugs (quinidine, disopyramide, and procainamide; see p 255); type II drugs (beta blockers, p 92); type IV drugs (calcium antagonists, p 102); and the older type Ib drugs (lidocaine, p 64 and p 320; and phenytoin, p 240 and p 335). This section describes toxicity caused by newer antiarrhythmic drugs: type Ib (tocainide and mexiletine); type Ic (flecainide and encainide); and type III (bretylium and amiodarone).

I. Mechanism of toxicity

    A. Type I drugs in general act by inhibiting the fast sodium channel responsible for initial cardiac cell depolarization and impulse conduction. Type Ia and type Ic drugs slow depolarization and conduction in normal cardiac tissue, and even at normal therapeutic doses the QT (types Ia and Ic) and QRS intervals (type Ic) are prolonged. Type Ib drugs slow depolarization primarily in ischemic tissue and have little effect on normal tissue or on the ECG. In overdose, all type I drugs have the potential to markedly depress myocardial automaticity, conduction, and contractility.

    B. Type II and type IV drugs act by blocking beta-adrenergic receptors (type II) or calcium channels (type IV). Their actions are discussed elsewhere (type II, p 92; type IV, p 102).

    C. Type III drugs act primarily to prolong the duration of the action potential and the effective refractory period, resulting in QT interval prolongation at therapeutic doses.

        1. Intravenous administration of **bretylium** initially causes release of catecholamines from nerve endings, followed by inhibition of catecholamine release.

        2. Amiodarone is a noncompetitive beta-adrenergic blocker and sodium channel blocker, which may explain its tendency to cause bradyarrhythmias. Amiodarone may also release iodine, and chronic use has resulted in altered thyroid function.

    D. Relevant pharmacokinetics. Normal elimination half-lives are summarized in Table II-3. All drugs discussed in this section are widely distributed to body tissues. Most are extensively metabolized, but significant fractions of tocainide (40%), flecainide (30%), and bretylium (> 90%) are excreted unchanged by the kidneys.

II. Toxic dose. In general, these drugs have a narrow therapeutic index, and severe toxicity may occur slightly above or sometimes even within the therapeutic range, especially if combinations of antiarrhythmic drugs are taken together.

A. Ingestion of **twice the daily therapeutic dose** should be considered potentially life-threatening (usual therapeutic doses are given in Table II-3).

B. An exception to this rule of thumb is amiodarone, which is so extensively distributed to tissues that even massive single overdoses produce little or no toxicity (toxicity does not occur until equilibrium is established after chronic amiodarone dosing).

III. **Clinical presentation**

A. **Tocainide and mexiletine**

1. **Side effects** with therapeutic use may include dizziness, paresthesias, tremor, ataxia, and gastrointestinal disturbance.

2. **Overdose** may cause sedation, confusion, coma, seizures, respiratory arrest, and cardiac toxicity (sinus arrest, AV block, asystole, and hypotension). As with lidocaine, the QRS and QT intervals are usually normal, although they may be prolonged after massive overdose.

B. **Flecainide and encainide**

1. **Side effects** with therapeutic use include dizziness, blurred vision, headache, and gastrointestinal upset. Ventricular arrhythmias (monomorphic or polymorphic ventricular tachycardia; see p 13) may occur at therapeutic levels, especially in persons receiving high doses and those with reduced ventricular function.

2. **Overdose** causes hypotension, bradycardia, AV block, and asystole. The QRS and QT intervals are prolonged.

C. **Bretylium**

TABLE II-3. ANTIARRHYTHMIC DRUGS

Class	Drug	Usual Half-Life (hrs)	Therapeutic Daily Dose (mg)	Therapeutic Serum Levels (mg/L)	Major Toxicity
Ia	Quinidine (p 255)				
Ib	Tocainide	13	1200–2400	5–12	S, B, H
	Mexiletine	12	300–1200	0.8–2	S, B, H
	Lidocaine (p 320)				
	Phenytoin (p 240)				
Ic	Flecainide	15	200–600	0.2–1	B, V, H
	Encainide[a]	12	75–300	[a]	S, B, V, H
II	Beta Blockers (p 92)				
III	Aminodarone	50 days	200–600	0.5–3	B, V, H
	Bretylium	14	5–10 mg/kg (IV loading dose)	0.7–1.5	H
IV	Calcium Antagonists (p 102)				

Major toxicity: S = Seizures   H = Hypotension
                B = Bradyarrhythmias   V = Ventricular arrhythmias

[a] Active metabolite may contribute to toxicity; level not established.

        1. The major toxic **side effect** of bretylium is hypotension due to inhibition of catecholamine release. Orthostatic hypotension may persist for several hours.

        2. After **rapid intravenous injection,** transient hypertension, nausea, and vomiting may occur.

  D. Amiodarone

        1. **Acute overdose** in a person not already on amiodarone is not expected to cause toxicity.

        2. With **chronic use,** amiodarone may cause ventricular arrhythmias (monomorphic or polymorphic ventricular tachycardia; see p 13) or bradyarrhythmias (sinus arrest, AV block). Amiodarone may aggravate cardiac failure and may cause pneumonitis or pulmonary fibrosis, photosensitivity dermatitis, corneal deposits, hypothyroidism or hyperthyroidism, tremor, and ataxia.

IV. Diagnosis. Diagnosis is usually based on a history of antiarrhythmic drug use and typical cardiac and electrocardiographic findings. Syncope in any patient taking these drugs should suggest possible drug-induced arrhythmia.

  A. Specific levels. Serum levels are available for most type Ia and type Ib drugs (Table II–3); however, because toxicity is immediately life-threatening, measurement of drug levels is primarily to confirm the diagnosis rather than to determine emergency treatment.

  B. Other useful laboratory studies. CBC, electrolytes, glucose, BUN and creatinine, thyroid panel (chronic amiodarone), ECG, electrocardiographic monitoring.

V. Treatment

  A. Emergency and supportive measures

        1. Maintain the airway and assist ventilation if necessary (see p 2).

        2. Treat coma (p 17), seizures (p 21), hypotension (p 14), and arrhythmias (p 13) if they occur. *Note:* Type Ia antiarrhythmic agents should not be used to treat cardiotoxicity due to type Ia, type Ic, or type III drugs.

        3. Continuously monitor vital signs and ECG for a minimum of 6 hours after exposure, and admit the patient for 24 hours of intensive monitoring if there is evidence of toxicity.

  B. Specific drugs and antidotes. In patients with intoxication by type Ia or type Ic drugs, QRS prolongation, bradyarrhythmias, and hypotension may respond to **sodium bicarbonate,** 1–2 meq/kg IV (see p 296). The sodium bicarbonate probably reverses cardiac-depressant effects caused by inhibition of the fast sodium channel.

  C. Decontamination

        1. Do *not* induce emesis because of the risk of abrupt onset of seizures, coma, or cardiotoxicity. Perform gastric lavage (see p 43).

        2. Administer activated charcoal and a cathartic (see p 45).

        3. Gut emptying is probably not necessary following small ingestions if activated charcoal is given promptly.

  D. Enhanced elimination. Owing to extensive tissue binding with resulting large volumes of distribution, dialysis and hemoperfusion are not likely to be effective for most of these agents. Hemodialysis may be of possible benefit for tocainide or flecainide overdose in patients with renal failure, but prolonged and repeated dialysis would be necessary. No data are available on the effectiveness of repeat-dose charcoal.

Reference

Pentel PR et al: Effect of hypertonic sodium bicarbonate in encainide overdose. *Am J Cardiol* 1986;57:878.

ANTIBIOTICS
Olga F. Woo, PharmD

ANTIDOTE   IPECAC   LAVAGE   CHARCOAL

The antibiotic class of drugs has proliferated immensely since the first clinical use of sulfonamide in 1936 and the mass production of penicillin in 1941. In general, harmful effects have resulted from allergic reactions or inadvertent intravenous overdose. Serious toxicity from single acute ingestion is rare. Table II-4 lists common antibiotics and their toxicities.

I. **Mechanism of toxicity.** The precise mechanisms underlying toxic effects vary depending on the agent and are not well understood. In some cases, toxicity is due to an extension of pharmacologic effects, while in other cases allergic or idiosyncratic reactions are responsible.

II. **Toxic dose.** The toxic dose is highly variable, depending on the agent. Life-threatening allergic reactions may occur after subtherapeutic doses in hypersensitive individuals.

III. **Clinical presentation.** After acute oral overdose, most agents cause only nausea, vomiting, and diarrhea. Specific features of toxicity are described in Table II-4.

IV. **Diagnosis.** Diagnosis is usually based on the history of exposure.
  A. **Specific levels.** Serum levels for most commonly used antibiotics are usually available. Serum levels are particularly useful for predicting toxic effects of **aminoglycosides, chloramphenicol,** and **vancomycin.**
  B. **Other useful laboratory studies.** CBC, electrolytes, glucose, BUN and creatinine, liver function tests, urinalysis, methemoglobin level (for patients with **dapsone** overdose).

TABLE II-4. COMMON ANTIBIOTICS AND THEIR TOXICITIES

Drug	Toxic Dose or Serum Level	Toxicity
Aminoglycosides Amikacin	> 35 mg/L	Ototoxicity to vestibular and cochlear cells; nephrotoxicity due to proximal tubular damage and acute tubular necrosis; competitive neuromuscular blockade if given rapidly intravenously with other neuromuscular blocking drugs.
Gentamicin	> 12 mg/L	
Kanamycin	> 30 mg/L	
Neomycin	0.5–1 g/d	
Streptomycin	> 40–50 mg/L	
Tobramycin	> 10 mg/L	
Bacitracin	Unknown	Ototoxicity and nephrotoxicity.
Cephalosporins Cefazolin, cephalothin	Unknown	Convulsions reported in patients with renal insufficiency.
Cephaloridine	6 g/d	Proximal tubular necrosis.
Cefoperazone, cefamandole, moxalactam	Unknown	Disulfiramlike interaction with ethanol; coagulopathy (inhibition of vitamin K_1 production).
Cefazolin, cefmetazole	Unknown	Coagulopathy (inhibition of vitamin K_1 production).

continued

TABLE II–4. COMMON ANTIBIOTICS AND THEIR TOXICITIES (Continued)

Drug	Toxic Dose or Serum Level	Toxicity
Chloramphenicol	> 50 mg/L	Leukopenia, reticulocytopenia; circulatory collapse (gray baby syndrome).
Dapsone	As little as 100 mg in 18-month-old	Methemoglobinemia, sulfhemoglobinemia, hemolysis; metabolic acidosis; hallucinations, confusion; hepatitis.
Erythromycin	Unknown	Abdominal pain; idiosyncratic hepatotoxicity with estolate salt.
Gramicidin	Unknown	Hemolysis.
Isonazid	1–2 g orally	Convulsions, metabolic acidosis (see p 180); hepatotoxicity with chronic use.
Lincomycin, clindamycin	Unknown	Hypotension and cardiopulmonary arrest after rapid intravenous administration.
Metronidazole	5 g/d	Convulsions; at therapeutic doses may cause disulfiramlike interaction with ethanol (see p 143).
Nalidixic acid	50 mg/kg/d	Seizures, hallucinations, confusion; visual disturbances; metabolic acidosis; intracranial hypertension.
Nitrofurantoin	Unknown	Hemolysis in G6PD-deficient patients.
Penicillins Penicillin	10 million units/d IV, or CSF > 5 mg/L	Seizures with single high dose or chronic excessive doses in patients with renal dysfunction.
Methicillin	Unknown	Interstitial nephritis, leukopenia.
Nafcillin	Unknown	Neutropenia.
Ampicillin, amoxicillin	Unknown	Acute renal failure caused by crystal deposition.
Polymyxins Polymyxin B	30,000 units/kg/d	Nephrotoxicity and noncompetitive neuromuscular blockade.
Polymyxin E	250 mg IM in a 10-month-old	
Rifampin	100 mg/kg/d	Facial edema, pruritus; headache, vomiting, diarrhea; red urine and tears.
Spectinomycin		Acute toxicity not reported.
Tetracyclines	> 1 g/d in infants	Benign intracranial hypertension.
	> 4 g/d in pregnancy	Acute fatty liver.
Demeclocycline	Unknown	Nephrogenic diabetes insipidus.
Minocycline	Unknown	Vestibular symptoms.
Sulfonamide	Unknown	Acute renal failure caused by crystal deposition.
Trimethoprim	Unknown	Bone marrow depression.
Vancomycin	> 80 mg/L	Ototoxic and nephrotoxic.

V. Treatment
A. Emergency and supportive measures
1. Maintain the airway and assist ventilation if necessary (see p 2).
2. Treat coma (p 17), seizures (p 21), hypotension (p 14), anaphylaxis (p 25), and hemolysis if they occur.
3. Replace fluid losses due to gastroenteritis with intravenous crystalloids (p 14).

B. Specific drugs and antidotes
1. **Trimethoprim** poisoning. Administer **leucovorin** (folinic acid; see p 319). Folic acid is not effective.
2. **Dapsone** overdose. Administer **methylene blue** (see p 322) if methemoglobinemia occurs.

C. Decontamination
1. Induce emesis or perform gastric lavage (see p 42).
2. Administer activated charcoal and cathartic (see p 45).
3. Gut emptying is probably not necessary following small ingestions if activated charcoal is given promptly.

D. Enhanced elimination
1. Most antibiotics are excreted unchanged in the urine, so maintenance of adequate urine flow is important. The role of forced diuresis is unclear. Hemodialysis is not usually indicated, except perhaps in patients with renal dysfunction and a high level of a toxic agent.
2. Charcoal hemoperfusion effectively removes **chloramphenicol** and is indicated after a severe overdose with a high serum level and metabolic acidosis.
3. **Dapsone** undergoes enterohepatic recirculation and is more rapidly eliminated with repeat-dose activated charcoal.

Reference
Kucers A, Bennett N: The Use of Antibiotics, 4th ed. Lippincott, 1987.

ANTICHOLINERGICS
Belle L. Lee, PharmD

ANTIDOTE   IPECAC   LAVAGE   CHARCOAL

Anticholinergic intoxication can occur with a wide variety of prescription and over-the-counter medications and numerous plants and mushrooms. Common drugs that possess anticholinergic acitivity include antihistamines, antipsychotics, antispasmodics, skeletal muscle relaxants, and cyclic antidepressants (Table II–5). Plants and mushrooms containing anticholinergic alkaloids include jimsonweed *(Datura stramonium),* deadly nightshade *(Atropa belladonna),* and the fly agaric *(Amanita muscaria).*

I. **Mechanism of toxicity.** Anticholinergic agents competitively antagonize the effects of acetylcholine at peripheral muscarinic and central receptors. Exocrine glands, such as those responsible for sweating and salivation, and smooth and cardiac muscle are mostly affected. Tertiary amines such as atropine are well absorbed centrally, whereas quaternary amines such as glycopyrrolate have less central effect.

II. **Toxic dose.** The range of toxicity is highly variable and unpredictable. Fatal atropine poisoning has occurred after as little as 1–2 mg was instilled in the eye of a young child. Intramuscular injection of 32 mg of atropine was fatal in an adult.

TABLE II-5. COMMON ANTIMUSCARINIC ANTICHOLINERGIC DRUGS[a]

Tertiary Amines	Usual Adult Single Dose (mg)	Quarternary Amines	Usual Adult Single Dose (mg)
Atropine	0.4–1	Anisotropine	50
Dicyclomine	10–20	Glycopyrrolate	1
Hyoscyamine	0.15–0.3	Methantheline	50
Oxyphencyclimine	10	Methscopolamine	2.5
Scopolamine	0.4–1	Propantheline	15
Trihexyphenidyl	6–10		
Benztropine	1–6		

[a] Adapted and reproduced, with permission, from Katzung BG: Cholinoceptor-blocking drugs. Table 8-2 in: *Basic & Clinical Pharmacology*, 4th ed. Katzung BG (editor). Appleton & Lange, 1989.

III. **Clinical presentation.** The anticholinergic syndrome is characterized by warm, dry, flushed skin; dry mouth; mydriasis; delirium; tachycardia; ileus; and urinary retention. Jerky myoclonic movements and choreoathetosis are common. Hyperthermia, coma, and respiratory arrest may occur. Seizures are rare.

IV. **Diagnosis.** Diagnosis is based on a history of exposure and the presence of typical features such as dilated pupils and flushed skin. A trial dose of physostigmine (see **V. B,** below) can be used to confirm the presence of anticholinergic toxicity: rapid reversal of signs and symptoms is consistent with the diagnosis.

    A. **Specific levels.** Not generally available.

    B. **Other useful laboratory studies.** CBC, electrolytes, glucose, arterial blood gases, ECG.

V. **Treatment**

    A. **Emergency and supportive measures**

        1. Maintain the airway and assist ventilation if needed (see p 2).

        2. Treat hyperthermia (p 19), coma (p 17), and seizures (p 21) if they occur.

    B. **Specific drugs and antidotes.** If a pure anticholinergic poisoning is suspected, a small dose of **physostigmine** (see p 336), 0.5–1 mg IV in an adult, can be given to patients with severe toxicity (eg, hyperthermia, severe delirium, or tachycardia). *Caution:* Physostigmine is capable of causing atrioventricular block, asystole, and seizures, especially in patients with cyclic antidepressant overdose.

    C. **Decontamination**

        1. Induce emesis or perform gastric lavage (see p 42).

        2. Administer activated charcoal and cathartic (see p 45).

        3. Gut emptying is probably not necessary following small ingestions if activated charcoal is given promptly.

    D. **Enhanced elimination.** Hemodialysis, hemoperfusion, peritoneal dialysis, and repeat-dose charcoal are not effective in removing anticholinergic agents.

Reference

Klein-Schwartz W, Oderda GM: Jimsonweed intoxication in adolescents and young adults. *Am J Dis Child* 1984;**138**:737.

ANTIHISTAMINES
Belle L. Lee, PharmD

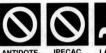

| ANTIDOTE | IPECAC | LAVAGE | CHARCOAL |

Antihistamines (H$_1$ receptor antagonists) are commonly found in over-the-counter and prescription medications used for motion sickness, control of allergy-related itching, and cough and cold palliation and as sleep aids (Table II-6). Acute intoxication with antihistamines results in symptoms very similar to those of anticholinergic poisoning. H$_2$ receptor blockers (cimetidine, ranitidine and famotidine) inhibit gastric acid secretion but otherwise share no effects with H$_1$ agents, do not produce significant intoxication, and are not discussed here.

I. **Mechanism of toxicity.** H$_1$ blocker antihistamines are structurally related to histamine and antagonize the effects of histamine on H$_1$ receptor sites. They possess anticholinergic effects. They may also stimulate or depress the central nervous system, and some agents (eg, diphenhydramine, pro-

TABLE II-6. COMMON H$_1$ RECEPTOR ANTAGONIST ANTIHISTAMINES[a]

Drug	Usual Duration of Action (hr)	Usual Single Adult Dose (mg)	Sedation
Ethanolamines			
Carbinoxamine	3–4	4–8	+ +
Dimenhydrinate	4–6	50	+ + +
Diphenhydramine	4–6	25–50	+ + +
Doxylamine	4–6	25	+ + +
Ethylenediamines			
Pyrilamine	4–6	25–50	+ +
Tripelennamine	4–6	25–50	+ +
Alkylamines			
Brompheniramine	4–6	4–8	+
Chlorpheniramine	4–6	4–8	+
Piperazines			
Cyclizine	4–6	25–50	+
Meclizine	12–24	25–50	+
Hydroxyzine	6–24	25–50	+
Others			
Promethazine	4–6	25	+ + +
Terfenadine	8–12	60	—

[a] Adapted and reproduced, with permission, from Douglas WW: Histamine and 5-hydroxytryptamine (serotonin) and their antagonists. Table 26–3 in: *Goodman and Gilman's The Pharmacological Basis of Therapeutics,* 7th ed. Gilman AG et al (editors). Macmillan, 1985; and Burkhalter A, Frick OL: Histamine, serotonin, and the ergot alkaloids. Table 16–1 in *Basic & Clinical Pharmacology,* 4th ed. Katzung BG (editor). Appleton & Lange, 1989.

methazine) have local anesthetic and membrane-depressant effects in large doses.

II. **Toxic dose.** The estimated fatal oral dose of diphenhydramine is 20–40 mg/kg. In general, toxicity occurs after ingestion of 3–5 times the usual daily dose. Children are more sensitive to the toxic effects of antihistamines than adults.

III. **Clinical presentation.** Overdose with antihistamines results in many symptoms similar to anticholinergic poisoning: drowsiness, dilated pupils, flushed dry skin, fever, tachycardia, hallucinations, choreoathetoid movements, and delirium. Convulsions and hyperthermia may occur with serious overdose. Massive diphenhydramine overdose has been reported to cause QRS widening and myocardial depression.

IV. **Diagnosis.** Diagnosis is usually based on the history of ingestion and can usually be readily confirmed by the presence of typical anticholinergic syndrome. Toxicology screening will detect most common antihistamines.
  A. **Specific levels.** Not generally available or useful.
  B. **Other useful laboratory studies.** CBC, electrolytes, glucose, arterial blood gases, ECG.

V. **Treatment**
  A. **Emergency and supportive measures**
    1. Maintain the airway and assist ventilation if necessary (see p 2).
    2. Treat coma (p 17), seizures (p 21), and hyperthermia (p 19) if they occur.
    3. Monitor the patient for at least 6–8 hours after ingestion.
  B. **Specific drugs and antidotes.** There is no specific antidote for antihistamine overdose. As for anticholinergic poisoning (see p 71), **physostigmine** (see p 336) has been used for treatment of severe delirium or tachycardia. However, because antihistamine overdose carries a greater risk for seizures, physostigmine is not recommended.
  C. **Decontamination**
    1. Perform gastric lavage (see p 43). Do *not* induce emesis because of the risk of abrupt onset of seizures and coma.
    2. Administer activated charcoal and cathartic (see p 45).
    3. Gut emptying is probably not necessary following small ingestions if activated charcoal is given promptly.
  D. **Enhanced elimination.** Hemodialysis, hemoperfusion, peritoneal dialysis, and repeat-dose activated charcoal are not effective in removing antihistamines.

Reference

Krenzelok EP, Anderson GM, Mirick M: Massive diphenhydramine overdose resulting in death. *Ann Emerg Med* 1982;**11**:212

ANTIMONY AND STIBINE
Peter Wald, MD

ANTIDOTE   IPECAC   LAVAGE   CHARCOAL

Antimony is widely used as a hardening agent in soft metal alloys; for compounding rubber; in flameproofing compounds; and as a coloring agent in dyes, varnishes, paints, and glazes. Exposure to antimony dusts and fumes may also occur during mining and refining of ores and from the discharge of firearms. Organic antimony compounds are used as antiparasitic drugs.

Stibine (antimony hydride, SbH_3) is a colorless gas with the odor of rotten eggs that is produced as a by-product when antimony-containing ores or furnace slag is treated with acid.

I. **Mechanism of toxicity.** The mechanism of antimony and stibine toxicity is not known. Because these compounds are chemically similar to arsenic and arsine, their modes of action may be similar.
   A. **Antimony** compounds probably act by binding to sulfhydryl groups and inactivating key enzymes.
   B. **Stibine,** like arsine, may cause hemolysis. It is also an irritant gas.

II. **Toxic dose**
   A. The lethal oral dose of **antimony** in mice is 100 mg/kg; at these doses mice developed eosinophilia and cardiac failure. The OSHA occupational permissible exposure limit (PEL) for antimony is 0.5 mg/m^3 as an 8-hour time-weighted average.
   B. The OSHA permissible exposure limit (PEL) for **stibine** is 0.1 ppm as an 8-hour time-weighted average. The air level considered immediately dangerous to life or health (IDLH) is 40 ppm.

III. **Clinical presentation**
   A. **Acute ingestion of antimony** causes nausea, vomiting, and diarrhea (often bloody). Hepatitis and renal insufficiency may occur. Death is rare if the patient survives the initial gastroenteritis.
   B. **Acute stibine inhalation** causes acute hemolysis, resulting in anemia, jaundice, hemoglobinuria, and renal failure.
   C. **Chronic exposure to antimony dusts and fumes** in the workplace is the most common type of exposure and may result in headache, anorexia, pneumoconiosis, peptic ulcers, and dermatitis (antimony spots). Sudden death presumably due to a direct cardiotoxic effect has been reported in workers exposed to antimony trisulfide.

IV. **Diagnosis.** Diagnosis is based on a history of exposure and typical clinical presentation.
   A. **Specific levels.** Normal serum and urine antimony levels are below 10 mcg/L. Serum and urine concentrations correlate poorly with workplace exposure. Urinary antimony is increased after firearm discharge exposure. There is no established toxic antimony level after stibine exposure.
   B. **Other useful laboratory studies.** CBC, plasma free hemoglobin, electrolytes, BUN, creatinine, urinalysis, liver function tests.

V. **Treatment**
   A. **Emergency and supportive measures**
      1. **Antimony.** Large-volume intravenous fluid resuscitation may be necessary for shock caused by gastroenteritis (see p 14).
      2. **Stibine.** Blood transfusion may be necessary after massive hemolysis. Treat hemoglobinuria with fluids and bicarbonate as for rhabdomyolysis (see p 24).
   B. **Specific drugs and antidotes.** There is no specific antidote. BAL (dimercaprol) and penicillamine are not effective chelators for antimony, nor are they expected to be effective for stibine.
   C. **Decontamination**
      1. **Inhalation.** Remove from exposure, and give supplemental oxygen if available. Protect rescuer from exposure.
      2. **Ingestion**
         a. Induce emesis or perform gastric lavage (see p 42).
         b. Administer activated charcoal (see p 45), although there is no evidence for its effectiveness. Do *not* use cathartics.
   D. **Enhanced elimination.** Hemodialysis, hemoperfusion, and forced diuresis are *not* effective at removing antimony or stibine. Exchange transfusion may be effective in treating massive hemolysis caused by stibine.

Reference

NIOSH: *Criteria for a Recommended Standard: Occupational Exposure to Antimony.* Department of Health, Education, and Welfare Publication No. 78-216. US Government Printing Office, 1978.

ANTINEOPLASTIC AGENTS
Susan Kim, PharmD

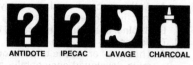

ANTIDOTE IPECAC LAVAGE CHARCOAL

Because of the inherently cytotoxic nature of most chemotherapeutic antineoplastic agents, overdoses are likely to be extremely serious. These agents are classified into 6 categories (Table II-7). Relatively few acute overdoses have been reported for these agents.

I. **Mechanism of toxicity.** In general, toxic effects are extensions of the pharmacologic properties of these drugs.
- A. **Alkylating agents.** These drugs provide highly charged carbon atoms that attack nucleophilic sites on DNA, resulting in alkylation and cross-stranding and thus inhibiting replication and transcription. Binding to RNA or protein moieties appears to contribute little to cytotoxic effects.
- B. **Antibiotics.** These drugs intercalate within base pairs in DNA, inhibiting DNA-directed RNA synthesis. Another potential mechanism may be generation of cytotoxic free radicals.
- C. **Antimetabolites.** These agents interfere with DNA synthesis at various stages. For example, methotrexate binds reversibly to dihydrofolate reductase, preventing synthesis of purine and pyrimidine nucleotides.
- D. **Hormones.** Steroid hormones regulate the synthesis of steroid-specific proteins. The exact mechanism of antineoplastic action is unknown.
- E. **Mitotic inhibitors.** These agents act in various ways to inhibit orderly mitosis, thereby arresting cell division.
- F. **Others.** The cytotoxic actions of other antineoplastic drugs result from a variety of mechanisms, including DNA alkylation, blockade of protein synthesis, and inhibition of hormone release.

II. **Toxic dose.** Because of the highly toxic nature of these agents (except for hormones), exposure to even therapeutic amounts should be considered potentially serious. Most oral antineoplastic agents are readily absorbed, with peak levels reached within 1–2 hours of ingestion.

III. **Clinical presentation.** The organ systems affected by the various agents are listed in Table II-7. The most common sites of toxicity are the hematopoietic and gastrointestinal systems.
- A. **Leukopenia** is the most common manifestation of bone marrow depression. Thrombocytopenia and anemia may also occur. Death may result from overwhelming infections or hemorrhagic diathesis. With alkylating agents, nadirs occur 1–4 weeks after exposure; while with antibiotics, antimetabolites, and mitotic inhibitors, the nadirs occur 1–2 weeks after exposure.
- B. **Gastrointestinal toxicity** is also very common. Nausea and vomiting often accompany therapeutic administration, and severe ulcerative gastroenteritis may occur.
- C. **Extravasation** of some antineoplastic drugs at the intravenous injection site may cause severe local injury, with skin necrosis and sloughing.

IV. **Diagnosis.** Diagnosis is usually based on the history. Because some of the most serious toxic effects may be delayed until several days after exposure, early clinical symptoms and signs may not be dramatic.
- A. **Specific levels.** Not generally available. For methotrexate, see Table III-5, p. 320.

TABLE II-7. COMMON ANTINEOPLASTIC AGENTS AND THEIR TOXICITIES

Drug	Major Site(s) of Toxicity[a]	Comments
Alkylating agents		
Busulfan	D+, En+, M+, P++	Pulmonary fibrosis with chronic use.
Carmustine	D+, G+, H+, M+, Ex+	Flushing, hypotension, and tachycardia with rapid IV injection.
Chlorambucil	D+, G+, H+, M+, N++	Seizures, confusion, coma reported after overdose.
Cisplatin	An+, G++, M+, N+, P+, R++	Ototoxic, nephrotoxic. Good hydration essential. Hemodialysis not effective.
Cyclophosphamide	Al++, C+, D+, En+, G++, M++, R+	Hemodialysis effective. Acetylcysteine and 2-mercaptoethanesulfonate have been used investigationally to reduce hemorrhagic cystitis.
Lomustine	Al+, G+, H+, M+	Thrombocytopenia, leukopenia, liver and lymph node enlargement after overdose.
Mechlorethamine	D+, G++, M++, N+, Ex+	Lymphocytopenia may occur within 24 hours.
Melphalan	G+, M+	Hemodialysis effective although of questionable need (half-life only 90 minutes).
Pipobroman	G+, M+	
Thiotepa	An+, G++, M++	Bone marrow suppression usually very severe.
Uracil mustard	G+, M++	Bone marrow suppression first noted as thrombocytopenia, leukopenia.
Antibiotics		
Bleomycin	An++, D++, G+, P++	Pulmonary fibrosis with chronic use.
Dactinomycin	Al++, D+, G++, M++, Ex++	Severe inflammatory reaction may occur at previously irradiated sites.
Daunorubicin	Al++, An+, C++, G++, M++, Ex++	Congestive cardiomyopathy may occur after total cumulative dose > 600 mg/m².
Doxorubicin	Al++, An+, C++, D+, G++, M++, Ex++	Cardiotoxicity and cardiomyopathy may occur after total cumulative dose > 55 mg/m². Arrhythmias after acute overdose. Hemoperfusion may be effective.

continued

TABLE II-7. COMMON ANTINEOPLASTIC AGENTS AND THEIR TOXICITIES (Continued)

Drug	Major Site(s) of Toxicity[a]	Comments
Mitomycin	Al+, D+, G++, H+, M+, P+, R+, Ex++	Hemolytic anemia reported with therapeutic doses.
Mitoxantrone	An+, C+, G++, M++	Four reported overdosed patients died from severe leukopenia and infection.
Plicamycin	An+, D+, G++, H++, M++, N+, Ex+	Coagulopathy, electrolyte disturbances may occur. Check calcium frequently.
Antimetabolites		
Cytarabine	An+, E+, G+, H+, M+	"Cytarabine syndrome": fever, myalgia, bone pain, rash, malaise.
5-Fluorouracil	Al+, D+, G++, M++, N+	Uridine has been used investigationally as a "rescue"agent.
6-Mercaptopurine	G+, H++, M+	Hemodialysis removes drug but of questionable need (half-life 20–60 minutes).
Methotrexate	Al+, D+, G++, H+, M++, N+, P+, R+	Folinic acid (leucovorin; see p 319) is specific antidote. Hemoperfusion effective.
6-Thioguanine	G+, H+, M+, R+	Hemodialysis probably ineffective owing to rapid intracellular incorporation.
Hormones		
Androgens		
Testolactone	En±, G±	Toxicity unlikely after single acute overdose.
Estrogens		
Diethylstilbestrol	En±, G±	Possible carcinogenic effect on fetus if taken during early pregnancy.
Estramustine	En±, G±, H±, M±	Has both weak estrogenic and alkylating activity.
Polyestradiol	En±, G±	Toxicity unlikely after single acute overdose.
Antiestrogens		
Tamoxifen	Al±, D±, En±, G±	Acute toxic effects unlikely. Hot flashes, vaginal bleeding with chronic use.

Drug	Toxicity	Comments
Progestins		
Medroxyprogesterone	An±, En±, G±	Acute toxic effects unlikely. May induce porphyria in susceptible patients.
Megestrol	En±, G±	Acute toxic effects unlikely. May induce porphyria in susceptible patients.
Other hormones		
Leuprolide	En+	Acute toxic effects unlikely. Initial increase in luteinizing hormone, follicle-stimulating hormone levels.
Mitotic inhibitors		
Etoposide	An+, G+, M++	Myelosuppression major toxicity. Dystonic reaction reported.
Vinblastine	G+, M++, N+, Ex++	Myelosuppression, ileus, syndrome of inappropriate antidiuretic hormone reported after overdose.
Vincristine sulfate	G+, M±, N++, Ex++	Delayed (up to 9 days) seizures, delirium, coma reported after overdoses.
Miscellaneous		
Asparaginase	An++, En+, G+, H++, N++, R+	Bleeding diathesis. Hyperglycemia.
Dacarbazine	AI+, An+, En+, G++, H+, M+, N+, Ex±	May produce flulike syndrome. Photosensitivity reported.
Hydroxyurea	D+, G+, M++	Leukopenia, anemia more common than thrombocytopenia.
Mitotane	AI+, D+, En+, G++, N++	Adrenal suppression; glucocorticoid replacement essential during stress.
Procarbazine hydrochloride	An+, D+, En+, G++, M++, N++	Monoamine oxidase inhibitor activity. Disulfiramlike ethanol interaction.
Streptozocin	En+, G+, H+, M+, R++	Destroys pancreatic beta islet cells, may produce acute diabetes mellitus. Niacinamide (see p 327) may be effective in preventing islet cell destruction.

*AI = alopecia; An = anaphalaxis allergy or drug fever; C = cardiac; D = dermatologic; En = endocrine; G = gastrointestinal; H = hepatic; M = myelosuppressive; N = neurologic; P = pulmonary; R = renal; Ex = extravasation risk. + = mild to moderate severity; ++ = severe toxicity. ± = minimal.

   B. Other useful laboratory studies. CBC, platelet count, electrolytes, glucose, BUN and creatinine, liver enzymes, and prothrombin time. ECG may be indicated for cardiotoxic agents, and pulmonary function tests are indicated for agents with known pulmonary toxicity.

V. Treatment

  A. Emergency and supportive measures

    1. Maintain the airway and assist ventilation if necessary (see p 2).

    2. Treat coma (p 17), seizures (p 19), hypotension (p 14), and arrhythmias (pp 9–13) if they occur.

    3. **Bone marrow depression** should be treated with the assistance of an experienced hematologist or oncologist.

    4. Treat nausea and vomiting with metoclopamide (p 322) and fluid loss due to gastroenteritis with intravenous crystalloid fluids.

    5. **Extravasation.** Immediately stop the infusion and withdraw as much fluid as possible by negative pressure on the syringe. Then give the following specific treatment:

      a. **Dactinomycin, daunorubicin, mitomycin-C, plicamycin, mitoxantrone.** Apply ice compresses to extravasation site for 15 minutes 4 times daily for 3 days.

      b. **Mechlorethamine.** Infiltrate site of extravasation with 10–15 mL of sterile 0.15 molar sodium thiosulfate (dilute 4 mL of 10% thiosulfate with sterile water to a volume of 15 mL); apply ice compresses for 6–12 hours.

      c. **Vincristine** or **vinblastine.** Place heating pad over the area on and off for 24 hours; elevate limb.

  B. Specific drugs and antidotes. Very few specific treatments or antidotes are available (Table II–7).

  C. Decontamination

    1. Induce emesis or perform gastric lavage (see p 42).

    2. Administer activated charcoal and a cathartic (see p 45).

    3. Gut emptying is probably not necessary following small ingestions if activated charcoal is given promptly.

  D. Enhanced elimination. Because of the rapid intracellular incorporation of most agents, dialysis and other extracorporeal removal procedures are generally not effective (see Table II–7 for exceptions).

Reference

Banerjee A et al: Cancer chemotherapy agent-induced perivenous extravasation injuries. *Postgrad Med J* 1987;**63**:5.

ANTISEPTICS AND DISINFECTANTS
Olga F. Woo, PharmD

ANTIDOTE   IPECAC   LAVAGE   CHARCOAL

Antiseptics are applied to living tissue to kill or prevent the growth of microorganisms. **Disinfectants** are applied to inanimate objects to destroy pathogenic microorganisms. Despite their unproved worth, they are widely used in the household, food industry, and hospitals. This chapter describes toxicity due to **hydrogen peroxide, potassium permanganate, hexylresorcinol,** and **ichthammol.** All these agents are generally used as dilute solutions and cause little or no toxicity. Hexylresorcinol is commonly found in throat lozenges. For toxicity of other antiseptics and disinfectants, see Iodine (p 174); Mercurochrome (p 197); Isopropyl alcohol (p 181); Pine oil (p 165); and Hypochlorite (p 119).

I. **Mechanism of toxicity**
   A. **Hydrogen peroxide** is an oxidizing agent, but it is very unstable and readily breaks down to oxygen and water. Generation of oxygen gas in closed body cavities can potentially cause mechanical distention resulting in gastric or intestinal perforation.
   B. **Potassium permanganate** is an oxidant, and the crystalline form or concentrated solutions are corrosive.
   C. **Hexylresorcinol** is related to phenol but is much less toxic, although alcohol-based solutions possess vesicant properties.
   D. **Ichthammol** contains about 10% sulfur in the form of organic sulfonates, and it is keratolytic to tissues.

II. **Toxic dose**
   A. **Hydrogen peroxide** for household use is available in 3–5% solutions and is mildly irritating; concentrations above 10% are found in some hair-bleaching solutions and are potentially corrosive. A 3-year-old child died after ingesting 40% hydrogen peroxide.
   B. **Potassium permanganate** solutions of greater than 1:5000 strength may cause corrosive burns.

III. **Clinical presentation.** Most antiseptic ingestions are benign, and mild irritation is self-limited. Spontaneous emesis and diarrhea may occur, especially after a large-volume ingestion.
   A. Exposure to **concentrated** solutions may cause corrosive burns on the skin and mucous membranes, and oropharyngeal, esophageal, or gastric injury may occur. Glottic edema has been reported after ingestion of concentrated potassium permanganate.
   B. Permanganate may also cause **methemoglobinemia** (see p 204).
   C. Hydrogen peroxide ingestion may cause gastric distention and, rarely, perforation.

IV. **Diagnosis.** Diagnosis is based on a history of exposure and the presence of mild gastrointestinal upset or frank corrosive injury. Solutions of potassium permanganate are dark purple, and skin and mucous membranes are often characteristically stained.
   A. **Specific levels.** Serum drug levels are not useful or available.
   B. **Other useful laboratory studies.** CBC, electrolytes, glucose, methemoglobin level (for potassium permanganate exposure).

V. **Treatment**
   A. **Emergency and supportive measures**
      1. After ingestion of concentrated solutions, monitor the airway for swelling and intubate if necessary.
      2. Consult a gastroenterologist for possible endoscopy. Most ingestions are benign, and mild irritation is self-limited.
   B. **Specific drugs and antidotes.** No specific antidotes are available for irritant or corrosive effects. If methemoglobinemia occurs, administer **methylene blue** (see p 322).
   C. **Decontamination**
      1. **Ingestion**
         a. Dilute immediately with water or milk.
         b. Perform gastric lavage (see p 43) cautiously. Do *not* induce emesis because of the risk of corrosive injury.
         c. Activated charcoal and cathartics are not effective.
      2. **Eyes and skin.** Irrigate the eyes and skin with copious amounts of tepid water. Remove contaminated clothing.
   D. **Enhanced elimination.** Enhanced elimination methods are neither necessary nor effective.

Reference

Sleigh JW, Linter SP: Hazards of hydrogen peroxide. *Br Med J* 1985;**291**:1706.

ARSENIC
Donna E. Foliart, MD, MPH

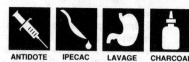

ANTIDOTE   IPECAC   LAVAGE   CHARCOAL

Arsenic (As) compounds are widely distributed in soil and are used in a variety of industries and commercial products, including weed killers, wood preservatives, pesticides, rodenticides, and hardening agents in metal alloys. Exposure to arsenic may occur during production of pigments, glass, and silicon chips and the smelting of copper ores. Arsine gas, a product of arsenic, is discussed on p 83.

I. **Mechanism of toxicity.** Arsenic compounds are irritants of the skin, mucous membranes, and respiratory and gastrointestinal tracts. Once absorbed, arsenic disrupts cellular metabolism by binding to sulfhydryl groups on a variety of enzymes.

   A. Arsenic compounds may be organic or inorganic and may contain arsenic in either a pentavalent (arsenate) or trivalent (arsenite) form. Organic pentavalent arsenates are ubiquitous in nature, rapidly excreted by the kidneys, and relatively nontoxic. In contrast, trivalent organic and inorganic arsenite compounds are highly toxic.

   B. Arsenic is also a known human carcinogen (see Table IV–13).

II. **Toxic dose**

   A. Acute ingestion of as little as 120 mg of arsenic trioxide (an inorganic trivalent compound) is reported to be fatal.

   B. In contrast, pentavalent arsenate compounds are far less toxic than trivalent arsenic compounds, by several orders of magnitude. Organic pentavalent forms are essentially nontoxic.

III. **Clinical presentation**

   A. **Acute exposure.** Symptoms occur rapidly after acute ingestion of toxic arsenic compounds and include throat and abdominal pain, vomiting, and profuse watery diarrhea; profound fluid and electrolyte loss may cause death within 24 hours. Delirium, coma, and QT interval prolongation with polymorphous ventricular tachycardia (see p 13) have also been reported. Survivors may develop peripheral sensory neuropathy, exfoliative dermatitis, and hair loss.

   B. **Chronic exposure.** Chronic exposure to arsenic dust or fumes causes irritation of the skin, mucous membranes, and respiratory tract and occasionally perforation of the nasal septum. Systemic effects of chronic exposure include weakness, anorexia, nausea, vomiting, diarrhea, hepatitis, peripheral sensory neuropathy (in a glove-stocking pattern), and alopecia. Skin hyperpigmentation and transverse white lines on the nails (Mees' lines) may be noted. Lung and skin cancer have been associated with chronic exposure.

IV. **Diagnosis.** Diagnosis is usually based on a history of exposure and typical presentation. Suspect acute arsenic poisoning in any patient with abrupt onset of severe vomiting and watery diarrhea and chronic poisoning in any patient with alopecia, sensory neuropathy, or both. Arsenic salts are radiopaque and may be visible on x-ray.

   A. **Specific levels.** Serum arsenic levels are highly variable and are rarely of value in emergency treatment. Arsenic levels higher than 50 mcg/L in a 24-hour urine specimen are considered abnormal. Because assays measure total arsenic, very high levels with little or no associated symptoms may be encountered in patients who have recently consumed a meal high in organic arsenate compounds (eg, seafood, liver, etc).

   B. **Other useful laboratory studies.** CBC, electrolytes, glucose, BUN and creatinine, liver enzymes, urinalysis, ECG and electrocardiographic monitoring, abdominal x-ray.

V. Treatment

A. Emergency and supportive measures

1. Maintain the airway and assist ventilation if neccessary (see p 2).
2. Treat coma (p 17), shock (p 14), and arrhythmias (p 13) if they occur.
3. Treat fluid and electrolyte loss due to gastroenteritis with aggressive use of intravenous crystalloid solutions (p 14).
4. Monitor vital signs and ECG for a minimum of 24 hours after significant acute exposure.

B. Specific drugs and antidotes

1. In symptomatic patients, administer **BAL (dimercaprol;** see p 294), 3–5 mg/kg IM every 4–6 hours.
2. Oral chelation therapy with **penicillamine** (p 322) or **2,3-DMSA** (p 306) may be used after the patient has stabilized or in chronically intoxicated patients.

C. Decontamination

1. Induce emesis or perform gastric lavage (see p 42).
2. Administer activated charcoal (see p 45). Do not use cathartics if the patient already has diarrhea.
3. Gut emptying is probably not necessary following small ingestions if activated charcoal is given promptly.

D. Enhanced elimination. There is no known role for diuresis, dialysis, hemoperfusion, or repeat-dose charcoal.

Reference

Levin-Scherz JK et al: Acute arsenic ingestion. *Ann Emerg Med* 1987;**16**:702.

ARSINE
Donna E. Foliart, MD, MPH

ANTIDOTE   IPECAC   LAVAGE   CHARCOAL

Arsine is a colorless gas formed when arsenic comes into contact with hydrogen or with reducing agents in aqueous solution. Typically, exposure occurs in metal smelting and refining industries when metals containing arsenic as an alloy react with an acid. Arsine is also used as a dopant in the microelectronics industry.

I. **Mechanism of toxicity.** Arsine enters red blood cells and forms a complex that results in massive intravascular hemolysis. Several explanations are postulated for the hemolysis, including liberation of elemental arsenic and the formation of complexes with sulfhydryl groups essential to erythrocyte enzymes. **Renal failure** is the most common cause of death after arsine exposure. Renal failure is probably secondary to massive hemolysis and hemoglobinuria, but it may also be due to direct toxic effects on renal tubular cells or deposition of the arsine-hemoglobin-haptoglobin complex.

II. **Toxic dose.** Arsine is the most toxic form of arsenic. The air level considered immediately dangerous to life or health (IDLH) is 6 ppm. Exposure to 250 ppm may be instantly lethal, and exposure to 25–50 ppm for 30 minutes is usually lethal. The OSHA permissible exposure limit (PEL) is 0.05 ppm as an 8-hour time-weighted average. The odor threshold is approximately 0.5 ppm.

III. **Clinical presentation**

A. Because arsine gas is not acutely irritating, inhalation causes **no immediate symptoms.** Those exposed to high concentrations may describe a garliclike odor in the air but more typically are unaware that significant exposure has occurred.

B. **After a latent period of 2–24 hours** (depending on the intensity of exposure), massive hemolysis occurs, with early symptoms of malaise, headache, weakness, dyspnea, nausea, vomiting, abdominal pain, hemoglobinuria, and jaundice. Oliguria and acute renal failure often occur 1–3 days after exposure.

IV. **Diagnosis.** Diagnosis is based on a history of exposure; it should be suspected in any worker potentially exposed to arsine who develops acute hemolysis. Laboratory evidence of hemolysis includes acute anemia, anisocytosis, and fragmented red cells. Plasma free hemoglobin levels may exceed 2 g/dL, and haptoglobin levels are lowered. Routine urinalysis reveals hemoglobinuria but few intact red blood cells.

A. **Specific levels.** The urine arsenic concentration may be elevated, but this does not assist in emergency management. Whole blood arsenic concentrations of greater than 0.4 mg/L are associated with fatal cases.

B. **Other useful laboratory studies.** CBC, plasma free hemoglobin, haptoglobin, blood type and screen (cross-match if needed), BUN and creatinine, urinalysis.

V. **Treatment**

A. **Emergency and supportive measures**

1. Treat hemolysis with blood transfusions as needed.

2. Prevent deposition of hemoglobin and arsine complex in the kidney tubules by intravenously administering bicarbonate, fluids, and mannitol, if needed, to maintain an adequate (2–3 mL/kg/h) alkaline urine flow. (See discussion of treatment of rhabdomyolysis, p 24.)

B. **Specific drugs and antidotes.** BAL (dimercaprol) is **not** effective for arsine-induced intoxication.

C. **Decontamination.** Remove victim from area. Rescuers should wear self-contained breathing apparatus to protect themselves from exposure.

D. **Enhanced elimination.** The arsine-haptoglobin-hemoglobin complex is not significantly removed by hemodialysis. Forced alkaline diuresis may prevent renal tubular necrosis but does not enhance removal of the complex.

Reference

Fowler BA, Weissberg JB: Arsine poisoning. *N Engl J Med* 1974;**291**:1171.

ASBESTOS
Donna E. Foliart, MD, MPH

ANTIDOTE   IPECAC   LAVAGE   CHARCOAL

Asbestos is the name given to a group of naturally occurring silicates: chrysotile, amosite, and crocidolite and the asbestiform types of tremolite, actinolite, and anthophylite. Exposure to asbestos is a well-documented cause of restrictive lung disease, lung cancer, and mesothelioma, illnesses that may appear many years after exposure.

I. **Mechanism of toxicity.** Inhalation of fibers longer than 5 μ produces lung fibrosis and cancer in animals (shorter fibers are generally phagocytosed by macrophages and removed from the lungs). The exact mechanism of toxicity is unknown. Smoking cigarettes appears to enhance the likelihood of developing lung disease and malignancy.

II. **Toxic dose.** A safe threshold of exposure to asbestos has not been established. Balancing potential health risks against feasibility of workplace control, the 1986 OSHA federal asbestos standard set a permissible exposure limit (PEL) of 0.2 fibers per cubic centimeters (fibers/cc) as an 8-hour time-weighted average.

III. **Clinical presentation.** After a latent period of 15–20 years, the patient may develop one or more of the following clinical syndromes:

   A. **Asbestosis** is a slowly progressive restrictive lung disease characterized by pulmonary fibrosis; death occurs within 15 years of onset, owing to cardiorespiratory failure or concurrent lung cancer.

   B. **Pleural plaques** are usually asymptomatic but provide a marker for asbestos exposure.

   C. **Pleural effusions** are uncommon and are usually asymptomatic.

   D. **Lung cancer** is a common cause of death in patients with asbestos exposure, especially in cigarette smokers. **Mesothelioma** is a malignancy that may affect the pleura or the peritoneum. The incidence of **gastrointestinal cancer** may be increased in asbestos-exposed workers.

IV. **Diagnosis.** Diagnosis is based on a history of exposure to asbestos (usually at least 15–20 years before onset of symptoms) and clinical presentation of one or more of the syndromes described above. Chest x-ray typically shows small, irregular, round opacities distributed primarily in the lower lung fields. Pleural plaques, thickening, or calcifications may be present. Pulmonary function tests reveal decreased vital capacity and total lung capacity and impairment of carbon monoxide diffusion.

   A. **Specific tests.** There are no specific blood or urine tests.

   B. **Other useful laboratory studies.** Chest x-ray, arterial blood gases, pulmonary function tests.

V. **Treatment**

   A. **Emergency and supportive measures.** Emphasis should be placed on **prevention** of exposure. All asbestos workers should be encouraged to stop smoking and to observe workplace control measures stringently.

   B. **Specific drugs and antidotes.** There are none.

   C. **Decontamination**

      1. **Inhalation.** Persons exposed to asbestos dust and those assisting victims should wear protective equipment, including disposable gowns, caps, and masks. Watering down any dried material will help to prevent its dispersion into the air as dust.

      2. **Skin exposure.** Asbestos is not absorbed through the skin. However, it may be inhaled from skin and clothes, so removal of clothes and washing the skin are recommended.

      3. **Ingestion.** Asbestos is not known to be harmful by ingestion, so no decontamination is necessary.

   D. **Enhanced elimination.** There is no role for these procedures.

Reference

Wheater RH: A physician's guide to asbestos-related diseases. *JAMA* 1984;252:2593.

BARBITURATES
Kent R. Olson, MD

ANTIDOTE   IPECAC   LAVAGE   CHARCOAL

Barbiturates are used as hypnotic and sedative agents, for the induction of anesthesia, and for the treatment of epilepsy and status epilepticus. They are often divided into 4 major groups by their pharmacologic activity and clinical use: **ultrashort-acting, short-acting, intermediating-acting,** and **long-acting** (Table II–8).

I. **Mechanism of toxicity**
   A. All barbiturates cause generalized **depression of neuronal activity** in the brain. These effects are primarily mediated through enhanced GABA-mediated synaptic inhibition. Hypotension that occurs with large doses is caused by depression of central sympathetic tone as well as by direct depression of cardiac contractility.
   B. The various agents have different pharmacokinetic properties:
      1. **Ultrashort-acting** barbiturates are highly lipid-soluble and rapidly penetrate the brain to induce anesthesia, then are quickly redistributed to other tissues. For this reason, the duration of effect is much shorter than the elimination half-life for these compounds.
      2. **Long-acting barbiturates** are distributed more evenly and have long elimination half-lives, making them useful for once-daily treatment of epilepsy.
II. **Toxic dose.** The toxic dose of barbiturates varies widely and depends on the drug, the route and rate of administration, and individual patient tolerance. In general, toxicity is likely when the dose exceeds 5–10 times the hypnotic dose. Chronic users or abusers may have striking tolerance to depressant effects.
   A. The potentially fatal **oral dose** of the shorter-acting agents is 2–3 g, compared with 6–10 g for phenobarbital.
   B. Several deaths were reported in young women undergoing therapeutic abortion after they received rapid **intravenous injections** of 1–3 mg/kg of methohexital.
III. **Clinical presentation.** The onset of symptoms depends on the drug and the route of administration.

TABLE II-8. COMMON BARBITURATES[a]

Drug	Normal Elimination Half-Life (h)	Usual Duration of Effect (h)	Usual Hypnotic Dose (Adult) (mg)	Minimum Toxic Level (mg/L)
Ultrashort-acting				
Methohexital	1–2	< 0.5	50–120	> 5
Thiopental	6–46	< 0.5	50–75	> 5
Short-acting				
Pentobarbital	15–48	> 3–4	100–200	> 10
Secobarbital	15–40	> 3–4	100–200	> 10
Intermediate-acting				
Amobarbital	8–42	> 4–6	65–200	> 10
Aprobarbital	14–34	> 4–6	40–160	> 10
Butabarbital	34–42	> 4–6	50–100	> 10
Long-acting				
Mephobarbital	11–67	> 6–12	50–100	> 30
Phenobarbital	80–120	> 6–12	100–320	> 30

[a] References: Harvey SC: Hypnotics and sedatives. Chap 17, pp 339–371, in: *Goodman & Gilman's The Pharmacological Basis of Therapeutics,* 7th ed. Gilman AG et al (editors). Macmillan, 1985; and Ellenhorn MJ, Barceloux DG: *Medical Toxicology.* Pages 576–577. Elsevier, 1988.

    A. With mild intoxication, lethargy, slurred speech, nystagmus, and ataxia are common.

    B. With higher doses, hypotension, coma, and respiratory arrest commonly occur. With deep coma, the pupils are usually small; the patient may lose all reflex activity and may appear to be dead.

    C. Hypothermia is common in patients with deep coma, especially if the victim has suffered exposure to a cool environment. Hypotension and bradycardia commonly accompany hypothermia.

IV. Diagnosis. Diagnosis is usually based on a history of ingestion and should be suspected in any epileptic patient with stupor or coma. Although skin bullae are sometimes seen with barbiturate overdose, these are not specific for barbiturates. Other causes of coma should be considered (see p 17).

    A. Specific levels. Serum levels of phenobarbital are usually readily available from hospital clinical laboratories; concentrations greater than 60–80 mg/L are usually associated with coma and those greater than 150–200 mg/L with severe hypotension. For short-acting barbiturates, coma is likely when the serum concentration exceeds 20–30 mg/L. Barbiturates are easily detected in routine toxicologic screening.

    B. Other useful laboratory studies. CBC, electrolytes, glucose, BUN, creatinine, arterial blood gases, chest x-ray.

V. Treatment

    A. Emergency and supportive measures

        1. Protect the airway and assist ventilation (see p 2) if necessary.

        2. Treat coma (p 17), hypothermia (p 18), and hypotension (p 14) if they occur.

    B. Specific drugs and antidotes. There is no specific antidote.

    C. Decontamination

        1. Induce emesis or perform gastric lavage (see p 42). Lavage is preferred because of the risk of coma.

        2. Administer activated charcoal and cathartic (see p 45).

        3. Gut emptying is probably not necessary following small ingestions if activated charcoal is given promptly.

    D. Enhanced elimination

        1. **Alkalinization** of the urine (see p 47) increases the elimination of phenobarbital but not other barbiturates. Its value in acute overdose is unproved, and it may potentially contribute to fluid overload and pulmonary edema.

        2. **Repeat-dose activated charcoal** has been shown to decrease the half-life of phenobarbital, but there is no evidence that it actually shortens duration of coma.

        3. **Hemoperfusion** may be indicated for severely intoxicated patients not responding to supportive care.

Reference

Goodman JM et al: Barbiturate intoxication: Morbidity and mortality. *West J Med* 1976;**124**:179.

BARIUM
Olga F. Woo, PharmD

| ANTIDOTE | IPECAC | LAVAGE | CHARCOAL |

Barium poisonings are uncommon and are usually due to accidental contamination of food sources or suicidal ingestion. The water-soluble barium salts (acetate, carbonate, chloride, hydroxide, nitrate, sulfide) are highly toxic, whereas the insoluble salt barium sulfate is nontoxic because it is not absorbed. Soluble barium salts are found in depilatories, fireworks, and rodenticides and are used in the manufacture of glass and in dyeing textiles. Barium sulfide and polysulfide may also produce hydrogen sulfide toxicity (see p 169).

I. **Mechanism of toxicity.** Barium poisoning is characterized by profound hypokalemia, leading to respiratory and cardiac arrest. The mechanism for the rapid onset of severe hypokalemia is not known; studies have excluded intracellular sequestration of potassium, enhanced renal elimination, and adrenergic stimulation. It is proposed that barium ions have a direct action on muscle cell potassium permeability, which stimulates smooth, striated, and cardiac muscles, resulting in peristalsis, arterial hypertension, muscle twitching, and cardiac arrhythmias.

II. **Toxic dose.** The minimum oral toxic dose of soluble barium salts is undetermined but may be as low as 200 mg. Lethal doses range between 1–30 g for various barium salts because absorption is influenced by gastric pH and foods high in sulfate.

III. **Clinical presentation.** Within minutes to a few hours after ingestion, victims develop profound hypokalemia and skeletal muscle weakness progressing to flaccid paralysis of the limbs and respiratory muscles. Ventricular arrhythmias also occur. Gastroenteritis with severe watery diarrhea, mydriasis with impaired visual accommodation, and central nervous system depression are sometimes present. More often, patients remain conscious even when severely intoxicated.

IV. **Diagnosis.** Diagnosis is based on a history of exposure, accompanied by rapidly progressive hypokalemia and muscle weakness.
   A. **Specific levels.** Blood barium levels are not routinely available.
   B. **Other useful laboratory studies.** CBC, electrolytes, BUN, creatinine, arterial blood gases, ECG.

V. **Treatment**
   A. **Emergency and supportive measures**
      1. Maintain the airway and assist ventilation if necessary (see p 2).
      2. Treat fluid losses from gastroenteritis with intravenous crystalloids.
      3. Attach a cardiac monitor and observe patient closely for several hours after ingestion.
   B. **Specific drugs and antidotes.** Administer **potassium chloride** (KCl) at 10–15 meq/h IV to treat symptomatic or severe hypokalemia (see p 32). Large doses of potassium may be necessary (doses as high as 420 meq over 24 hours have been given).
   C. **Decontamination**
      1. Induce emesis or perform gastric lavage (see p 42). *Caution:* Rapidly progressive weakness may increase the risk of pulmonary aspiration.
      2. Administer activated charcoal and cathartic (see p 45).
      3. Magnesium sulfate or sodium sulfate (60–100 mL) may be administered orally to precipitate ingested barium as the insoluble sulfate salt.
   D. **Enhanced elimination**
      1. **Diuresis with saline and furosemide** to obtain a urine flow of 4–6 mL/kg/h may enhance barium elimination.
      2. Hemodialysis and hemoperfusion have not been evaluated in the treatment of serious barium poisoning.

Reference

Gould DB, Sorrell MR, Lupariello AD: Barium sulfide poisoning: Some factors contributing to survival. *Arch Intern Med* 1973;**132**:891.

BENZENE
Gary Pasternak, MD

| ANTIDOTE | IPECAC | LAVAGE | CHARCOAL |

Benzene, a clear volatile liquid with a characteristic pleasant odor, is one of the most widely used industrial chemicals, with more than 2 million workers potentially exposed. It is used as a constituent in gasoline; as a solvent for fats, inks, paints, and plastics; and as a chemical intermediate in the synthesis of a variety of materials. It is generally not present in household products.

I. **Mechanism of toxicity.** Like other hydrocarbons, benzene can cause a chemical pneumonia if it is aspirated. See p 165 for a general discussion of hydrocarbon toxicity.
   A. Once absorbed, benzene causes central nervous system depression and may sensitize the myocardium to the arrhythmogenic effects of catecholamines.
   B. Benzene is also known for its chronic effects on the hematopoetic system, which are thought to be due to the phenolic metabolite.
   C. Benzene is a suspected human carcinogen (see Table IV–13).

II. **Toxic dose.** Benzene is rapidly absorbed by inhalation and ingestion and, to a limited extent, percutaneously.
   A. The estimated lethal **oral** dose is 100 mL, but as little as 15 mL has caused death.
   B. The OSHA permissible exposure limit (PEL) for benzene **vapor** is 10 ppm as an 8-hour time-weighted average. A single exposure to 20,000 ppm can be fatal. Chronic exposure to air concentrations well below the threshold for smell are associated with hematopoietic toxicity.

III. **Clinical presentation**
   A. **Acute exposure** may cause immediate central nervous system effects, including headache, nausea, dizziness, convulsions, and coma. Symptoms of CNS toxicity should be apparent immediately after inhalation or within 30–60 minutes after ingestion. Ventricular arrhythmias may result from sensitization of the myocardium.
   B. After **chronic exposure,** hematologic disorders such as aplastic anemia, thrombocytopenia, myelofibrosis, preleukemia, and acute leukemia may occur. Chromosomal abnormalities have been reported, although no effects on fertility have been described in women following occupational exposure.

IV. **Diagnosis.** Diagnosis of benzene poisoning is based on a history of exposure and typical clinical findings. With chronic hematologic toxicity, erythrocyte, leukocyte, and thrombocyte counts may first increase before the onset of aplastic anemia.
   A. **Specific levels**
      1. Increased urine phenol levels may be useful for following workers' exposure (if diet is carefully controlled for phenol products). Spot urine phenol higher than 20 mg/L suggests excessive occupational exposure.
      2. Benzene can also be measured in expired air.
      3. Blood levels of benzene or metabolites are not clinically useful.
   B. **Other useful laboratory studies.** CBC, electrolytes, BUN, creatinine, liver function tests, electrocardiographic monitoring, chest x-ray (if aspiration suspected).

V. **Treatment**
   A. **Emergency and supportive measures**
      1. Maintain the airway and assist ventilation if necessary (see p 2).

2. Treat coma (p 17), seizures (p 21), arrhythmias (p 13), and other complications if they occur.
3. Do not give epinephrine because of the possibility of myocardial sensitization.
4. Monitor vital signs and ECG for 12–24 hours after significant exposure.

B. Specific drugs and antidotes. There is no specific antidote.

C. Decontamination
1. **Inhalation.** Immediately move the victim to fresh air and administer oxygen, if available.
2. **Skin and eyes.** Remove clothing and wash the skin; irrigate exposed eyes with copious amounts of water or saline.
3. **Ingestion**
   a. Perform gastric lavage (see p 43). Do *not* induce emesis because of the risk of abrupt seizures or coma.
   b. Administer activated charcoal and cathartic (see p 45).
   c. Lavage and charcoal are most effective if initiated within the first 30 minutes.
   d. Gut emptying is probably not necessary following small ingestions if activated charcoal is given promptly.

D. Enhanced elimination. Dialysis and hemoperfusion are not effective.

Reference

Aksoy M: Benzene as a leukemogenic and carcinogenic agent. *Am J Ind Med* 1985;8:9.

BENZODIAZEPINES
James F. Buchanan, PharmD

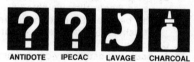

The drug class of benzodiazepines contains many compounds that vary widely in potency, duration of effect, presence or absence of active metabolites, and clinical use (Table II–9). In general, death from benzodiazepine overdose is rare, unless the drugs are combined with other central nervous system depressant agents such as alcohol or barbiturates. Newer potent short-acting agents have been considered the sole cause of death in recent forensic cases.

I. **Mechanism of toxicity.** Benzodiazepines enhance the action of the inhibitory neurotransmitter gamma-aminobutyric acid (GABA). They also inhibit other neuronal systems by poorly defined mechanisms. The result is generalized depression of spinal reflexes and the reticular activating system. This may cause coma and respiratory arrest.
   A. Respiratory arrest is more likely with newer short-acting triazolobenzodiazepines such as triazolam (Halcion), alprazolam (Xanax), and midazolam (Versed).
   B. Cardiopulmonary arrest has occurred after rapid injection of diazepam, possibly because of CNS-depressant effects or because of the toxic effects of the diluent propylene glycol.

II. **Toxic dose.** In general, the toxic-therapeutic ratio for benzodiazepines is very high. For example, oral overdoses of diazepam have been reported in excess of 15–20 times the therapeutic dose without serious depression of consciousness. In contrast, respiratory arrest has been reported after ingestion of 5 mg of triazolam and after rapid intravenous injection of diazepam, midazolam, and many other benzodiazepines.

III. **Clinical presentation.** Onset of CNS depression may be observed within

TABLE II-9. BENZODIAZEPINES FOR ORAL USE[a]

Drug	Half-Life (h)	Active Metabolite	Oral Adult Dose Sedative (mg)	Hypnotic (mg)
Alprazolam	10	Yes	0.25-0.5	—
Chlordiazepoxide	5-15	Yes	5-20	25-50
Clorazepate	50-80[b]	Yes	3.75-15	15-30
Diazepam	30-60	Yes	5-10	5-10
Flurazepam	50-100[b]	Yes	—	15-30
Lorazepam	10-20	No	0.5-2	2-4
Oxazepam	5-10	No	10-15	15-30
Temazepam	10-17	Slight	—	15-30
Triazolam	1.5-3	?	—	0.125-0.5

[a] Adapted with permission, in part from Harvey SC: Hypnotics and sedatives. Table 17-4 in *Goodman and Gilman's The Pharmacological Basis of Therapeutics,* 7th ed. Gilman AG et al (editors). Macmillan, 1985.
[b] Half-life of active metabolite, to which effects can be attributed.

30–120 minutes of ingestion, depending on the compound. Lethargy, slurred speech, ataxia, coma, and respiratory arrest may occur. Generally, patients with benzodiazepine-induced coma have hyporeflexia and mid-position or small pupils. Hypothermia may occur. Serious complications are more likely when newer short-acting agents are involved or whenever other depressant drugs have been ingested.

IV. **Diagnosis.** Diagnosis is usually based on the history of ingestion or recent injection. The differential diagnosis should include other sedative-hypnotic agents, antidepressants, antipsychotics, and narcotics. Coma and small pupils do not respond to naloxone but will reverse with administration of flumazenil (see p 313), a new benzodiazepine antagonist.

    A. **Specific levels.** Serum drug levels are often available from regional commercial toxicology laboratories but are rarely of value in emergency management. Urine and blood qualitative screening may provide rapid confirmation of exposure.

    B. **Other useful laboratory studies.** CBC, electrolytes, glucose, BUN, creatinine, arterial blood gases.

V. **Treatment**

    A. **Emergency and supportive measures**

        1. Protect the airway and assist ventilation if necessary (see p 2).

        2. Treat coma (p 17), hypotension (p 14), and hypothermia (p 18) if they occur. Hypotension usually responds promptly to supine position and intravenous fluids.

    B. **Specific drugs and antidotes.** The specific benzodiazepine antagonist **flumazenil** (see p 313) is not yet commercially available in the USA but is undergoing clinical trials. It is reported to rapidly reverse coma caused by benzodiazepine overdose. However, because benzodiazepine overdose by itself is rarely fatal or even extremely serious, the role of a specific antagonist is questionable. Seizures or other acute withdrawal reactions might be precipitated in patients with benzodiazepine addiction.

    C. **Decontamination**

1. Induce emesis or perform gastric lavage (see p 42). Do **not** induce emesis in patients who have ingested newer ultrashort-acting agents such as triazolam, because onset of coma may be rapid and abrupt.
2. Administer activated charcoal and cathartic (see p 45).
3. Gut emptying is probably not necessary following small ingestions if activated charcoal is given promptly.

D. **Enhanced elimination.** There is no role for diuresis, dialysis, or hemoperfusion. Repeat-dose charcoal has not been studied.

Reference

Olson KR et al: Coma caused by trivial triazolam overdose. *Am J Emerg Med* 1985;**3**:210.

BETA-ADRENERGIC BLOCKERS
Neal L. Benowitz, MD

ANTIDOTE   IPECAC   LAVAGE   CHARCOAL

Beta-adrenergic blocking agents are widely used for the treatment of hypertension, arrhythmias, angina pectoris, migraine headaches, and glaucoma. Many patients with beta-blocker overdose will have underlying cardiovascular diseases or will be taking other cardioactive medications, both of which may aggravate beta-blocker overdose. A variety of beta blockers are available, with varying pharmacologic effects and clinical uses (Table II–10).

I. **Mechanism of toxicity.** Excessive beta-adrenergic blockade is common to overdose with all drugs in this category. Although beta-receptor specificity is seen at low doses, it is lost in overdose.
  A. Propranolol and other agents with membrane-depressant (quinidine-like) effects further depress myocardial contractility and conduction.
  B. Propranolol and other agents with high lipid solubility cause seizures and coma.
  C. Some drugs (eg, pindolol) have partial beta-agonist activity and may cause hypertension.
II. **Toxic dose.** The response to beta-blocker overdose is highly variable depending on underlying medical disease or other medications. Susceptible patients may have severe or even fatal reactions to therapeutic doses. There are no clear guidelines, but ingestion of only 2–3 times the therapeutic dose (Table II–10) should be considered potentially life-threatening in all patients. Atenolol and pindolol appear to be less toxic than other agents.
III. **Clinical presentation.** The pharmacokinetics of beta blockers vary considerably, and duration of poisoning may range from minutes to days.
  A. **Cardiac disturbances,** including hypotension and sinus bradycardia, are the most common manifestations of poisoning. Atrioventricular block, intraventricular conduction disturbances, cardiogenic shock, and asystole may occur with severe overdose, especially with membrane-depressant drugs such as propranolol. The ECG usually shows a normal QRS duration with increased PR interval; QRS widening occurs with massive intoxication.
  B. **Central nervous system toxicity** including convulsions, coma, and respiratory arrest may be seen with membrane-depressant drugs.
  C. **Bronchospasm** is most common in patients with preexisting asthma or chronic bronchospastic disease.
  D. **Hypoglycemia** and **hyperkalemia** may occur.
IV. **Diagnosis.** Diagnosis is based on the history of ingestion, accompanied by

TABLE II-10. COMPARISON OF BETA-ADRENERGIC BLOCKING AGENTS

Drug	Usual Daily Adult Dose (mg/24 h)	Cardio-selective	Membrane Depression	Partial Agonist	Normal Half-Life (h)
Acebutolol	400–800	+	+	+	7
Alprenolol	200–800	0	+	+ +	2–3
Atenolol	50–100	+	0	0	6–9
Betaxolol[a]		+	0	0	14–22
Esmolol[b]		+	0	0	9 min
Labetolol[c]	200–800	0	+	0	3–5
Levobunolol[a]		0	0	0	5–6
Metoprolol	100–450	+	+/-	0	3–4
Nadolol	80–240	0	0	0	14–24
Oxyprenolol	40–480	0	+	+ +	2
Pindolol	2.5–45	0	+	+ + +	3–4
Propranolol	40–360	0	+ +	0	2–6
Timolol[a]		0	0	+/-	4–5

[a] Ophthalmic preparation.
[b] Intravenous infusion 50–200 mcg/kg/min.
[c] Alpha-adrenergic blocking activity.

bradycardia and hypotension. Other drugs that may cause a similar presentation after overdose include sympatholytic antihypertensive drugs, digitalis, cyclic antidepressants, and calcium channel blockers.

A. **Specific levels.** Measurement of beta-blocker serum levels may confirm the diagnosis but does not contribute to emergency management.

B. **Other useful laboratory studies.** CBC, electrolytes, glucose, BUN, creatinine, arterial blood gases, ECG and electrocardiographic monitoring, chest x-ray.

V. **Treatment**

A. **Emergency and supportive measures**
   1. Maintain the airway and assist ventilation if necessary (see p 2).
   2. Treat coma (p 17), seizures (p 21), hypotension (p 14), hyperkalemia (p 32), and hypoglycemia (p 31) if they occur.
   3. Treat bradycardia (p 9) with atropine, 0.01–0.03 mg/kg IV; isoproterenol (start with 4 mcg/min and increase infusion as needed); or cardiac pacing.
   4. Treat bronchospasm with nebulized bronchodilators (p 8).
   5. Continuously monitor the vital signs and ECG for at least 6 hours after ingestion.

B. **Specific drugs and antidotes**
   1. Bradycardia and hypotension resistant to the above measures should be treated with **glucagon,** 0.1–0.3 mg/kg IV bolus, repeated as needed (see p 314).
   2. Wide complex conduction defects due to membrane-depressant poisoning may respond to **hypertonic sodium bicarbonate** as given for cyclic antidepressant overdose (see p 296).

C. **Decontamination**
1. Perform gastric lavage (see p 43). Emesis is not recommended, especially with propranolol overdose, because of the risk of seizures and coma.
2. Administer activated charcoal and cathartic (see p 45).
3. Gut emptying is probably not necessary following small ingestions if activated charcoal is given promptly.
D. **Enhanced elimination.** Most beta blockers, especially the more toxic drugs such as propranolol, are highly lipophilic, have a large volume of distribution, and are not effectively removed by dialysis procedures. For those with a small volume of distribution (eg, atenolol), a very long half-life, or low intrinsic clearance (eg, nadolol), hemoperfusion, hemodialysis, or repeat-dose charcoal may be attempted if toxicity is severe.

Reference

Weinstein RS: Recognition and management of poisoning with beta-adrenergic blocking agents. *Ann Emerg Med* 1984;**13**:1123.

BORIC ACID AND BORATES
Olga F. Woo, PharmD

ANTIDOTE   IPECAC   LAVAGE   CHARCOAL

Boric acid has been used for many years in a variety of products as an antiseptic and as a fungistatic agent in baby talcum powder. Boric acid powder (99%) is still used as a pesticide against ants and cockroaches. In the past, widespread and indiscriminate use resulted in many cases of severe poisoning due to chronic absorption of boric acid through abraded skin. Epidemics have also occurred in which boric acid was added to infant formula. Although such cases of chronic toxicity seldom occur now, acute ingestion by children at home is common.

I. **Mechanism of toxicity.** The mechanism of borate poisoning is unknown. Boric acid is not highly corrosive. It is distributed in all tissues and probably acts as a generalized cellular poison. Organ systems most commonly affected are the gastrointestinal tract, brain, liver, and kidney.
II. **Toxic dose**
A. The **acute** single oral toxic dose is highly variable, but serious poisoning is reported to occur with 1–3 g in newborns, 5 g in infants, and 20 g in adults. A teaspoon of 99% boric acid contains 3–4 g. Most accidental ingestions in children result in minimal or no toxicity.
B. **Chronic** ingestion or application to abraded skin is much more serious than acute single ingestion. Serious toxicity and death occurred in infants ingesting 5–15 g in formula over several days; serum borate levels were 400–1600 mg/L.
III. **Clinical presentation**
A. Following oral or dermal absorption, the earliest symptoms are gastrointestinal with vomiting and diarrhea. Emesis and diarrhea may have a blue-green color. Significant dehydration and renal failure can occur, with death caused by profound shock.
B. Neurologic symptoms of hyperactivity, agitation, and seizures may occur early.
C. An erythrodermic rash (boiled lobster appearance) is followed by exfoliation after 2–5 days. Alopecia totalis has been reported.

IV. Diagnosis. Diagnosis is based on a history of exposure, the presence of gastroenteritis (possibly with blue-green emesis), exfoliative rash, and elevated serum borate levels.

   A. Specific levels. Analysis of blood for borates can be obtained free of charge from the US Borax & Chemical Co. Send 10 mL of heparinized blood in a polyethylene bottle by express courier service prepaid to: US Borax Laboratories, 412 Crescent Way, Anaheim, CA 92801; telephone (714) 774–2673 (collect calls accepted); or consult a local laboratory. Normal blood levels are less than 5 mg/L. Serum boric acid levels may not correlate accurately with the severity of intoxication.

   B. Other useful laboratory studies. CBC, electrolytes, glucose, BUN, creatinine, urinalysis.

V. Treatment

   A. Emergency and supportive measures

   1. Maintain the airway and assist ventilation if necessary (see p 2).
   2. Treat coma (p 17), seizures (p 21), hypotension (p 14), and renal failure (p 33) if they occur.

   B. Specific drugs and antidotes. There is no specific antidote.

   C. Decontamination

   1. Induce emesis or perform gastric lavage (see p 42).
   2. Administer activated charcoal (although boric acid is not well adsorbed by activated charcoal) and cathartic (unless diarrhea is already present; see p 45).

   D. Enhanced elimination. Hemodialysis is effective and is indicated after massive ingestions and for supportive care of renal failure. Peritoneal dialysis has not proved effective in enhancing elimination in infants.

Reference

Litovitz TL et al: Clinical manifestations of toxicity in a series of 784 boric acid ingestions. *Am J Emerg Med* 1988;**6**:209.

BOTULISM
Olga F. Woo, PharmD

ANTIDOTE   IPECAC   LAVAGE   CHARCOAL

Botulism dates back to the 1700s as a recognized cause of fatal food poisoning. Rare outbreaks still occur in the USA, usually associated with improper home canning of foods. Recently, new sources of botulism have been discovered, such as improperly prepared or stored pot pies, fried onions, and baked potatoes; **wound botulism** in parenteral drug abusers; and **infant botulism.**

   I. Mechanism of toxicity

   A. Botulism is caused by a heat-labile neurotoxin (botulin) produced by the bacteria *Clostridium botulinum.* Different strains of the bacterium produce 6 distinct exotoxins: A, B, C, D, E, and F; types A, B, E, and F are most frequently involved in human disease. Botulin toxin irreversibly binds to cholinergic nerve terminals and prevents acetylcholine release from the axon. Severe muscle weakness results, and death is due to respiratory failure.

   B. Botulinum spores are ubiquitous in nature but are not dangerous unless they are allowed to germinate in an anaerobic environment with a pH greater than 4.6. Incompletely cooked foods left out at ambient temperatures for more than 16 hours may produce lethal amounts of botulin toxin. The spores can be destroyed by pressure cooking at a temperature of at least 120 °C (250 °F) for 30 minutes. The toxin can be de-

stroyed by boiling at 100 °C (212 °F) for one minute or heating at 80 °C (176 °F) for 20 minutes.
  II. Toxic dose. Botulin toxin is extremely potent; as little as one taste of botulin-contaminated food (approximately 0.05 mcg of toxin) may be fatal.
 III. Clinical presentation
   A. Classic botulism occurs after ingestion of preformed toxin in contaminated food. The incubation period is usually 18 to 36 hours after ingestion but can vary from a few hours to 8 days. The earlier the onset of symtoms, the more severe the illness. Initial symptoms may suggest a flulike syndrome: sore throat, dry mouth, and gastrointestinal upset. Later, diplopia, ptosis, dysarthria, and other cranial nerve weaknesses occur, followed by progressive descending paralysis and finally respiratory arrest. The patient's mentation is clear, and there is no sensory loss. Pupils may be dilated and unreactive or normal. Constipation may occur.
   B. Infant botulism is not caused by ingestion of preformed toxin but by in vivo production of toxin in the immature infant gut. Infants who are breast-fed and those given honey may have a higher risk of developing the disease, which is characterized by hypotonia, constipation, tachycardia, difficulty in feeding, head lag, and diminished gag reflex. It is rarely fatal, and infants usually recover strength within 4–6 weeks.
   C. Wound botulism occurs mostly in young adult intravenous drug abusers. The organism germinates in an infected injection site and produces toxin in vivo. Typical manifestations of botulism occur after an incubation period of 4–14 days.
 IV. Diagnosis. Diagnosis is based on a high index of suspicion in any patient with a dry sore throat, clinical findings of descending cranial nerve palsies or gastroenteritis, and a history of ingestion of home-canned food. Symptoms may be slow in onset but are sometimes rapidly progressive. Electromyography may reveal normal conduction velocity but decreased motor action potential and no incremental response to repetitive stimulation.
   A. Specific levels. Diagnosis is confirmed by determination of the toxin in serum or stool; although these tests are useful for public health investigation, they cannot be used to determine initial treatment because analysis takes more than 24 hours to perform. Obtain serum, stool, vomitus, gastric contents, and suspect food for toxin analysis by the local or state health department. The results may be negative if the samples were collected late or the quantity of toxin is small.
   B. Other useful laboratory studies. CBC, electrolytes, blood sugar, arterial blood gases, electromyogram, CSF if CNS infection is suspected.
  V. Treatment
   A. Emergency and supportive measures
     1. Obtain arterial blood gases and observe closely for respiratory weakness; respiratory arrest can occur abruptly.
     2. Maintain the airway and assist ventilation if necessary (see p 2).
   B. Specific drugs and antidotes
     1. Classic and wound botulism
       a. Botulin **antitoxin** (see p 297) binds the circulating free toxin and prevents the progression of illness; however, it does not reverse established neurologic manifestations. Available antitoxins are bivalent (AB) and trivalent (ABE); trivalent antitoxin is preferred unless the exact toxin is known.
         (1) Consult the local health department or Centers for Disease Control, Atlanta, Ga; telephone (404) 329–2888 (24-hour number).
         (2) Determine sensitivity to horse serum prior to treatment.
         (3) Administer 1 vial every 4 hours for at least 4–5 doses or until no toxin is present in serum.
       b. Guanidine may be useful as adjunctive therapy in enhancing re-

lease of acetylcholine at the nerve terminal and improving ocular and limb paralysis but not respiratory paralysis. The dose is 15–50 mg/kg/d divided into 4–5 doses.

    2. Infant botulism. Antitoxin is not recommended for infant botulism. The use of oral antibiotics and cathartics is controversial.

C. Decontamination

    1. Induce emesis or perform gastric lavage (see p 42) if recent known ingestion has occurred.

    2. Administer activated charcoal and a cathartic (see p 45).

D. Enhanced elimination. There is no role for enhanced elimination; the toxin binds rapidly to nerve endings, and any free toxin can be readily detoxified with antitoxin.

References

Hughes JM et al: Clinical features of types A and B foodborne botulism. *Ann Intern Med* 1981;**95**:442.
Johnson RO, Clay SA, Arnon SS: Diagnosis and management of infant botulism. *Am J Dis Child* 1979;**133**:586.

BROMATES
Kathryn H. Keller, PharmD

ANTIDOTE   IPECAC   LAVAGE   CHARCOAL

Bromate poisoning was more common during the 1940s and 1950s when it was a popular ingredient in home permanent neutralizers. Less toxic substances have been substituted for bromates in kits for home use, but poisonings still occur occasionally from professional products. Commercial bakeries often use bromate salts to improve bread texture, and bromates are components of fusing material for some explosives. Bromates were previously used in matchstick heads. Bromate-contaminated sugar was the cause of one reported epidemic of bromate poisoning.

I. Mechanism of toxicity. The mechanism of bromate intoxication is unknown. Bromates are oxidizing agents capable of oxidizing hemoglobin to methemoglobin (see p 204). The bromate ion is toxic to the cochlea, causing irreversible hearing loss, and nephrotoxic, causing acute tubular necrosis. Bromates may be converted to hydrobromic acid in the stomach, causing gastritis.

II. Toxic dose. The acute ingestion of 200–500 mg/kg of potassium bromate is likely to cause serious poisoning. Ingestion of 2–4 oz of 2% potassium bromate solution caused serious toxicity in children. The sodium salt is believed to be less toxic.

III. Clinical presentation

    A. Within 2 hours of ingestion, victims develop gastrointestinal symptoms, including vomiting, diarrhea, and epigastric pain. This may be accompanied by restlessness, lethargy, coma, and convulsions. An asymptomatic phase of a few hours may follow before overt renal failure occurs, usually 1–2 days after ingestion.

    B. Tinnitus and irreversible sensorineural deafness occurs **between 4–16 hours after ingestion.**

    C. Hemolysis and thrombocytopenia have been reported in some pediatric cases.

    D. Methemoglobinemia (see p 204) has been reported, but is rare.

IV. Diagnosis. Diagnosis depends on a history of ingestion accompanied by signs of gastroenteritis and renal failure.

    A. Specific levels. Bromates may liberate bromine or bromide in the serum, but bromide levels do not correlate with the severity of poisoning. Bromate concentrations are not available.

   B. Other useful laboratory studies. CBC, electrolytes, glucose, BUN, creatinine, urinalysis, audiometry, methemoglobin.

V. Treatment

   A. Emergency and supportive measures

      1. Maintain the airway and assist ventilation if necessary (see p 2).

      2. Treat coma (p 17) and seizures (p 21) if they occur.

      3. Replace fluid losses, treat electrolyte disturbances due to vomiting and diarrhea, and monitor renal function.

   B. Specific drugs and antidotes

      1. Sodium thiosulfate (see p 340) may theoretically reduce bromate to the less toxic bromide ion. There are few data to support the use of thiosulfate, but in the recommended dose it is benign. Administer 10% thiosulfate solution, 10–50 mL (0.2–1 mL/kg) IV.

      2. Treat methemoglobinemia with **methylene blue** (see p 322).

   C. Decontamination

      1. Induce emesis or perform gastric lavage (see p 42).

      2. Administer activated charcoal and cathartic (see p 45).

      3. Thiosulfate 1%, 100–200 mL, may be given orally or by gastric tube.

   D. Enhanced elimination. The bromate ion may be removed by hemodialysis, but this treatment has not been carefully evaluated. It may be prudent therapy in documented massive ingestions.

Reference

Warshaw BL et al: Bromate poisoning from hair permanent preparations. *Pediatrics* 1985;76:975.

BROMIDES
James F. Buchanan, PharmD

ANTIDOTE   IPECAC   LAVAGE   CHARCOAL

Bromide was once used as a sedative agent and was found in a variety of prescription and over-the-counter products such as Bromo-Seltzer and Dr. Miles' Nervine. However, when its potential for toxicity was recognized, it was removed from these products and is now rarely used. Bromide may still be found as salts or constituents of other drugs (eg, dextromethorphan hydrobromide, brompheniramine), but bromide toxicity is not seen with overdose of these compounds. Bromide is also found in some sources of well water, and it may be released from some bromide-containing hydrocarbons (eg, methyl bromide, ethylene dibromide, and halothane).

   I. Mechanism of toxicity. Bromide ion substitutes for chloride in various membrane transport systems, particularly within the nervous system. With high bromide levels, the membrane-depressant effect progressively impairs neuronal transmission.

  II. Toxic dose. The adult therapeutic dose of bromide is 3–5 g. Oral doses of more than 10–20 g may be fatal. Before its reformulation in 1972, one dose of Bromo-Seltzer contained 150 mg of bromide. Chronic consumption of well water containing as little as 20 mg/L of bromide has reportedly caused toxicity.

 III. Clinical presentation. Acute oral overdose usually causes nausea and vomiting due to gastric irritation. Once absorbed, bromide causes the clinical syndrome of "bromism," characterized by neurologic, gastrointestinal, and dermatologic effects.

    A. **Neurologic** effects include lethargy, ataxia, confusion, hallucinations, psychosis, weakness, stupor, and coma. At one time bromism was responsible for a large number of admissions to psychiatric facilities.

    B. **Gastrointestinal** effects include anorexia and constipation.

    C. **Dermatologic** effects include acneiform, pustular, or erythematous rashes.

IV. **Diagnosis.** Consider bromism in any confused or psychotic patient, especially if there is a history of bromide use. The serum chloride level may be falsely elevated owing to interference by bromide in the analytic test: the serum chloride is elevated by 0.8 meq/L for each 1 meq/L (or 8 mg/dL) of bromide present.

    A. **Specific levels.** A specific serum bromide level may be obtained. Therapeutic levels are 5–10 mg/dL (0.6–1.2 meq/L). Sedation may occur with levels of 10–50 mg/dL (1.2–6 meq/L); bromide levels above 50–80 mg/dL (6–10 meq/L) may cause lethargy and confusion; and levels above 300 mg/dL (40 meq/L) may be fatal.

    B. **Other useful laboratory studies.** CBC, electrolytes, glucose, BUN, creatinine.

V. **Treatment**

    A. **Emergency and supportive measures**

        1. Protect the airway and assist ventilation if needed (see p 2).

        2. Treat coma if it occurs (see p 17).

    B. **Specific drugs and antidotes.** There is no specific antidote. However, administering chloride will promote bromide excretion (see below).

    C. **Decontamination**

        1. After recent ingestion, induce emesis or perform gastric lavage (see p 42).

        2. Administer a cathartic (see p 45).

        3. Activated charcoal does not adsorb bromide ion, but it may be used if other drug ingestion is suspected.

    D. **Enhanced elimination.** Bromide is eliminated entirely by the kidney. Administer **sodium chloride** intravenously as half-normal saline (D50.5NS) at a rate sufficient to obtain a urine output of 4–6 mL/kg/h. Hemodialysis may rarely be indicated in patients with renal insufficiency or severe toxicity. Hemoperfusion is not effective.

Reference

Trump DL, Hochberg MC: Bromide intoxication. *Johns Hopkins Med J* 1976;**138**:119.

CADMIUM
Gail M. Gullickson, MD

ANTIDOTE   IPECAC   LAVAGE   CHARCOAL

Cadmium (Cd) is found in sulfide ores, along with zinc and lead. The metallic form is used in electroplating because of its anticorrosive properties; the metallic salts are used as pigments and stabilizers in plastics; and cadmium alloys are used in soldering and welding and in nickel-cadmium batteries. Cadmium solder in water pipes and cadmium pigments in pottery can be sources of contamination of water and acidic foods.

   I. **Mechanism of toxicity.** Inhaled cadmium is at least 60 times more toxic than the ingested form. Fumes and dust may cause delayed chemical pneumonitis and resultant pulmonary edema and hemorrhage. Ingested cadmium is a gastrointestinal tract irritant. Once absorbed, cadmium is bound to metallothionein and filtered by the kidney, where renal tubule damage may occur.

II. **Toxic dose.** The ACGIH-recommended threshold limit value (TLV) for **air exposure** to cadmium dusts, salts, and fumes is 0.05 mg/m^3 as an 8-hour time-weighted average. Exposure to 5 mg/m^3 inhaled for 8 hours may be lethal. Cadmium salts in solutions of greater than 15 mg/L may induce vomiting. The lethal **oral** dose ranges from 350 to 8900 mg.

III. **Clinical presentation**

A. **Acute inhalation** may cause cough, wheezing, headache, fever, and, if severe, pulmonary edema within 12–24 hours after exposure.

B. **Acute oral ingestion** of cadmium salts causes nausea, vomiting, abdominal cramps, and diarrhea, sometimes bloody, within minutes after exposure. Deaths after oral ingestion result from shock or acute renal failure.

IV. **Diagnosis.** Diagnosis is based on a history of exposure and the presence of respiratory complaints (after inhalation) or gastroenteritis (after ingestion).

A. **Specific levels.** Whole blood cadmium levels may confirm the exposure. Very little cadmium is excreted in the urine, although urine determinations are sometimes used to monitor occupational exposures. Measures of tubular microproteinuria (beta-microglobulin, retinol-binding protein, albumin, metallothionein) are used to monitor the toxic effect of cadmium on the kidney.

B. **Other useful laboratory studies.** CBC, electrolytes, glucose, BUN, creatinine, arterial blood gases, chest x-ray.

V. **Treatment**

A. **Emergency and supportive measures**

1. **Inhalation.** Monitor arterial blood gases and obtain chest x-ray. Observe for at least 6–8 hours and treat wheezing and pulmonary edema (see pp 7–8) if they occur. After significant exposure, it may be necessary to observe for 1–2 days for delayed-onset pulmonary edema.

2. **Ingestion.** Treat fluid loss caused by gastroenteritis with intravenous crystalloid fluids (see p 14). Avoid overhydration because of the potential for pulmonary edema.

B. **Specific drugs and antidotes.** There is no evidence that chelation therapy (eg, with BAL, EDTA, or penicillamine) is effective.

C. **Decontamination**

1. **Inhalation.** Remove the victim from exposure and give supplemental oxygen, if available.

2. **Ingestion.** Perform gastric lavage (see p 43). Do **not** induce emesis because of the irritant nature of cadmium salts.

3. Administer activated charcoal (see p 45), although the efficacy of charcoal is unknown. Do not give cathartics if the patient has diarrhea.

D. **Enhanced elimination.** There is no role for dialysis, hemoperfusion, or repeat-dose charcoal.

Reference

Shaikh ZA, Smith LM: Biological indicators of cadmium exposure and toxicity. *Experientia (Suppl)* 1986;**50**:124.

CAFFEINE

Christopher R. Brown, MD

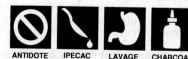

ANTIDOTE   IPECAC   LAVAGE   CHARCOAL

Caffeine is the most widely used psychoactive substance. Besides its well-known presence in coffee, it is available in many over-the-counter and prescription oral medications and as injectable caffeine sodium benzoate (occasionally used for neonatal apnea). Caffeine is widely used as an anorexiant, a coanalgesic, a diuretic, and a sleep suppressant. Although caffeine has a wide therapeutic index and rarely causes serious toxicity, there are many documented cases of accidental, suicidal, and iatrogenic intoxication, some resulting in death.

I. **Mechanism of toxicity.** Caffeine is a trimethylxanthine closely related to theophylline. It acts primarily through inhibition of the adenosine receptor. In addition, with overdose there is considerable β_1- and β_2-adrenergic stimulation secondary to release of endogenous catecholamines.

Caffeine is 100% absorbed orally with a volume of distribution of 0.7–0.8 L/kg. Its elimination half-life ranges from 3 hours in healthy smokers to 10 hours in nonsmokers. In infants less than 2–3 months old, metabolism is extremely slow and the half-life may exceed 24 hours.

II. **Toxic dose.** The reported lethal oral dose is 10 g (150–200 mg/kg), although one case report documents survival after a 24-g ingestion. In children, ingestion of 35 mg/kg may lead to moderate toxicity. Coffee contains 50–200 mg of caffeine per cup depending on how it is brewed. Infants younger than 2–3 months of age metabolize caffeine very slowly and may become toxic after repeated doses. As with theophylline, chronic administration of excessive doses may cause serious toxicity with relatively low serum concentrations compared with acute single ingestion.

III. **Clinical presentation**
   A. The earliest symptoms with **acute** caffeine poisoning are usually anorexia, tremor, and restlessness. These are followed by nausea, vomiting, tachycardia, and confusion. With serious intoxication, delirium, seizures, supraventricular and ventricular tachyarrhythmias, hypokalemia, and hyperglycemia may occur. Hypotension is caused by excessive β_2-mediated vasodilation and is characterized by a low diastolic pressure and a wide pulse pressure.
   B. **Chronic** high-dose caffeine intake can lead to "caffeinism" (nervousness, irritability, anxiety, tremulousness, muscle twitching, insomnia, palpitations, and hyperreflexia).

IV. **Diagnosis.** The diagnosis is suggested by the history of caffeine exposure or the constellation of nausea, vomiting, tremor, tachycardia, seizures, and hypokalemia.
   A. **Specific levels.** Serum caffeine levels are not routinely available in hospital laboratories but can be determined at regional commercial toxicology laboratories. Toxic concentrations may be detected by cross-reaction with theophylline assays (see Table I–31, p 38). Coffee drinkers have caffeine levels of 1–10 mg/L, while levels of 80 mg/L have been associated with death. The level associated with a high likelihood of seizures is unknown.
   B. **Other useful laboratory studies.** CBC, electrolytes, glucose, ECG.

V. **Treatment**
   A. **Emergency and supportive measures**
      1. Maintain the airway and assist ventilation if necessary (see p 2).
      2. Treat seizures (p 21) and hypotension (p 14) if they occur.
      3. Hypokalemia usually resolves without aggressive treatment.
      4. Monitor ECG and vital signs for at least 6 hours after ingestion or until serum level is documented to be decreasing.
   B. **Specific drugs and antidotes. Beta blockers** effectively reverse cardiotoxic effects mediated by excessive beta-adrenergic stimulation. Treat tachyarrhythmias or hypotension with intravenous **propranolol**, 0.01–0.02 mg/kg (see p 338), or **esmolol**, 0.05 mg/kg/min (see p 311), carefully titrated beginning with low doses. Because of its short half-life and cardioselectivity, esmolol is preferred.
   C. **Decontamination**

1. Induce emesis or perform gastric lavage (see p 42). (If the patient is already vomiting, give an antiemetic and perform gastric lavage.)
2. Administer activated charcoal and cathartic (see p 45).
3. Gut emptying is probably not necessary following small ingestions if activated charcoal is given promptly.
D. **Enhanced elimination. Repeat-dose activated charcoal** (see p 49 and p 299) may enhance caffeine elimination. Seriously intoxicated patients (with multiple seizures, significant tachyarrhythmias, or intractable hypotension) may require **charcoal hemoperfusion** (see p 48).

Reference

Benowitz NL et al: Massive catecholamine release from caffeine poisoning. *JAMA* 1982;**248**:1097.

CALCIUM ANTAGONISTS
Neal L. Benowitz, MD

ANTIDOTE   IPECAC   LAVAGE   CHARCOAL

Calcium antagonists (also known as calcium channel blockers) are widely used to treat angina pectoris, coronary spasm, hypertension, hypertrophic cardiomyopathy, supraventricular cardiac arrhythmias, and migraine headache. Toxicity from calcium antagonists may occur with therapeutic use (often owing to drug interactions) and as a result of accidental or intentional overdose.

I. **Mechanism of toxicity**
   A. Calcium antagonists slow the influx of calcium through cellular calcium channels. Currently marketed agents act primarily on vascular smooth muscle and the heart. They result in coronary and peripheral vasodilation, reduced cardiac contractility, slowed (AV) nodal conduction, and depressed sinus node activity. Lowering of blood pressure through a fall in peripheral vascular resistance may be offset by reflex tachycardia, although this reflex response may be blunted by depressant effects on contractility and sinus node activity.
   B. In usual therapeutic doses, nifedipine and nitrendipine act primarily on blood vessels, whereas verapamil and diltiazem act on both the heart and blood vessels. However, in overdose this selectivity may be lost (Table II-11 summarizes usual doses, sites of activity, and half-lives of common calcium antagonists).
   C. Important **drug interactions** may result in toxicity. Hypotension is more likely to occur in patients taking beta blockers, nitrates, or both, especially if they are hypovolemic after diuretic therapy. Patients taking

TABLE II-11. COMMON CALCIUM ANTAGONISTS[a]

Drug	Usual Adult Daily Dose (mg)	Elimination Half-Life (h)	Primary Site (S) of Activity[a]
Diltiazem	90–360	4	M, V
Nifedipine	30–120	4	V
Nitrendipine	40–80	12	V
Verapamil	240–480 (PO) 0.075–0.15 mg/kg (IV)	3–7	M, V

[a]Major toxicity: M = myocardial (decreased contractility, AV block); V = vascular (vasodilation).

disopyramide or other depressant cardioactive drugs and those with severe underlying myocardial disease are also at risk for hypotension. Life-threatening bradyarrhythmias, including asystole, may occur when beta blockers and verapamil are given together, especially after parenteral administration.

II. **Toxic dose.** Usual therapeutic daily doses for each agent are listed in Table II–11. The toxic/therapeutic ratio is relatively small, and serious toxicity may occur with therapeutic doses. Any dose greater than the usual therapeutic range should be considered potentially life-threatening.

III. **Clinical presentation**

   A. The primary features of calcium antagonist intoxication are **hypotension** and **bradycardia.** Hypotension may be caused by peripheral vasodilation, reduced cardiac contractility, slowed heart rate, or a combination of all of these. Bradycardia may be due to sinus bradycardia, second- or third-degree atrioventricular block, or sinus arrest with junctional escape rhythm. Calcium antagonists do not affect intraventricular conduction, so the QRS duration is usually unaffected. The PR interval is prolonged even with therapeutic doses of verapamil.

   B. **Noncardiac manifestations** of intoxication include nausea and vomiting, abnormal mental status (stupor, confusion), metabolic acidosis (probably resulting from hypotension), and hyperglycemia (owing to blockade of insulin release).

IV. **Diagnosis.** The findings of hypotension and bradycardia, particularly with sinus arrest or AV block, in the absence of QRS interval prolongation should suggest calcium antagonist intoxication. The differential diagnosis should include beta blockers and other sympatholytic drugs.

   A. **Specific levels.** Serum drug levels are not widely available.

   B. **Other useful laboratory studies.** CBC, electrolytes, glucose, BUN, creatinine, arterial blood gases, ECG and electrocardiographic monitoring.

V. **Treatment**

   A. **Emergency and supportive measures**

      1. Maintain the airway and assist ventilation if necessary (see p 2).

      2. Treat coma (p 17), hypotension (p 14), and bradyarrhythmias (p 9) if they occur.

      3. Monitor the vital signs and ECG for at least 6 hours after alleged ingestion. Admit symptomatic patients for at least 24 hours.

   B. **Specific drugs and antidotes**

      1. **Calcium** (see p 298) usually promptly reverses the depression of cardiac contractility, but it does *not* affect sinus node depression or peripheral vasodilation and has variable effects on AV nodal conduction. Administer **calcium chloride** 10%, 10 mL (0.1–0.2 mL/kg) IV, or **calcium gluconate** 10%, 20 mL (0.3–0.4 mL/kg) IV.

      2. Outside the USA, **4-aminopyridine** may be available as an antidote for calcium antagonist intoxication.

   C. **Decontamination**

      1. Induce emesis or perform gastric lavage (see p 42). Lavage is preferred because of the risk of abrupt hypotension or cardiac arrhythmias.

      2. Administer activated charcoal and cathartic (see p 45).

      3. Gut emptying is probably not necessary following small ingestions if activated charcoal is given promptly.

   D. **Enhanced elimination.** Owing to extensive protein binding, dialysis and hemoperfusion are not effective. Repeat-dose activated charcoal has not been evaluated.

Reference

Zoghbi W, Schwartz JB: Verapamil overdose: Report of a case and review of the literature. *Cardiovasc Rev Rep* 1984;5:356.

CAMPHOR AND OTHER ESSENTIAL OILS
Ilene B. Anderson, PharmD

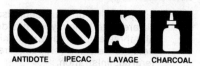

ANTIDOTE   IPECAC   LAVAGE   CHARCOAL

Camphor is one of several essential oils (volatile oils) derived from natural plant products that have been used for centuries as topical rubefacients and counter-irritant agents for analgesic and antipruritic purposes (Table II–12). Camphor and other essential oils are found in many over-the-counter remedies such as Campho-Phenique (10.8% camphor, 4.66% phenol), Vicks Vaporub (4.73% camphor, 2.6% menthol, 1.2% eucalyptus oil, 4.5% turpentine spirits), camphorated oil (20% camphor), and Mentholatum (9% camphor, 1.35% menthol, 1.96% eucalyptus oil, 1.4% turpentine spirits). Accidental ingestion has occurred when camphorated oil was mistakenly ingested instead of castor oil.

I. **Mechanism of toxicity.** After topical application, essential oils produce inflammation followed by a feeling of comfort, but if ingested they can cause systemic toxicity. Camphor is a central nervous system stimulant that causes seizures shortly after ingestion. The underlying mechanism is unknown, but neuronal necrosis involving the cortex, basal ganglia, and hippocampus was described in one case at autopsy. Camphor is rapidly

TABLE II–12. SOME ESSENTIAL OILS

Name	Comments
Birch oil	Contains 98% methyl salicylate (see p 261).
Camphor	Pediatric toxic dose 1 g (see text).
Clove oil	Contains 80–90% eugenol. Clove cigarettes may cause irritant tracheobronchitis.
Cinnamon oil	Stomatitis and skin burns can result from prolonged contact. Potent antigen. Smoked as a hallucinogen.
Eugenol	A phenol derived from clove oil; used in dentistry for its disinfectant property.
Eucalyptus oil	Contains 70% eucalyptol. Toxic dose is 5 mL.
Guaiacol	Nontoxic.
Lavender oil	Used in doses of 0.1 mL as a carminative. Contains trace amounts of coumarin (see p 132).
Menthol	An alcohol derived from various mint oils. Toxic dose is 2 gm.
Myristica oil	Nutmeg oil. A carminative in a dose of 0.03 mL. Used as a hallucinogen.
Pennyroyal oil	Fatal hepatic necrosis occurred after ingestion of 30 mL by an 18-year-old woman. Ingestion of 10 mL produces gastroenteritis.
Peppermint oil	Contains 50% menthol. Toxic dose is 5–10 g.
Thymol	Used as an antiseptic (see phenol, p 234).
Turpentine oils	Toxic dose 15 mL in children; 140 mL in adults may be fatal.
Wintergreen oil	Contains methyl salicylate 98% wt/wt.

absorbed from the gastrointestinal tract and is metabolized by the liver. It is not known whether metabolites contribute to toxicity.

II.

Toxic dose. Serious poisonings and death have occurred in children after ingestion of as little as 1 g of camphor. This is equivalent to just 10 mL of Campho-Phenique or 5 mL of camphorated oil. Recovery after ingestion of 42 g in an adult has been reported. The concentrations of other essential oils range from 1 to 20%; doses of 5-15 mL are considered potentially toxic.

III. **Clinical presentation**

   A. Manifestations of **acute oral overdose** usually occur within 5-30 minutes after ingestion. Burning in the mouth and throat occurs immediately, followed by nausea and vomiting. Ataxia, drowsiness, confusion, restlessness, delirium, muscle twitching, and coma may occur. Camphor typically causes abrupt onset of seizures about 20-30 minutes after ingestion. Death may be due to CNS depression and respiratory arrest or secondary to status epilepticus.

   B. Prolonged **skin contact** may result in a burn.

   C. **Smoking** (eg, clove cigarettes) or inhaling essential oils may cause tracheobronchitis.

IV. **Diagnosis.** Diagnosis is usually based on a history of exposure. The pungent odor of camphor and other volatile oils is usually apparent.

   A. **Specific levels.** Serum drug levels are not available.

   B. **Other useful laboratory studies.** CBC, electrolytes, glucose, arterial blood gases (if patient is comatose or in status epilepticus).

V. **Treatment**

   A. **Emergency and supportive measures**

      1. Maintain the airway and assist ventilation if necessary (see p 2).

      2. Treat seizures (p 21) and coma (p 17) if they occur.

   B. **Specific drugs and antidotes.** There are no specific antidotes.

   C. **Decontamination**

      1. Perform prompt gastric lavage (see p 43). Do **not** induce emesis because of the risk of abrupt onset of seizures.

      2. Administer activated charcoal as soon as the gastric tube is placed (see p 45).

      3. Gut emptying is probably not necessary following small ingestions if activated charcoal is given promptly.

   D. **Enhanced elimination.** The volumes of distribution of camphor and other essential oils are extremely large, and it is unlikely that any enhanced removal procedure will remove significant amounts of camphor. Poorly substantiated case reports have recommended resin hemoperfusion.

Reference

Autman E et al: Camphor overdosage: Therapeutic considerations. *N Y State J Med* 1978;**78:**896.

CAPTOPRIL AND RELATED DRUGS
Olga F. Woo, PharmD

ANTIDOTE   IPECAC   LAVAGE   CHARCOAL

Captopril, enalapril, and lisinopril are angiotensin-converting enzyme (ACE) inhibitors introduced recently for the treatment of renovascular and resistant idiopathic hypertension. The few reports of acute overdose with these drugs suggest that toxicity is mild.

I. **Mechanism of toxicity.** These agents inhibit vasoconstriction by inhibiting the enzyme peptidyldipeptide carboxyhydrolase, which converts angiotensin I to angiotensin II. Enalapril must be metabolized to its active moiety, enalaprilat. Enalaprilat is now available in a parenteral formulation.

II. Toxic dose. Only mild toxicity has resulted from large overdoses of up to 5 g of captopril and 300 mg of enalapril. Bradycardia has been reported with therapeutic doses of enalapril. No fatalities have been reported from acute poisonings.

III. Clinical presentation. Mild hypotension, usually responsive to fluid therapy, has been the only toxic effect seen with acute overdose. Bradycardia may also occur. Hyperkalemia has been reported with therapeutic use, especially in patients with renal insufficiency and those taking nonsteroidal anti-inflammatory drugs.

IV. Diagnosis. Diagnosis is based on a history of exposure.
  A. Specific levels. A radioimmunoassay is available to measure serum levels of ACE inhibitors, but blood levels do not correlate with clinical effects.
  B. Other useful laboratory studies. CBC, electrolytes, glucose, BUN, and creatinine.

V. Treatment
  A. Emergency and supportive measures. Treat hypotension with supine positioning and intravenous fluids (see p 14) if it occurs. Vasopressors are rarely necessary.
  B. Specific drugs and antidotes. No specific antidote is available.
  C. Decontamination
    1. Induce emesis or perform gastric lavage (see p 42). Gut emptying is not necessary following small ingestions.
    2. Administer activated charcoal and a cathartic (see p 45) orally or by gastric tube.
  D. Enhanced elimination. Hemodialysis may effectively remove these drugs but is not likely to be indicated clinically.

Reference

Waeber B, Nussberger J, Bonner HR: Self-poisoning with enalapril. *Br Med J* 1984;**288**:287.

CARBAMATE INSECTICIDES
Olga F. Woo, PharmD

ANTIDOTE   IPECAC   LAVAGE   CHARCOAL

Carbamate insecticides are less toxic than organophosphates, although their clinical effects are similar. They are found in a variety of commercial veterinary and pesticide products widely used in agriculture. Many household insect sprays contain carbamates. An acute outbreak of aldicarb poisoning occurred in California in 1985 after ingestion of contaminated watermelons.

  I. Mechanism of toxicity. Like organophosphates, carbamates inhibit acetylcholinesterase enzyme, which allows excessive accumulation of acetylcholine at muscarinic, nicotinic, and central nervous system receptors. Unlike the case with organophosphates, this inhibition is short-lived and reversible. Carbamates are absorbed by inhalation, ingestion, and through the skin (with the exception of aldicarb, most carbamates are relatively poorly absorbed dermally compared with organophosphates).

  II. Toxic dose. There is wide variability in the potency of carbamates (Table II–13). Carbamates are not highly lipophilic and do not cause delayed or persistent toxicity. Aldicarb is an important carbamate because it is rela-

TABLE II-13. CARBAMATE INSECTICIDES[a]

Highly Toxic (LD_{50} < 50 mg/kg)	Moderately Toxic (LD_{50} > 50 mg/Kg)	Low Toxicity (LD_{50} > 1 g/kg)
Aldicarb	Dioxacarb	Metam sodium
Oxamyl	Bendiocar	
Carbofuran	Promecarb	
Methomyl	Bufencarb	
Formetanate	MTMC (Metacrate)	
Aminocarb	Propoxur	
Dimetilan	Pirimicarb	
	MPMC (Meobal)	
	Isoprocarb	
	Carbaryl	

[a] Listed in decreasing order of potency.

tively more potent, undergoes extensive enterohepatic recirculation, and is translocated systemically by certain plants (eg, melons) and concentrated in their fruit.

III. **Clinical presentation.** Signs and symptoms of cholinergic excess usually occur within 30 minutes but may not develop until 1–2 hours after exposure. Clinical manifestations are the same as those seen with organophosphates (see p 255), but the duration of toxicity is usually shorter (< 6 hours) and symptoms are self-limited.

IV. **Diagnosis.** Diagnosis is based on a history of exposure and the characteristic presentation of muscarinic, nicotinic, and central nervous system acetylcholine excess.

A. **Specific levels.** Red blood cell cholinesterase and plasma pseudocholinesterase are not reliable indicators of carbamate poisoning because enzyme activity rapidly and spontaneously recovers within several minutes or hours. Thus, normal levels do not rule out intoxication. Also, because the range of normal enzyme activity is broad and interindividual variability is high, intoxication may be present despite normal enzyme activity. However, a depression of 25% or more from an individual's baseline value is indicative of exposure. Samples should be analyzed immediately, because in vitro degradation hydrolysis of the carbamate can occur.

B. **Other useful laboratory studies.** Arterial blood bases, CBC, electrolytes, glucose, BUN, creatinine.

V. **Treatment**

A. **Emergency and supportive measures**
   1. Maintain the airway and assist ventilation if necessary (see p 2).
   2. Treat coma (p 17) and seizures (p 21) if they occur.
   3. Observe for 4–6 hours. Few patients require prolonged observation.

B. **Specific treatment**
   1. Administer **atropine**, 0.5–2 mg (0.01–0.04 mg/kg) IV or IM every 15 minutes until manifestations of muscarinic toxicity (eg, symptomatic bradycardia, bronchorrhea, or wheezing) are reversed (see p 293).
   2. **Pralidoxime** (see p 337) is not generally recommended, because atropine alone is sufficient and cholinesterase enzyme inhibition is reversible. However, if a combination of carbamate and organophosphate poisoning has occurred, pralidoxime should be given.

C. **Decontamination**
   1. **Skin and eyes.** Remove all contaminated clothing and wash affected skin copiously with soap and water, including the hair and under the nails. Irrigate exposed eyes with copious tepid water or saline.
   2. **Ingestion**

     a. Perform gastric lavage (see p 43). Do **not** induce emesis because of the risk of sudden seizures, coma, or respiratory depression.

     b. Administer activated charcoal (see p 45). Do not give a cathartic if diarrhea is present.

     c. Gut emptying is probably not necessary following small ingestions if activated charcoal is given promptly.

  D. Enhanced elimination. Dialysis and hemoperfusion are not indicated because the duration of toxicity is brief and effective antidotal therapy is available. Repeat-dose activated charcoal is theoretically applicable to aldicarb poisoning, because aldicarb undergoes enterohepatic recirculation.

Reference

Willis JH et al: Effects of oral doses of carbaryl on man. *Clin Toxicol* 1968;**1**:265.

CARBAMAZEPINE
Olga F. Woo, PharmD

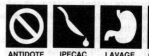

ANTIDOTE   IPECAC   LAVAGE   CHARCOAL

Carbamazepine has been a popular anticonvulsant in Europe for many years, but reports of bone marrow depression and leukopenia delayed its entry into the US market until 1974, when it was approved for the treatment of trigeminal neuralgia. Since then it has become a first-line drug for the treatment of temporal lobe epilepsies and a variety of other seizure disorders.

  I. Mechanism of toxicity. Presumably because its chemical structure is similar to that of the the tricyclic antidepressant imipramine, acute carbamazepine overdose can cause anticholinergic effects, seizures, and cardiac conduction disturbances.

 II. Toxic dose. Acute ingestion of over 10 mg/kg will result in a blood level above the maximum therapeutic range of 5–10 mg/L. Serious poisoning is likely with ingestion of more than 50 mg/kg.

III. Clinical presentation

  A. Ataxia, nystagmus, ophthalmoplegia, mydriasis, and sinus tachycardia are common with mild to moderate overdose. With more serious intoxication, myoclonus, seizures, hyperthermia, coma, and respiratory arrest may occur. Atrioventricular block and bradycardia have been reported, although QRS and QT widening are uncommon.

  B. After an acute overdose, manifestations of intoxication may be delayed for a few hours because of anticholinergic effects causing slowed gastric emptying and absorption. Cyclic coma and rebound relapse of symptoms may be due to continued absorption and enterohepatic circulation of the drug.

IV. Diagnosis. Diagnosis is based on a history of exposure and clinical signs such as ataxia, stupor, and tachycardia, along with elevated serum levels.

  A. Specific levels. Obtain a **stat serum carbamazepine** level and repeat levels every 4–6 hours to rule out delayed or prolonged absorption. Serious intoxication occurs with levels greater than 40 mg/L. Death occurred in a patient who had a peak concentration of 120 mcg/mL. The metabolite carbamazepine epoxide is nearly equipotent, and specific epoxide levels may be useful.

  B. Other useful laboratory studies. CBC, electrolytes, glucose, arterial blood gases, ECG.

 V. Treatment

A. Emergency and supportive measures
1. Maintain the airway and assist ventilation if necessary (see p 2).
2. Treat seizures (p 21), coma (p 17), and arrhythmias (pp 9–13) if they occur. Most patients with serum levels below 60 mg/L will recover with supportive care alone.
3. Asymptomatic patients should be observed for a minimum of 6 hours after ingestion.

B. Specific drugs and antidotes. There is no specific antidote. Physostigmine is *not* recommended.

C. Decontamination
1. Induce emesis or perform gastric lavage (see p 42). Lavage is the preferred method, especially with very large ingestions.
2. Administer activated charcoal and a cathartic (see p 45).
3. Gut emptying is probably not necessary following small ingestions if activated charcoal is given promptly.

D. Enhanced elimination. In contrast to tricyclic antidepressants, the volume of distribution of carbamazepine is small (1 L/kg), making it accessible to enhanced removal procedures.
1. **Repeat-dose activated charcoal** is very effective and may increase clearance by up to 50%.
2. **Peritoneal dialysis and hemodialysis** do not effectively remove carbamazepine because it is 80% protein-bound.
3. **Charcoal hemoperfusion** is highly effective and is indicated for severe intoxication (eg, status epilepticus, cardiotoxicity) unresponsive to standard treatment.

Reference

Sullivan JB et al: Acute carbamazepine toxicity resulting from overdose. *Neurology* 1981;**31**:621.

CARBON MONOXIDE
Evan T. Wythe, MD

ANTIDOTE   IPECAC   LAVAGE   CHARCOAL

Carbon monoxide (CO) is a nonirritating, tasteless, colorless, odorless gas produced by the incomplete combustion of any carbon-containing material. Common sources of human exposure include smoke inhalation in fires; automobile exhaust fumes; faulty or poorly ventilated charcoal, kerosene, or gas stoves; cigarette smoke; and methylene chloride (see p 207).

I. Mechanism of toxicity. Toxicity is a consequence of cellular hypoxia.
   A. Carbon monoxide binds to hemoglobin with an affinity 250 times that of oxygen, resulting in reduced oxyhemoglobin saturation and decreased blood oxygen-carrying capacity. In addition, the oxyhemoglobin dissociation curve is displaced to the left, impairing oxygen delivery at the tissues.
   B. Carbon monoxide may also directly inhibit cytochrome oxidase, further disrupting cellular function, and it is known to bind to myoglobin, possibly contributing to impaired myocardial contractility.

II. Toxic dose. The OSHA permissible exposure limit (PEL) for carbon monoxide is 35 ppm as an 8-hour time-weighted average. The level considered immediately dangerous to life or health (IDLH) is 1500 ppm (0.15%). Several minutes of exposure to 1000 ppm (0.1%) may result in 50% saturation of carboxyhemoglobin and fatal poisoning.

III. Clinical presentation. Symptoms of intoxication are predominantly in organs with high oxygen consumption such as the brain and heart.
  A. The majority of patients complain of headache, dizziness, and nausea. Patients with coronary disease may experience angina or myocardial infarction. With more severe exposures, impaired thinking, syncope, coma, convulsions, cardiac arrhythmias, hypotension, and death may occur (Table II–14).
  B. Survivors of serious poisoning may suffer numerous neurologic sequelae such as parkinsonism and personality and memory disorders.
IV. Diagnosis. Diagnosis is not difficult if there is a history of exposure (eg, patient found in car in locked garage) but may be elusive if not suspected in less obvious cases. There are no specific reliable clinical findings; cherry red skin coloration or bright red venous blood is highly suggestive but not frequently noted. The routine arterial blood gas measures oxygen dissolved in plasma but does not directly measure oxygen saturation or oxygen content and therefore is usually misleadingly normal. Pulse oximetry gives a falsely normal saturation.
  A. Specific levels. Obtain a specific blood carboxyhemoglobin concentration.
  B. Other useful laboratory studies. CBC, electrolytes, glucose, BUN, creatinine, ECG, arterial blood gases.
V. Treatment
  A. Emergency and supportive measures
    1. Maintain the airway and assist ventilation if necessary (see p 2). If smoke inhalation has also occurred, consider early intubation for airway protection (p 4).
    2. Treat coma (p 17) and seizures (p 21) if they occur.
    3. Continuously monitor the ECG for several hours after exposure.
    4. Because smoke often contains other toxic gases, consider the possibility of cyanide poisoning (p 134), methemoglobinemia (p 204), and irritant gas injury (p 163).
  B. Specific drugs and antidotes. Administer **oxygen** in the highest possible concentration (100%). Breathing 100% oxygen reduces the half-time of the carboxyhemoglobin complex from 6 hours (in room air) to approximately 1 hour. Use a tight-fitting mask and high-flow oxygen with a reservoir (nonrebreather) or administer the oxygen by endotracheal tube.

TABLE II-14. CARBON MONOXIDE POISONING[a]

Estimated Carbon Monoxide Concentration	Carboxy-hemoglobin (%)	Symptoms
Less than 35 ppm (cigarette smoking)	5	None, or mild headache.
0.005% (50 ppm)	10	Slight headache, dyspnea on vigorous exertion.
0.01% (100 ppm)	20	Throbbing headache, dyspnea with moderate exertion.
0.02% (200 ppm)	30	Severe headache, irritability, fatigue, dimness of vision.
0.03–0.05% (300–500 ppm)	40–50	Headache, tachycardia, confusion, lethargy, collapse.
0.08–0.12% (800–1200 ppm)	60–70	Coma, convulsions.
0.19% (1900 ppm)	80	Rapidly fatal.

[a] Reproduced, with permission, from *Current Emergency Diagnosis & Treatment*, 3rd ed. Ho MT, Saunders CE (editors). Appleton & Lange, 1990.

C. **Decontamination.** Remove the patient immediately from exposure and give supplemental oxygen. Rescuers exposed to high concentrations of carbon monoxide should wear self-contained breathing apparatus.

D. **Enhanced elimination. Hyperbaric oxygen** provides 100% oxygen under 2–3 atm of pressure and can enhance elimination of carbon monoxide (half-time reduced to 20–30 minutes). It may be useful in patients with very high carbon monoxide levels and ready access to a chamber. However, long-distance transport of an unstable patient for hyperbaric treatment may be risky, and it remains controversial whether hyperbaric oxygen is more effective than 100% oxygen administered at atmospheric pressure. Consult a regional poison center (see p 50) for information regarding local hyperbaric chambers.

Reference

Olson KR: Carbon monoxide poisoning: Mechanisms, presentation, and controversies in management. *J Emerg Med* 1984;1:233.

CARBON TETRACHLORIDE
Margaret Atterbury, MD

| ANTIDOTE | IPECAC | LAVAGE | CHARCOAL |

Carbon tetrachloride (CCl_4) was formerly widely used as a dry cleaning solvent, degreaser, spot remover, fire extinguisher agent, and anthelmintic. Because of its liver toxicity and known carcinogenicity in animals, its role has been limited and it is now used mainly as a fumigant and as an intermediate in chemical manufacturing.

I. **Mechanism of toxicity.** Carbon tetrachloride is a central nervous system depressant and a potent hepatic and renal toxin. It may also sensitize the myocardium to arrhythmogenic effects of catecholamines. The mechanism of hepatic and renal toxicity is thought to be due to a toxic free radical intermediate of metabolism. Chronic use of metabolic enzyme inducers such as phenobarbital and ethanol increase the toxicity of carbon tetrachloride. Carbon tetrachloride is a known animal carcinogen.

II. **Toxic dose**

A. Toxicity from **inhalation** is dependent on the concentration in air and the duration of exposure. Symptoms have occurred after exposure to 160 ppm for 30 minutes. The OSHA workplace permissible exposure limit (PEL) is 2 ppm as an 8-hour time-weighted average, and the air level considered immediately dangerous to life or health (IDLH) is 300 ppm.

B. **Ingestion** of as little as 5 mL has been reported to be fatal.

III. **Clinical presentation**

A. Persons exposed to carbon tetrachloride from acute inhalation, skin absorption, or ingestion may present with nausea, vomiting, dizziness, and confusion. With serious intoxication, coma and cardiac arrhythmias may occur.

B. Severe and sometimes fatal renal and hepatic damage may become apparent after 1–3 days.

IV. **Diagnosis.** Diagnosis is based on a history of exposure and the clinical presentation of central nervous system depression, arrhythmias, and hepatic necrosis. The liquid is radiopaque and may be visible on abdominal x-ray.

A. **Specific levels.** Serum levels are not available in most commercial laboratories.

B. **Other useful laboratory studies.** CBC, electrolytes, glucose, BUN, creatinine, liver transaminases, prothrombin time, ECG.

V. Treatment
  #### A. Emergency and supportive measures
  1. Maintain the airway and assist ventilation if necessary (see p 2).
  2. Treat coma (p 17) and arrhythmias (p 13) if they occur. *Caution:* Avoid use of epinephrine because it may induce or aggravate arrhythmias.
  #### B. Specific treatment. **Acetylcysteine** (NAC; see p 289) may minimize hepatic and renal toxicity by providing a scavenger for the toxic intermediate. Although its use for carbon tetrachloride poisoning has not been studied in humans, acetylcysteine is widely used without serious side effects for treatment of acetaminophen overdose. If possible, it should be given within the first 12 hours after exposure.
  #### C. Decontamination
  1. **Inhalation.** Remove from exposure and give supplemental oxygen, if available.
  2. **Skin and eyes.** Remove contaminated clothing and wash affected skin with copious soap and water. Irrigate exposed eyes with copious saline or water.
  3. **Ingestion**
      a. Perform gastric lavage (see p 43). Do **not** induce emesis because of rapid absorption and the risk of CNS depression.
      b. Administer activated charcoal and cathartic (see p 45).
  #### D. Enhanced elimination. There is no role for dialysis, hemoperfusion, or other enhanced removal procedures.

Reference

Ruprah M, Mant TG, Flanagan RJ: Acute carbon tetrachloride poisoning in 19 patients: Implications for diagnosis and treatment. *Lancet* 1985;**1**:1027.

CARDIAC GLYCOSIDES
James F. Buchanan, PharmD

ANTIDOTE   IPECAC   LAVAGE   CHARCOAL

Cardiac glycosides are found in several plants, including oleander, foxglove, and rhododendron. They are used therapeutically in tablet form as digoxin and digitoxin. Digoxin is also available in liquid-filled capsules with greater bioavailability. Intoxication may occur after acute accidental or suicidal ingestion or with chronic therapy. Toxicity after acute ingestion is clinically different from that seen with chronic therapy.

  I. Mechanism of toxicity. Cardiac glycosides inhibit the function of the sodium-potassium-ATPase pump. After acute overdose, this results in hyperkalemia. In contrast, with chronic intoxication, the serum potassium level is usually normal or low owing to concurrent diuretic therapy. Vagal tone is potentiated, and sinus and atrioventricular node conduction velocity is decreased. Automaticity in Purkinje fibers is increased.
  II. Toxic dose. Acute ingestion of less than 2 mg of digoxin in a child and 5 mg of digoxin in an adult rarely results in serious poisoning. However, this amount of digoxin and other cardiac glycosides may be found in just a few leaves of oleander or foxglove. Generally, children appear to be more resistant than adults to the cardiotoxic effects of cardiac glycosides.
  III. Clinical presentation. Signs and symptoms depend on the chronicity of the intoxication.
  A. With **acute overdose,** vomiting, hyperkalemia, and sinus and atrioven-

tricular block are common, whereas ventricular tachyarrhythmias are seen only with severe poisoning.

B. In contrast, with **chronic intoxication,** visual disturbances, weakness, and ventricular tachyarrhythmias (ventricular tachycardia, bidirectional tachycardia, and ventricular fibrillation) are common. In patients with chronic atrial fibrillation, accelerated junctional tachycardia and paroxysmal atrial tachycardia with block are frequently seen. Hypokalemia and hypomagnesemia due to chronic diuretic use may be evident and appear to worsen the tachyarrhythmias.

IV. **Diagnosis.** Diagnosis is based on a history of recent overdose or characteristic arrhythmias (bidirectional tachycardia, accelerated junctional rhythym) in a patient receiving chronic therapy. Hyperkalemia suggests acute ingestion but may also be seen with very severe chronic poisoning. Serum potassium levels higher than 5.5 meq/L are associated with a poor prognosis.

A. **Specific levels. Stat digoxin** or **digitoxin levels** are recommended, although they may not correlate accurately with severity of intoxication. This is especially true after acute ingestion, when the level may be falsely high for 6–12 hours before tissue distribution is complete. After use of digitalis-specific antibodies, the radioimmunoassay digoxin level is falsely markedly elevated. Therapeutic levels of digoxin are 0.5–2 ng/mL; of digitoxin, 10–30 ng/mL.

B. **Other useful laboratory studies.** CBC, electrolytes, BUN, creatinine, serum magnesium, ECG and electrocardiographic monitoring.

V. **Treatment**

A. **Emergency and supportive measures**

1. Maintain the airway and assist ventilation if necessary (see p 2).
2. Monitor the patient closely for at least 12–24 hours after significant ingestion because of delayed tissue distribution.
3. Treat **hyperkalemia** (p 32), if greater than 5.5 meq/L, with sodium bicarbonate (1 meq/kg), glucose (0.5 g/kg IV) with insulin (0.1 unit/kg IV), or sodium polystyrene sulfonate (Kayexalate, 0.5 g/kg orally). Do **not** use calcium; it may worsen ventricular arrhythmias. Mild hyperkalemia may actually protect against tachyarrhythmias.
4. Treat **bradycardia** or **heart block** with atropine, 0.5–2 mg IV (p 9); a pacemaker may be needed for persistent symptomatic bradycardia.
5. **Ventricular tachyarrhythmias** may respond to lidocaine (p 320) or phenytoin (p 335), or to potassium or magnesium replacement. Avoid quinidine, procainamide, and bretylium.

B. **Specific drugs and antidotes.** Fab fragments of digoxin-specific antibodies are now available **(Digibind)** and are indicated for severe toxicity unresponsive to standard care described above. Digibind rapidly binds to digoxin and, to a lesser extent, digitoxin and other cardiac glycosides. The inactive complex that is formed is rapidly excreted in the urine. Details of Digibind dose calculation and infusion rate are given on p 304.

C. **Decontamination**

1. Induce emesis or perform gastric lavage (see p 42). *Caution:* Vagal stimulation due to emesis or lavage may exacerbate bradycardia and heart block.
2. Administer activated charcoal and cathartic (see p 45).
3. Gut emptying is probably not necessary following small ingestions if activated charcoal is given promptly.

D. **Enhanced elimination**

1. Because of its large volume of distribution, **digoxin** is not effectively removed by dialysis, hemoperfusion, or repeat-dose activated charcoal.
2. In contrast, **digitoxin** has a small volume of distribution and also

undergoes extensive enterohepatic recirculation, and its elimination is markedly enhanced by **repeat-dose charcoal** (see p 49 and p 299).

Reference

Bhatia SJ: Digitalis toxicity: Turning over a new leaf? *West J Med* 1986;**145**:74.

CAUSTIC AND CORROSIVE AGENTS
Kent R. Olson, MD

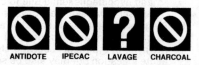

ANTIDOTE   IPECAC   LAVAGE   CHARCOAL

A wide variety of chemical and physical agents may cause corrosive injury. These include mineral and organic acids, alkalies, oxidizing agents, denaturants, some hydrocarbons, and agents causing exothermic reactions. Although the mechanism and the severity of injury may vary, the consequences of mucosal damage and permanent scarring are shared by all agents. **Button batteries** are small disk-shaped batteries used in watches, calculators, and cameras. They contain caustic metals salts such as mercuric chloride that may cause corrosive injury.

I. **Mechanism of toxicity**
   A. **Acids** cause an immediate coagulation-type necrosis that tends to self-limit further damage.
   B. In contrast, **alkalies** cause a liquefactive necrosis with saponification and continued penetration of deeper tissues, resulting in extensive damage.
   C. **Other agents** may act by denaturing cellular proteins or by defatting surface tissues.
   D. **Button batteries** cause injury by caustic effects resulting from leakage of the corrosive metals salts, by direct impaction of the disk-shaped foreign body, and possibly by discharge of the electrical current at the site of impaction.

II. **Toxic dose.** There is no specific toxic dose or level, because the concentration of solutions and the potency of corrosive effect vary widely. The concentration or the pH of the solution may indicate the potential for serious injury.

III. **Clinical presentation**
   A. **Inhalation** of corrosive gases (eg, chlorine, ammonia) may cause upper respiratory tract injury, with stridor, hoarseness, wheezing, and non-cardiogenic pulmonary edema. Pulmonary symptoms may be delayed after exposure to gases with low water solubility (eg, nitrogen dioxide, phosgene; see p 163).
   B. **Eye or skin** exposure to corrosive agents usually results in immediate pain and redness, followed by blistering. Conjunctivitis and lacrimation are common. Serious full-thickness burns and blindness can occur.
   C. **Ingestion** of corrosives can cause oral pain, dysphagia, drooling, and pain in the throat, chest or abdomen. Esophageal or gastric perforation may occur, manifested by severe chest or abdominal pain, signs of peritoneal irritation, or pancreatitis. Free air may be visible in the mediastinum or abdomen on x-ray. Hematemesis may occur. Systemic acidosis has been reported following acid ingestion and is thought to be due to absorption of hydrogen ion. Scarring of the esophagus or stomach may result in stricture formation and chronic dysphagia.
   D. **Systemic symptoms** can occur after inhalation, skin exposure, or ingestion of a variety of agents (Table II–15).
   E. **Button batteries** usually cause serious injury only if they become im-

TABLE II–15. EXAMPLES OF SYSTEMIC SYMPTOMS FROM CORROSIVE AGENTS[a]

Corrosive Agent	Systemic Symptoms
Formaldehyde	Metabolic acidosis; formate poisoning
Hydrofluoric acid	Hypocalcemia; hyperkalemia
Oxalic acid	Hypocalcemia; renal failure
Paraquat	Pulmonary fibrosis
Permanganate	Methemoglobinemia
Phenol	Seizures, coma; hepatic and renal damage
Phosphorus	Hepatic and renal injury
Picric acid	Renal injury
Tannic acid	Hepatic injury

[a] Reference: Edelman PA: Chemical and electrical burns. Pages 183–202 in: *Management of the Burned Patient.* Achauer BM (editor). Appleton & Lange, 1987.

pacted in the esophagus, leading to perforation into the aorta or mediastinum. Most cases involve large (25 mm in diameter) batteries. If they reach the stomach without impaction in the esophagus, they nearly always pass uneventfully into the stools within several days.

IV. **Diagnosis.** Diagnosis is based on a history of exposure to a corrosive agent and characteristic findings of skin, eye, or mucosal irritation or redness and the presence of injury to the gastrointestinal tract. Victims with oral or esophageal injury nearly always have drooling and pain on swallowing.

   A. **Endoscopy.** Esophageal or gastric injury is unlikely after ingestion if the patient is completely asymptomatic, but studies have repeatedly shown that a small number of patients will have injury in the absence of oral burns or obvious dysphagia. For this reason, many authorities recommend endoscopy for all patients regardless of symptoms.

   B. **X-ray.** X-ray of the chest will reveal impacted button batteries, as well as air in the mediastinum resulting from esophageal perforation.

   C. **Specific levels.** There are no specific serum levels available.

   D. **Other useful laboratory studies.** CBC, electrolytes, glucose, arterial blood gases, upright abdominal x-ray.

V. **Treatment**

   A. **Emergency and supportive measures**

      1. **Inhalation.** Give supplemental oxygen, and observe closely for signs of progressive airway obstruction or noncardiogenic pulmonary edema (see pp 7–8).

      2. **Ingestion**

         a. Immediately give water or milk to drink.

         b. If esophageal or gastric perforation is suspected, obtain immediate surgical or endoscopic consultation.

   B. **Specific drugs and antidotes.** For most agents, there is no specific antidote. (See p 167 for hydrofluoric acid burns and p 234 for phenol burns.) Corticosteroids are used by many clinicians in the hope of reducing scarring, but there is no credible evidence that they are effective. Moreover, steroids may be harmful in the patient with perforation by masking early signs of inflammation and inhibiting resistance to infection.

   C. **Decontamination**

1. **Inhalation.** Remove from exposure; give supplemental oxygen if available.
2. **Skin and eyes.** Remove all clothing; wash skin and irrigate eyes with copious water or saline.
3. **Ingestion**
   a. Immediately give water or milk to drink. Do **not** induce emesis. Gastric lavage (see p 43) to remove the corrosive material is controversial but is probably beneficial in acute liquid caustic ingestion, and it will be required before endoscopy anyway. Use a soft flexible tube and lavage with repeated aliquots of water or saline, frequently checking the fluid pH.
   b. Do **not** give activated charcoal, as it may interfere with visibility at endoscopy.
   c. **Button batteries** lodged in the esophagus must be removed immediately by endoscopy to prevent rapid perforation. Batteries in the stomach or intestine should not be removed unless signs of perforation or obstruction develop.
D. **Enhanced elimination.** There is no role for any of these procedures.

Reference

Crain EF et al: Caustic ingestions: Symptoms as predictors of esophageal injury. *Am J Dis Child* 1984;**138**:863.

CHLORATES
Kathryn H. Keller, PharmD

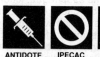

ANTIDOTE   IPECAC   LAVAGE   CHARCOAL

Potassium chlorate is used in some matchheads; barium chlorate (see also p 87) is used in the manufacture of fireworks and explosives; and other chlorate salts are used in dye production. Safer and more effective compounds have replaced chlorate in toothpaste, antiseptic mouthwashes, and weedkillers. Chlorate poisoning is similar to bromate intoxication (see p 97), but intravascular hemolysis and methemoglobinemia are more prominent features with the former.

I. **Mechanism of toxicity.** Chlorates are potent oxidizing agents that may produce severe methemoglobinemia, intravascular hemolysis, and gastrointestinal irritation. Renal failure is probably due to hemolysis.
II. **Toxic dose.** The minimum toxic dose in children is not established. Children may ingest up to 1–2 matchbooks without toxic effect (each matchhead may contain 10–12 mg of chlorate). The adult lethal dose was estimated to be 7.5 g in one case but is probably closer to 20–35 g. A 26-year-old woman survived a 150- to 200-g ingestion.
III. **Clinical presentation.** Within a few minutes to hours after ingestion, abdominal pain, vomiting, and diarrhea may occur. Methemoglobinemia is common (see p 204). Massive hemolysis, hemoglobinuria, and acute tubular necrosis may occur over 1–2 days after ingestion. Coagulopathy and hepatic injury have been described.
IV. **Diagnosis.** Diagnosis is usually based on a history of exposure and the presence of methemoglobinemia and hemolysis.
   A. **Specific levels.** Serum levels are not available, nor are they useful.
   B. **Other useful laboratory studies.** CBC, plasma free hemoglobin, electrolytes, glucose, BUN, creatinine, methemoglobin level, prothrombin time, urinalysis.
V. **Treatment**

A. **Emergency and supportive measures**
   1. Maintain the airway and assist ventilation if necessary (see p 2).
   2. Treat coma (p 17), hyperkalemia (p 32), and renal (p 33) or hepatic failure (p 34) if they occur.
   3. Massive hemolysis may require blood transfusions. To prevent renal failure resulting from deposition of free hemoglobin in the kidney tubules, administer intravenous fluids and sodium bicarbonate.
B. **Specific drugs and antidotes**
   1. Treat methemoglobinemia with **methylene blue** (see p 322), 1–2 mg/kg (0.1–0.2 mL/kg) of 1% solution.
   2. **Sodium thiosulfate** (see p 340) may inactivate the chlorate ion and has been reported successful in anecdotal reports. However, this treatment has not been clinically tested; administration as a lavage fluid may potentially produce some hydrogen sulfide.
C. **Decontamination**
   1. Induce emesis or perform gastric lavage (see p 42). *Note:* Spontaneous emesis is common after significant ingestion.
   2. Administer activated charcoal and cathartic (see p 45).
   3. Gut emptying is probably not necessary following small ingestions if activated charcoal is given promptly.
D. **Enhanced elimination.** Chlorate elimination may be hastened by **hemodialysis,** especially in patients with renal insufficiency.

Reference

Steffen C, Seitz R: Severe chlorate posioning: Report of a case. *Arch Toxicol* 1981;**48**:282.

CHLORINATED HYDROCARBON PESTICIDES
Olga F. Woo, PharmD

| ANTIDOTE | IPECAC | LAVAGE | CHARCOAL |

Chlorinated hydrocarbon pesticides are widely used in agriculture, structural insect control, and malaria control programs around the world. Lindane is used medicinally for the treatment of lice and scabies. Chlorinated hydrocarbons are of major toxicologic concern, and many (eg, DDT, chlordane) are now banned from commercial use because they persist in the environment and accumulate in biologic systems.

  I. **Mechanism of toxicity.** Chlorinated hydrocarbons are well absorbed from the gastrointestinal tract, across the skin, and by inhalation. They are highly lipid-soluble and accumulate with repeated exposure.
   A. Chlorinated hydrocarbons interfere with transmission of nerve impulses, especially in the brain, resulting in behavioral changes, involuntary muscle activity, and depression of the respiratory center.
   B. In addition, they may sensitize the myocardium to arrhythmogenic effects of catecholamines, and many can cause liver or renal injury, possibly owing to generation of toxic metabolites.
   C. Some chlorinated hydrocarbons may be carcinogenic (see Table IV–13).
 II. **Toxic dose.** The acute toxic doses of these compounds are highly variable, and reports of acute human poisonings are limited. Table II–16 ranks the relative toxicity of several common compounds.
   A. **Ingestion** of as little as 1 g of lindane can produce seizures in a child, and 10–30 g is considered lethal in an adult. The estimated adult lethal oral dose of aldrin and chlordane is 3–7 g; of dieldrin, 2–5 g.

TABLE II-16. COMMON CHLORINATED HYDROCARBONS

Highly Toxic (animal oral LD$_{50}$ < 50 mg/kg)	Moderately Toxic (animal oral LD$_{50}$ > 50 mg/kg)	Low Toxicity (animal oral LD$_{50}$ > 1 g/kg)
Aldrin	Chlordane	Ethylan (Perthane)
Dieldrin	DDT	Hexachlorobenzene
Endrin	Heptachlor	Methoxychlor
Endosulfan	Kepone	
	Lindane	
	Mirex	
	Toxaphene	

  B. **Skin absorption** is a significant route of exposure, especially with aldrin, dieldrin, and endrin. Extensive or repeated whole-body application of lindane to infants has resulted in seizures and death.
III. **Clinical presentation.** Shortly after acute ingestion, nausea and vomiting occur, followed by confusion, tremor, obtundation, coma, seizures, and respiratory depression. Because chlorinated hydrocarbons are highly lipid-soluble, the duration of toxicity may be prolonged.
  A. Recurrent or delayed-onset seizures have been reported.
  B. Arrhythmias may occur owing to myocardial sensitivity to catecholamines.
  C. Signs of hepatitis or renal injury may develop.
IV. **Diagnosis.** Diagnosis is based on the history of exposure and clinical presentation.
  A. **Specific levels.** Chlorinated hydrocarbons can be measured in the serum, but levels are not routinely available. A poison control center (see Table I–41) or the nearest US Environmental Protection Agency branch may be consulted to help locate a laboratory that can perform these assays.
  B. **Other useful laboratory studies.** CBC, electrolytes, glucose, BUN, creatinine, hepatic transaminases, prothrombin time, ECG.
V. **Treatment**
  A. **Emergency and supportive measures**
    1. Maintain the airway and assist ventilation if necessary (see p 2).
    2. Treat seizures (p 21), coma (p 17), and respiratory depression (p 6) if they occur. Ventricular arrhythmias may respond to propranolol (p 338).
    3. Attach electrocardiographic monitor, and observe the patient for at least 6–8 hours.
  B. **Specific drugs and antidotes.** There is no specific antidote.
  C. **Decontamination**
    1. **Skin and eyes.** Remove contaminated clothing and wash affected skin with copious soap and water, including hair and nails. Irrigate exposed eyes with copious tepid water or saline. Rescuers must take precautions to avoid personal exposure.
    2. **Ingestion**
      a. Perform gastric lavage (see p 43). Do **not** induce emesis because of the risk of sudden onset of seizures.
      b. Administer activated charcoal and cathartic (see p 45).
      c. Gut emptying is probably not necessary following small ingestions if activated charcoal is given promptly.
  D. **Enhanced elimination**
    1. **Repeated doses of activated charcoal** (see p 49 and p 299) **or cholestyramine** resin may be administered to enhance elimination by interrupting enterohepatic circulation.
    2. Exchange transfusion, peritoneal dialysis, hemodialysis, and

hemoperfusion are not likely to be beneficial because of the large volume of distribution of these chemicals.

Reference

Davies JE et al: Lindane poisonings. *Arch Dermatol* 1983;**119**:142.

CHLORINE
Kent R. Olson, MD

ANTIDOTE   IPECAC   LAVAGE   CHARCOAL

Chlorine is a yellowish-green gas with an irritating odor, used widely in chemical manufacturing, bleaching, and (as hypochlorite) in swimming pool disinfectant and cleaning agents. **Hypochlorite** is an aqueous solution produced by the reaction of chlorine gas with water; most household bleach solutions contain 3–5% hypochlorite; swimming pool disinfectants and industrial strength cleaners may contain up to 20% hypochlorite. Addition of acid to hypochlorite solution may release chlorine gas. Addition of ammonia to hypochlorite solution may release chloramine, a gas with similar properties.

I. **Mechanism of toxicity.** Chlorine gas is highly water-soluble and rapidly produces a corrosive effect on contact with moist tissues such as the eyes and upper respiratory tract. Exposure to aqueous solutions causes corrosive injury to the eyes, skin, or gastrointestinal tract (see p 114).

II. **Toxic dose**
   A. **Chlorine gas.** The OSHA permissible exposure limit (PEL) for chlorine gas is 0.5 ppm (3 mg/m^3) as an 8-hour time-weighted average. The level considered immediately dangerous to life or health (IDLH) is 25 ppm.
   B. **Aqueous solutions.** Dilute aqueous hypochlorite solutions (3–5%) rarely cause serious burns but are moderately irritating. More concentrated industrial cleaners (20% hypochlorite) are much more likely to cause serious corrosive injury.

III. **Clinical presentation**
   A. **Inhalation of chlorine gas.** Symptoms are rapid in onset owing to the high water solubility of chlorine. Immediate burning of the eyes, nose, and throat occurs, accompanied by coughing. Wheezing may also occur, especially in patients with preexisting bronchospastic disease. With serious exposure, upper airway swelling may rapidly cause airway obstruction, preceded by croupy cough, hoarseness, and stridor. With very great exposure, noncardiogenic pulmonary edema may also occur.
   B. **Skin or eye contact with gas or concentrated solution.** Serious corrosive burns may occur. Manifestations are similar to those of other caustic exposures (see p 114).
   C. **Ingestion of aqueous solutions.** Immediate burning in the mouth and throat is common, but no further injury is expected after ingestion of 3–5% hypochlorite. With more concentrated solutions, serious esophageal and gastric burns may occur, and victims often have dysphagia; drooling; and severe throat, chest, and abdominal pain. Hematemesis and perforation of the esophagus or stomach may occur.

IV. **Diagnosis.** Diagnosis is based on a history of exposure and description of the typical irritating odor, accompanied by irritative or corrosive effects on the eyes, skin, or upper respiratory or gastrointestinal tract.
   A. **Specific levels.** There are no specific serum levels.
   B. **Other useful laboratory studies.** CBC, electrolytes, arterial blood gases, chest x-ray.

V. **Treatment**
   A. **Emergency and supportive measures**

1. **Inhalation of chlorine gas**
    a. Immediately give humidified supplemental oxygen. Observe carefully for signs of progressive upper airway obstruction, and intubate the trachea if necessary (see p 4).
    b. Use bronchodilators for wheezing (p 8), and treat noncardiogenic pulmonary edema (p 7) if it occurs.
2. **Ingestion of hypochlorite solution.** If solution of 10% or greater has been ingested, or if there are any symptoms of corrosive injury (dysphagia, drooling, pain), flexible endoscopy is recommended to evaluate for serious esophageal or gastric injury. Obtain a chest x-ray to look for mediastinal air, which suggests esophageal perforation.
B. **Specific drugs and antidotes.** There is no proved specific treatment for this or other common caustic burns. Administration of corticosteroids is favored by many toxicologists in the hope of limiting esophageal scarring, but this treatment is unproved and may be harmful in patients with perforation or serious infection.
C. **Decontamination**
1. **Inhalation.** Remove immediately from exposure, and give supplemental oxygen if available.
2. **Skin and eyes.** Remove contaminated clothing, and flush exposed skin immediately with copious water. Irrigate exposed eyes with water or saline.
3. **Ingestion of hypochlorite solution**
    a. Immediately give water or milk by mouth.
    b. Do *not* induce emesis. Gastric lavage (see p 43) is recommended after concentrated liquid ingestion, in order to remove any liquid caustic in the stomach and to prepare for endoscopy; use a small flexible tube to avoid injury to damaged mucosa.
    c. Do *not* use activated charcoal; it may obscure the endoscopist's view.
D. **Enhanced elimination.** There is no role for enhanced elimination.

Reference

Hedges JR, Morrissey WL: Acute chlorine gas exposure. *JACEP* 1979;8:59.

CHLOROFORM
Peter Wald, MD

ANTIDOTE   IPECAC   LAVAGE   CHARCOAL

Chloroform (trichloromethane) is a chlorinated hydrocarbon solvent used as a raw material in the production of Freon and as an extractant and solvent in the chemical and pharmaceutical industry. Because of its hepatic toxicity, it is no longer used as a general anesthetic or anthelmintic agent. Chronic low-level exposure may occur in some municipal water supplies owing to chlorination of biologic methanes.

I. **Mechanism of toxicity.** Chloroform is a direct central nervous system depressant. In addition, as with other chlorinated hydrocarbons, it may potentiate cardiac arrhythmias by sensitizing the myocardium to catecholamines. Hepatic and renal toxicity is probably due to metabolism to a highly reactive intermediate, possibly a free radical or phosgene. Chloroform is embryotoxic and is a suspected human carcinogen.
II. **Toxic dose**
    A. The fatal **oral** dose of chloroform may be as little as 10 mL, although survival after ingestion of more than 100 mL has been reported. The oral LD_{50} in rats is 2000 mg/kg.
    B. The **air level** considered immediately dangerous to life or health (IDLH)

is 1000 ppm. The OSHA permissible exposure limit (PEL) for inhalation is 2 ppm as an 8-hour time-weighted average.

III. Clinical presentation

A. Skin or eye contact results in irritation and defatting. Mucous membrane irritation is seen with ingestion or inhalation.

B. Inhalation or ingestion. Mild to moderate systemic toxicity includes headache, nausea, vomiting, confusion, and drunkenness. More severe exposures may cause coma, respiratory arrest, and ventricular arrhythmias. Hepatic and renal injury may be apparent 1–3 days after exposure.

IV. Diagnosis.
Diagnosis is based on history and clinical presentation. Be aware that hepatic and renal toxicity may be delayed.

A. Specific levels. Blood, urine, or breath concentrations may document exposure but are rarely available and are not useful for acute management.

B. Other useful laboratory studies. CBC, electrolytes, BUN, creatinine, hepatic transaminases, prothrombin time, urinalysis, electrocardiographic monitoring.

V. Treatment

A. Emergency and supportive measures

1. Maintain the airway and assist ventilation if necessary (see p 2).
2. Treat coma (p 17) and arrhythmias (p 13) if they occur. Avoid use of epinephrine or other sympathomimetic amines, which may precipitate arrhythmias.
3. Monitor ECG for at least 4–6 hours after exposure.

B. Specific drugs and antidotes. Acetylcysteine (NAC; see p 289) may be helpful in preventing hepatic and renal damage by scavenging toxic metabolic intermediates, but no controlled study has been performed.

C. Decontamination

1. **Inhalation.** Remove victim from exposure and give supplemental oxygen if available.
2. **Skin and eyes.** Remove contaminated clothing and wash exposed skin with soap and water. Irrigate exposed eyes with copious tepid water or saline.
3. **Ingestion**
   a. Perform gastric lavage (see p 43). Do **not** induce emesis because chloroform is rapidly absorbed and may cause abrupt central nervous system depression.
   b. Administer activated charcoal and cathartic (see p 45).
   c. Gut emptying is probably not necessary following small ingestions if activated charcoal is given promptly.

D. Enhanced elimination. There is no documented efficacy for forced diuresis, hemodialysis, hemoperfusion, or repeat-dose charcoal.

Reference

NIOSH: *Criteria Document for a Recommended Standard: Occupational Exposure to Chloroform.* NIOSH Publication No. 75-114. US Department of Health, Education, & Welfare, 1974.

CHLOROPHENOXY HERBICIDES
Kent R. Olson, MD

ANTIDOTE   IPECAC   LAVAGE   CHARCOAL

Chlorophenoxy compounds have been widely used as herbicides. Agent Orange was a mixture of the chlorophenoxy herbicides 2,4-D (dichlorophenoxyacetic acid) and 2,4,5-T (trichlorophenoxyacetic acid) that also contained small amounts of the highly toxic contaminant TCDD (2,3,7,8-tetrachlorodibenzo-*p*-dioxin; see p 142). Commercially available 2,4-D no longer contains TCDD.

I. **Mechanism of toxicity.** In plants, the compounds act as growth hormone stimulators. Their mechanism of toxicity in animals is not known. In animal studies, widespread muscle damage occurs and the cause of death is usually ventricular fibrillation. Massive rhabdomyolysis has been described in human cases.

II. **Toxic dose.** The minimum toxic dose of 2,4-D in humans is 3–4 g or 40–50 mg/kg, and death has occurred after adult ingestion of 6.5 g.

III. **Clinical presentation.** Tachycardia, muscle weakness, and muscle spasms occur shortly after ingestion and may progress to profound muscle weakness and coma. Massive rhabdomyolysis and severe and intractable hypotension have been reported, resulting in death within 24 hours. Hepatitis and renal injury may occur.

IV. **Diagnosis.** Diagnosis depends on a history of exposure and the presence of muscle weakness and elevated serum creatine phosphokinase (CPK).

    A. **Specific levels.** Serum levels are not routinely available.

    B. **Other useful laboratory studies.** CBC, electrolytes, glucose, BUN, creatinine, creatine phosphokinase (CPK), urinalysis (for myoglobin), liver enzymes, ECG and electrocardiographic monitoring.

V. **Treatment**

    A. **Emergency and supportive measures**

        1. Maintain the airway and assist ventilation if necessary (see p 2).

        2. Treat coma (p 17), hypotension (p 14), and rhabdomyolysis (p 24) if they occur.

        3. Monitor the patient closely for at least 6–12 hours after ingestion because of the potential for delayed onset of symptoms.

    B. **Specific drugs and antidotes.** There is no specific antidote.

    C. **Decontamination**

        1. Induce emesis or perform gastric lavage (see p 42).

        2. Administer activated charcoal and cathartic (see p 45).

        3. Gut emptying is probably not necessary following small ingestions if activated charcoal is given promptly.

    D. **Enhanced elimination.** There is no proved role for these procedures, although alkalinization of the urine may promote excretion of 2,4-D.

Reference

Osterloh J, Lotti M, Pond SM: Toxicologic studies in a fatal overdose of 2,4-D, MCPP, and chlorpyrifos. *J Anal Toxicol* 1983;7:125.

CHLOROQUINE AND OTHER AMINOQUINOLINES
Neal L. Benowitz, MD

ANTIDOTE   IPECAC   LAVAGE   CHARCOAL

Chloroquine and other aminoquinolines are used in the prophylaxis or therapy of malaria and other parasitic diseases. Chloroquine and hydroxychloroquine are also used in the treatment of rheumatoid arthritis. Drugs in this class include chloroquine phosphate (Aralen), amodiaquine hydrochloride (Camoquin), hydroxychloroquine sulfate (Plaquenil), primaquine phosphate, and quinacrine hydrochloride (Atabrine). Chloroquine overdose is common, especially in countries where malaria is prevalent, and the mortality rate is 10–30%.

I. **Mechanism of toxicity.** Chloroquine and related drugs are highly tissue-bound (volume of distribution is 200 L/kg) and are eliminated very slowly from the body (half-life of 280 hours).

      A. Chloroquine blocks the synthesis of DNA and RNA and also has some quinidinelike cardiotoxicity.

      B. Primaquine and **quinacrine** are oxidizing agents and can cause methemoglobinemia or hemolytic anemia (especially in patients with G6PD deficiency).

II. Toxic dose. The therapeutic dose of chloroquine for malaria prophylaxis is 500 mg once a week, or 500 mg/d to a total dose of 2.5 g for treatment of malaria. Deaths have been reported in children after doses as low as 300 mg; the lethal dose of chloroquine for an adult is estimated at 30–50 mg/kg.

III. Clinical presentation

      A. Mild to moderate chloroquine overdose results in dizziness, nausea and vomiting, abdominal pain, headache and visual disturbances (sometimes including irreversible blindness), agitation, and neuromuscular excitability.

      B. More severe overdose may cause convulsions, coma, shock, and respiratory or cardiac arrest. Quinidinelike cardiotoxicity may be seen, including sinoatrial arrest, depressed myocardial contractility, QRS or QT interval prolongation, and ventricular arrhythmias. Severe hypokalemia sometimes occurs and may contribute to arrhythmias.

      C. Primaquine and **quinacrine** intoxication commonly cause gastrointestinal upset and may also cause severe methemoglobinemia (see p 204) or hemolysis; chronic treatment can cause ototoxicity and retinopathy.

IV. Diagnosis. The findings of gastritis, visual disturbances, and neuromuscular excitability, especially if accompanied by hypotension, QRS or QT interval widening, or ventricular arrhythmias, should suggest chloroquine overdose. Hemolysis or methemoglobinemia should suggest primaquine or quinacrine overdose.

      A. Specific levels. Chloroquine levels can be measured in blood but are not generally available. Because chloroquine is concentrated intracellularly, whole blood measurements are 2-fold higher than serum or plasma levels.

        1. Plasma (trough) concentrations of 10–20 ng/mL (0.01–0.02 mg/L) are effective in the treatment of malaria.

        2. Cardiotoxicity may be seen with serum levels of 5 mg/L; serum levels reported in fatal cases have ranged from 1–210 mg/L (average, 55 mg/L).

      B. Other useful laboratory studies. CBC, free plasma hemoglobin, electrolytes, glucose, BUN, creatinine, methemoglobin, ECG and electrocardiographic monitoring.

V. Treatment

      A. Emergency and supportive measures

        1. Maintain the airway and assist ventilation if necessary (see p 2).

        2. Treat seizures (p 21), coma (p 17), hypotension (p 14), and methemoglobinemia (p 204) if they occur.

        3. Treat massive hemolysis with blood transfusions if needed, and prevent hemoglobin deposition in the kidney tubules by alkaline diuresis (as for rhabdomyolysis; see p 24).

        4. Continuously monitor the ECG for at least 6 hours.

      B. Specific drugs and antidotes

        1. Treat cardiotoxicity as for quinidine poisoning (see p 255) with **sodium bicarbonate** (see p 296), 1–2 meq/kg IV.

        2. High-dose **diazepam** (0.5–1 mg/kg IV) has been reported to reduce mortality in animals and ameliorate cardiotoxicity in a few anecdotal human cases. However, the mechanism of protection is unknown and its routine use is not recommended.

      C. Decontamination

        1. Perform gastric lavage (see p 43). Do *not* induce emesis because of the risk of rapid onset of coma or seizures.

        2. Administer activated charcoal and a cathartic (see p 45).

    3. Gut emptying is probably not necessary following small ingestions if activated charcoal is given promptly.

   D. Enhanced elimination. Because of extensive tissue distribution, enhanced removal procedures are ineffective.

Reference

Jaeger A et al: Clinical features and management of poisoning due to antimalarial drugs. *Med Toxicol Adverse Drug Exp* 1987;**2**:242.

CHROMIUM
Peter Yip, MD

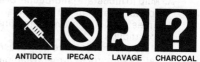

ANTIDOTE   IPECAC   LAVAGE   CHARCOAL

Chromium is a hard silver-colored metal used in chrome plating, pigments, and oxidizing agents. Electroplaters, welders, lithographers, and metal and textile workers are among those potentially exposed. Chromium salts occur in 2 valence states: trivalent (chromic oxide, chromic sulfate) and hexavalent (chromium trioxide, chromic anhydride, chromic acid, and dichromate salts).

I. Mechanism of toxicity

  A. Trivalent chromium compounds and chromate salts of lead, zinc, barium, bismuth, and silver are relatively insoluble and poorly absorbed, and have low toxicity.

  B. Hexavalent compounds are soluble and are more readily absorbed from the gastrointestinal tract, skin, and lungs. Hexavalent chromium salts are strong oxidizing agents that may oxidize hemoglobin to produce methemoglobinemia. They also produce corrosive burns by denaturation of tissue protein. Some hexavalent chromium compounds are carcinogenic (see Table IV-13).

  C. Chromic acid is a strong acid, while some chromate salts are strong bases.

II. Toxic dose

  A. Inhalation. The OSHA permissible exposure limit (PEL) for chromic acid and chromates is 0.1 mg/m^3 as an 8-hour time-weighted average.

  B. Skin. Skin burns may enhance systemic absorption, and death has occurred after a 10% surface area burn.

  C. Ingestion. Serious toxicity has occurred from ingestion of as little as 500 mg of hexavalent chromium. The estimated lethal dose of chromic acid is 1–2 g; of potassium dichromate, 6–8 g.

III. Clinical presentation

  A. Inhalation. Inhalation can cause upper respiratory tract irritation, wheezing, and pulmonary edema (which may be delayed for several hours after exposure).

  B. Skin and eyes. Acute contact may cause severe corneal injury, deep skin burns, and oral or esophageal burns. Hypersensitivity dermatitis may result.

  C. Ingestion. Ingestion may cause immediate hemorrhagic gastroenteritis; resulting massive fluid and blood loss may cause shock and oliguric renal failure. Hemolysis, hepatitis, and cerebral edema have been reported. Chromates are capable of oxidizing hemoglobin, but clinically significant methemoglobinemia is relatively uncommon after acute overdose.

IV. Diagnosis. Diagnosis is based on a history of exposure and clinical manifestations of skin and mucous membrane burns, gastroenteritis, and shock.

    A. Specific levels. Blood levels are not useful in emergency management, nor are they widely available. Detection in the urine may confirm exposure.

    B. Other useful laboratory studies. CBC, electrolytes, glucose, BUN, creatinine, liver function tests, arterial blood gas, methemoglobin level, chest x-ray.

V. Treatment

  A. Emergency and supportive measures

    1. Inhalation. Give supplemental oxygen. Treat wheezing (see p 8), and monitor closely for several hours for development of noncardiogenic pulmonary edema (p 7).

    2. Ingestion

      a. Treat hemorrhagic gastroenteritis with aggressive fluid and blood replacement (p 14). Consider endoscopy to rule out esophageal or gastric burns.

      b. Treat hemoglobinuria due to hemolysis with alkaline diuresis as for rhabdomyolysis (p 24).

  B. Specific drugs and antidotes

    1. Chelation therapy (eg, with BAL) is not effective.

    2. After oral ingestion of hexavalent compounds, **ascorbic acid** may assist the conversion of hexavalent to less toxic trivalent compounds. For each 0.135 g of chromium compound ingested, give 1 g of ascorbic acid orally.

    3. Acetylcysteine (see p 289) has been used in animals and one human case of dichromate poisoning.

  C. Decontamination

    1. Inhalation. Remove victim from exposure and give supplemental oxygen, if available.

    2. Skin. Remove contaminated clothing and wash exposed areas with copious soap and water. EDTA (see p 308) 10% ointment may facilitate removal of chromate scabs.

    3. Eyes. Irrigate copiously with tepid water or saline and perform fluorescein examination to rule out corneal injury if pain or irritation persists.

    4. Ingestion

      a. Give milk or water to dilute corrosive effects.

      b. Perform gastric lavage (see p 43). Do *not* induce emesis owing to the potential for corrosive injury.

      c. Administer activated charcoal (see p 45), although there is no evidence for its efficacy. Do *not* give charcoal if endoscopy is planned.

  D. Enhanced elimination. There is no evidence for efficacy of enhanced removal procedures such as dialysis or hemoperfusion.

Reference

Korallus U, Harzdorf C, Lewalter J: Experimental bases for ascorbic acid therapy of poisoning by hexavalent chromium compounds. *Int Arch Occup Environ Health* 1984;53:247.

CLONIDINE AND RELATED DRUGS
Olga F. Woo, PharmD

ANTIDOTE   IPECAC   LAVAGE   CHARCOAL

Clonidine and the related centrally acting adrenergic inhibitors guanabenz and methyldopa are commonly used for the treatment of hypertension. Clonidine has also been used to alleviate opioid and nicotine withdrawal symptoms. Clonidine overdose is a common pediatric problem that may occur after ingestion of pills or the newer long-acting skin patches. A few cases of methyldopa ingestion have been reported, usually without serious complications. Guanabenz is a newer agent, and there is very little information on its effect in acute overdose.

I. **Mechanism of toxicity.** All agents decrease central sympathetic outflow by stimulating α_2-adrenergic (inhibitory) receptors in the brain.
   A. **Clonidine** may also stimulate peripheral α_1-receptors, resulting in vasoconstriction and transient hypertension.
   B. **Oxymetazoline** and **tetrahydrozoline** are nasal decongestants that may cause toxicity similar to that of clonidine.
   C. **Methyldopa** may further decrease sympathetic outflow by metabolism to a false neurotransmitter (alpha-methylnorepinephrine) or by decreasing plasma renin activity.
   D. **Guanabenz** is structurally similar to guanethidine, a ganglionic blocker, and has some neuron-blocking action.

II. **Toxic dose**
   A. **Clonidine.** As little as one tablet of 0.1 mg clonidine has produced toxic effects in children; however, 10 mg shared by twin 34-month-old girls was not lethal. Adults have survived acute ingestions with as much as 18.8 mg. No fatalities from acute overdoses have been reported.
   B. **Methyldopa.** More than 2 g in adults is considered a toxic dose, and death was reported in an adult after ingesting 25 g. The therapeutic dose of methyldopa for children is 10–65 mg/kg/d, and the higher dose is expected to cause mild symptoms.
   C. **Guanabenz.** Mild toxicity developed in adults who ingested 160–320 mg and in a 3-year-old who ingested 12 mg. Severe toxicity developed in a 19-month-old who ingested 28 mg. A 3-year-old child had moderate symptoms after ingesting 480 mg. All these children had recovered by 24 hours.

III. **Clinical presentation.** Manifestations of intoxication are due to generalized sympathetic depression and include pupillary constriction, lethargy, coma, apnea, bradycardia, hypotension, and hypothermia. Paradoxic hypertension, caused by stimulation of peripheral α_1-receptors, may occur with clonidine (and possibly guanabenz) and is usually transient. The onset of symptoms is usually within 30–60 minutes, although peak effects may occur 6–12 hours after ingestion, with full recovery within 24 hours.

IV. **Diagnosis.** The diagnosis should be suspected in patients with pinpoint pupils, apnea, hypotension, and bradycardia. Clonidine overdose may mimic opioid overdose but does not respond to administration of naloxone.
   A. **Specific levels.** Serum drug levels are not routinely available or clinically useful.
   B. **Other useful laboratory studies.** CBC, electrolytes, glucose, arterial blood gases, ECG.

V. **Treatment.** Recovery is usually complete within 24 hours with supportive care.
   A. **Emergency and supportive measures**
      1. Protect the airway and assist ventilation if necessary (see p 2).
      2. Treat coma (p 17), hypotension (p 14), bradycardia (p 9), and hypothermia (p 18) if they occur. These signs usually resolve with supportive measures such as fluids, atropine, dopamine, and warming. Hypertension is usually transient but may require brief treatment (p 16).
      3. Symptomatic patients should be admitted for 24-hour observation.
   B. **Specific drugs and antidotes**
      1. **Naloxone** (see p 325) has been reported to reverse signs and symp-

toms of clonidine overdose, but this has not been confirmed. However, because the overdose mimics opioid intoxication, naloxone is indicated because narcotics may also have been ingested.

2. **Tolazoline,** a central α₂-receptor antagonist, has been recommended by some, but the response is highly variable and it should not be used.

C. **Decontamination**

1. Induce emesis or perform gastric lavage (see p 42). Lavage is preferred because of the risk of coma, apnea, and aspiration.
2. Administer activated charcoal and a cathartic (see p 45).
3. Gut emptying is probably not necessary following small ingestions if activated charcoal is given promptly.

D. **Enhanced elimination.** There is no evidence that enhanced removal procedures are effective.

References

Hall AH et al: Guanabenz overdose. *Ann Intern Med* 1985;**102**:787.
Olsson JM, Pruitt AW: Management of clonidine ingestion in children. *J Pediatr* 1983;**103**:646.

COCAINE
Neal L. Benowitz, MD

| ANTIDOTE | IPECAC | LAVAGE | CHARCOAL |

Cocaine is one of the most popular drugs of abuse. It may be sniffed into the nose (snorted), smoked, or injected intravenously. Occasionally it is combined with heroin and injected (speedball). Cocaine purchased on the street is usually of high purity, but it may occasionally contain substitute stimulants such as caffeine (see p 100), phenylpropanolamine (p 238), ephedrine (p 238), or phencyclidine (p 233).

The "free base" form of cocaine is preferred for smoking because it volatilizes at a lower temperature and is not as easily destroyed by heat as the crystalline hydrochoride salt. Free base (also known as "crack") is made by dissolving cocaine salt in an aqueous alkaline solution and then extracting the free base form with a solvent such as ether. Heat is often applied to hasten solvent evaporation, creating a fire hazard.

I. **Mechanism of toxicity.** The primary actions of cocaine are local anesthetic effects (see p 64), central nervous system stimulation, and inhibition of neuronal uptake of catecholamines.

A. Central nervous system stimulation and inhibition of catecholamine uptake result in a state of generalized sympathetic stimulation very similar to that of amphetamine intoxication (see p 62).

B. Cocaine is well absorbed from all routes, and toxicity has been described after mucosal application as a local anesthetic. Smoking and intravenous injection produce maximum effects within 1–2 minutes, while oral or mucosal absorption may take up to 20–30 minutes. Once absorbed, cocaine is eliminated by metabolism and hydrolysis with a half-life of about 60 minutes.

II. **Toxic dose.** The toxic dose is highly variable and depends on individual tolerance, the route of administration, and the presence of other drugs, as well as other factors. Rapid intravenous injection or smoking may produce transient high brain and heart levels resulting in convulsions or cardiac arrhythmias, whereas the same dose swallowed or snorted may produce only euphoria.

A. The usual maximum recommended dose for intranasal local anesthesia is 100–200 mg (1–2 mL of 10% solution).

B. A typical "line" of cocaine to be snorted contains 20–30 mg or more. Crack is usually sold in pellets or "rocks" containing 100–150 mg.

C. Ingestion of 1 g or more of cocaine is likely to be fatal.

III. Clinical presentation

A. Central nervous system manifestations of toxicity may occur within minutes after smoking or intravenous injection or may be delayed for 30–60 minutes after snorting, mucosal application, or oral ingestion.

1. Initial euphoria may be followed by anxiety, agitation, delirium, psychosis, tremulousness, muscle rigidity or hyperactivity, and seizures.
2. Seizures are usually brief and self-limited; status epilepticus should suggest continued drug absorption (as from ruptured cocaine-filled packets or condoms in the gastrointestinal tract) or hyperthermia.
3. Coma may be caused by a postictal state, hyperthermia, or intracranial hemorrhage resulting from cocaine-induced hypertension.
4. With chronic cocaine use, insomnia, weight loss, and paranoid psychosis may occur.

B. Cardiovascular toxicity may also occur rapidly after smoking or intravenous injection and is mediated by sympathetic overactivity.

1. Fatal ventricular tachycardia or fibrillation may occur.
2. Severe hypertension may cause hemorrhagic stroke or aortic dissection.
3. Coronary artery spasm or thrombosis may result in myocardial infarction, even in patients with no coronary disease. Diffuse myocardial necrosis similar to catecholamine myocarditis, and chronic cardiomyopathy have been described.
4. Shock may be caused by myocardial, intestinal, or brain infarction, hyperthermia, tachyarrhythmias, or hypovolemia produced by extravascular fluid sequestration due to vasoconstriction.
5. Renal failure may result from shock, renal arterial spasm, or rhabdomyolysis with myoglobinuria.

C. Death is usually caused by a sudden fatal arrhythmia, status epilepticus, intracranial hemorrhage, or hyperthermia. Hyperthermia is usually caused by seizures, muscular hyperactivity, or rigidity and is typically associated with rhabdomyolysis, myoglobinuric renal failure, coagulopathy, and multiple organ failure.

D. A variety of **other effects** have occurred after smoking or snorting cocaine.

1. Pneumothorax and pneumomediastinum cause pleuritic chest pain, and the latter is often recognized by a "crunching" sound (Hammond's "crunch") heard over the anterior chest.
2. Nasal septal perforation may occur after chronic snorting.
3. Accidental subcutaneous injection of cocaine may cause localized necrotic ulcers ("coke burns"), and wound botulism (see p 95) has been reported.

E. Body "packers" or "stuffers." Persons attempting to smuggle cocaine may swallow large numbers of tightly packed cocaine-filled condoms ("body packers"). Street vendors suddenly surprised by a police raid may quickly swallow their wares, often without carefully wrapping the packets ("body stuffers"). The swallowed condoms or packets may break open, releasing massive quantities of cocaine. The packages are sometimes, but not always, visible on plain abdominal x-ray.

IV. Diagnosis.
Diagnosis is based on a history of cocaine use or typical features of sympathomimetic intoxication. Skin marks of chronic intravenous drug abuse, especially with scarring due to coke burns, and nasal septal perforation after chronic snorting suggest cocaine use. Chest pain with

electrocardiographic evidence of ischemia or infarction in a young, otherwise healthy person also suggests cocaine use.

    A. Specific levels. Serum cocaine levels are not routinely available and do not assist in emergency management. Cocaine and its metabolite benzoylecgonine are easily detected in the urine and provide qualitative confirmation of cocaine use.

    B. Other useful laboratory studies. CBC, electrolytes, glucose, BUN, creatinine, creatine phosphokinase (CPK), urinalysis, urine myoglobin, ECG and electrocardiographic monitoring, CT head scan (if hemorrhage is suspected), abdominal x-ray (if cocaine-filled condom or packet ingestion is suspected).

V. Treatment

    A. Emergency and supportive measures

        1. Maintain the airway and assist ventilation if necessary (see p 2).

        2. Treat coma (p 17), agitation (p 22), seizures (p 21), hyperthermia (p 19), arrhythmias (pp 12–13), and hypotension (p 14) if they occur.

        3. Angina pectoris or myocardial infarction may be treated with nitrates or calcium channel blockers such as nifedipine (p 328).

        4. Monitor vital signs and ECG for several hours.

    B. Specific drugs and antidotes. There is no specific antidote. Although propranolol has previously been recommended for treatment of cocaine-induced hypertension, it may in fact produce paradoxic worsening of hypertension because of blockade of β_2-mediated vasodilation; **propranolol** (see p 338) or **esmolol** (p 311) may be used **in combination** with a vasodilator such as **phentolamine** (p 335). Beta blockers may be used alone for treatment of tachyarrhythmias.

    C. Decontamination. Decontamination is not necessary after smoking, snorting, or intravenous injection. After **ingestion:**

        1. Perform gastric lavage (see p 43). Do **not** induce emesis because of the risk of seizures.

        2. Administer activated charcoal and cathartic (see p 45).

        3. Gut emptying is probably not necessary following small ingestions if activated charcoal is given promptly.

        4. For ingestion of cocaine-filled condoms or packets, give repeated doses of activated charcoal and consider whole gut lavage (see p 46). If large ingested packets (ie, Ziploc bags) are not removed by these procedures, laparotomy and surgical removal may be necessary.

    D. Enhanced elimination. Because cocaine is extensively distributed to tissues and rapidly metabolized, dialysis and hemoperfusion procedures are not effective. Acidification of the urine does not significantly enhance elimination and may aggravate myoglobinuric renal failure.

Reference

Cregler LL, Mark H: Medical complications of cocaine abuse. *N Engl J Med* 1986;**315**:1495.

COLCHICINE
Neal L. Benowitz, MD

ANTIDOTE   IPECAC   LAVAGE   CHARCOAL

Colchicine is marketed in tablets used for treatment of gout and familial Mediterranean fever and is found in certain plants: autumn crocus or meadow saffron *(Colchicum autumnale)* and glory lily *(Gloriosa superba)*. Colchicine overdose is extremely serious, with considerable mortality that is often delayed.

I. **Mechanism of toxicity.** Colchicine inhibits mitosis of dividing cells and, in high concentration, is a general cellular poison. Colchicine is rapidly absorbed and extensively distributed to body tissues.

II. **Toxic dose.** The maximum therapeutic dose of colchicine is 8–10 mg in one day. Tablets contain 0.5–0.6 mg. Fatalities have been reported with single ingestions of as little as 7 mg. In a series of 150 cases, doses of 0.5 mg/kg were associated with diarrhea and vomiting but not death; 0.5–0.8 mg/kg with marrow aplasia and 10% mortality. Ingestions of parts of colchicine-containing plants have resulted in severe toxicity and death.

III. **Clinical presentation.** Colchicine poisoning affects many organ systems, with toxic effects occurring over days to weeks.

   A. Following **acute overdose,** symptoms are typically delayed for 2–12 hours and include nausea, vomiting, abdominal pain, and severe bloody diarrhea. Shock is due to depressed cardiac contractality and fluid loss into the gastrointestinal tract and other tissues. **Death** usually occurs after 8–36 hours and is due to respiratory failure, intractable shock, or sudden cardiac arrest. Other manifestations of acute colchicine poisoning include acute myocardial injury, rhabdomyolysis with myoglobinuria, disseminated intravascular coagulation, and acute renal failure.

   B. **Late complications** include bone marrow suppression, particularly leukopenia and thrombocytopenia (4–5 days) and alopecia (2–3 weeks). Chronic colchicine therapy may produce myopathy (proximal muscle weakness and elevated creatinine kinase levels) and polyneuropathy.

IV. **Diagnosis.** A syndrome beginning with severe gastroenteritis, shock, rhabdomyolysis, and acute renal failure and, several days later, leukopenia and thrombocytopenia should suggest colchicine poisoning. A history of gout or familial Mediterranean fever in the patient or family member is also suggestive.

   A. **Specific levels.** Measurement of levels in blood and urine is not available nor clinically useful.

   B. **Other useful laboratory studies.** CBC, electrolytes, glucose, BUN, creatinine, creatine phosphokinase (CPK), prothrombin time, urinalysis, ECG.

V. **Treatment**

   A. **Emergency and supportive measures.** Provide aggressive supportive care, with careful monitoring and treatment of fluid and electrolyte disturbances.

   1. Anticipate sudden respiratory or cardiac arrest, and maintain the airway and assist ventilation if necessary (see p 2).

   2. Treatment of shock (p 14) may require large amounts of crystalloid fluids, possibly blood (to replace loss from hemorrhagic gastroenteritis), and pressor agents such as dopamine (p 307).

   3. Infusion of sodium bicarbonate and mannitol is recommended if there is evidence of rhabdomyolysis (p 24).

   4. Bone marrow depression requires specialized intensive care. Severe neutropenia requires patient isolation and management of febrile episodes as for other neutropenic conditions. Platelet transfusions may be required to control bleeding.

   B. **Specific drugs and antidotes.** No specific antidotes are available.

   C. **Decontamination**

   1. Induce emesis or perform gastric lavage (see p 42).

   2. Administer activated charcoal (see p 45), by gastric tube if necessary.

   D. **Enhanced elimination.** Because colchicine is highly bound to tissues, with a large volume of distribution, hemodialysis and hemoperfusion are ineffective. Colchicine undergoes enterohepatic recirculation, so

repeat-dose charcoal might be expected to accelerate elimination, although this has not been documented.

Reference

Murray SS et al: Acute toxicity after excessive ingestion of colchicine. *Mayo Clin Proc* 1983;**58**:528.

COPPER
Gail M. Gullickson, MD, and
Kent R. Olson, MD

ANTIDOTE   IPECAC   LAVAGE   CHARCOAL

Copper is widely used in its elemental metal form, in metal alloys, and in the form of copper salts. Elemental metallic copper is used in electrical wiring and plumbing materials, and copper salts are used as pesticides and algicides. Because of its toxicity, copper sulfate is no longer used as an emetic. The copper alloy brass is an important source of exposure because of leaching of copper ions into acidic beverages stored in brass containers.

I. **Mechanism of toxicity**
   A. **Elemental metalic copper** is poorly absorbed orally and has little toxicity. However, inhalation of copper dust or fumes may cause chemical pneumonitis or metal fumes fever (see p 201).
   B. **Copper sulfate** salt is highly irritating, depending on the concentration, and may produce mucous membrane irritation and gastroenteritis.
   C. **Systemic absorption** can produce hepatic and renal tubular injury. Hemolysis has been associated with copper exposure from hemodialysis equipment or absorption through burned skin.

II. **Toxic dose**
   A. **Inhalation.** The OSHA permissible exposure limit (PEL) for copper fumes is 0.1 mg/m³; for dusts and mists, it is 1 mg/m³.
   B. **Ingestion** of more than 250 mg of copper sulfate can produce vomiting, and larger ingestions can potentially cause hepatic and renal injury.

III. **Clinical presentation**
   A. **Inhalation of copper fumes** or **dusts** may cause cough, dyspnea, fever, and pulmonary infiltrates (see Metal fumes fever, p 201).
   B. **Ingestion of copper salts** rapidly causes metallic taste, epigastric burning, vomiting, and diarrhea. The vomitus may be blue-green. Hypotension may occur acutely, presumably owing to fluid loss from gastroenteritis, and oliguric renal failure may follow. Hepatitis has been reported. Deaths within the first 24 hours after ingestion have been due to shock.

IV. **Diagnosis.** Diagnosis is based on a history of ingestion of copper salts accompanied by gastroenteritis, of inhalation of copper fumes, or of welding accompanied by fever and respiratory complaints.
   A. **Specific levels.** If copper salt ingestion is suspected, a serum copper level should be obtained. Normal serum copper concentrations average 1 mg/L, and this doubles during pregnancy. Serum copper levels above 5 mg/L are considered very toxic. Whole blood copper levels may correlate better with acute intoxication because acute excess copper is carried in the red blood cell; however, blood copper levels are not as widely available.
   B. **Other useful laboratory studies.** BUN, creatinine, hepatic transaminases, arterial blood gases, chest x-ray.

V. **Treatment**
   A. **Emergency and supportive measures**

1. **Inhalation of copper fumes** or **dusts.** Give supplemental oxygen if indicated by arterial blood gases, and treat bronchspasm (see p 8) and chemical pneumonia (p 7) if they occur. Symptoms are usually short-lived and resolve without specific treatment.
2. **Ingestion of copper salts**
   a. Treat shock due to gastroenteritis with aggressive intravenous fluid replacement and, if necessary, pressor drugs (p 14).
   b. Consider endoscopy to rule out corrosive esophageal or stomach injury, depending on the concentration of the solution and the patient's symptoms.
B. **Specific drugs and antidotes.** BAL (dimercaprol; see p 294) and **penicillamine** (see p 332) are effective chelating agents and should be used in seriously ill patients with large ingestion.
C. **Decontamination**
   1. **Inhalation.** Remove victim from exposure and give supplemental oxygen if available.
   2. **Ingestion**
      a. Perform gastric lavage (see p 43). Do **not** induce emesis because it may worsen gastroenteritis.
      b. Administer activated charcoal (see p 45), although there is no documentation of its effectiveness.
D. **Enhanced elimination.** Dialysis, hemoperfusion, and repeat-dose charcoal are not effective in enhancing elimination. Hemodialysis may be required for supportive care of patients with acute renal failure, and it can marginally increase the elimination of the copper-chelator complex.

Reference

Schwartz E, Schmidt E: Refractory shock secondary to copper sulfate ingestion. *Ann Emerg Med* 1986;15:952.

COUMARIN AND RELATED RODENTICIDES
Chris Dutra, MD

ANTIDOTE   IPECAC   LAVAGE   CHARCOAL

Dicumarol and other natural anticoagulants are found in sweet clover. Coumarin derivatives (warfarin [Coumadin]) are used therapeutically and as rodenticides. Some of the newer superwarfarin products (indandione and related compounds) have profound and prolonged anticoagulant effects. Other rodenticides (eg, thallium, phosphorus, arsenic) are discussed elsewhere.

I. **Mechanism of toxicity.** All these compounds inhibit hepatic synthesis of vitamin K-dependent coagulation factors (II, IV, IX, and X). Only the synthesis of new factors is affected, and the anticoagulant effect is delayed until currently circulating factors have been degraded. Because the half-life of factor VII is the shortest (approximately 6 hours), anticoagulant effects may be seen as early as 8–12 hours after ingestion; however, peak effects are usually not observed for 1–3 days because of the longer half-lives of the other vitamin K-dependent factors (24–60 hours).
   A. The duration of anticoagulant effect after a single dose of **warfarin** is usually 5–7 days.
   B. Newer **"superwarfarin"** products (Table II–17) may continue to produce

TABLE II-17. "SUPERWARFARIN" RODENTICIDES

Brodifacoum	Difenacoum	Pindone
Bromadiolone	Diphacinone	Valone
Chlorophacinone		

significant anticoagulation for weeks to months after a single ingestion.

II. **Toxic dose.** The toxic dose is highly variable.
  A. Generally, a single small ingestion of **warfarin** (eg, 10–20 mg) will not cause serious intoxication (most warfarin-based rodenticides contain 0.05% warfarin). In contrast, chronic or repeated ingestion of even small amounts (eg, 2 mg/d) can produce significant anticoagulation. Patients with hepatic dysfunction, malnutrition, interacting drugs, or a bleeding diathesis are at greater risk.
  B. New **superwarfarins** are extremely potent and have prolonged effects even after a single small ingestion (ie, as little as 1 mg in an adult).
  C. Multiple **drug interactions** are known to alter the anticoagulation effect of warfarin (Table II-18).

III. **Clinical presentation.** Excessive anticoagulation may cause ecchymoses, subconjunctival hemorrhage, bleeding gums, or evidence of internal hemorrhage (eg, hematemesis, melena, or hematuria). The most immediately life-threatening complications are massive gastrointestinal bleeding and intracranial hemorrhage.
  A. Because anticoagulant effects are delayed up to 8–12 hours or more, patients with a single ingestion may be asymptomatic shortly after.
  B. Evidence of continuing anticoagulant effect may persist for days, weeks, or even months, especially with superwarfarin products.

IV. **Diagnosis.** Diagnosis is based on the history and evidence of anticoagulant effect. It is important to identify the exact product ingested to ascertain whether a superwarfarin is involved.
  A. **Specific levels.** Blood levels of anticoagulants are not available, nor are they helpful. Anticoagulant effect is best quantified by baseline and repeated measurement of the **prothrombin time,** which will begin to be prolonged 8–12 hours after ingestion, with peak prolongation at 24–48 hours.
  B. **Other useful laboratory studies.** CBC, blood type and cross-match.

V. **Treatment**
  A. **Emergency and supportive measures.** If significant bleeding occurs, be prepared to treat shock with transfusions and fresh-frozen plasma, and obtain immediate neurosurgical consultation if intracranial bleeding is suspected.
    1. Take care not to precipitate hemorrhage in greatly anticoagulated patients; prevent falls and other trauma. If possible, avoid use of nasogastric or endotracheal tubes, arterial punctures, or central intravenous lines.
    2. Avoid drugs that may enhance bleeding or decrease metabolism of the anticoagulant (Table II-18).
  B. **Specific drugs and antidotes.** Vitamin K_1 **(phytonadione),** but *not* vitamin K_3 (menadione), effectively competes with the coumarins to restore production of clotting factors. It should be given if there is evidence of significant anticoagulation. *Note,* however, that if it is given prophylactically after an acute ingestion, the prothrombin time cannot be used to determine severity of the overdose.
    1. Give 5–10 mg of **vitamin K_1** very slowly IV or SC (see p 341). *Caution:* Vitamin K-mediated reversal of anticoagulation may be dangerous

TABLE II–18. EXAMPLES OF DRUG INTERACTIONS WITH COUMARIN.[a]

Increased anticoagulant effect	Decreased anticoagulant effect
Allopurinol	Barbiturates
Chloral hydrate	Carbamazepine
Cimetidine	Cholestyramine
Disulfiram	Glutethimide
Indomethacin and other nonsteroidal	Oral contraceptives
anti-inflammatory agents	Rifampin
Quinidine	
Salicylates	
Sulfonamides	

[a] Adapted and reproduced, with permission, from Olson KR, Becker CE: Poisoning. In: *Current Emergency Diagnosis & Treatment*, 3rd ed. Ho MT, Saunders CE (editors). Appleton & Lange, 1990.

for patients who require constant anticoagulation (eg, for prosthetic heart valves). Very minute doses should be given to titrate for partial effect. **Repeated doses** of vitamin K may be required, especially in patients who have ingested a long-acting superwarfarin product.

2. Because vitamin K will not restore clotting factors for several hours, patients with active hemorrhage may require **fresh-frozen plasma or fresh whole blood.**

C. Decontamination

1. Induce emesis or perform gastric lavage (see p 42) if the patient is not already anticoagulated. In patients who are already anticoagulated, do **not** induce emesis; gentle orogastric lavage may be necessary after significant ingestion despite the risk of inducing hemorrhage.

2. Administer activated charcoal and a cathartic (see p 45).

3. Gut emptying is probably not necessary following small ingestions if activated charcoal is given promptly.

D. Enhanced elimination. There is no role for enhanced elimination procedures.

Reference

Jones EC, Growe GH, Naiman SC: Prolonged anticoagulation in rat poisoning. *JAMA* 1984;252:3005.

CYANIDE
Paul D. Blanc, MD

ANTIDOTE IPECAC LAVAGE CHARCOAL

Cyanide is a highly reactive chemical with a variety of uses, including chemical synthesis, laboratory analysis, and metal plating. Aliphatic nitriles (acrylonitrile, propionitrile) used in plastics manufacturing are metabolized to cyanide. The vasodilator drug nitroprusside releases cyanide on exposure to light. Natural sources of cyanide (amygdalin and many other cyanogenic glycosides) are found in apricot pits, cassava, and many other plants and seeds.

Hydrogen cyanide is a gas easily generated by mixing acid with cyanide salts and is a common combustion by-product of burning plastics, wool, and many other natural and synthetic products. Hydrogen cyanide poisoning is an important cause of death in fires, and deliberate cyanide exposure remains an important instrument of homicide and suicide.

I. Mechanism of toxicity. Cyanide is a chemical asphyxiant; by irreversibly binding to cellular cytochrome oxidase, it blocks the aerobic utilization of oxygen. Unbound cyanide is detoxified by metabolism to thiocyanate, a much less toxic compound that is slowly excreted in the urine.

II. Toxic dose

A. Exposure to hydrogen cyanide **gas** (HCN) at low levels (150–200 ppm) can be rapidly fatal. The OSHA permissible exposure limit (PEL) for HCN is 10 ppm (11 mg/m^3) as an 8-hour time-weighted average.

B. Adult **ingestion** of as little as 200 mg of the sodium or potassium salt may be fatal.

C. Acute cyanide poisoning is relatively rare with nitroprusside **infusion** (at normal infusion rates) or after ingestion of amygdalin-containing seeds (unless they have been pulverized).

III. Clinical presentation.
Abrupt onset of profound toxic effects shortly after exposure is the hallmark of cyanide poisoning. Symptoms include headache, nausea, dyspnea, and confusion. Syncope, seizures, coma, agonal respirations, and cardiovascular collapse ensue rapidly.

A. Brief delay may occur if the cyanide is ingested as a salt, especially if it is in a capsule or if there is food in the stomach.

B. Delayed symptoms may also occur after acrylonitrile exposure because of metabolism to cyanide.

C. Chronic neurologic sequelae may follow severe cyanide poisoning.

IV. Diagnosis.
Diagnosis is based on a history of exposure or the presence of rapidly progressive symptoms and signs. Lactic acidosis is often present. The **measured venous oxygen saturation** may be elevated owing to blocked cellular oxygen consumption. The classic bitter almond aroma of hydrogen cyanide may or may not be noted, because of genetic variability in the ability to appreciate the smell.

A. **Specific levels.** Cyanide determinations are rarely of use in emergency management, because they cannot be performed rapidly enough to alter initial treatment. They must be interpreted with caution because of a variety of complicating technical factors.
   1. Levels higher than 0.5–1 mg/L are considered toxic.
   2. Smokers may have levels up to 0.1 mg/L.
   3. Rapid nitroprusside infusion may produce levels as high as 1 mg/L.

B. **Other useful laboratory studies.** CBC, electrolytes, glucose, arterial blood gas, carboxyhemoglobin (if smoke inhalation exposure), ECG.

V. Treatment

A. **Emergency and supportive measures.** Treat all cyanide exposures as potentially lethal.
   1. Maintain the airway and assist ventilation if necessary (see p 2). Administer supplemental oxygen
   2. Treat coma (p 17), hypotension (p 14), and seizures (p 21) if they occur.
   3. Start an intravenous line and monitor the patient's vital signs and ECG closely.

B. **Specific drugs and antidotes**
   1. The **Lilly cyanide antidote kit** consists of amyl and sodium nitrites (see p 328), which produce cyanide-scavenging methemoglobinemia, and sodium thiosulfate (see p 340), which accelerates the conversion of cyanide to thiocyanate.
      a. Break a pearl of **amyl nitrite** under the nose of the victim; and administer **sodium nitrite,** 300 mg IV (6 mg/kg for children). *Caution:* Nitrite-induced methemoglobinemia can be extremely dangerous and even lethal. Nitrite should *not* be given if the symptoms are mild or if the diagnosis is uncertain.
      b. Administer **sodium thiosulfate,** 12.5 g IV. Thiosulfate is relatively benign and may be given empirically if the diagnosis is uncertain.
   2. The most promising alternative antidote is **hydroxocobalamin** (see p 316). It is currently undergoing investigational trials in the USA.

3. Hyperbaric oxygen has no established role in cyanide poisoning treatment.

C. Decontamination

1. **Inhalation.** Remove victim from hydrogen cyanide exposure and give supplemental oxygen, if available. Rescuers should wear protective self-contained breathing apparatus.

2. **Skin.** Remove all contaminated clothing and wash affected areas with copious soap and water.

3. **Ingestion**

   a. Immediately place a gastric tube and administer activated charcoal, then perform gastric lavage (see p 43). Do **not** induce emesis unless victim is more than 20 minutes from a medical facililty.

   b. Administer additional activated charcoal and a cathartic (see p 45) after the lavage. Even though charcoal has a relatively low affinity for cyanide, it is effective for the doses of cyanide (100–300 mg) often ingested.

D. Enhanced elimination. There is no role for hemodialysis or hemoperfusion in cyanide poisoning treatment. Hemodialysis may be indicated in patients with renal insufficiency who develop high thiocyanate levels while on extended nitroprusside therapy.

Reference

Hall AH, Rumack BH: Clinical toxicology of cyanide. *Ann Emerg Med* 1986;**15:**1067.

CYCLIC ANTIDEPRESSANTS
Neal L. Benowitz, MD

ANTIDOTE   IPECAC   LAVAGE   CHARCOAL

Cyclic antidepressants, also called tricyclic antidepressants, are commonly taken in overdose by suicidal patients and represent a major cause of poisoning hospitalizations and deaths. Currently available cyclic antidepressants are described in Table II–19. Amitriptyline is also marketed in combination with chlordiazepoxide (Limbitrol) or perphenazine (Etrafon, Triavil).

Trazodone and **fluoxetine** (newer antidepressants) and **cyclobenzaprine** (a centrally acting muscle relaxant) are structurally related to the cyclic antidepressants but exhibit minimal cardiotoxic and variable CNS effects. Monoamine oxidase inhibitors are discussed on page 208.

I. Mechanism of toxicity. Cyclic antidepressant toxicity affects primarily the cardiovascular and central nervous systems.

A. Several mechanisms contribute to **cardiovascular toxicity.**

1. Anticholinergic effects and inhibition of neuronal reuptake of catecholamines result in tachycardia and mild hypertension.

2. Peripheral alpha-adrenergic blockade induces vasodilation.

3. Membrane-depressant (quinidinelike) effects cause myocardial depression and cardiac conduction disturbances by inhibition of the fast sodium channel that initiates the cardiac cell action potential. Metabolic acidosis may contribute to cardiotoxicity by further depressing the fast sodium channel.

B. Central nervous system effects are due in part to anticholinergic toxicity (eg, sedation and coma), but seizures are probably a result of inhibition of reuptake of norepinephrine or serotonin in the central nervous system or other central effects.

C. Relevant pharmacokinetics

1. Anticholinergic effects of the drugs may retard gastric emptying, resulting in slow or erratic absorption.
2. Cyclic antidepressants are primarily metabolized by the liver, with only a small fraction excreted unchanged in the urine. Active metabolites may contribute to toxicity; several drugs are metabolized to other well-known cyclic antidepressants (eg, amitriptyline to nortriptyline, imipramine to desipramine).
3. Most of these drugs are extensively bound to body tissues and plasma proteins, resulting in very large volumes of distribution and long elimination half-lives (Table II–19).

II. Toxic dose.
Most of the cyclic antidepressants have a narrow therapeutic index so that doses of less than 10 times the therapeutic daily dose may produce severe intoxication. In general, ingestion of 10–20 mg/kg is potentially life-threatening.

III. Clinical presentation.
Cyclic antidepressant poisoning may produce 3 major toxic syndromes: anticholinergic, cardiovascular, and seizures. Depending on the dose and the drug, patients may experience some or all of these toxic effects. Symptoms usually begin within 30–40 minutes of ingestion but may be delayed owing to erratic gut absorption. Patients who are initially awake may abruptly lose consciousness or develop seizures without warning.

A. Anticholinergic effects include sedation, delirium, coma, dilated pupils, dry skin and mucous membranes, diminished sweating, tachycardia, diminished or absent bowel sounds, and urinary retention. Myoclonic or myokymic jerking is common with anticholinergic intoxication and may be mistaken for seizure activity.

TABLE II-19. CYCLIC AND RELATED ANTIDEPRESSANTS

Drug	Type[a]	Usual Adult Daily Dose (mg)	Usual Half-Life (h)	Toxicity[b]
Amitriptyline	Tri	75–200	19	A, C, S
Amoxapine	DiB	150–300	8	S
Cyclobenzaprine	Tri	20–40	24	A
Desipramine	Tri	75–200	22	A, C, S
Doxepin	Tri	75–300	17	A, C, S
Fluoxetine	Oth	30–60	70	S
Imipramine	Tri	75–200	18	A, C, S
Maprotiline	Tet	75–300	40	C, S
Nortriptyline	Tri	75–150	28	A, C, S
Protriptyline	Tri	20–40	78	A, C, S
Trazodone	Oth	50–600	8	Minimal
Trimipramine	Tri	75–200	23	A, C, S

[a]Tri = tricyclic; Tet = tetracyclic; DiB = dibenzoxazepine; Oth = structurally unrelated to other cyclic antidepressants; toxicity generally mild.
[b]A = anticholinergic; C = cardiovascular; S = seizures.

B. Cardiovascular toxicity manifests as abnormal cardiac conduction, arrhythmias, and hypotension.

1. Typical electrocardiographic findings include sinus tachycardia with prolongation of the PR, QRS, and QT intervals. Varying degrees of atrioventricular block may be seen. Prolongation of the QRS complex to 0.12 s or longer is a fairly reliable predictor of serious cardiovascular and neurologic toxicity (except in the case of amoxapine, which causes seizures and coma with no change in the QRS interval).

2. Sinus tachycardia accompanied by QRS interval prolongation may resemble ventricular tachycardia (see Fig I-4). True ventricular tachycardia and fibrillation may also occur. Atypical or polymorphous ventricular tachycardia (torsades de pointes; see Fig I-5) associated with QT interval prolongation may oocur. Development of bradyarrhythmias usually indicates a severely poisoned heart and carries a poor prognosis.

3. Hypotension due to venodilation is common and usually mild. In severe cases, hypotension is due to myocardial depression and may be refractory to treatment; some patients die with progressive intractable cardiogenic shock. Pulmonary edema is also common in severe intoxication.

C. Seizures are common with cyclic antidepressant toxicity and may be recurrent or persistent. The muscular hyperactivity from seizures and myoclonic jerking, combined with diminished sweating, can lead to severe hyperthermia (see p 19), resulting in rhabdomyolysis, brain damage, multisystem failure, and death.

D. Death due to cyclic antidepressant overdose usually occurs within a few hours of admission and may be due to ventricular fibrillation, intractable cardiogenic shock, or status epilepticus with hyperthermia. Sudden death several days after apparent recovery has occasionally been reported, but in all such cases there was evidence of continuing cardiac toxicity within 24 hours of death.

IV. Diagnosis. Cyclic antidepressant poisoning should be suspected in any patient with lethargy, coma, or seizures accompanied by QRS interval prolongation. QRS interval prolongation greater than 0.12 s in the limb leads suggests severe poisoning. However, with some newer drugs such as amoxapine and fluoxetine, seizures and coma may occur with no widening of the QRS interval.

A. Specific levels. Plasma levels of some of the cyclic antidepressants can be measured by clinical laboratories. Therapeutic concentrations are usually less than 0.3 mcg/mL (300 ng/mL). Total concentrations of parent drug plus metabolite of 1 mcg/mL (1000 ng/mL) or greater are usually associated with serious poisoning. Generally, plasma levels are not used in emergency management because the QRS interval and clinical manifestations of overdose are reliable and more readily available indicators of toxicity.

Newer antidepressants (such as amoxapine, maprotiline, trazodone, and fluoxetine) may not appear on routine toxicology screening of urine and gastric aspirates.

B. Other useful laboratory studies. CBC, electrolytes, glucose, BUN, creatinine, creatine phosphokinase (CPK), urinalysis for myoglobin, arterial blood gases, 12-lead ECG and continuous electrocardiographic monitoring, chest x-ray.

V. Treatment

A. Emergency and supportive measures

1. Maintain the airway and assist ventilation if necessary (see p 2). *Caution:* Respiratory arrest can occur abruptly and without warning.

2. Treat coma (p 17), seizures (p 21), hyperthermia (p 19), hypotension (p 14), and arrhythmias (pp 9–13) if they occur.

3. If seizures are not immediately controlled with usual anticonvulsants, paralyze the patient with pancuronium (p 326) to prevent hyperthermia, which may induce further seizures, and lactic acidosis, which aggravates cardiotoxicity.

4. Continuously monitor the temperature, other vital signs, and ECG in asymptomatic patients for a minimum of 6 hours, and admit patients to an intensive care setting for at least 24 hours if there are any signs of toxicity.

B. Specific drugs and antidotes

1. In patients with QRS interval prolongation or hypotension, administer **sodium bicarbonate** (see p 296), 1–2 meq/kg IV, and repeat as needed to maintain the arterial pH between 7.45–7.55. Sodium bicarbonate may reverse membrane-depressant effects by increasing extracelluar sodium concentrations and by a direct effect of pH on the fast sodium channel.

2. Although **physostigmine** has been widely advocated in the past, it should **not** be routinely administered to patients with cyclic antidepressant poisoning; it may aggravate conduction disturbances, causing asystole, and may contribute to seizures.

C. Decontamination

1. Perform gastric lavage (see p 43). Do **not** induce emesis because of the risk of abrupt onset of seizures or coma.

2. Administer activated charcoal and cathartic (see p 45).

D. Enhanced elimination. Owing to extensive tissue and protein binding with resulting large volume of distribution, dialysis and hemoperfusion are not effective. Although repeat-dose charcoal has been reported to accelerate cyclic antidepressant elimination, the data are not convincing.

Reference

Pentel PR, Benowitz NL: Tricyclic antidepressant poisoning: Management of arrhythmias. *Med Toxicol* 1986;1:101.

DETERGENTS
Olga F. Woo, PharmD

| ANTIDOTE | IPECAC | LAVAGE | CHARCOAL |

Detergents, familiar and indispensable products in the home, are synthetic surface-active agents chemically classified as **anionic, nonionic,** or **cationic** (Table II–20). Most products also contain bleaching (chlorine-releasing), bacteriostatic (low concentration of quaternary ammonium compound), or enzymatic agents. Accidental ingestion of detergents by children is very common, but severe toxicity rarely occurs.

I. Mechanism of toxicity. Detergents may precipitate and denature protein, are irritating to tissues, and possess keratolytic and corrosive actions.

A. Anionic and **nonionic** detergents are only mildly irritating, but **cationic** detergents are more hazardous because quaternary ammonium compounds may be caustic (benzalkonium chloride solutions of 10% have been reported to cause corrosive burns).

B. Low-phosphate detergents and **electric dishwasher** soaps often contain alkaline corrosive agents such as sodium metasilicate, sodium carbonate, and sodium tripolyphosphate.

C. The **enzyme-containing** detergents may cause skin irritation and have

TABLE II–20. COMMON CATIONIC DETERGENTS

Pyridinium compounds	Quaternary ammonium compounds	Quinolinium compounds
Cetalkonium chloride	Benzalkonium chloride	Dequalinium chloride
Cetrimide	Benzethonium chloride	
Cetrimonium bromide		
Cetylpyridinium chloride		
Stearalkonium chloride		

sensitizing properties; they may release bradykinin and histamine, causing bronchospasm.

II. **Toxic dose.** No minimum or lethal toxic doses have been established. Mortality and serious morbidity are rare. Cationic and dishwasher detergents are more dangerous than anionic and nonionic products.

III. **Clinical presentation.** Immediate spontaneous emesis often occurs after oral ingestion. Large ingestions may produce intractable vomiting, diarrhea, and hematemesis. Exposures to the eye may cause mild to serious corrosive injury depending on the specific product. Dermal contact generally causes a mild erythema or rash.

    A. Phosphate-containing products may produce hypocalcemia and tetany.

    B. Methemoglobinemia was reported in a 45-year-old woman after copious irrigation of a hydatid cyst with a 0.1% solution of cetrimide, a cationic detergent.

IV. **Diagnosis.** Diagnosis is based on a history of exposure and prompt onset of vomiting. A sudsy or foaming mouth may also suggest exposure.

    A. **Specific levels.** There are no specific blood or urine levels.

    B. **Other useful laboratory studies.** CBC, electrolytes, glucose, calcium and phosphate (after ingestion of phosphate-containing products), methemoglobin (cationic detergents).

V. **Treatment**

    A. **Emergency and supportive measures**

        1. In patients with protracted vomiting or diarrhea, administer intravenous fluids to correct dehydration and electrolyte imbalance (see p 14).

        2. If corrosive injury is suspected, consult a gastroenterologist for possible endoscopy.

    B. **Specific drugs and antidotes.** If symptomatic hypocalcemia occurs after ingestion of a phosphate-containing product, administer intravenous **calcium** (see p 298). If methemoglobinemia occurs, administer **methylene blue** (see p 322).

    C. **Decontamination**

        1. **Ingestion.** Dilute orally with small amounts of water or milk. A significant ingestion is unlikely if spontaneous emesis has not already occurred.

            a. Do **not** induce emesis because of the risk for corrosive injury.

            b. Perform gastric lavage after large ingestions of cationic, corrosive, or phosphate-containing detergents.

            c. Activated charcoal is not effective.

        2. **Eyes and skin.** Irrigate with copious amounts of tepid water or saline. Consult an ophthalmologist if eye pain persists or if there is significant corneal injury on fluorescein examination.

    D. **Enhanced elimination.** There is no role for these procedures.

Reference

Lawrence RA, Haggerty RJ: Household agents and their potential toxicity. *Mod Treat* 1971;8:511.

DEXTROMETHORPHAN
Kent R. Olson, MD

| ANTIDOTE | IPECAC | LAVAGE | CHARCOAL |

Dextromethorphan is a common antitussive agent found in many over-the-counter cough and cold preparations. Many ingestions occur in children, but severe intoxication is rare. Dextromethorphan is often found in combination products containing antihistamines (see p 73), decongestants (p 238), ethanol (p 148), or acetaminophen (p 57).

I. **Mechanism of toxicity.** Dextromethorphan is the *d*-isomer of the opioid analgesic levorphanol. Although it has approximately equal antitussive efficacy as codeine, dextromethorphan has no apparent analgesic or addictive properties and produces relatively mild opioid effects in overdose. It also is reported to have anticholinergic properties.

   Dextromethorphan is well absorbed orally, and effects are apparent within 15–30 minutes. The duration of effects is normally 3–6 hours.

II. **Toxic dose.** The toxic dose is highly variable and depends largely on other ingredients in the ingested product. Symptoms usually occur when the amount of dextromethorphan ingested exceeds 10 mg/kg. The usual recommended adult daily dose of dextromethorphan is 60–120 mg/d; in children age 2–5 years, up to 30 mg/d.

III. **Clinical presentation**
   A. **Mild intoxication** produces clumsiness, ataxia, nystagmus, and restlessness. Visual and auditory hallucinations have been reported.
   B. With **severe poisoning,** stupor, coma, and respiratory depression may occur, especially if alcohol has been coingested. The pupils may be constricted or dilated. A few cases of seizures have been reported after ingestions of more than 20–30 mg/kg.
   C. Severe hyperthermia and hypertension may occur with **therapeutic doses** in patients taking **monoamine oxidase inhibitors** (see p 208). The mechanism is not known.

IV. **Diagnosis.** Diagnosis should be considered with ingestion of any over-the-counter cough suppressant, especially when there is nystagmus, ataxia, and lethargy. Because dextromethorphan is often combined with other ingredients, suspect mixed ingestion.
   A. **Specific levels.** Serum levels are not generally available, nor are they clinically useful. Serum levels of dextromethorphan and its metabolites are in the range of 200–400 ng/mL 2–4 hours after a therapeutic dose. Blood ethanol and acetaminophen levels should be obtained if those drugs are contained in the ingested product.
   B. **Other useful laboratory studies.** CBC, electrolytes, glucose, ethanol, acetaminophen, arterial blood gases (if respiratory depression suspected).

V. **Treatment**
   A. **Emergency and supportive measures.** Most patients with mild symptoms (ie, restlessness, ataxia, mild drowsiness) can be observed for 4–6 hours and discharged if they are improving.
      1. Maintain the airway and assist ventilation if needed (see p 2).
      2. Treat seizures (p 21) and coma (p 17) if they occur.
   B. **Specific drugs and antidotes.** Although **naloxone** (see p 325) has been reported effective in doses of 0.06–0.4 mg, other cases have failed to respond to as much as 2.4 mg. If the patient exhibits signs of opioid intoxication (eg, coma, pinpoint pupils), administer 0.4–2 mg naloxone IV, with repeat doses as needed.
   C. **Decontamination**

1. Induce emesis or perform gastric lavage (see p 42).
2. Administer activated charcoal and cathartic (see p 45).
3. Gut emptying is probably not necessary following small ingestions if activated charcoal is given promptly.

D. Enhanced elimination. The volume of distribution of dextromethorphan is very large, and there is no role for enhanced removal procedures.

Reference

Katona B, Wason S: Dextromethorphan danger. (Letter.) *N Engl J Med* 1986;**314**:993.

DIOXINS
Bruce Bernard, MD, and
Kent R. Olson, MD

ANTIDOTE   IPECAC   LAVAGE   CHARCOAL

Polychlorinated dibenzodioxins (PCDDs) and dibenzofurans (PCDFs) are a group of highly toxic substances commonly known as dioxins. PCDDs are formed during the production of certain organochlorines (trichlorophenoxy-acetic acid [2,4,5-T], silvex, hexachlorophene, pentachlorophenol, etc), and PCDFs are formed by the combustion of these and other compounds such as polychlorinated biphenyls (PCBs; see p 252). Agent Orange, a herbicide used in Vietnam, contained small quantities of a dioxin (2,3,7,8-tetrachlorodibenzo-*p*-dioxin, TCDD) as a contaminant.

I. **Mechanism of toxicity.** Dioxins are highly lipid-soluble and are concentrated in the fat and the thymus. Dioxins are known to induce porphyrinogen synthesis and oxidative cytochrome P-450 metabolism and have a variety of effects on various organ systems. The actual mechanism of toxicity is unknown. They are mutagenic and are suspected human carcinogens.

II. **Toxic dose.** Dioxins are extremely potent animal toxins. The FDA-suggested "no effect" level for inhalation is 70 ng/d per person. The oral 50% lethal dose (LD$_{50}$) in animals varies from 0.0006 to 0.045 mg/kg. Daily dermal exposure to 10–30 ppm in oil or 100–3000 ppm in soil produces toxicity in animals. Chloracne is likely with daily dermal exposure exceeding 100 ppm.

III. **Clinical presentation**
   A. **Acute symptoms** after exposure include irritation of the skin, eyes, and mucous membranes and nausea, vomiting, and myalgias.
   B. **After a latency period** of up to several weeks, chloracne, porphyria cutanea tarda, hirsutism, or hyperpigmentation may occur. Elevated levels of hepatic transaminases and blood lipids may be found. Polyneuropathies with sensory impairment and lower extremity motor weakness have been reported.
   C. **Death** in laboratory animals occurs a few weeks after a lethal dose and is due to a "wasting syndrome" characterized by reduced food intake and loss of body weight.

IV. **Diagnosis.** Diagnosis is difficult and rests mainly on history of exposure. Although 2,4,5-T no longer contains TCDD as a contaminant, possible exposures to PCDDs and PCDFs occur during many types of chemical fires (eg, PCBs), and the possibility of exposure results in considerable public and individual anxiety.
   A. **Specific levels.** It is difficult and expensive to detect dioxins in human blood or tissue, and there is no established correlation with symptoms.
   B. **Other useful laboratory studies.** CBC, glucose, electrolytes, BUN, creatinine, liver transaminases and liver function tests.

V. Treatment
A. Emergency and supportive measures. Treat skin, eye, and respiratory irritation symptomatically.

B. Specific drugs and antidotes. There is no specific antidote.

C. Decontamination
1. **Inhalation.** Remove victim from exposure and give supplemental oxygen, if available.
2. **Eyes and skin.** Remove contaminated clothing and wash affected skin with copious soap and water; irrigate exposed eyes with copious tepid water or saline. Personnel involved in decontamination should wear gowns and gloves.
3. **Ingestion**
   a. Induce emesis or perform gastric lavage (see p 42).
   b. Administer activated charcoal and cathartic (see p 45).

D. Enhanced elimination. There is no known role for these procedures.

Reference

Weber LW, Greim H, Rozman KK: Metabolism and distribution of [14C]glucose in rats treated with 2,3,7,8-tetrachlorodibenzo-*p*-dioxin (TCDD). *J Toxicol Environ Health* 1987;**22**:195.

DISULFIRAM
Bruce Bernard, MD

ANTIDOTE   IPECAC   LAVAGE   CHARCOAL

Disulfiram (Antabuse) is an antioxidant drug used in the treatment of alcoholism. When a person taking disulfiram ingests alcohol, a well-defined unpleasant reaction occurs, the fear of which provides a negative incentive to drink.

I. Mechanism of toxicity.
Disulfiram is usually taken orally and is well absorbed and highly fat-soluble. Its mechanisms of toxicity include:
A. Irreversible inhibition of aldehyde dehydrogenase, resulting in accumulation of acetaldehyde after ethanol ingestion.
B. Depletion of norepinephrine in terminal presynaptic nerve endings, causing orthostatic hypotension.
C. Long-term use of disulfiram may cause peripheral neuropathy, thought to be mediated by its metabolite carbon disulfide.

II. Toxic dose
A. Disulfiram overdose. Ingestion of 3 g or more may cause toxicity.
B. Disulfiram-ethanol interaction. Ingestion of as little as 7 mL of ethanol can cause a severe reaction in patients taking as little as 200 mg/d of disulfiram. Reactions have been reported after use of cough syrup, after-shave lotions, and other alcohol-containing products.

III. Clinical presentation
A. Acute disulfiram overdose may cause vomiting, ataxia, confusion, lethargy, seizures, and coma. Peripheral neuropathy has been reported. Hypersensitivity hepatitis has occurred, including several deaths resulting from hepatic failure.
B. Disulfiram-ethanol interaction. Shortly after ingestion of ethanol, the patient receiving chronic disulfiram therapy develops flushing, throbbing headache, dyspnea, anxiety, vertigo, vomiting, and confusion. Orthostatic hypotension with warm extremities is very common. The severity of the reaction usually depends on the dose of disulfiram and ethanol. Reactions do not usually occur unless the patient has been on disulfiram therapy for at least 1 day; the reaction may occur up to several days after the last dose of disulfiram.

IV. Diagnosis. Diagnosis of disulfiram overdose is based on a history of acute ingestion and the presence of central nervous system symptoms. The disulfiram-ethanol interaction is diagnosed in a patient with a history of chronic disulfiram use and possible exposure to ethanol who exhibits a characteristic hypotensive flushing reaction.

  A. Specific levels. Blood disulfiram levels are not of value in diagnosis or treatment. Blood acetaldehyde levels may be elevated during the disulfiram-ethanol reaction, but this information is of little value in acute management.

  B. Other useful laboratory studies. CBC, electrolytes, glucose, BUN, creatinine, liver function tests, ECG.

V. Treatment

  A. Emergency and supportive measures

   1. Acute disulfiram overdose

     a. Maintain the airway and assist ventilation if necessary (see p 2).

     b. Treat coma (p 17) and seizures (p 21) if they occur.

   2. Disulfiram-ethanol interaction

     a. Maintain the airway and assist ventilation if necessary (see p 2).

     b. Treat orthostatic hypotension with supine position and large quantities of intravenous fluids (eg, saline). If a pressor agent is needed, norepinephrine (see p 330) is preferred over dopamine.

  B. Specific drugs and antidotes. There is no specific antidote.

  C. Decontamination

   1. Disulfiram overdose

     a. Induce emesis or perform gastric lavage (see p 42).

     b. Administer activated charcoal and cathartic (see p 45).

     c. Gut emptying is probably not necessary following small ingestions if activated charcoal is given promptly.

   2. Disulfiram-ethanol interaction. Decontamination procedures are not likely to be of benefit once the reaction begins (unless a very large ethanol ingestion has occurred, in which case gastric lavage should be performed, followed by administration of activated charcoal).

  D. Enhanced elimination. Hemodialysis is not indicated for disulfiram overdose, but it may remove ethanol and acetaldehyde and has been reported to be effective in treating the acute disulfiram-ethanol interaction. This is not likely to be necessary in patients receiving adequate fluid and pressor support. There are no data to support the use of repeat-dose activated charcoal for any of the disulfiram syndromes.

Reference

Motte S et al: Refractory hyperdynamic shock associated with alcohol and disulfiram. *Am J Emerg Med* 1986;4:323.

DIURETICS
Olga F. Woo, PharmD

ANTIDOTE IPECAC LAVAGE CHARCOAL

Diuretics are the most commonly prescribed drugs for the management of essential hypertension. Adverse effects from chronic use or misuse are more frequently encountered than those from acute overdose. Overdoses are generally benign, and no serious outcomes have resulted from acute ingestion. Historically, the organic mercurials were the first diuretics used clinically, but systemic mercury poisoning was a toxic consequence and safer diuretics have since replaced them. Common currently available diuretics are listed in Table II–21.

I. **Mechanism of toxicity.** The toxicity of these drugs is associated with their pharmacologic effects to decrease fluid volume and promote electrolyte loss: dehydration, hypokalemia or hyperkalemia, and hypochloremic alkalosis. Electrolyte imbalance may lead to cardiac arrhythmias and may enhance digitalis toxicity (see p 112). Diuretics are classified according to the pharmacologic mechanisms by which they affect solute and water loss (Table II–21).

TABLE II-21. COMMON DIURETICS

Drug	Maximum Adult Daily Dose (mg)
Carbonic anhydrase inhibitors	
Acetazolamide	1000
Dichlorphenamide	200
Methazolamide	300
Loop diuretics	
Bumetanide	2
Ethacrynic acid	200
Furosemide	600
Mercurial	
Mersalyl	200
Potassium-sparing	
Amiloride	20
Spironolactone	200
Triamterene	300
Thiazides	
Bendroflumethiazide	20
Benzthiadiazide	200
Chlorthalidone	200
Chlorothiazide	2000
Cyclothiazide	6
Flumethiazide	2000
Hydrochlorothiazide	200
Hydroflumethiazide	200
Indapamide	5
Methyclothiazide	10
Metolazone	20
Polythiazide	4
Quinethazone	200
Trichlormethiazide	4

II. Toxic dose. Minimum toxic doses have not been established. Significant dehydration or electrolyte imbalance is unlikely if the amount ingested is less than the usual recommended daily dose (Table II–21). High doses of intravenous ethacrynic acid and furosemide can cause ototoxicity, especially when administered rapidly and in patients with renal failure.

III. Clinical presentation. Symptoms of lethargy, weakness, hyporeflexia, and dehydration may be present. Orthostatic hypotension suggests significant volume loss. The onset of symptoms may be delayed for 2–4 hours until diuretic action is obtained. Spironolactone is very slow, with maximal effects after the third day. Spironolactone and other potassium-sparing agents may cause hyperkalemia. Hyperglycemia and hyperuricemia may occur, especially with thiazide diuretics. Carbonic anhydrase inhibitors may induce metabolic acidosis.

IV. Diagnosis. Diagnosis is based on a history of exposure and evidence of dehydration and acid-base or electrolyte imbalance.

  A. Specific levels are not routinely available nor clinically useful.

  B. Other useful laboratory studies. CBC, electrolytes, glucose, BUN, creatinine, ECG.

V. Treatment

  A. Emergency and supportive measures

    1. Replace fluid loss with intravenous crystalloid solutions (see p 14), and correct electrolyte abnormalities (see Potassium, p 32).

    2. Monitor the ECG until the potassium level is normalized.

  B. Specific drugs and antidotes. There are no specific antidotes.

  C. Decontamination

    1. Induce emesis or perform gastric lavage (see p 42).

    2. Administer activated charcoal and cathartic (see p 45). Do not use cathartics if the patient is dehydrated.

    3. Gut emptying is not necessary following small ingestions if activated charcoal is given promptly.

  D. Enhanced elimination. No experience with extracorporeal removal of diuretics has been reported.

Reference

Moser M: Diuretics in the management of hypertension. *Med Clin North Am* 1987;**71**:935.

ERGOT DERIVATIVES
Neal L. Benowitz, MD

ANTIDOTE   IPECAC   LAVAGE   CHARCOAL

Ergot derivatives are used primarily to treat migraine headache and to a lesser extent to enhance uterine contraction postpartum. Ergots are produced by the fungus *Claviceps purpurea,* which may grow on rye and other grains. Specific ergot-containing drugs include ergotamine (Cafergot, Ergomar, Gynergen, Ergostat), methysergide (Sansert), dihydroergotamine (DHE-45), and ergonovine (Ergotrate). Some ergoloid derivatives (dihydroergocornine, dihydroergocristine, and dihydroergocryptine) have been used in combination (Hydergine, Deapril-ST) for the treatment of dementia.

  I. Mechanism of toxicity. Ergot derivatives directly stimulate vasoconstriction and uterine contraction, antagonize alpha-adrenergic and serotonin receptors, and may also dilate some blood vessels via a central nervous system sympatholytic action. The relative contribution of each of these mechanisms to toxicity depends on the particular ergot alkaloid and its dose.

Sustained **vasoconstriction** causes most of the serious toxicity; reduced blood flow causes local tissue hypoxia and ischemic injury, resulting in tissue edema and local thrombosis, worsening ischemia and causing further injury. At a certain point, reversible vasospasm progresses to irreversible vascular insufficiency and limb gangrene.

II. **Toxic dose.** Death has been reported in a 14-month-old child after acute ingestion of 12 mg of ergotamine. However, most cases of severe poisoning occur with chronic overmedication for migraine headaches rather than acute single overdose. Daily doses of 10 mg or more of ergotamine are usually associated with toxicity. There are many case reports of vasospastic complications with normal therapeutic dosing.

III. **Clinical presentation.** Mild intoxication causes nausea and vomiting. Serious poisoning results in vasoconstriction that may involve many parts of the body. Owing to persistence of ergots in tissues, vasospasm may continue for up to 10–14 days.

    A. Involvement of the **extremities** causes paresthesias, pain, pallor, coolness, and loss of peripheral pulses in the hands and feet; gangrene may ensue.

    B. **Other complications of vasospasm** include coronary ischemia and myocardial infarction, abdominal angina and bowel infarction, renal infarction and failure, visual disturbances and blindness, and stroke. Psychosis, seizures, and coma occur rarely.

    C. Chronic use of **methysergide** occasionally causes retroperitoneal fibrosis.

IV. **Diagnosis.** Diagnosis is based on a history of ergot use and clinical findings of vasospasm.

    A. **Specific levels.** Ergotamine levels are not widely available, and blood concentrations do not correlate well with toxicity, although ergotamine levels higher than 1.8 ng/mL have been associated with minor toxicity.

    B. **Other useful laboratory studies.** CBC, BUN, creatinine, ECG. Arteriography of the affected vascular bed is occasionally indicated.

V. **Treatment**

    A. **Emergency and supportive measures**

        1. Maintain the airway and assist ventilation if necessary (see p 2).

        2. Treat coma (p 17) and convulsions (p 21) if they occur.

        3. Immediately discontinue ergot treatment. Hospitalize patients with vasospastic symptoms and treat promptly to prevent complications.

    B. **Specific drugs and antidotes**

        1. **Peripheral ischemia** requires prompt vasodilator therapy and anticoagulation (to prevent local thrombosis).

          a. Administer **intravenous nitroprusside** (see p 330), starting with 1–2 mcg/kg/min, or **intravenous phentolamine** (p 335), starting with 0.5 mg/min, increasing the infusion rate until ischemia is improved or systemic hypotension occurs. Intra-arterial infusion is occasionally required. **Nifedipine** (p 328) may also enhance peripheral blood flow.

          b. Administer **heparin,** 5000 units IV followed by 1000 units/h (in adults), with adjustments in the infusion rate to maintain the activated coagulation time (ACT) or the activated partial thromboplastin time (APTT) approximately 2 times baseline.

        2. **Coronary spasm.** Adult doses only: Administer **nitroglycerin,** 0.15–0.6 mg sublingually or 5–20 mcg/min IV; or **nifedipine** (see p 328), 10–20 mg orally. Intracoronary artery nitroglycerin may be required if there is no response to intravenous infusion.

    C. **Decontamination**

        1. Induce emesis or perform gastric lavage (see p 42).

        2. Administer activated charcoal and cathartic (see p 45).

        3. Gut emptying is probably not necessary following small ingestions if activated charcoal is given promptly.

D. Enhanced elimination. Dialysis and hemoperfusion are not effective. Repeat-dose charcoal has not been studied, but because of extensive tissue distribution of ergots it is not likely to be useful.

Reference

Graham AN et al: Ergotamine toxicity and serum concentrations of ergotamine in migraine patients. *Hum Toxicol* 1984;3:193.

ETHANOL
Chris Dutra, MD

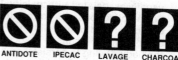

ANTIDOTE   IPECAC   LAVAGE   CHARCOAL

Ethanol is found in a variety of commercial liquors, colognes, perfumes, after-shaves, mouthwashes, some rubbing alcohols, many food flavorings (eg, vanilla, almond, and lemon extracts), pharmaceutical preparations (eg, elixirs), and many other products. Ethanol is frequently ingested recreationally and is also a common coingestant with other drugs in suicide attempts.

I. **Mechanism of toxicity**
   A. **Central nervous system depression** is the principal effect of acute ethanol intoxication. Ethanol has additive effects with other central nervous system depressants such as barbiturates, benzodiazepines, antidepressants, and antipsychotics.
   B. **Hypoglycemia** may be due to impaired gluconeogenesis in patients with depleted glycogen stores (particularly small children and poorly nourished persons).
   C. Ethanol intoxication also predisposes patients to trauma, exposure-induced hypothermia, and a number of metabolic derangements that may easily be overlooked in the "drunk" patient.

II. **Toxic dose.** The volume of distribution of ethanol is 0.7 L/kg, or about 50 liters in the average adult. Generally, 0.7 g/kg pure ethanol (approximately 3–4 drinks) will produce a blood ethanol concentration of 100 mg/dL (0.1 g/dL), considered legally drunk in most communities.
   A. A level of 100 mg/dL is enough to inhibit gluconeogensis and cause hypoglycemia but by itself is not enough to cause coma.
   B. The level sufficient to cause deep coma or respiratory depression is highly variable, depending on the individual's degree of tolerance to ethanol: Although levels above 300 mg/dL usually cause coma in novice drinkers, chronic alcoholics may be awake with levels in the 500–600 mg/dL range.

III. **Clinical presentation**
   A. **Acute intoxication**
      1. With **mild to moderate intoxication,** patients exhibit euphoria, mild incoordination, ataxia, nystagmus, and impaired judgment and reflexes. Social inhibitions are decreased, and boisterous or aggressive behavior is common. Hypoglycemia may occur.
      2. With **deep intoxication,** coma, respiratory depression, and pulmonary aspiration may occur. In these patients, the pupils are usually small and the temperature, blood pressure, and pulse rate are often decreased. Rhabdomyolysis may result from prolonged immobilization.
   B. **Chronic ethanol abuse** produces gastrointestinal bleeding from gastritis, ulcers, Mallory-Weiss tears, or esophageal varices; pancreatitis; hepatitis, cirrhosis and hepatic encephalopathy; hypokalemia, hypophosphatemia, and hypomagnesemia; thiamine deficiency (Wernicke's encephalopathy); alcoholic ketoacidosis; and decreased resistance to infections.
   C. **Alcohol withdrawal** from chronic high-level use usually causes tremu-

lousness, anxiety, sympathetic nervous system overactivity, and convulsions. Occasionally, this may progress to **delirium tremens,** a life-threatening syndrome of severe autonomic hyperactivity, hyperthermia, and delirium, which has significant morbidity and mortality if untreated.

D. Other problems. Ethanol abusers sometimes intentionally or accidentally ingest ethanol substitutes such as isopropyl alcohol (see p 181), methanol (p 202), or ethylene glycol (p 151). In addition, ethanol may serve as the vehicle for swallowing large numbers of pills in a suicide attempt. Disulfiram (Antabuse, p 143) may cause acute reactions.

IV. Diagnosis. The diagnosis of ethanol intoxication is usually simple, based on the history of ingestion, the characteristic smell of fresh alcohol or the fetid odor of metabolic products, and the presence of nystagmus, ataxia, and altered mental status. It is imperative to consider other etiologies that may accompany or mimic intoxication, such as hypoglycemia, head trauma, hypothermia, meningitis, or intoxication with other drugs or poisons.

A. Specific levels. Ethanol levels are easily and rapidly determined by most hospital laboratories and, depending on the method used, are accurate and specific.

1. In general, there is poor correlation between blood levels and clinical presentation; however, an ethanol level below 300 mg/dL in a comatose patient should initiate a search for alternative causes.
2. If ethanol levels are not readily available, the ethanol concentration may be estimated by calculating the osmolar gap (see p 29).

B. Suggested laboratory studies. CBC, glucose, electrolytes, BUN, creatinine, hepatic transaminases, prothrombin time (PT), magnesium, arterial blood gases, chest x-ray.

V. Treatment

A. Emergency and supportive measures

1. **Acute intoxication.** Treatment is mainly supportive.
   a. Protect the airway to prevent aspiration (see p 1), and intubate and assist ventilation if needed (p 4).
   b. Give glucose and thiamine (p 340), and treat coma (p 17) and seizures (p 21) if they occur.
   c. Correct hypothermia with gradual rewarming (p 18).
   d. Most patients will recover within 4–6 hours.
2. **Alcohol withdrawal.** Treat with benzodiazepines (diazepam, 2–5 mg IV, repeated as needed; see p 302) or phenobarbital (130 mg IV slowly, repeated as needed; see p 334).

B. Specific drugs and antidotes. There is no commercially available specific ethanol receptor antagonist, but there are anecdotal reports of arousal after administration of naloxone, 2–5 mg IV (see p 325).

C. Decontamination. Because ethanol is rapidly absorbed, emesis or gastric lavage is usually not indicated unless a substantial ingestion has occurred within 30 minutes of presentation or other drug ingestion is suspected.

1. Induce emesis or perform gastric lavage (see p 42) if the ingestion was recent (within 30–45 minutes).
2. Activated charcoal (see p 45) does not efficiently adsorb ethanol but may be given, especially if other toxins were ingested.

D. Enhanced elimination. Elimination normally occurs at a fixed rate, between 20–40 mg/dL/h. Hemodialysis efficiently removes ethanol, but enhanced removal is rarely needed because supportive care is usually sufficient. Hemoperfusion and forced diuresis are not effective.

References

Sellers EM, Kalant H: Alcohol intoxication and withdrawal. *N Engl J Med* 1976;**294**:757.
Young GP et al: Intravenous phenobarbital for alcohol withdrawal and convulsions. *Ann Emerg Med* 1987;**16**:847.

ETHYLENE DIBROMIDE
Gail M. Gullickson, MD

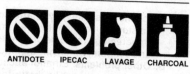

Ethylene dibromide (EDB, dibromoethane) is a volatile liquid produced by the bromination of ethylene. EDB is used as a lead scavanger in leaded gasoline and as a pesticide and fumigant in soil and on fruits and vegetables. Because EDB has been found to be a suspected human carcinogen, its use as a pesticide has been restricted since 1984.

I. **Mechanism of toxicity**
   A. **Liquid EDB is an irritant** capable of causing chemical burns. Inhalation of EDB vapor produces respiratory tract irritation and delayed-onset pulmonary edema.
   B. **Once absorbed systemically,** EDB acts as an alkylating agent and can cause disruption of cellular metabolism and multisystem failure.

II. **Toxic dose**
   A. **Inhalation.** Because EDB is a suspected carcinogen (ACGIH class A2), no safe workplace exposure limit has been determined. Exposure to vapor concentrations greater than 200 ppm can produce lung irritation, and 400 ppm may be immediately dangerous to life or health (IDLH).
   B. **Ingestion** of 4.5 mL of liquid EDB has resulted in death.

III. **Clinical presentation**
   A. **Inhalation of EDB vapor** causes irritation of the eyes and upper respiratory tract. Pulmonary edema usually occurs within 1–6 hours but may be delayed as long as 48 hours after exposure.
   B. **Oral ingestion** causes prompt vomiting and diarrhea.
   C. **Systemic** manifestations of intoxication include central nervous system depression, seizures, and metabolic acidosis. Skeletal muscle necrosis, acute renal failure, and hepatic necrosis have also been reported in fatal cases.

IV. **Diagnosis.** Diagnosis of EDB poisoning is based on a history of exposure and evidence of upper airway and eye irritation (in case of inhalation) or gastroenteritis (after ingestion). EDB vapor has a strong chemical odor.
   A. **Specific levels.** EDB is detectable in expired air, blood, and tissues, although levels are not useful in emergency management. Serum bromide levels may be elevated (> 0.1 meq/L) in severe cases, because bromide is released from EDB in the body.
   B. **Other useful laboratory studies.** CBC, electrolytes, glucose, BUN, creatinine, liver transaminases and function tests, creatine phosphokinase (CPK), arterial blood gases, chest x-ray.

V. **Treatment**
   A. **Emergency and supportive measures**
      1. Maintain the airway and assist ventilation if necessary (see p 2).
      2. After inhalation exposure, anticipate and treat wheezing, airway obstruction, and pulmonary edema (p 7). Monitor blood gases, provide supplemental oxygen if needed, and avoid fluid overload.
      3. Treat coma (p 17), seizures (p 21), rhabdomyolysis (p 24), and metabolic acidosis (p 30) if they occur.
   B. **Specific drugs and antidotes.** There is no specific antidote.
   C. **Decontamination**
      1. **Inhalation.** Remove the victim from exposure and provide supplemental oxygen, if available. Rescuers must use self-contained breathing apparatus and wear protective clothing to avoid personal exposure.
      2. **Skin and eyes.** Remove and safely discard all contaminated clothing,

and wash exposed skin with copious soap and water. Irrigate exposed eyes with tepid saline or water.

3. **Ingestion**
    a. Perform gastric lavage (see p 43). Do **not** induce emesis because of corrosive effects and the risk of rapid onset of coma or seizures.
    b. Administer activated charcoal and a cathartic (see p 45).
    c. Gut emptying is probably not necessary following small ingestions if activated charcoal is given promptly.

D. **Enhanced elimination.** There is no role for dialysis or hemoperfusion, diuresis, or repeat-dose charcoal.

Reference

Letz GA et al: Two fatalities after acute occupational exposure to ethylene dibromide. *JAMA* 1984;**252**:2428.

ETHYLENE GLYCOL AND OTHER GLYCOLS
Ilene B. Anderson, PharmD

ANTIDOTE   IPECAC   LAVAGE   CHARCOAL

Ethylene glycol is the primary ingredient (up to 95%) in antifreeze. It is sometimes intentionally consumed as an alcohol substitute by alcoholics and is tempting to children because of its sweet taste. Intoxication by ethylene glycol itself causes inebriation and mild gastritis; however, its metabolic products cause metabolic acidosis, renal failure, and death after a delay of 4–12 hours. Other glycols may also produce toxicity (Table II–22).

I. **Mechanism of toxicity**
   A. **Ethylene glycol** is metabolized by alcohol dehydrogenase to glycoaldehyde, which is then metabolized to glycolic, glyoxylic, and oxalic acids. These acids, along with excess lactic acid, are responsible for the anion gap metabolic acidosis. Oxalate readily precipitates with calcium to form insoluble calcium oxalate crystals. Tissue injury is caused by widespread deposition of oxalate crystals and the toxic effects of glycolic and glyoxylic acids.
   B. **Other glycols** (Table II–22). Propylene and butylene glycols are of relatively low toxicity, and polypropylene glycol is virtually nontoxic. However, diethylene glycol and glycol ethers produce toxic metabolites with toxicity similar to that of ethylene glycol.

II. **Toxic dose.** The approximate lethal oral dose of 95% ethylene glycol (eg, antifreeze) is 1.5 mL/kg; however, survival has been reported following ingestion of 2 L in a patient who received treatment within 1 hour of ingestion.

III. **Clinical presentation**
   A. **Ethylene glycol**
      1. **During the first 3–4 hours** after acute ingestion, the victim may appear intoxicated as if by ethanol. The osmolar gap (see p 29) is increased, but there is no initial acidosis. Gastritis with vomiting may also occur.
      2. **After a delay of 4–12 hours,** evidence of intoxication by metabolic products occurs, with anion gap acidosis, hyperventilation, convulsions, coma, cardiac conduction disturbances, and arrhythmias. Renal failure is common but usually reversible. Pulmonary edema

and cerebral edema may also occur. Hypocalcemia with tetany has been reported.

B. Other glycols (Table II–22). Diethylene glycol and glycol ethers are extremely toxic and may produce acute renal failure and metabolic acidosis, usually without oxalate crystals.

IV. Diagnosis. The diagnosis of ethylene glycol poisoning is usually based on the history of antifreeze ingestion, typical symptoms, and elevation of the osmolar and anion gaps. Oxalate or hippurate crystals may be present in the urine. Because many antifreeze products also contain fluorescein, the urine may fluoresce under Wood's lamp.

A. Specific levels. Tests for ethylene glycol levels are usually available from regional commercial toxicology laboratories but are difficult to perform accurately. Calculation of the osmolar gap (see p 29) may be used to estimate the ethylene glycol level. Serum levels higher than 50 mg/dL are usually associated with serious intoxication, although lower levels do not rule out poisoning if the parent compound has already been metabolized. In such a case, the anion gap should be markedly elevated. If the osmolar and anion gaps are both normal and the patient is asymptomatic, then serious ingestion has not occurred.

B. Other useful laboratory studies. CBC, electrolytes, glucose, BUN, creatinine, calcium, hepatic transaminases, urinalysis (for crystals and Wood's lamp examination), serum osmolality and osmolar gap, arterial blood gases, ECG, chest x-ray.

V. Treatment

A. Emergency and supportive measures

1. Maintain the airway and assist ventilation if necessary (see p 2).
2. Treat coma (p 17), convulsions (p 21), cardiac arrhythmias (p 9), and metabolic acidosis (p 30) if they occur. Observe patient for several hours to monitor for development of metabolic acidosis.
3. Treat hypocalcemia with intravenous calcium gluconate or calcium chloride (p 298).

B. Specific drugs and antidotes

TABLE II-22. TOXICITY OF OTHER GLYCOLS[a]

Compound	Toxicity and Comments
Propylene glycol	Relatively low toxicity; osmolar gap elevated, but acidosis, coma, seizures, and hypoglycemia are rare. Metabolized to lactate and acetate.
Polyethylene glycols	High-molecular-weight compounds; poorly absorbed, rapidly excreted by kidneys; virtually nontoxic.
Diethylene glycol	Highly nephrotoxic; metabolic acidosis may occur, but there are no oxalate crystals. Lethal dose approximately 1 mL/kg.
Glycol ethers (cellosolves)	Many agents are highly nephrotoxic; ethylene glycol monomethyl ether (methyl cellosolve) may hydrolyze to ethylene glycol and methanol, resulting in acidosis and oxaluria; ethylene glycol monoethyl ether (cellosolve) and ethylene glycol monobutyl ether (butyl cellosolve) cause kidney injury without oxalate formation.
Dioxane	Dimer of ethylene glycol; toxicity may cause coma, liver and kidney damage. Metabolites not known. Workplace air exposure limit is 25 ppm.
Glycols used in cosmetics (hexylene, dipropylene glycols)	Full-strength hexylene glycol is a skin and eye irritant; both can cause kidney damage with large overdose.

[a] References: Ellenhorn MJ, Barceloux DG: Alcohols and glycols. Pages 809–811 in: *Medical Toxicology: Diagnosis & Treatment of Human Poisoning.* Elsevier, 1988; and Cornish H: Solvents and vapors. Pages 481–485 in: *Casarett & Doull's Toxicology: The Basic Science of Poisons,* 2nd ed. Doull J et al (editors). MacMillan, 1980.

1. Administer **ethanol** (see p 312) to saturate the enzyme alcohol dehydrogenase and prevent metabolism of ethylene glycol to its toxic metabolites. Indications for ethanol therapy include:
   a. Ethylene glycol level higher than 20 mg/dL.
   b. History of ethylene glycol ingestion accompanied by an osmolar gap greater than 5 mosm/L not accounted for by ethanol or other alcohols.
   c. Anion gap acidosis accompanied by history of glycol ingestion or presence of oxalate crystalluria.
2. Administer **pyridoxine** (see p 339), **folate** (p 314), and **thiamine** (p 340), cofactors required for the metabolism of ethylene glycol that may decrease toxicity by enhancing metabolism of glyoxylic acid to nontoxic metabolites.

C. **Decontamination**
   1. Induce emesis or perform gastric lavage (see p 42). Immediate lavage is preferred for hospital treatment because ethylene glycol is rapidly absorbed.
   2. Activated charcoal is probably not effective, and it may delay the absorption of orally administered ethanol used for treatment.
D. **Enhanced elimination.** The volume of distribution of ethylene glycol is 0.7–0.8 L/kg, making it accessible to enhanced elimination procedures. **Hemodialysis** efficiently removes ethylene glycol and its toxic metabolites and rapidly corrects acidosis and electrolyte and fluid abnormalities.
   1. Indications for hemodialysis:
      a. Suspected ethylene glycol poisoning with osmolar gap greater than 10 mosm/L not accounted for by ethanol or other alcohols.
      b. Any ethylene glycol intoxication accompanied by renal failure.
      c. Ethylene glycol serum concentration greater than 20–50 mg/dL.
   2. The minimum serum concentration of ethylene glycol associated with serious toxicity is not known; dialysis should be continued until the osmolar and anion gaps are normalized. Ethanol infusion must be increased during dialysis (see p 312) and should be continued for at least 24 hours after the last dialysis because of possible rebound elevation of ethylene glycol levels.

Reference

Jacobsen D, McMartin KE: Methanol and ethylene glycol poisoning: Mechanism of toxicity, clinical course, diagnosis and treatment. *Med Toxicol* 1986;1:309.

ETHYLENE OXIDE
Charles E. Becker, MD

| ANTIDOTE | IPECAC | LAVAGE | CHARCOAL |

Ethylene oxide is a highly penetrating gas, widely used in hospitals as a sterilizer of medical equipment and supplies. It is also an important industrial chemical, used as a solvent, plasticizer, and chemical intermediate.

I. **Mechanism of toxicity.** Ethylene oxide is an alkylating agent and reacts directly with proteins and DNA to cause cell death. Direct contact with the gas causes irritation of the eyes, mucous membranes, and lungs. Ethylene oxide is probably mutagenic, teratogenic, and carcinogenic in humans.
II. **Toxic dose.** The permissible exposure limit (PEL) in air is 1 ppm as an 8-hour time-weighted average. The air level considered immediately dangerous to life or health (IDLH) is 800 ppm. The odor threshold is about 700 ppm, giving the gas poor warning properties. High levels of ethylene oxide

can occur when sterilizers malfunction or simply with the opening or replacing of ethylene oxide tanks.

III. **Clinical presentation**
   A. Ethylene oxide is a potent mucous membrane irritant, and high levels can cause eye and oropharyngeal irritation, bronchospasm, and pulmonary edema. Cataract formation has been described after significant eye exposure. Exposure to the liquid can cause vesicant injury to the skin.
   B. Neurotoxicity, including convulsions and delayed peripheral neuropathy, may occur after great exposure.
   C. Other systemic effects include cardiac arrhythmias when ethylene oxide is used with the carrier gas Freon.
   D. Leukemia has been described in workers chronically exposed to ethylene oxide.

IV. **Diagnosis.** Diagnosis is based on a history of exposure and typical upper airway irritant effects. Detection of ethylene oxide odor indicates significant exposure. Industrial hygiene sampling may be necessary to document levels of exposure.
   A. **Specific levels.** Serum levels are not available.
   B. **Other useful laboratory studies.** Arterial blood gases, chest x-ray.

V. **Treatment**
   A. **Emergency and supportive measures.** Monitor closely for several hours after exposure.
      1. Maintain the airway and assist ventilation if necessary (see p 2). Treat bronchospasm (p 8) and pulmonary edema (p 7) if they occur.
      2. Treat coma (p 17), convulsions (p 21), and arrhythmias (p 9) if they occur.
   B. **Specific drugs and antidotes.** There is no specific antidote.
   C. **Decontamination**
      1. Remove the victim from the contaminated environment immediately and administer oxygen. Rescuers should wear self-contained breathing apparatus and protective skin covering.
      2. Remove all contaminated clothing and wash exposed skin. For eye exposures, irrigate copiously with tepid water or saline.
   D. **Enhanced elimination.** There is no role for these procedures.

Reference

Estrin WJ et al: Evidence of neurologic dysfunction related to long-term ethylene oxide exposure. *Arch Neurol* 1987;**44**:1283.

FLUORIDE
James F. Buchanan, PharmD

ANTIDOTE   IPECAC   LAVAGE   CHARCOAL

Fluoride is a constituent of various insecticides, rodenticides, dental products, and vitamins or dietary supplements. It is commonly added to community drinking water. It is also found in hydrofluoric acid (see p 167). Soluble fluoride salts (eg, sodium fluoride) are rapidly absorbed within 30 minutes. Serum fluoride binds to calcium ion and bone and is only slowly eliminated by renal excretion.

   I. **Mechanism of toxicity.** Fluoride interferes with a number of cellular metabolic processes. Oxidative phosphorylation is impaired, proteolytic processes are enhanced, and blood coagulation is inhibited. The binding of fluoride to calcium causes systemic hypocalcemia and inhibits various calcium ion-mediated reactions in nervous and muscle tissue.

II. Toxic dose. Vomiting and abdominal pain occur commonly with ingestions of 3–5 mg/kg elemental fluoride; hypocalcemia and muscular symptoms appear with ingestions of 5–10 mg/kg. Death has been reported in a 3-year-old child following ingestion of 16 mg/kg and in adults with doses in excess of 32 mg/kg.

III. Clinical presentation. Nausea and vomiting frequently occur within 30–60 minutes of ingestion. Symptoms of more serious intoxication include skeletal muscle weakness, tetanic contractions, respiratory muscle weakness, and respiratory arrest. Cardiac arrhythmias may be associated with hypocalcemia and hyperkalemia.

IV. Diagnosis. The diagnosis is usually based on a history of ingestion. Symptoms of abdominal distress, muscle weakness, hypocalcemia, and hyperkalemia suggest fluoride intoxication.

    A. Specific levels. The normal serum fluoride concentration is less than 20 mcg/L (ng/mL) but varies considerably with diet and water source. Serum fluoride concentrations are generally difficult to obtain and thus are of limited utility for acute overdose management.

    B. Other useful laboratory studies. CBC, electrolytes, glucose, BUN, creatinine, calcium, ECG.

V. Treatment

    A. Emergency and supportive measures

      1. Maintain the airway and assist ventilation if necessary (see p 2).

      2. Monitor ECG and serum calcium for at least 4–6 hours, and admit symptomatic patients to an intensive care setting.

    B. Specific drugs and antidotes. When clinically significant hypocalcemia is present, administer intravenous **calcium chloride** (see p 298), 10–20 mL (0.1–0.2 mL/kg).

    C. Decontamination

      1. Following recent ingestion, induce emesis or perform gastric lavage (see p 42).

      2. Administer **calcium** salts (eg, calcium carbonate, calcium lactate, or milk) orally to form insoluble complexes with fluoride, minimizing absorption.

      3. Activated charcoal does not adsorb fluoride and is not likely to be beneficial.

    D. Enhanced elimination. Although fluoride is a small ion with minimal protein binding, it rapidly binds to free calcium ion and bone; therefore, hemodialysis and hemoperfusion are unlikely to be beneficial.

Reference

Eichler HG et al: Accidental ingestion of NaF tablets by children: Report of a poison control center and one case. *Int J Clin Pharmacol Ther Toxicol* 1982;**20**:334.

FLUOROACETATE
James F. Buchanan, PharmD

ANTIDOTE   IPECAC   LAVAGE   CHARCOAL

Fluoroacetate, also known as compound 1080, is one of the most toxic substances known. In the past, it was used primarily as a rodenticide by licensed pest control companies, but it has been removed from the US market because of its hazard.

    I. Mechanism of toxicity. Fluoroacetate is metabolized to the toxic compound fluorocitric acid, which blocks cellular metabolism by inhibiting the Krebs cycle. Clinical effects of poisoning are delayed (from 30 minutes to several hours) until fluoroacetate is metabolized to fluorocitrate.

II. Toxic dose. As little as 1 mg of fluoroacetate is sufficient to cause serious toxicity. Death is likely after ingestion of more than 5 mg/kg.

III. Clinical presentation. After a delay of minutes to several hours, manifestations of diffuse cellular poisoning become apparent: nausea, vomiting, diarrhea, metabolic acidosis, agitation, confusion, seizures, coma, respiratory arrest, and ventricular arrhythmias may occur.

IV. Diagnosis. Diagnosis is based on a history of ingestion and clinical findings, which may be delayed for several hours. Poisoning with fluoroacetate may mimic poisoning with other cellular toxins such as cyanide and hydrogen sulfide, although with these poisons the onset of symptoms is usually very rapid.

  A. Specific levels. There is no assay available.

  B. Other useful laboratory studies. BUN, creatinine, arterial blood gases, ECG.

V. Treatment

  A. Emergency and supportive measures

    1. Maintain the airway and assist ventilation if necessary (see p 2). Administer supplemental oxygen.

    2. Replace fluid losses from gastroenteritis with intravenous saline or other crystalloids.

    3. Treat shock (p 14), seizures (p 21), and coma (p 17) if they occur. Monitor the ECG for at least 4–6 hours.

  B. Specific treatment. There is **no available antidote.** Monoacetin has been used experimentally in monkeys but is not available or recommended for human use.

  C. Decontamination

    1. Perform gastric lavage (see p 43). Do *not* induce emesis, because seizures may occur as early as 30 minutes after ingestion.

    2. Administer activated charcoal and a cathartic (p 45).

  D. Enhanced elimination. There is no role for any enhanced removal procedure.

Reference

Egekeze JO, Oehme FW: Sodium monofluoroacetate (SMFA, compound 1080): A literature review. *Vet Hum Toxicol* 1979;21:411.

FOOD POISONING: BACTERIAL
James F. Buchanan, PharmD

ANTIDOTE   IPECAC   LAVAGE   CHARCOAL

Foodborne illness is one of the most common causes of epidemic gastroenteritis. In general, common bacterial food poisoning is relatively mild and self-limited, with recovery within 24 hours. However, severe and even fatal poisoning may occur with botulism (see p 95). Poisoning following consumption of fish and shellfish is discussed on p 158.

  I. Mechanism of toxicity. Gastroenteritis may be caused by invasive bacterial infection of the intestinal mucosa or by a toxin elaborated by bacteria. Bacterial toxins may be preformed in food that is improperly prepared and improperly stored before use or may be produced in the gut by the bacteria after they are ingested (Table II–23).

  II. Toxic dose. The toxic dose depends on the type of bacteria or toxin and its concentration in the ingested food, as well as individual susceptibility or resistance. Some of the preformed toxins (eg, staphylococcal toxin) are heat-resistant and once in the food are not removed by cooking or boiling.

III. **Clinical presentation.** Commonly, a delay or "incubation period" of from 2 hours to 3 days precedes the onset of symptoms (Table II–23).

   A. **Gastroenteritis** is the most common finding, with nausea, vomiting, abdominal cramps, and diarrhea. Significant fluid and electrolyte abnormalities may occur, especially in young children or elderly patients.

   B. **Fever, bloody stools,** and **fecal leukocytosis** are common with invasive bacterial infections.

IV. **Diagnosis.** Bacterial food poisoning is often difficult to distinguish from common viral gastroenteritis, unless the incubation period is short and there are multiple victims who ate similar foods at one large gathering. The presence of many white blood cells in a stool smear suggests invasive bacterial infection. With any epidemic gastroenteritis, consider other foodborne illnesses, such as seafood (see below), botulism (p 95), and mushrooms (p 210).

   A. **Specific levels.** There are no specific assays that will assist clinical management.

      1. Stool culture may differentiate *Salmonella, Shigella,* and *Campylobacter* infections.

      2. Food samples should be saved for bacterial culture and toxin analysis, primarily for use by public health investigators.

   B. **Other useful laboratory studies.** CBC, electrolytes, glucose, BUN, creatinine, liver function tests.

V. **Treatment**

   A. **Emergency and supportive measures**

      1. Replace fluid and electrolyte losses with intravenous saline or other crystalloid solutions (patients with mild illness may tolerate oral rehydration). Patients with hypotension may require large-volume intravenous fluid resuscitation (see p 14).

      2. Antiemetic agents are acceptable for symptomatic treatment, but antidiarrheal agents such as Lomotil (diphenoxylate plus atropine; see p 190) should *not* be used because they may prolong the course of the infection.

   B. **Specific drugs and antidotes.** There are no specific antidotes. In patients with invasive bacterial infection, antibiotics may be used once the stool culture reveals the specific bacteria responsible.

TABLE II-23. SUMMARY OF BACTERIAL FOOD POISONING

Organism	Incubation Period	Mechanism	Common Foods
Bacillus cereus	1–6 h	Toxin produced in food and patient	Reheated fried rice.
Campylobacter	1–2 days	Invasive	Water; direct contact.
Clostridium perfringens	6–16 h	Toxin produced in food and patient	Meats, gravy.
Escherichia coli (toxigenic)	12–72 h	Toxin produced in patient	Water
Salmonella	12–36 h	Invasive	Meat, dairy, bakery foods; water; direct contact.
Shigella	1–7 days	Invasive	Water; fruits, vegetables.
Staphylococcus aureus	1–6 h	Toxin preformed in food; heat-resistant	Very common; meats, dairy, bakery foods.
Vibrio parahemolyticus	8–30 h	Invasive *and* toxin produced in patient	Shellfish; water.

C. Decontamination. There is no role for gut decontamination.

D. Enhanced elimination. There is no role for enhanced removal procedures.

Reference

Mills J: Acute gastroenteritis: The when, what and how of treatment. *Mod Med* 1979;**47**:20.

FOOD POISONING: FISH AND SHELLFISH
James F. Buchanan, PharmD

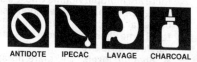

ANTIDOTE   IPECAC   LAVAGE   CHARCOAL

A variety of toxins may produce illness after ingestion of fish or shellfish. The most common types of seafood-related toxins include **ciguatera, scombroid, neurotoxic shellfish poisoning, paralytic shellfish poisoning,** and **tetrodotoxin.** Shellfish-induced bacterial diarrhea is described below.

I. **Mechanism of toxicity.** The mechanism varies with each toxin. The toxins are all heat-stable; therefore, cooking the seafood does not prevent illness.

A. **Ciguatera.** The toxin is produced by dinoflagellates that are then consumed by reef fish. The mechanism of intoxication is unknown.

B. **Scombroid.** Scombrotoxin is a mixture of histamine and other histamine-like compounds produced when histidine in fish tissue decomposes.

C. **Neurotoxic shellfish.** The mechanism is unknown. Neurotoxins are thought to stimulate postganglionic cholinergic neurons.

D. **Paralytic shellfish.** Dinoflagellates ("red tide") produce saxitoxin, which is concentrated by filter-feeding clams and mussels. Saxitoxin blocks sodium conductance and neuronal transmission in skeletal muscles.

E. **Tetrodotoxin.** Tetrodotoxin, produced in the skin of puffer fish, California newts, and some South American frogs, is similar to saxitoxin and blocks sodium conductance and neuronal transmission in skeletal muscles.

II. **Toxic dose.** The concentration of toxin varies widely depending on geographic and seasonal factors. The amount of toxin necessary to produce symptoms is unknown. Saxitoxin is extremely potent; the estimated lethal dose in humans is 0.3–1 mg, and contaminated mussels may contain 15–20 mg.

III. **Clinical presentation.** The onset of symptoms and clinical manifestations vary with each toxin (Table II–24). In the majority of cases, the seafood appears normal with no adverse smell or taste (scombroid may have a peppery taste).

A. **Ciguatera.** Intoxication produces vomiting and watery diarrhea 1–6 hours after ingestion, followed by headache, malaise, myalgias, paresthesias of the mouth and extremities, ataxia, blurred vision, photophobia, reversal of hot and cold sensation, hypotension, bradycardia, and rarely, seizures and respiratory arrest.

B. **Scombroid.** Symptoms begin rapidly (minutes to 3 hours) after ingestion. Gastroenteritis, headache, and skin flushing are sometimes accompanied by urticaria and bronchospasm.

C. **Neurotoxic shellfish.** Onset is within a few minutes to 3 hours. Gastroenteritis is accompanied by paresthesias of the mouth, face, and extremities; muscular weakness; and respiratory arrest.

D. **Paralytic shellfish.** Vomiting, diarrhea, and facial paresthesias usually begin within 30 minutes of ingestion. Headache, myalgias, dysphagia,

TABLE II-24. SUMMARY OF FISH AND SHELLFISH INTOXICATIONS

Type	Onset	Common Sources	Syndrome
Ciguatera	1-6 h	Barracuda, red snapper, grouper	Gastroenteritis, hot and cold reversal, paresthesias, myalgias, weakness.
Scombroid	Minutes to hours	Tuna, mahi mahi, bonita, mackerel	Gastroenteritis, flushed skin, urticaria, wheezing.
Neurotoxic shellfish	Minutes to 3 h	Mussels	Gastroenteritis, ataxia, paresthesias.
Paralytic shellfish	Within 30 minutes	Mussels and clams, "red tide"	Gastroenteritis, paresthesias, ataxia, respiratory paralysis.
Tetrodotoxin	Within 30-40 minutes	Puffer fish, sun fish, porcupine fish, California newt	Vomiting, paresthesias, muscle twitching, diaphoresis, weakness, respiratory paralysis.

weakness, and ataxia have been reported. In serious cases respiratory arrest may occur after 1–12 hours.

   E. Tetrodotoxin. Symptoms occur within 30–40 minutes after ingestion, with vomiting and paresthesias. Salivation, twitching, diaphoresis, weakness, and dysphagia are reported. Hypotension, bradycardia, and respiratory arrest may occur up to 6–24 hours after ingestion.

IV. **Diagnosis.** The diagnosis depends on a history of ingestion and is more likely to be recognized when multiple victims present after consumption of a common meal. Scombroid may be confused with an allergic reaction because of the histamine-induced urticaria.

   A. Specific levels are not generally available. However, when epidemic poisoning is suspected, state public health departments or the Centers for Disease Control can analyze suspect for toxins.

   B. Suggested laboratory tests: CBC, electrolytes, glucose, BUN, creatinine, arterial blood gases, electrocardiographic monitoring.

V. **Treatment**

   A. Emergency and supportive measures. Most cases of mild poisoning are self-limited and require no specific treatment. However, because of the risk of respiratory arrest, all patients should be observed for several hours.

   1. Maintain the airway and assist ventilation if necessary (see p 2).
   2. Replace fluid and electrolyte losses from gastroenteritis with intravenous crystalloid fluids (see p 14).

   B. Specific drugs and antidotes

   1. **Antihistamines** (eg, diphenhydramine; see p 73) provide effective symptomatic relief for **scombroid** intoxication. Rarely, bronchodilators may also be required.
   2. There are anecdotal reports of successful treatment of ciguatera with intravenous mannitol and of scombroid with cimetidine.

   C. Decontamination

   1. Induce emesis or perform gastric lavage (see p 42) if ingestion occurred within the preceding hour. Lavage is preferred if there is evidence of respiratory weakness or dysphagia.
   2. Administer activated charcoal and a cathartic (see p 45).

   D. Enhanced elimination. There is no role for enhanced elimination procedures.

Reference

Hughes JM, Merson MH: Fish and shellfish poisoning. *N Engl J Med* 1976;**295**:1117.

FORMALDEHYDE
Gail M. Gullickson, MD

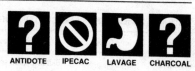

Formaldehyde is a gas with a pungent odor commonly used in the processing of paper, fabrics, and wood products and for the production of urea foam insulation. Low-level formaldehyde exposure has been found in clothing stores selling clothing treated with formaldehyde-containing crease-resistant resins, in mobile homes, and in tightly enclosed rooms built with large quantities of formaldehyde-containing products used in construction materials. Formaldehyde aqueous solution (formalin) is used in varying concentrations (usually 37%) as a disinfectant and tissue fixative. Stabilized formalin may also contain 6–15% **methanol.**

I. Mechanism of toxicity
A. Formaldehyde causes precipitation of proteins and will cause coagulation necrosis of exposed tissue. The gas is highly water-soluble and when inhaled produces immediate local irritation of the upper respiratory tract and has been reported to cause spasm and edema of the larynx.

B. Metabolism of formaldehyde produces formic acid, which may accumulate and produce metabolic acidosis (see p 202).

C. Formaldehyde is a known animal and suspected human carcinogen.

II. Toxic dose
A. Inhalation. The OSHA permissible exposure limit (PEL) is 1 ppm and the 15-minute short-term exposure limit (STEL) is 2 ppm. The air level considered immediately dangerous to life or health (IDLH) is 100 ppm.

B. Ingestion of as little as 30 mL of 37% formaldehyde solution has been reported to cause death in an adult.

III. Clinical presentation
A. Formaldehyde gas exposure produces irritation of the eyes, and inhalation can produce cough, wheezing, and pulmonary edema.

B. Ingestion of formaldehyde solutions may cause severe corrosive esophageal and gastric injury, depending on the concentration. Lethargy and coma have been reported. Metabolic (anion gap) acidosis may be caused by formic acid accumulation from metabolism of formaldehyde or methanol.

C. Hemolysis has occurred when formalin was accidentally introduced into the blood through contaminated hemodialysis equipment.

IV. Diagnosis. Diagnosis is based on a history of exposure and evidence of mucous membrane, respiratory, or gastrointestinal tract irritation.
A. Specific levels
1. Plasma formaldehyde levels are not useful, but formate levels may indicate severity of intoxication.
2. Methanol (see p 202) and formate levels may be helpful in cases of intoxication by formalin solutions containing methanol.

B. Other useful laboratory studies. CBC, electrolytes, BUN, creatinine, liver function tests, osmolar gap.

V. Treatment
A. Emergency and supportive measures
1. Maintain the airway and assist ventilation if necessary (see p 2). Administer supplemental oxygen, and observe for at least 4–6 hours.
2. **Inhalation.** Treat bronchospasm (p 8) and pulmonary edema (p 7) if they occur.

    3. Ingestion
      a. Treat coma (p 17) and shock (p 14) if they occur.
      b. Administer intravenous saline or other crystalloids to replace fluid losses caused by gastroenteritis. Avoid fluid overload in patients with inhalation exposure because of the risk of pulmonary edema.
      c. Treat metabolic acidosis with sodium bicarbonate (p 30).
  B. Specific drugs and antidotes
    1. If a **methanol-containing solution** has been ingested, then evaluate and treat with **ethanol and folic acid** as for methanol poisoning (see p 202).
    2. Formate intoxication due to formaldehyde alone should be treated with **folic acid** (see p 314), but ethanol infusion is not effective.
  C. Decontamination
    1. Inhalation. Remove from exposure and give supplemental oxygen, if available.
    2. Skin and eyes. Remove contaminated clothing and wash exposed skin with soap and water. Irrigate exposed eyes with copious tepid water or saline; perform fluorescein examination to rule out corneal injury if pain and lacrimation persist.
    3. Ingestion. Depending on concentration of solution and patient symptoms, consider endoscopy to rule out esophageal or gastric injury.
      a. Perform gastric lavage (see p 43). Do *not* induce emesis because of the risk of corrosive injury.
      b. Administer activated charcoal. Do *not* use charcoal if endoscopy is planned.
  D. Enhanced elimination
    1. Hemodialysis is effective in removing methanol and formate (see p 202) and in correcting severe metabolic acidosis. Indications for hemodialysis include severe acidosis or osmolar gap (see p 29) greater than 10 mosm/L.
    2. Alkalinization of the urine helps promote excretion of formate.

Reference

Kochhar R et al: Formaldehyde-induced corrosive gastric cicatrization: Case report. *Hum Toxicol* 1986;**5**:381.

FREONS (FLUORINATED HYDROCARBONS)
Peter Wald, MD

ANTIDOTE   IPECAC   LAVAGE   CHARCOAL

Freons (fluorinated hydrocarbons) are widely used as aerosol propellants, in refrigeration units, and as degreasing agents. Some fire extinguishers contain Freons. Most of these compounds are gases at room temperature, but some are liquids (Freons 11, 21, 113, 114) and may be ingested. Many Freons contain chlorine in addition to fluorine.

I. Mechanism of toxicity
  A. Freons are mild central nervous system depressants. They are well absorbed by inhalation or ingestion and are usually rapidly excreted in the breath within 15–60 minutes.

B. As with chlorinated hydrocarbons, Freons may potentiate cardiac arrhythmias by sensitizing the myocardium to catecholamines.

C. Direct freezing of the skin, with frostbite, may occur if the skin is exposed to rapidly expanding gas as it escapes from a pressurized tank.

D. Freons containing chlorine may decompose to the irritant gases phosgene and hydrogen chloride (see p 163), and those containing fluorine may produce hydrogen fluoride (p 167), if they are burned at high temperature, as may happen in a fire or if a refrigeration line is cut by a welding torch or electric arc.

II. **Toxic dose**

A. **Inhalation.** The toxic air level is quite variable (see Table IV-12). The OSHA occupational permissible exposure limit (PEL) for fluorotrichloromethane is 1000 ppm as an 8-hour time-weighted average, and its level considered immediately dangerous to life or health (IDLH) is 10,000 ppm.

B. **Ingestion.** The toxic dose by ingestion is not known.

III. **Clinical presentation**

A. **Skin or mucous membrane** exposure may result in skin defatting and erythema. Frostbite may occur after exposure to rapidly expanding compressed gas.

B. **Systemic effects** of moderate exposure include headache, nausea and vomiting, confusion, and drunkenness. More severe intoxication may result in coma or respiratory arrest. Ventricular arrhythmias may occur even with moderate exposures. A number of deaths, presumably caused by ventricular fibrillation, have been reported after Freon abuse by "sniffing" or "huffing" Freon products from plastic bags.

IV. **Diagnosis.** Diagnosis is based on a history of exposure and clinical presentation. Many chlorinated and aromatic hydrocarbon solvents may cause identical symptoms.

A. **Specific levels.** Expired-breath monitoring is possible, and blood levels may be obtained to document exposure, but these are not useful in emergency clinical management.

B. **Other useful laboratory studies.** Arterial blood gases, electrocardiographic monitoring.

V. **Treatment**

A. **Emergency and supportive measures**

1. Maintain the airway and assist ventilation if necessary (see p 2).

2. Treat coma (p 17) and arrhythmias (p 13) if they occur. Avoid epinephrine or other sympathomimetic amines that may precipitate ventricular arrhythmias.

3. Monitor the ECG for 4–6 hours.

B. **Specific drugs and antidotes.** There is no specific antidote.

C. **Decontamination**

1. **Inhalation.** Remove victim from exposure, and give supplemental oxygen if available.

2. **Ingestion**

a. Perform gastric lavage (see p 43). Do **not** induce emesis because of rapid absorption and the risk of abrupt onset of central nervous system depression.

b. Administer activated charcoal and cathartic (see p 45), although the efficacy of charcoal is unknown.

D. **Enhanced elimination.** There is no documented efficacy for diuresis, hemodialysis, hemoperfusion, or repeat-dose charcoal.

Reference

Harris WS: Toxic effects of aerosol propellants on the heart. *Arch Intern Med* 1973;**131**:162.

GASES, IRRITANT
Peter Wald, MD

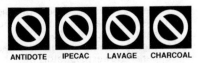

A vast number of compounds produce irritant effects when inhaled in their gaseous form. The most common souce of exposure to irritant gases is in industry, but significant exposures may occur in a variety of circumstances, such as after mixing cleaning agents at home, with smoke inhalation in structural fires, or after highway tanker spills.

- I. **Mechanism of toxicity.** Irritant gases are often divided into 2 major groups based on their water solubility (Table II–25).
    - A. **Highly soluble gases** (eg, ammonia, chlorine) are rapidly adsorbed by the upper respiratory tract and rapidly produce their primary effects on moist mucous membranes in the eyes, nose, and throat.
    - B. **Less soluble gases** (eg, phosgene, nitrogen dioxide) are not rapidly adsorbed by the upper respiratory tract and can be inhaled deeply into the lower respiratory tract to produce delayed-onset pulmonary toxicity.
- II. **Toxic dose.** The toxic dose varies depending on the properties of the gas.

TABLE II-25. CHARACTERISTICS OF SOME COMMON IRRITANT TOXIC GASES

Gas	PEL[a] (ppm)	IDLH[b] (ppm)
High water solubility		
Ammonia	50	500
Formaldehyde	3	100
Hydrogen chloride	5	100
Hydrogen fluoride	3	20
Nitric acid	2	100
Sulfuric acid	1	80
Sulfur dioxide	2	100
Moderate water solubility		
Acrolein	0.1	5
Chlorine	0.5	25
Fluorine	0.1	25
Low water solubility		
Nitric oxide	25	100
Nitrogen dioxide	5	50
Ozone	0.1	10
Phosgene	0.1	2

[a]PEL = OSHA workplace permissible exposure limit as an 8-hour time-weighted average for a 40-hour workweek.
[b]IDLH = Air level considered immediately dangerous to life or health, defined as the maximum air concentration from which one could reasonably escape within 30 minutes without any escape-impairing symptoms or any irreversible health effects.

Table II–25 illustrates the permissible exposure limits (PEL) and the levels immediately dangerous to life or health (IDLH) for several common irritant gases (see also Table IV–12).

III. **Clinical presentation.** All these gases may produce irritant effects to the upper and lower respiratory tract, but warning properties and the onset and location of primary symptoms depend largely on their water solubility and the concentration of exposure.

   A. **Highly soluble gases.** Because of the good warning properties (upper respiratory tract irritation) of highly soluble gases, voluntary prolonged exposure to even low concentrations is unlikely.

      1. Low-level exposure causes rapid onset of mucous membrane and upper respiratory tract irritation; conjunctivitis, rhinitis, skin erythema and burns, sore throat, cough, wheezing, and hoarseness are common.

      2. With great exposure, tracheobronchitis, laryngeal edema, and abrupt airway obstruction may occur. Irritation of the lower respiratory tract and lung parenchyma causes tracheobroncheal mucosal sloughing, chemical pneumonia, and noncardiogenic pulmonary edema.

   B. **Less soluble gases.** Because of poor warning properties owing to minimal upper respiratory tract effects, prolonged exposure to moderate levels of these gases often occurs; therefore, chemical pneumonia and pulmonary edema are more common. The onset of pulmonary edema is frequently delayed up to 12–24 hours or even longer.

IV. **Diagnosis** is based on a history of exposure or the presence of typical irritant upper and lower respiratory effects. Arterial blood gases and chest x-ray may reveal early evidence of chemical pneumonia or pulmonary edema. Whereas highly soluble gases have good warning properties and the diagnosis is not difficult, less soluble gases may produce minimal symptoms shortly after exposure; therefore, a high index of suspicion and repeated examinations are required.

   A. **Specific levels.** There are no specific blood levels.

   B. **Other useful laboratory studies.** Arterial blood gases, chest x-ray, pulmonary function tests.

V. **Treatment**

   A. **Emergency and supportive measures**

      1. Immediately assess the airway: hoarseness or stridor suggests laryngeal edema, which necessitates direct laryngoscopy and endotracheal intubation if swelling is present (see p 4). Assist ventilation if necessary (p 6).

      2. Give supplemental oxygen, and treat bronchospasm with humidified air and aerosolized bronchodilators (p 8).

      3. Monitor arterial blood gases and chest x-ray, and treat pulmonary edema if it occurs (p 7).

      4. For victims of smoke inhalation, consider the possibility of concurrent intoxication by carbon monoxide (p 109) or cyanide (p 134).

   B. **Specific drugs and antidotes.** There is no specific antidote for any of these gases.

   C. **Decontamination.** Remove victim from exposure and give supplemental oxygen if available. Rescuers should take care to avoid personal exposure; in most cases, self-contained breathing apparatus should be worn.

   D. **Enhanced elimination.** There is no role for enhanced elimination.

Reference

Wald PW et al: Respiratory effects of acute toxic inhalations: Smoke, gases, and fumes. *J Intensive Care Med* 1987;2:260.

HYDROCARBONS
Peter Yip, MD, and
Kent R. Olson, MD

ANTIDOTE   IPECAC   LAVAGE   CHARCOAL

Hydrocarbons, or petroleum distillates, are a group of organic compounds widely used in the petroleum, plastic, agricultural, and chemical industries as solvents, degreasers, fuels, and pesticides. There are 4 major groups of hydrocarbons: aliphatic (saturated carbon structure); alicyclic (ring compounds); aromatic (containing one or more benzene ring structures); and halogenated (containing chlorine, bromine, or fluoride atoms).

I. **Mechanism of toxicity.** Toxicity from hydrocarbons may be due to direct injury from **pulmonary aspiration,** or **systemic intoxication** after **ingestion** or **inhalation** (Table II-26). Many hydrocarbons are also irritating to the eyes and skin.

   A. **Pulmonary aspiration.** Hydrocarbons are capable of inducing chemical pneumonia if aspirated. The risk of aspiration is increased for agents that have a low viscosity (eg, mineral seal oil, furniture polish).

   B. **Ingestion.** Most **aliphatic hydrocarbons** are poorly absorbed from the gastrointestinal tract and do not pose significant risk of systemic toxicity after ingestion. In contrast, many **aromatic** and **halogenated hydrocarbons** are capable of causing serious systemic toxicity after ingestion, such as coma, seizures, and cardiac arrhythmias.

   C. **Inhalation** of any hydrocarbon vapors in an enclosed space may cause intoxication as a result of systemic absorption or by displacing oxygen from the atmosphere.

II. **Toxic dose.** The toxic dose is highly variable depending on the agent involved and whether it is aspirated, ingested, or inhaled.

   A. **Pulmonary aspiration** of as little as a few milliliters of any hydrocarbon may produce chemical pneumonia.

   B. **Ingestion** of as little as 10–20 mL of systemic toxins such as camphor or carbon tetrachloride may cause serious poisoning.

   C. For recommended **inhalation** exposure limits for common hydrocarbons, see Table IV-12.

III. **Clinical presentation**

   A. If **pulmonary aspiration** has occurred, there is usually immediate onset of coughing, gagging, or choking. This may progress within a few hours to tachypnea, wheezing, and severe chemical pneumonia. Death may ensue from secondary bacterial infection and other respiratory complications.

   B. **Ingestion** often causes abrupt nausea and vomiting, occasionally with hemorrhagic gastroenteritis. Some compounds will be absorbed and produce systemic toxicity.

   C. **Systemic toxicity** caused by ingestion of a toxic hydrocarbon or inhalation of any hydrocarbon is highly variable depending on the compound but usually includes confusion, ataxia, lethargy, and headache. With significant exposure, syncope, coma, and respiratory arrest may occur. Cardiac arrhythmias may occur owing to myocardial sensitization by halogenated hydrocarbons. With many agents, hepatic and renal injury may occur.

   D. **Skin or eye contact** may cause local irritation, burns, or corneal injury.

IV. **Diagnosis**

   A. Diagnosis of **aspiration pneumonia** is based on a history of exposure and the presence of respiratory symptoms such as coughing, choking, and wheezing. If these symptoms are not present within 4–6 hours of exposure, it is very unlikely that chemical pneumonia will occur. Chest

TABLE II–26. RISK OF TOXICITY FROM HYDROCARBON INGESTION

Toxicity	Risk of Systemic Toxicity After Ingestion	Risk of Chemical Aspiration Pneumonia	Treatment
No systemic toxicity, high viscosity Petrolatum jelly, motor oil	Low	Low	None.
No systemic toxicity, low viscosity Gasoline, kerosene, petroleum naphtha, mineral seal oil, petroleum ether	Low	High	Observe for pneumonia; do not empty stomach.
Unknown or uncertain systemic toxicity Turpentine, pine oil	Uncertain	High	Observe for pneumonia; do **not** empty stomach if ingestion is < 2 mL/kg.
Systemic toxins Camphor, phenol, halogenated, or aromatic compounds	High	High	Observe for pneumonia; perform gastric lavage or give activated charcoal or do both.

    x-ray and arterial blood gases may assist in the diagnosis of chemical pneumonia.

  B. The diagnosis of **systemic intoxication** is based on a history of ingestion or inhalation, accompanied by the appropriate systemic clinical manifestations.

  C. Specific levels. Specific levels are generally not available or useful. See additional discussion of individual compounds described elsewhere in this book (eg, benzene, p 89; toluene, p 281; trichloroethane and trichloroethylene, p 282).

  D. Other useful laboratory studies. CBC, electrolytes, glucose, BUN, creatinine, liver function tests, arterial blood gases, chest x-ray, electrocardiographic monitoring.

V. Treatment

  A. Emergency and supportive measures

    1. General. Provide basic supportive care for all symptomatic patients, whether from aspiration, ingestion, or inhalation:

      a. Maintain the airway and assist ventilation if necessary (see p 2).

      b. Monitor arterial blood gases, chest x-ray, and ECG and admit symptomatic patients to an intensive care setting.

      c. If possible, avoid use of epinephrine and other sympathomimetic amines in patients with halogenated hydrocarbon intoxication, because arrhythmias may be induced.

    2. Pulmonary aspiration. Patients who remain asymptomatic after 4–6 hours of observation may be discharged. In contrast, if the patient is coughing on arrival, aspiration has probably occurred.

      a. Administer supplemental oxygen, and treat bronchospasm (see p 8), hypoxia (p 7), and pneumonia (p 7) if they occur.

      b. Do **not** use steroids or prophylactic antibiotics.

    3. Ingestion. In the vast majority of accidental ingestions, less than

5–10 mL is actually swallowed and systemic toxicity is rare. Treatment is primarily supportive.

B. Specific drugs and antidotes
  1. There is no specific antidote for general hydrocarbon aspiration pneumonia; corticosteroids are of no proved value.
  2. Specific drugs or antidotes may be available for systemic toxicity of some hydrocarbons (eg, acetylcysteine for carbon tetrachloride, p 111; methylene blue for methemoglobin formers; etc); see the discussion of individual topics elsewhere in this book.

C. Decontamination
  1. **Inhalation.** Move the victim to fresh air and administer oxygen, if available.
  2. **Skin and eyes.** Remove contaminated clothing and wash exposed skin with water and soap. Irrigate exposed eyes with copious tepid water or saline, and perform fluorescein examination for corneal injury.
  3. **Ingestion.** For agents with no known systemic toxicity, gut decontamination is neither necessary nor desirable because any gut-emptying procedure may increase the risk of aspiration. For systemic toxins:
     a. Perform gastric lavage (see p 43), taking care to protect the airway. Do *not* induce emesis, because systemic complications such as seizures and coma may occur rapidly or abruptly.
     b. Administer activated charcoal and cathartic (see p 45).
     c. For small ingestions of systemic toxins known to be adsorbed by charcoal, activated charcoal may be given alone without first performing lavage.

D. Enhanced elimination. There is no known role for any of these procedures.

Reference

Machado B, Cross K, Snodgrass WR: Accidental hydrocarbon ingestion cases telephoned to a regional poison center. *Ann Emerg Med* 1988;**17**:804.

HYDROGEN FLUORIDE AND HYDROFLUORIC ACID
Kent R. Olson, MD

ANTIDOTE   IPECAC   LAVAGE   CHARCOAL

Hydrogen fluoride (HF) is an irritant gas that liquifies at 19.5 °C; in aqueous solution it produces hydrofluoric acid. HF gas is used in chemical manufacturing. In addition, it may be released from fluorosilicates, fluorocarbons, or Teflon when heated over 350 °C. Hydrofluoric acid (aqueous HF solution) is widely used as a rust remover, in glass etching, and in the manufacture of silicon semiconductor chips. Hydrofluoric acid poisoning usually occurs after skin contact, although ingestions occasionally occur.

  I. Mechanism of toxicity. Hydrogen fluoride is a skin and respiratory irritant. Hydrofluoric acid is actually a relatively weak acid (the dissociation constant is about 1000 times less than that of hydrochloric acid), and toxic effects are due primarily to the highly reactive fluoride ion.
  A. HF is able to penetrate tissues deeply, where the highly cytotoxic fluoride ion is released and cellular destruction occurs.
  B. In addition, fluoride readily precipitates with calcium; this may cause local bone demineralization and systemic hypocalcemia.

 II. **Toxic dose.** Toxicity depends on the air levels of hydrogen fluoride or concentration of aqueous HF solutions.
- **A. Hydrogen fluoride gas.** The OSHA permissible exposure limit (PEL) for HF gas is 3 ppm; 20 ppm is considered immediately dangerous to life or health (IDLH). A 5-minute exposure to air concentrations of 50–250 ppm is likely to be lethal.
- **B. Aqueous solutions.** Solutions of 50–70% are highly toxic and produce immediate pain; intermediate concentrations (20–40%) may cause little pain initially but result in deep injury after 1–8 hours; weak solutions (5–15%) cause almost no pain on contact but may cause delayed serious injury after 12–24 hours. Most household products containing aqeous HF are 5–8% solutions.
III. **Clinical presentation.** Symptoms and signs depend on the type of exposure (gas or liquid) and the concentration.
- **A. Inhalation of HF gas.** Inhalation of HF produces eye and nose irritation, sore throat, coughing, and bronchospasm. After a delay of up to several hours, chemical penumonia and pulmonary edema may occur.
- **B. Skin exposure.** After acute exposure to weak (5–15%) or intermediate (20–40%) solutions, there may be no symptoms because the pH effect is relatively weak. Strong (50–70%) solutions have better warning properties because of immediate pain. After a delay of 1–12 hours, progressive redness, swelling, skin blanching, and pain occur owing to deep penetration by the fluoride ion. The exposure is typically through a pinhole-sized defect in a rubber glove, and the fingertip is the most common site of injury. The pain is progressive and unrelenting. Severe deep-tissue destruction may occur, including full-thickness skin loss and destruction of underlying bone.
- **C. Ingestion** of HF may cause corrosive injury to the mouth, esophagus, and stomach.
- **D. Systemic hypocalcemia** and **hyperkalemia** may occur after ingestion or following skin burns involving a large body surface area or highly concentrated solutions.
IV. **Diagnosis.** Diagnosis is based on a history of exposure and typical findings. Immediately after exposure to weak or intermediate solutions, there may be few or no symptoms even though potentially severe injury may develop later.
- **A. Specific levels.** Serum fluoride concentrations are not useful after acute exposure but may be used in evaluating chronic occupational exposure. Normal serum fluoride is less than 0.1 mg/L.
- **B. Other useful laboratory studies.** CBC, electrolytes, calcium, ECG.
 V. **Treatment**
- **A. Emergency and supportive measures**
  1. Maintain the airway and assist ventilation if necessary (see p 2). Administer supplemental oxygen. Treat pulmonary edema (p 7) if it occurs.
  2. Patients with HF ingestion should be evaluated for corrosive injury, with consultation by a gastroenterologist or surgeon for possible endoscopy.
  3. Monitor the ECG and serum calcium and potassium levels; give intravenous calcium (p 298 and below) if there is evidence of hypocalcemia.
- **B. Specific drugs and antidotes. Calcium** (see p 298) rapidly precipitates fluoride ion and is an effective antidote for fluoride skin exposure and for systemic hypocalcemia resulting from absorbed fluoride.
  1. **Skin burns.** For exposures involving the hands or fingers, consult an experienced hand surgeon, medical toxicologist, or Poison Control Center (see Table I–41, p 51). This is especially important if pain is not relieved with initial injections. The nail may need to be removed, and occasionally calcium may need to be given intra-arterially. *Cau-*

tion: Calcium itself can cause tissue necrosis. Do *not* use calcium *chloride* for subcutaneous or intra-arterial injections.

a. Topical treatment. Apply a gel containing calcium gluconate or carbonate (p 298); or soak in Epsom salt (Mg) solution. If pain is not relieved in 30–60 minutes, consider SQ or intra-arterial treatment.

b. Subcutaneous injection. Inject calcium gluconate 10% subcutaneously (p 298) in affected areas, using a 27- or 30-guage needle and no more than 0.5 mL per digit or 1 mL/cm² in other regions.

c. Intra-arterial injection may be necessary for burns involving several digits or subungual areas (p 298).

2. **Systemic hypocalcemia or hyperkalemia.** Administer **calcium gluconate** 10%, 2–4 mL/kg IV, or **calcium chloride** 10%, 1–2 mL/kg IV.

C. **Decontamination**

1. **Inhalation.** Immediately remove from exposure and give supplemental oxygen, if available. Rescuers should wear self-contained breathing apparatus and protective gear to avoid personal exposure.

2. **Skin.** Immediately flood exposed areas with water. Then soak in solution of Epsom salts (magnesium sulfate) or calcium; immediate topical use of calcium or magnesium may prevent deep burns. After skin penetration by HF, topical treatment is relatively ineffective and calcium injections (see above) may be required.

3. **Eyes.** Flush with copious water or saline. The use of weak (1–2%) calcium solution is not established.

4. **Ingestion**

a. Perform gastric lavage (see p 43). Do *not* induce emesis because of the risk of corrosive injury.

b. Immediately give magnesium-containing preparation (Epsom salts, magnesium hydroxide, etc) or calcium-containing preparation (calcium carbonate or milk) by mouth or gastric tube. Activated charcoal is not effective.

D. **Enhanced elimination.** There is no role for enhanced elimination procedures.

References

Caravati EM: Acute hydrofluoric acid exposure. *Am J Emerg Med* 1988;**6:**143.

Edelman PA: Chemical and electrical burns. Pages 183–202 in: *Management of the Burned Patient.* Achauer BM (editor). Appleton & Lange, 1987.

HYDROGEN SULFIDE
Peter Yip, MD

ANTIDOTE   IPECAC   LAVAGE   CHARCOAL

Hydrogen sulfide is a highly toxic, flammable, colorless gas that is heavier than air. It is produced naturally by decaying organic matter and is also a by-product of many industrial processes. Hazardous levels may be found in petroleum refineries, tanneries, mines, pulp-making factories, sulfur hot springs, carbon disulfide production, hot asphalt fumes, and pools of sewage sludge or liquid manure.

I. **Mechanism of toxicity.** Hydrogen sulfide causes cellular asphyxia by inhibition of the cytochrome oxidase system, similar to the action of cyanide. Because it is rapidly absorbed by inhalation, symptoms occur nearly immediately after exposure. Hydrogen sulfide is also a mucous membrane irritant.

II. **Toxic dose.** The characteristic rotten egg odor of hydrogen sulfide is de-

170   POISONING AND DRUG OVERDOSE

tectable at concentrations as low as 0.025 ppm. The OSHA workplace permissible exposure limit (PEL) is 10 ppm as an 8-hour time-weighted average, with a short-term exposure limit (STEL) of 15 ppm. Marked respiratory tract irritation occurs with levels of 50–100 ppm. Olfactory nerve paralysis occurs with levels of 100–150 ppm. Pulmonary edema occurs at levels of 300–500 ppm. Levels of 600–800 ppm are rapidly fatal.

III. **Clinical presentation**
   A. **Irritant effects.** Upper airway irritation, burning eyes, and blepharospasm may occur at relatively low levels. Skin exposure can cause painful dermatitis. Chemical pneumonitis and noncardiogenic pulmonary edema may occur after a delay of several hours.
   B. Acute **systemic effects** include headache, nausea and vomiting, dizziness, confusion, seizures, and coma. Massive exposure may cause immediate cardiovascular collapse, respiratory arrest, and death.

IV. **Diagnosis.** Diagnosis is based on a history of exposure and rapidly progressive manifestations of airway irritation and cellular asphyxia, with sudden collapse. The victim may describe the smell of rotten eggs, but because of olfactory nerve paralysis the absence of this smell does not rule out exposure.
   A. **Specific levels.** Serum levels are not commonly available. Sulfhemoglobin is not thought to be produced after hydrogen sulfide exposure.
   B. **Other useful laboratory studies.** CBC, electrolytes, glucose, arterial blood gases, chest x-ray.

V. **Treatment**
   A. **Emergency and supportive measures**
      1. Maintain the airway and assist ventilation if necessary (see p 2). Administer high-flow humidified supplemental oxygen. Observe for several hours for delayed-onset chemical pneumonia or pulmonary edema (p 7).
      2. Treat coma (p 17), seizures (p 21), and hypotension (p 14) if they occur.
   B. **Specific drugs and antidotes.** Theoretically, administration of nitrites (see p 328) to produce methemoglobinemia may promote conversion of sulfide ion to sulfhemoglobin, which is far less toxic. However, there is no credible evidence that this is effective.
   C. **Decontamination.** Remove the victim from exposure and give supplemental oxygen, if available. Rescuers should use self-contained breathing apparatus to prevent personal exposure.
   D. **Enhanced elimination.** There is no role for enhanced elimination procedures. Although hyperbaric oxygen therapy has been promoted for treatment of hydrogen sulfide poisoning, this is based on anecdotal evidence and there is no convincing rationale or scientific evidence for its effectiveness.

Reference

Hoidal CR et al: Hydrogen sulfide poisoning from toxic inhalations of roofing asphalt fumes. *Ann Emerg Med* 1986;**15**:826

HYMENOPTERA
Howard E. McKinney, PharmD

ANTIDOTE   IPECAC   LAVAGE   CHARCOAL

Venomous insects are grouped into 4 families of the order Hymenoptera: Apidae (honeybees), Bombidae (bumblebees), Vespidae (wasps, hornets, and yellow jackets), and Formicidae (ants).

I. **Mechanism of toxicity.** The venoms of the Hymenoptera are complex mixtures of enzymes and are delivered by various methods. The venom apparatus is located in the posterior abdomen of the females.
   A. **Apidae, Bombidae, Vespidae.** The terminal end of the stinger of the honeybee is barbed, so the stinger remains in the victim and some or all of the venom apparatus will be torn from the body of the bee, resulting in its death as it flies away. The musculature surrounding the venom sac continues to contract for several minutes, causing venom to be ejected. The Bombidae and Vespidae have nonbarbed stingers that remain functionally intact after a sting, resulting in their ability to inflict multiple stings.
   B. **Formicidae.** The envenomating Formicidae have secretory venom glands in the posterior abdomen and envenomate either by injecting venom through a stinger or by spraying venom from the posterior abdomen into a bite wound produced by their mandibles.
II. **Toxic dose.** The dose of venom delivered per sting may vary from none to the entire contents of the venom gland. The toxic response is highly variable depending on individual sensitivity.
III. **Clinical presentation.** The patient may present with signs of envenomation or an allergic reaction.
   A. **Envenomation.** Once venom is injected, there is usually immediate onset of severe pain followed by a local inflammatory reaction, which may include erythema, wheal formation, ecchymosis, edema, vesiculation and blisters, itching, and a sensation of warmth. Multiple stings, and very rarely severe single stings, may also produce vomiting, diarrhea, hypotension, syncope, cyanosis, dyspnea, rhabdomyolysis, coagulopathy, and death.
   B. **Allergic reactions.** About 50 deaths occur annually in the USA from immediate hypersensitivity (anaphylactic) reactions characterized by urticaria, angioedema, bronchospasm, and shock. Most anaphylactic reactions occur within 15 minutes of envenomation. Rarely, delayed-onset reactions may occur, including Arthus reactions (arthralgias, fever), nephritis, transverse myelitis, and Guillain-Barré syndrome.
IV. **Diagnosis.** The diagnosis is usually obvious from the history of exposure and typical findings. Patients should be observed for at least 30–60 minutes for any onset of allergic reaction.
   A. **Specific levels** are not available.
   B. **Other useful laboratory studies.** No specific laboratory studies are required.
V. **Treatment**
   A. **Emergency and supportive measures**
      1. Monitor the victim closely for at least 30–60 minutes.
      2. Treat anaphylaxis (see p 25), if it occurs, with epinephrine (p 309) and diphenhydramine (p 305). Persons known to be sensitive to Hymenoptera venom should wear medical alert jewelry and carry an epinephrine emergency kit at all times.
      3. In most cases the painful localized tissue response will resolve in a few hours without therapy. Some symptomatic relief may be obtained by topical application of ice, papain (meat tenderizer), or creams containing corticosteroids or antihistamines.
      4. Provide tetanus prophylaxis if appropriate.
   B. **Specific drugs and antidotes.** There is no available antidote.
   C. **Decontamination.** Examine the sting site carefully for any retained stingers; these can be removed by gentle scraping with a knife blade or key (do **not** squeeze the stinger with forceps or fingers; this will release more venom). Wash the area with soap and water.
   D. **Enhanced elimination.** These procedures are not applicable.

Reference

Green VA, Siegel CJ: Bites and stings of Hymenoptera, caterpillar and beetles. *J Toxicol Clin Toxicol* 1983–1984;**21**:491.

HYPOGLYCEMIC AGENTS
James F. Buchanan, PharmD

ANTIDOTE   IPECAC   LAVAGE   CHARCOAL

Agents used to lower blood glucose are divided into 2 groups: the oral hypoglycemics and insulin products. The **oral hypoglycemic agents** are sulfonylureas, and all produce qualitatively similar blood glucose-lowering effects; they differ primarily by potency and duration of action. All **insulin** products are given by the parenteral route, and all produce effects similar to those of endogenous insulin; they differ by antigenicity and by onset and duration of effect. Table II–27 lists the various available hypoglycemic agents.

I. Mechanism of toxicity

  A. Oral hypoglycemic agents. Hypoglycemia is produced primarily by stimulating endogenous pancreatic insulin secretion and secondarily by enhancing peripheral insulin receptor sensitivity and by reducing glycogenolysis. Chlorpropamide may inhibit free water clearance, resulting in hyponatremia. In contrast, glipizide and glyburide may produce a diuresis by enhancing free water clearance.

  B. Insulin. Blood glucose is lowered directly by stimulation of cellular uptake and metabolism of glucose. Cellular glucose uptake is accom-

TABLE II–27. PHARMACOLOGIC PROFILES OF HYPOGLYCEMIC AGENTS

Agent	Onset (h)	Peak (h)	Duration (h)
Insulins			
Regular insulin	0.5–1	2–3	5–7
Rapid insulin zinc	0.5–1	4–7	12–16
Insulin zinc	1–2	8–12	18–24
Isophane insulin (NPH)	1–2	8–12	18–24
Prolonged insulin zinc	4–8	16–18	36
Protamine zinc	4–8	14–20	36
Oral hypoglycemic agents			
Glipizide	0.25–0.5	0.5–2	< 24
Glyburide	0.25–1	1–2	24
Chlorpropamide	1	3–6	24–72
Tolazamide	1	4–6	14–20
Tolbutamide	1	5–8	6–12
Acetohexamide	2	4	12–24

panied by intracellular shift of potassium and magnesium. Insulin also promotes glycogen formation and lipogenesis.

II. Toxic dose

A. Oral hypoglycemic agents. Toxic dose depends on the agent and the total dose or duration of overdose. Toxicity may also occur owing to drug interactions, resulting in impaired elimination of the oral agent.

1. **Acetohexamide,** 500 mg/d for 5 days, has caused hypoglycemic coma in adults.
2. **Chlorpropamide,** 500–750 mg/d for 2 weeks, has caused hypoglycemia in adults.
3. **Glyburide,** 10–15 mg; acute overdose in a child produced profound hypoglycemic coma.
4. **Interactions** with the following drugs may increase the risk of hypoglycemia: other hypoglycemics, sulfonamides, propranolol, salicylates, clofibrate, phenylbutazone, probenecid, dicumarol, chloramphenicol, monoamine oxidase inhibitors, and alcohol. In addition, coingestion of alcohol may occasionally produce a disulfiramlike interaction (see p 143).
5. **Hepatic** or **renal insufficiency** may impair drug elimination and result in hypoglycemia.

B. Insulin. Severe hypoglycemic coma and permanent neurologic sequelae have occurred after injections of 800–3200 units of insulin. Orally administered insulin is not absorbed and is not toxic.

III. Clinical presentation.
All agents cause hypoglycemia, which may be delayed in onset depending on the agent used and the route of administration (ie, subcutaneous vs intravenous).

A. Manifestations of hypoglycemia include agitation, confusion, coma, seizures, tachycardia, and diaphoresis. The serum potassium and magnesium levels may be depressed.

B. With chlorpropamide intoxication, hyponatremia may occur; in contrast, glipizide and glyburide intoxication may cause dehydration and hypernatremia.

IV. Diagnosis.
The diagnosis should be suspected in any patient with hypoglycemia. Note that in patients receiving beta-adrenergic blocking agents many of the manifestations of hypoglycemia (tachycardia, diaphoresis) may be blunted or absent. Other causes of hypoglycemia that should be considered include alcohol ingestion (especially in children) and hepatic failure.

A. Specific levels

1. Tolazamide, tolbutamide, and chlorpropamide serum concentrations can be determined in most regional commercial toxicology laboratories.
2. Exogenously administered animal insulin can be distinguished from endogenous insulin (ie, in a patient with hypoglycemia caused by insulinoma) by determination of C peptide (present with endogenous insulin secretion).

B. Other useful laboratory studies. CBC, glucose, electrolytes, magnesium, ethanol, liver function tests.

V. Treatment

A. Emergency and supportive measures

1. Maintain the airway and assist ventilation if necessary (see p 2).
2. Treat coma (p 17) and seizures (p 21) if they occur.
3. Correct hyponatremia or hypernatremia if they occur.

B. Specific drugs and antidotes

1. Administer concentrated **glucose** (see p 315) as soon as possible after drawing a baseline blood sample for later blood glucose determination. Give 50% dextrose ($D_{50}W$), 1–2 mL/kg, in adults; 25% dextrose ($D_{25}W$), 2–4 mL/kg, in children. Repeat glucose boluses and

administer 5–10% dextrose (D_5–D_{10}) to maintain the serum glucose level at or above 100 mg/dL.
   2. For patients with oral hypoglycemic overdose, consider intravenous **diazoxide** (see p 303) if dextrose infusions do not maintain satisfactory glucose concentrations.
C. **Decontamination**
   1. **Oral hypoglycemic agents**
      a. Induce emesis or perform gastric lavage (see p 42).
      b. Administer activated charcoal and cathartic (see p 45).
      c. Gut emptying is probably not necessary following small ingestions if activated charcoal is given promptly.
   2. **Insulin**
      a. Orally ingested insulin is not absorbed and produces no toxicity, so gut decontamination is not necessary.
      b. Local excision of tissue at the site of massive intradermal injection has been performed, but the general utility of this procedure has not been established.
D. **Enhanced elimination. Alkalinization of the urine** (pH 8 or greater) increases the renal elimination of chlorpropamide. Forced diuresis and dialysis procedures are of no known value for other hypoglycemic agents. The high degree of protein binding of the sulfonylureas suggests that dialysis procedures would not be effective.

Reference

Bobzien WF III: Suicidal overdoses with hypoglycemic agents. *JACEP* 1979;**8**:467.

IODINE
Olga F. Woo, PharmD

ANTIDOTE   IPECAC   LAVAGE   CHARCOAL

The chief use of iodine is for its antiseptic property. It is bactericidal, sporicidal, protozoacidal, cysticidal, and virucidal. Because it is poorly soluble in water, liquid formulations are usually prepared as a tincture in ethanol (50% or higher). Iodoform, iodochlorhydroxyquin, iodophors (povidine-iodine), and sodium and potassium iodides also exert their bactericidal effect by liberating iodine. Lugol's solution (5% iodine and 10% potassium iodide) is used in the treatment of hyperthyroidism and for the prevention of radioactive iodine absorption after nuclear accidents. The antiarrhythmic drug amiodarone releases iodine and may cause thyrotoxicosis after prolonged use.

I. **Mechanism of toxicity.** Iodine is corrosive because of its oxidizing properties. When ingested, iodine is poorly absorbed but may cause severe gastroenteritis. Iodine is readily inactivated by starch to convert it to iodide, which is nontoxic. In the body, iodine is rapidly converted to iodide and stored in the thyroid gland.
II. **Toxic dose.** Toxic dose depends on the product and the route of exposure. Iodophors and iodoform liberate only small amounts of iodine and are generally nontoxic and noncaustic.
   A. **Iodine vapor.** The OSHA permissible exposure limit (PEL) for iodine vapor is 0.1 ppm as an 8-hour time-weighted average. The air level considered immediately dangerous to life or health (IDLH) is 10 ppm.
   B. **Skin and mucous membranes.** Strong iodine tincture (7% iodine and 5% potassium iodide in 83% ethanol) may cause burns, but USP iodine

tincture (2% iodine and 2% sodium iodide in 50% ethanol) is not likely to produce corrosive damage.
   C. **Ingestion.** Reported fatal doses vary from 200 mg to more than 20 g of iodine; an estimated mean lethal dose is approximately 2–4 g of free iodine. USP iodine tincture contains 100 mg iodine per 5 mL, and strong iodine tincture contains 350 mg of iodine per 5 mL. Iodine ointment contains 4% iodine.
III. **Clinical presentation.** The clinical manifestations of iodine poisoning are largely related to its corrosive effect on mucous membranes.
   A. **Inhalation** of iodine vapor can cause severe pulmonary irritation leading to pulmonary edema.
   B. **Skin and eye** exposures may result in severe corrosive burns. Exposures on the skin from strong iodine tincture may cause dermal necrosis and systemic absorption of iodine.
   C. **Ingestion** causes corrosive gastroenteritis with vomiting, hematemesis, and diarrhea, which can result in significant volume loss and circulatory collapse. Pharyngeal swelling and glottic edema have been reported. Mucous membranes are usually stained brown, and the vomitus may be blue if starchy foods are already present in the stomach.
   D. **Chronic ingestions or absorption** may result in hypothyroidism and goiter. Iodides cross the placenta, and neonatal hypothyroidism and death from respiratory distress secondary to goiter have been reported.
IV. **Diagnosis.** Diagnosis is based on a history of exposure and evidence of corrosive injury. Mucous membranes are usually stained brown, and vomitus may be blue.
   A. **Specific levels.** Iodide levels are not clinically useful but may confirm exposure.
   B. **Other useful laboratory studies.** CBC, electrolytes, glucose, BUN, creatinine, arterial blood gases, chest x-ray.
V. **Treatment**
   A. **Emergency and supportive measures**
      1. Maintain the airway and perform endotracheal intubation if airway edema is progressive (see p 4). Administer oxygen, and treat pulmonary edema (p 7) if it occurs.
      2. Treat fluid loss from gastroenteritis aggressively with intravenous crystalloid solutions (p 14).
      3. If caustic injury to the esophagus or stomach is suspected, consult a gastroenterologist to perform endoscopy.
   B. **Specific drugs and antidotes**
      1. **Cornstarch, flour,** or **milk** will convert iodine to nontoxic iodide in the stomach.
      2. **Sodium thiosulfate** will convert iodine to iodide and tetrathionate but is not recommended for intravenous use because iodine is rapidly converted to iodide in the body.
   C. **Enhanced elimination**
      1. **Inhalation.** Remove victim from exposure and administer oxygen, if available.
      2. **Skin and eyes.** Remove contaminated clothing and flush exposed skin with water. Irrigate exposed eyes copiously with tepid water for at least 15 minutes (see p 40).
      3. **Ingestion**
         a. Do *not* induce emesis because of the corrosive effects of iodine.
         b. After small ingestions of less corrosive products (eg, USP iodine tincture, povidone), administer a starchy food (potato, flour) or milk to lessen gastrointestinal irritation.
         c. In more serious exposures, perform gastric lavage (see p 43) using cornstarch or sodium thiosulfate.

    d. Activated charcoal should not be given until the decision whether to perform endoscopy has been made, because it may obscure endoscopic view.

  D. Enhanced elimination. Once absorbed into the circulation, iodine is rapidly converted to the far less toxic iodide. Therefore, there is no need for enhanced drug removal.

Reference

Moore M: The ingestion of iodine as a method of attempted suicide. *N Engl J Med* 1938;**219**:383.

IPECAC SYRUP
James F. Buchanan, PharmD

ANTIDOTE   IPECAC   LAVAGE   CHARCOAL

Ipecac syrup is an extract of the ipecacuanha plant. Its principle active ingredients are emetine and cephaeline. Syrup of ipecac is widely available over-the-counter as an effective, rapidly acting emetic agent. Presently, the major source of poisoning is chronic intoxication due to intentional misuse by patients with eating disorders.

  I. Mechanism of toxicity
    A. Acute ingestion of ipecac causes vomiting by stimulation of the gastric mucosa and by stimulation of the central chemoreceptor trigger zone.
    B. Chronic poisoning causes interstitial edema and necrosis of skeletal and myocardial muscle fibers. The normal cellular architecture is disrupted, and clinical myopathy occurs.
  II. Toxic dose. Toxicity depends on the formulation and whether the exposure is acute or chronic.
    A. Acute ingestion of 60–120 mL of **syrup of ipecac** is not likely to cause serious poisoning. However, the **fluid extract** is approximately 14 times more potent than syrup of ipecac; ingestion of as little as 10 mL of the fluid extract has been reported to cause death.
    B. Chronic daily ingestion of 90–120 mL of syrup of ipecac for 3 months has caused death due to cardiomyopathy.
  III. Clinical presentation
    A. Acute ingestion of ipecac causes nausea and vomiting. In patients with depressed airway protective reflexes, pulmonary aspiration of gastric contents may occur. Prolonged or forceful emesis may cause gastritis or Mallory-Weiss tears of the cardioesophageal junction.
    B. Chronic intoxication. In patients with chronic misuse, dehydration and electrolyte abnormalities (eg, hypokalemia) are common secondary to frequent vomiting, and myopathy or cardiomyopathy may occur. Symptoms of myopathy include muscle weakness and tenderness, hyporeflexia, and elevated serum creatine phosphokinase (CPK). Cardiomyopathy, with congestive heart failure and arryhthmias, is often fatal.
  IV. Diagnosis. Diagnosis is based on a history of ingestion. Chronic ipecac poisoning should be suspected in any patient with a known eating disorder and evidence of dehydration, electrolyte imbalance, or myopathy. The electrocardiogram may show prolonged QRS and QT intervals, flat or inverted T waves, and supraventricular and ventricular arrhythmias.
    A. Specific levels. Emetine may be detected in the urine, and its presence may provide qualitative confirmation of ipecac exposure. It is not part of a routine toxicology screen and must be specifically requested.

B. Other useful laboratory studies. CBC, electrolytes, BUN, creatinine, creatine phosphokinase (CPK), lactate dehydrogenase (LDH), ECG.

V. Treatment

A. Emergency and supportive measures

1. Correct fluid and electrolyte abnormalities with intravenous fluids and potassium as needed (see p 14 and p 32).

2. Diuretics and pressor support may be required in patients with congestive cardiomyopathy.

3. Treat arrhythmias, if they occur, with standard drugs (see p 9).

4. Monitor the ECG for 6–8 hours, and admit patients with evidence of myopathy or cardiomyopathy.

B. Specific drugs and antidotes. There is no specific antidote.

C. Decontamination

1. Perform gastric lavage (see p 43) if a large ingestion of fluid extract has occurred. Do *not* induce emesis.

2. Activated charcoal may inhibit the absorption of ipecac if given very shortly after a single ingestion. It is of no benefit in patients with chronic ingestion.

D. Enhanced elimination. There is no known role for enhanced elimination. The alkaloids are highly bound to muscle tissue.

Reference

Adler AG et al: Death resulting from ipecac syrup poisoning. *JAMA* 1980;**243:**1927.

IRON
Olga F. Woo, PharmD

ANTIDOTE   IPECAC   LAVAGE   CHARCOAL

Iron is widely used for treatment of anemia, for prenatal supplementation, and as a common daily vitamin supplement. Because of its wide availability (often in large nonchildproof containers) and its presumed innocence as a common over-the-counter product, it remains one of the most common childhood ingestions. Fortunately, since discovery of the antidote deferoxamine, death from iron poisoning has declined markedly. There are many different iron preparations, containing various amounts of iron salts. Most children's preparations contain 15–18 mg of elemental iron per dose, and most adult preparations contain 60–90 mg of elemental iron per dose.

I. Mechanism of toxicity. Toxicity is due to direct corrosive effects and cellular toxicity.

A. Iron has a direct **corrosive effect** on mucosal tissue and may cause hemorrhagic necrosis and perforation. Fluid loss from the gastrointestinal tract results in severe hypovolemia.

B. Absorbed iron (in excess of the iron-binding capacity) is distributed to tissues and causes cellular dysfunction, resulting in lactic acidosis and necrosis. The exact mechanism for cellular toxicity is not known.

II. Toxic dose. The acute lethal dose in animal studies is 150–200 mg/kg of elemental iron. The lowest reported lethal dose in a child was 600 mg. Symptoms are unlikely if less than 20–30 mg/kg of elemental iron has been ingested. Ingestion of more than 40 mg/kg is considered potentially serious and more than 60 mg/kg potentially lethal.

III. Clinical presentation. The manifestations of poisoning are usually described in 4 stages.

A. Shortly after ingestion, the corrosive effects of iron cause vomiting and diarrhea, often bloody. Massive fluid or blood loss into the gastrointestinal tract may result in shock, renal failure, and death.

B. Victims who survive this phase may experience a latent period of apparent improvement over 12 hours.

C. This may be followed by an abrupt relapse, with coma, shock, seizures, consumptive coagulopathy, hepatic failure, and death. *Yersinia enterocolitica* sepsis may occur.

D. If the victim survives, scarring from the initial corrosive injury may result in pyloric stricture or other intestinal obstruction.

IV. Diagnosis. Diagnosis is based on a history of exposure and the presence of vomiting, diarrhea, hypotension, and other clinical signs. Elevation of the white blood count (> 15,000) or blood glucose (> 150 mg/dL) or visible radiopaque pills on abdominal x-ray also suggest significant ingestion. Serious toxicity is very unlikely if the white count, glucose, and x-ray are normal and there is no spontaneous vomiting or diarrhea.

A. Specific levels. If the total serum iron level is higher than 450–500 mcg/dL or higher than the total iron-binding capacity (TIBC), then toxicity is likely to develop. Serum levels higher than 800–1000 mcg/dL are nearly always associated with severe poisoning. Determine the serum iron level at 4–6 hours after ingestion, and repeat determinations after 8–12 hours to rule out delayed absorption (eg, from a sustained-release tablet or a tablet bezoar).

B. Other useful laboratory studies. CBC, electrolytes, glucose, BUN, creatinine, liver function tests, abdominal x-ray.

V. Treatment. Patients who have self-limited mild gastrointestinal symptoms or who remain asymptomatic for 6 hours are unlikely to develop serious intoxication. On the other hand, those few with serious ingestion must be promptly and aggressively managed.

A. Emergency and supportive measures

   1. Maintain the airway and assist ventilation if necessary (see p 2).

   2. Treat shock caused by hemorrhagic gastroenteritis aggressively with intravenous crystalloid fluids (p 14), and replace blood if needed.

   3. Treat coma (p 17), seizures (p 21), and metabolic acidosis (p 30) if they occur.

B. Specific treatment. For seriously intoxicated victims (ie, shock, acidosis, serum iron greater than 500 μg/dL), administer **deferoxamine** (see p 301). Monitor the urine for the characteristic orange or pink-red ("vin rose") color of the chelated deferoxamine-iron complex. Therapy may be stopped when the urine color returns to normal or when the serum iron level decreases to the normal range.

   1. The intravenous route is preferred: give 10–15 mg/kg/h by constant infusion; faster rates (up to 45 mg/kg/h) have been reportedly well tolerated in single cases, but rapid boluses usually cause hypotension. The recommended maximum daily dose is 6 g, but larger amounts have been safely given in massive iron overdose.

   2. Deferoxamine has also been given intramuscularly, for example as a test dose in patients with mild symptoms (the usual dose is 50 mg/kg, maximum 1 g). However, hypotension can also occur with the intramuscular route, and this route is not recommended.

C. Decontamination

   1. Induce emesis or perform gastric lavage (see p 42).

   2. Obtain an abdominal x-ray to determine if radiopaque tablets persist after initial emesis or lavage; if so, repeat gastric lavage using a 2% bicarbonate solution to a total volume of 500–1000 mL. Leave 50–100 mL in the stomach.

   3. Do not use phosphate-containing solutions for lavage; these may result in fatal hypernatremia, hyperphosphatemia, and hypocalcemia.

4. Deferoxamine lavage is of doubtful efficacy and may actually enhance toxicity by promoting absorption.
5. **Activated charcoal does not adsorb iron** and is not recommended unless other drugs have been ingested.
6. Massive ingestions may result in tablet concretions or bezoars. Repeated saline lavage, cathartics, or whole gut lavage (see p 46) may remove the tablets, but occasionally endoscopy or even surgical gastrotomy is required.

D. Enhanced elimination
1. Hemodialysis and hemoperfusion are not effective at removing iron but may be necessary to remove deferoxamine-iron complex in patients with renal failure.
2. **Exchange transfusion** is occasionally employed for massive pediatric ingestion but is of questionable efficacy.

Reference

Lacouture PG et al: Emergency assessment of severity in iron overdose by clinical and laboratory methods. *J Pediatr* 1981;**99**:89.

ISOCYANATES
Paul D. Blanc, MD

ANTIDOTE   IPECAC   LAVAGE   CHARCOAL

Toluene diisocyanate (TDI) and related chemicals are industrial components in the polymerization of urethane coatings and insulation materials. Most 2-part urethane products contain some amount of one of these chemicals. **Methylene isocyanate** (the toxin released in the Bhopal, India, tragedy) is a carbamate insecticide precursor; it is not used in urethanes, has actions different from those of the TDI group of chemicals, and is not discussed here (see Table IV-12).

I. **Mechanism of toxicity.** Toluene diisocyanate and related isocyanates act as irritants and sensitizers at very low concentrations. The mechanism is poorly understood, but it is thought that they act as haptens. Once a person is sensitized to one isocyanate, cross-reactivity to others may occur.

II. **Toxic dose.** The OSHA workplace short-term exposure limit (STEL) for TDI is 0.02 ppm, with a permissible exposure limit (PEL) of 0.005 ppm as an 8-hour time-weighted average. This exposure limit seeks to prevent acute irritant effects. However, in individuals with prior TDI sensitivity, even this level may be hazardous. The level considered immediately dangerous to life or health is 10 ppm.

III. **Clinical presentation**
A. **Acute exposure** to irritant levels causes skin and upper respiratory tract toxicity. Burning eyes and skin, cough, and wheezing are common. Noncardiogenic pulmonary edema may occur with severe exposure. Symptoms may occur immediately with exposure or may occasionally be delayed several hours.
B. **Low-level chronic exposure** may produce dyspnea and wheezing, often diagnosed as asthma.

IV. **Diagnosis.** Diagnosis requires a careful occupational history. Pulmonary function testing may document obstructive lung disease or histamine reactivity.

A. **Specific levels.** There are no specific blood or urine tests for isocyanates.
   1. Test inhalation challenge to isocyanate is not advised except in experienced laboratories owing to the danger of severe asthma attack.
   2. Isocyanate antibody testing, although useful epidemiologically, is difficult to interpret in an individual patient.
B. **Other useful laboratory studies.** Arterial blood gases, chest x-ray, pulmonary function tests.
V. **Treatment**
   A. **Emergency and supportive measures**
      1. After acute inhalational exposure, maintain the airway (see p 2), give bronchodilators as needed for wheezing (p 8), and observe for 8–12 hours for pulmonary edema (p 7).
      2. When airway hyperreactivity has been documented, further exposure to isocyanate is contraindicated. Involve public health or OSHA agencies to determine if other workers are at risk.
   B. **Specific drugs and antidotes.** There is no specific antidote.
   C. **Decontamination**
      1. **Inhalation.** Remove the victim from exposure, and give supplemental oxygen if available.
      2. **Skin and eyes.** Remove contaminated clothing, and wash exposed skin with copious soap and water. Irrigate exposed eyes with copious saline or tepid water (see p 40).
   D. **Enhanced elimination.** There is no role for these procedures.

Reference

Chan-Yeung M, Lam S: Occupational asthma. *Am Rev Respir Dis* 1986;**133**:686.

ISONIAZID (INH)
Christopher R. Brown, MD

ANTIDOTE   IPECAC   LAVAGE   CHARCOAL

Isoniazid (INH), a hydrazide derivative of isonicotinic acid, is the bactericidal drug of choice for tuberculosis. INH is well known for its propensity to cause hepatitis with chronic use. Acute isoniazid overdose is a common cause of drug-induced seizures and metabolic acidosis.

I. **Mechanism of toxicity**
   A. **Acute overdose.** Isoniazid produces acute toxic effects by competing with brain pyridoxal 5-phosphate, the active form of vitamin B_6, for the enzyme glutamic acid decarboxylase. This results in lower levels of gamma-aminobutyric acid (GABA), an inhibitory neurotransmitter in the brain, which leads to uninhibited electrical activity manifested as seizures. INH also inhibits the hepatic conversion of lactate to pyruvate, resulting in lactic acidosis. Peripheral neuritis with chronic use is thought to be related to competition with pyridoxine.
   B. **Chronic toxicity.** The mechanism of chronic hepatic injury and INH-induced systemic lupus erythematosus (SLE) is not discussed here.
II. **Toxic dose**
   A. **Acute ingestion** of as little as 1.5 g can produce toxicity. Severe toxicity is common after ingestion of 80–150 mg/kg.
   B. With **chronic use,** 10–20% of patients will develop hepatic toxicity when the dose is 10 mg/kg/d, but less than 2% will develop this toxicity if the dose is 3–5 mg/kg/d. Older persons are more susceptible to chronic toxicity.

III. Clinical presentation
   A. After **acute overdose,** slurred speech, ataxia, coma, and seizures may occur rapidly (usually within 30–60 minutes). Profound anion gap metabolic acidosis (pH 6.8–6.9) often occurs after only one or 2 seizures, probably owing to muscle release of lactic acid. This usually clears slowly even after the seizure activity is controlled. Hemolysis may occur in patients with glucose-6-phosphate dehydrogenase (G6PD) deficiency.
   B. Chronic therapeutic INH use may cause peripheral neuritis, hepatitis, hypersensitivity reactions including drug-induced lupus erythematosus, and pyridoxine deficiency.

IV. Diagnosis.
The diagnosis is usually made by history and clinical presentation. INH should be considered in any patient with acute onset seizures, especially when accompanied by profound metabolic acidosis.
   A. Specific levels. Isoniazid is not usually detected in routine toxicology screening. A 5-mg/kg dose produces a peak INH concentration of 3 mg/L at 1 hour. Serum levels higher than 30 mg/L are associated with acute toxicity.
   B. Other useful laboratory studies. CBC, electrolytes, glucose, BUN, creatinine, liver function tests, arterial blood gases.

V. Treatment
   A. Emergency and supportive measures
   1. Maintain the airway and assist ventilation if necessary (see p 2).
   2. Treat coma (p 17), seizures (p 21), and metabolic acidosis (p 30) if they occur. Diazepam, 0.1–0.2 mg/kg IV, is usually effective for treatment of seizures.
   B. Specific drugs and antidotes. Pyridoxine (vitamin B) is a specific antidote and usually terminates diazepam-resistant seizures. Administer pyridoxine, 5 g IV (see p 339), if the amount of INH ingested is not known; if the amount is known, give an equivalent amount in grams of pyridoxine to grams of ingested INH. If no pyridoxine is available, high-dose diazepam (0.3–0.4 mg/kg) may be effective for status epilepticus. Pyridoxine treatment may also hasten the resolution of metabolic acidosis.
   C. Decontamination
   1. Perform gastric lavage (see p 43). Do **not** induce emesis because of the risk of rapid onset of coma and seizures.
   2. Administer activated charcoal and cathartic (see p 45).
   3. Gut emptying is probably not necessary following small ingestions if activated charcoal is given promptly.
   D. Enhanced elimination. The volume of distribution of INH is 0.6 L/kg, and forced diuresis and dialysis have been reported to be successful. There is probably no role for enhanced elimination because the half-life of INH is relatively short (1–5 hours, depending on acetylator status), and toxicity can usually be easily managed with pyridoxine or diazepam.

Reference

Wason S, Lacouture PG, Lovejoy FH Jr: Single high-dose pyridoxine treatment for isoniazid overdose. *JAMA* 1981;**246**:1102.

ISOPROPYL ALCOHOL
Kent R. Olson, MD

ANTIDOTE   IPECAC   LAVAGE   CHARCOAL

Isopropyl alcohol is widely used as a solvent, an antiseptic, and a disinfectant and is commonly available in the home as a 70% solution (rubbing alcohol). It is commonly ingested by alcoholics as a cheap substitute for liquor. Unlike the other common alcohol substitutes methanol and ethylene glycol, isopropyl alcohol is not metabolized to highly toxic organic acids.

I. **Mechanism of toxicity**
   A. Isopropyl alcohol is a potent depressant of the central nervous system, and intoxication by ingestion or inhalation may result in coma and respiratory arrest. It is metabolized to acetone, which may contribute to and prolong central nervous system depression.
   B. Very large doses of isopropyl alcohol may cause hypotension secondary to vasodilation and possibly myocardial depression.
   C. Isopropyl alcohol is irritating to the gastrointestinal tract and commonly causes gastritis.

II. **Toxic dose.** Isopropyl alcohol is approximately twice as potent a central nervous system depressant as ethanol.
   A. **Ingestion.** The toxic oral dose is about 0.5–1 mL/kg of rubbing alcohol (70% isopropyl alcohol) but varies depending on individual tolerance and whether any other depressants were ingested. Fatalities have occurred after adult ingestion of 240 mL, but patients with up to 1-L ingestions have recovered with supportive care.
   B. **Inhalation.** The OSHA permissible exposure limit (PEL) for isopropyl alcohol vapor is 400 ppm (980 mg/m^3) as an 8-hour time-weighted average. The air level considered immediately dangerous to life or health (IDLH) is 20,000 ppm. Toxicity has been reported in children after isopropyl alcohol sponge baths, probably due to a combination of inhalation and skin absorption.

III. **Clinical presentation.** Intoxication mimics drunkenness due to ethanol, with slurred speech, ataxia, and stupor followed in large ingestions by coma, hypotension, and respiratory arrest. Because of the gastric irritant properties of isopropyl alcohol, abdominal pain and vomiting are common, and hematemesis occasionally occurs. Isopropyl alcohol is metabolized to acetone, which contributes to central nervous system depression and gives a distinct odor to the breath. Metabolic acidosis may occur but is usually mild. The osmolar gap is elevated. Children are especially prone to hypoglycemia.

IV. **Diagnosis.** The diagnosis is usually based on a history of ingestion and the presence of an elevated osmolar gap (see p 29), the absence of severe acidosis, and the characteristic smell of isopropyl alcohol or its metabolite acetone.
   A. **Specific levels.** Serum isopropyl alcohol levels are usually available through commercial toxicology laboratories. The serum level may also be estimated by calculating the osmolar gap (see p 29). Isopropyl alcohol levels higher than 150 mg/dL usually cause coma, but patients with levels up to 560 mg/dL have survived with supportive care and dialysis. Serum acetone concentrations may be elevated.
   B. **Other useful laboratory studies.** CBC, electrolytes, glucose, BUN, creatinine, serum osmolality and osmolar gap, arterial blood gases.

V. **Treatment**
   A. **Emergency and supportive measures**
      1. Maintain the airway and assist ventilation if necessary (see p 2).
      2. Treat coma (p 17), hypotension (p 14), and hypoglycemia (p 31) if they occur.
      3. Admit and observe symptomatic patients for at least 6–12 hours.
   B. **Specific drugs and antidotes.** There is no specific antidote. Ethanol therapy is **not** indicated because isopropyl alcohol does not produce a toxic organic acid metabolite.
   C. **Decontamination.** Because isopropyl alcohol is rapidly absorbed after ingestion, gastric emptying procedures are not likely to be useful if the

ingestion is small (a few swallows) or if more than 30 minutes has passed. For large ingestions:

1. Perform gastric lavage (see p 43). Do *not* induce emesis because of the risk of rapidly developing coma.
2. Administer activated charcoal and cathartic (see p 45); although isopropyl alcohol adsorbs poorly to charcoal, approximately 1 g of charcoal will bind 1 mL of 70% alcohol.

D. Enhanced elimination. Hemodialysis effectively removes isopropyl alcohol and acetone but is rarely indicated because the majority of patients can be managed with supportive care alone. **Dialysis** is indicated when levels are extremely high (eg, > 500–600 mg/dL) or if hypotension does not respond to fluids and vasopressors. Hemoperfusion, repeat-dose charcoal, and forced diuresis are not effective.

Reference

Lacouture PG et al: Acute isopropyl alcohol intoxication: Diagnosis and management. *Am J Med* 1983;**75**:680.

JELLYFISH AND OTHER CNIDARIA
Howard E. McKinney, PharmD

ANTIDOTE   IPECAC   LAVAGE   CHARCOAL

The large phylum Cnidaria (coelenterates) includes **fire coral, Portuguese man-of-war, box jellyfish, sea wasps, sea nettle, and anemones.** Despite considerable morphologic variation, all these organisms have venom contained in microscopic balloonlike structures called **nematocysts.**

I. **Mechanism of toxicity.** Each nematocyst contains a small ejectable thread soaking in viscous venom. The thread has a barb on the tip and is fired from the nematocyst with enough velocity to pierce human skin. The nematocysts are contained in outer sacs (cnidoblasts) arranged along the tentacles stretched out in the water beneath the body of the jellyfish or along the surface of fire coral and the fingerlike projections of sea anemones. When the cnidoblasts are opened by hydrostatic pressure, physical contact, changes in osmolarity, or chemical stimulants as yet unidentified, they release their nematocysts, which eject the thread and spread venom along and into the skin of the victim. The venom contains numerous chemical components, including serotonin, hyaluronidases, and neurotoxins.

II. **Toxic dose.** Each time a nematocyst is opened, all the contained venom is released. The degree of effect will depend on the number of nematocysts that successfully discharge venom onto and into the victim's skin. Hundreds of thousands of nematocysts may be discharged with a single exposure.

III. **Clinical presentation**

A. Immediately upon nematocyst discharge, there is stinging, burning pain and a pruritic rash. Depending on the degree of envenomation, there may follow paresthesias, anaphylactoid symptoms, hypotension, muscle spasm, local edema and hemolysis, desquamation, chills, fever, nausea, vomiting, abdominal pain, myalgias, arthralgias, headache, dysphonia, ataxia, paralysis, coma, seizures, and cardiac arrhythmias. Lethal outcomes from box jellyfish envenomation are associated with rapid onset of cardiovascular collapse.

B. Potentially severe long-lasting effects include erythema multiforme, keloids, infections, cosmetic tissue damage (fat atrophy, pigmentation), contractures, paresthesias, neuritis, and paralysis.

IV. Diagnosis. Diagnosis is based on the history and observation of characteristic lines of inflammation along the sites of exposure ("tentacle tracks").

    A. Specific levels. Specific toxin levels are not available.

    B. Other useful laboratory studies. CBC, electrolytes, glucose, BUN, creatinine, creatine phosphokinase (CPK), ECG.

V. Treatment. Symptomatic care is sufficient for the majority of envenomations, even that of the box jellyfish.

    A. Emergency and supportive measures

        1. Maintain the airway and assist ventilation if necessary (see p 2). Administer supplemental oxygen.

        2. Treat hypotension (p 14), arrhythmias (p 9), coma (p 17), and seizures (p 21) if they occur.

    B. Specific drugs and antidotes. Box jellyfish antivenin from Australia terminates acute pain and cardiovascular symptoms, prevents tissue effects, and can be located by a regional poison control center (see Table I–41) for use in severe cases. Local marine biologists can help identify indigenous species for planning of specific therapy.

    C. Decontamination. Avoid thrashing about, scratching, scraping, or other mechanical maneuvers that may break open the nematocysts. **Do not use fresh water** to wash affected areas because it will cause nematocysts to be instantly discharged. Use vinegar or baking soda as described below; symptoms will not be relieved by these procedures, but they will allow careful removal of tentacles with forceps followed by shaving of the area to remove the undischarged nematocysts.

        1. For most cnidarian envenomations, spray or flood the affected area with **vinegar** for 30 seconds to disarm nematocysts.

        2. However, for *Chrysora quinquecirrha* (American sea nettle), *Pelagia noctiluca* (little mauve stinger jellyfish), and *Cyanea captillata* (hair jellyfish), **do not apply vinegar** because it may precipitate firing in these species; instead, apply a slurry of **baking soda.**

    D. Enhanced elimination. These procedures are not applicable.

Reference

Burnett JW, Calton GJ: Jellyfish envenomation syndromes updated. *Ann Emerg Med* 1987;**16**:1000.

LEAD

Kent R. Olson, MD, and
Bruce Bernard, MD

    ANTIDOTE   IPECAC   LAVAGE   CHARCOAL

Lead is a heavy metal that is found in all animal species but serves no useful physiologic purpose. Lead is widely distributed in the earth's crust and is found in a variety of products, including storage batteries, solder, electric cable insulation, bootleg whiskey, paints, pottery and ceramic glazes, water from lead pipes, and leaded gasoline.

In children, exposure occurs most commonly after repeated ingestion of house dust or paint chips containing lead salts. In adults, exposure is usually by inhalation and may occur occupationally (eg, welding, battery factories, radiator repair shops, metal smelting) or while heat-stripping or sanding paint from old houses. Exposure may also occur from use of lead-glazed pottery for cooking and eating.

    I. Mechanism of toxicity. Lead displaces other metals (eg, iron, zinc, copper) from normal binding sites to produce some of its biochemical effects (eg, interruption of heme synthesis). In addition, lead binds to sulfhydryl groups and disrupts cellular function. The primary organ systems affected are the nervous system, the kidneys, and the reproductive and hematopoietic systems.

II. **Toxic dose.** Elemental **(metallic) lead** is poorly absorbed after ingestion but when heated is vaporized to a fume that is well absorbed. **Lead salts** are better absorbed, but most products contain a relatively small percentage of lead and toxicity usually occurs only after chronic, repeated exposure. **Organic lead** compounds (eg, tetraethyl lead in gasoline) are well absorbed by inhalation as well as ingestion.

   A. **Ingestion.** Toxicity is rare after a single exposure, although intoxication has been reported after ingestion of several grams of lead acetate or tetraethyl lead or from lead curtain or fishing weights that remained in the intestinal tract for several days. Accumulation and toxicity are likely to occur when more than 0.5 mg/d is absorbed for several days.

   B. **Inhalation.** The OSHA permissible exposure limit (PEL) for airborne elemental lead fumes and dusts of inorganic lead compounds is 0.05 mg/m^3 as an 8-hour time-weighted average. For organic lead (tetraethyl or tetramethyl lead), the PEL is 0.075 mg/m^3.

III. **Clinical presentation**

   A. **Acute ingestion** of a very large amount of lead may cause abdominal pain, vomiting, and diarrhea.

   B. **Chronic intoxication** produces abdominal colic, constipation, anorexia, headache, irritability, and fatigue. Microcytic anemia (with or without basophilic stippling) may be found, although normocytic anemia is more common. Peripheral motor neuropathy (wrist- or footdrop) may occur.

   C. **Encephalopathy** is characterized by ataxia, delirium, coma, and convulsions; is more common in children; and represents a life-threatening emergency.

   D. Repeated intentional **inhalation of leaded gasoline** may cause ataxia, myoclonic jerking, delirium, and convulsions.

IV. **Diagnosis.** Lead poisoning may be difficult to diagnose because poisoned patients usually present with nonspecific gastrointestinal symptoms, and exposure is often not suspected. Consider lead poisoning in any patient with microcytic anemia, abdominal complaints, or neuropathy; or in any child with delirium or convulsions. X-rays of the abdomen may reveal radiopaque flecks of paint, and x-rays of the long bones may demonstrate lead lines (premature opacification of distal long bones) in children.

   A. **Specific levels.** There are a variety of tests that can be performed to determine the presence of lead. The **whole blood lead level** is the best indicator of cumulative exposure, although it may be misleadingly high soon after exposure before equilibration with tissues occurs.

      1. Blood lead levels below 25 mcg/dL are usually associated with no demonstrable toxic effects, although recent reports suggest the possibility of altered neural development and behavior in children at lower levels.

      2. Chronic levels of 25–50 mcg/dL may be associated with renal abnormalities and decreased nerve conduction velocity.

      3. With levels of 50–70 mcg/dL, gastrointestinal symptoms, anemia, and other hematologic effects are often seen.

      4. With chronic levels above 70 mcg/dL, serious intoxication may occur. Encephalopathy is unlikely with levels below 100 mcg/dL.

   B. Urinary **lead mobilization** by EDTA (calcium disodium EDTA; see p 308) may provide a useful measure of total body burden. The EDTA mobilization test is performed as follows: Administer 20–25 mg/kg (500 mg/m^2) EDTA in 100 mL 5% dextrose by intravenous infusion over 1 hour, then measure urinary lead excretion over the next 8 hours. A lead excretion ratio (excreted lead [in mcg] divided by the dose of EDTA [in mg]) of more than 0.6 is considered positive.

C. The **free erythrocyte protoporphyrin (FEP) or zinc protoporphyrin (ZPP) tests,** which reflect lead-induced inhibition of heme synthesis, are inexpensive, sensitive tests suitable for screening for chronic exposure. However, the FEP or ZPP may also be elevated with iron deficiency anemia. Also, the FEP and ZPP will not be elevated until a few weeks after a single acute exposure.

V. Treatment
A. Emergency and supportive measures
1. In most adult cases, patients do not present with acute life-threatening symptoms.
2. However, in children with delirium or encephalopathy, monitor closely and treat seizures (see p 21) and coma (see p 17) if they occur. Provide adequate fluids to maintain urine flow but avoid overhydration, which may aggravate encephalopathy.

B. Specific drugs and antidotes. The indications for **chelation therapy** and the choice of agents depend on the blood level and the patient's clinical status (Table II–28).
1. Although there is limited evidence for effectiveness of **BAL** (dimercaprol; see p 294), most experts recommend that patients with encephalopathy and all patients with blood lead levels higher than 70 mcg/dL receive BAL along with **EDTA** (p 308). BAL is given first because of suspicion that EDTA alone in the presence of high lead levels may increase lead toxicity.
2. Other symptomatic patients and asymptomatic patients with elevated blood lead levels between 55–69 mcg/dL or with positive urinary mobilization tests may be treated with **EDTA** alone.
3. An alternative therapy for asymptomatic patients and for follow-up treatment of symptomatic patients is **oral penicillamine** (p 332). DMSA (p 306), another promising new chelating agent effective by the oral and parenteral routes, is currently undergoing experimental study.

C. Decontamination
1. **Acute ingestion.** A single ingestion of lead-containing paint or gasoline does not require gastric decontamination because the amount of lead is very small.

TABLE II–28. TREATMENT OF LEAD POISONING[a]

Clinical Presentation	Treatment[b]
Acute encephalopathy	BAL, 75 mg/m.^{2} (approximately 3–5 mg/kg) IM every 4 hours; after 4 hours start EDTA, 1500 mg/m^2/d (60–75 mg/kg/d) as continuous IV infusion. Treat for 5 days, then wait 48 hours. Repeat 5-day course if lead level remains > 50 mcg/dL.
Other symptoms, or asymptomatic with lead level > 70 mcg/dL	BAL, 50 mg/m.^{2} (approximately 2–4 mg/kg) IM every 4 hours; after 4 hours start EDTA, 1000 mg/m^2/d (35–50 mg/kg/d) as continuous IV infusion. Treat for 5 days, then wait 48 hours. Repeat 5-day course if lead level remains > 50 mcg/dL.
Asymptomatic with lead level of 56–69 mcg/dL or positive EDTA mobilization test	EDTA alone, 1000 mg/m.^{2}/d (35–50 mg/kg/d) as continuous IV infusion for 5 days.

[a] Reference: Piomelli S et al: Management of childhood lead poisoning. *J Pediatr* 1984;**105**:523.
[b] See BAL, p 294; and EDTA, p 308. *Note:* EDTA is usually diluted to 0.5% in dextrose or saline for IV infusion. It may also be given IM if fluid overload is a concern.

      a. After ingestion of a very large dose (eg, > 1 g) of a lead salt or organic lead compound, induce emesis or perform gastric lavage (see p 42) and administer activated charcoal and cathartic (although there is no proved efficacy for charcoal).

      b. After ingestion of a metallic lead object (fishing or curtain weight), administer activated charcoal and cathartic (see p 45).

      c. Repeated cathartics, whole gut lavage (see p 46), or enemas should be given if radiopaque material remains on x-ray.

    2. Lead-containing buckshot, shrapnel, or bullets in or adjacent to synovial spaces should be surgically removed if possible, particularly if associated with evidence of systemic lead absorption.

D. Enhanced elimination. There is no role for dialysis, hemoperfusion, or repeat-dose charcoal.

E. Other required measures

    1. Remove the patient from the source of exposure, and institute control measures at home or at work, wherever the exposure occurred, to prevent repeated intoxication; in addition, other possibly exposed persons must be immediately evaluated.

    2. Detailed federal standards for workers exposed to lead have been established and include instructions for periodic blood lead monitoring and specific guidelines for removing the worker from exposure. Workers must be removed from exposure if a single blood lead level exceeds 60 mcg/dL (or if 3 successive monthly levels exceed 50 mcg/dL) and may not return to work until the blood lead level is below 40 mcg/dL.

References

Occupational Safety and Health Administration (OSHA), Department of Labor: Lead standard. Pages 746–783 US Government Printing Office 29 CFR Chapter XVII (July 1985 ed.) 1910.1025.

Piomelli S et al: Management of childhood lead poisoning. *J Pediatr* 1984;**105**:523.

LIONFISH AND OTHER SCORPAENIDAE
Howard E. McKinney, PharmD

ANTIDOTE   IPECAC   LAVAGE   CHARCOAL

The family Scorpaenidae are saltwater fish that are mostly bottom dwellers noted for their ability to camouflage themselves and disappear into the environment. There are 30 genera and about 300 species, some 30 of which have envenomated humans. Although they were once considered to be only an occupational hazard of commercial fishing, increasing contact with these fish by scuba divers and home aquarists has increased the frequency of envenomations.

I. Mechanism of toxicity. Envenomation usually occurs when the fish is being handled or stepped on or when the aquarist has hands in the tank. The dorsal, anal, and pectoral fins are supported by spines that are connected to venom glands. The fish will erect its spines and jab the victim, causing release of venom (and often sloughing of the integumentary sheath of the spine into the wound). The venom of all these organisms is a heat-labile mixture that is not completely characterized.

II. Toxic dose. The dose of venom involved in any sting is variable. Interspecies variation in the severity of envenomation is generally the result of the relation between the venom gland and the spines.

   A. The **Synanceja (Australian stonefish)** have short, strong spines with the venom gland located near the tip; therefore, large doses of venom are delivered and severe envenomation results.

   B. The **Pterois (lionfish, turkeyfish)** have long delicate spines with poorly developed venom glands near the base of the spine and therefore are capable of delivering only small doses of venom.

III. **Clinical presentation.** Envenomation typically produces immediate onset of excruciating, sharp, throbbing, intense pain. In untreated cases, the intensity of pain peaks at 60–90 minutes and may last for 1–2 days.

   A. The severe **systemic intoxication** typically associated with stonefish envenomation is characterized by the rapid onset of hypotension, tachycardia, cardiac arrhythmias, myocardial ischemia, syncope, diaphoresis, nausea, vomiting, abdominal cramping, dyspnea, pulmonary edema, cyanosis, headache, muscular weakness, and spasticity.

   B. **Local tissue effects** include erythema, ecchymosis, and swelling. Infection may occur owing to retained integumentary sheath. Hyperalgesia, anesthesia, or paresthesias of the affected extremity may occur, and persistent neuropathy has been reported.

IV. **Diagnosis.** The diagnosis is usually based on a history of exposure, and the severity of envenomation is usually readily apparent.

   A. **Specific levels.** There are no specific toxin levels available.

   B. **Other useful laboratory studies.** CBC, electrolytes, glucose, BUN, creatinine, creatine phosphokinase (CPK), urinalysis, ECG, chest x-ray.

V. **Treatment**

   A. **Emergency and supportive measures**

     1. **After severe stonefish envenomation**

       a. Maintain the airway and assist ventilation if needed (see p 2).

       b. Treat hypotension (p 14) and arrhythmias (p 9) if they occur.

     2. **General wound care**

       a. Clean the wound carefully and remove any visible integumentary sheath. Monitor wounds for development of infection.

       b. Give tetanus prophylaxis if needed.

   B. **Specific drugs and antidotes.** Immediately immerse the extremity in **hot water** (45 °C or 113 °F) for 30–60 minutes. This should result in prompt relief of pain. For stonefish envenomations, a specific antivenin can be located by a regional poison control center (see Table I-41, p 51), but most of these cases can be successfully managed with hot water immersion and supportive symptomatic care.

   C. **Decontamination.** Decontamination procedures are not applicable.

   D. **Enhanced elimination.** There is no role for these procedures.

Reference

Kizer KW, McKinney HE, Auerbach PS: Scorpaenidae envenomation: A five-year poison center experience. *JAMA* 1985;**253**:807.

LITHIUM
Belle L. Lee, PharmD

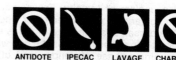

Lithium is used for the treatment of bipolar depression and other psychiatric disorders and occasionally to boost the white blood cell count in patients with leukopenia. Serious toxicity is most commonly caused by chronic overmedication in patients with renal impairment. Acute overdose, in contrast, is generally less severe.

I. **Mechanism of toxicity.** Lithium is a cation that enters cells and substitutes for sodium or potassium. Lithium is thought to stabilize cell membranes. With excessive levels, it depresses neural excitation and synaptic transmission. Entry into the brain is slow, which explains the delay between peak blood levels and central nervous system effects after acute overdose.

II. **Toxic dose.** The usual daily dose of lithium ranges from 300 to 2400 mg/d (8–64 meq/d), and the therapeutic serum lithium level is 0.6–1.2 meq/L. The toxicity of lithium depends on whether the overdose is acute or chronic.

A. **Acute ingestion** of 1 meq/kg (40 mg/kg) will produce a blood level at equilibrium of approximately 0.7 meq/L (the volume of distribution of lithium is 0.7 L/kg). Acute ingestion of more than 150–200 meq (6000–7000 mg) in an adult would potentially cause serious toxicity.

B. **Chronic intoxication** may occur in patients on stable therapeutic doses. Lithium is excreted by the kidney, where it is handled like sodium; any state that causes dehydration, sodium depletion, or excessive sodium reabsorption will result in increased lithium reabsorption, accumulation, and possibly intoxication. Common states causing lithium retention include gastroenteritis, diuretic use, and lithium-induced nephrogenic diabetes insipidus.

III. **Clinical presentation.** Mild to moderate intoxication results in lethargy, muscular weakness, slurred speech, ataxia, tremor, and myoclonic jerks. Rigidity and extrapyramidal effects may be seen. Severe intoxication may result in agitated delirium, coma, convulsions, and hyperthermia. Recovery is often very slow, and patients may remain confused or obtunded for several days to weeks. The ECG commonly shows T-wave inversions; less commonly, bradycardia and sinus node arrest may occur. The white cell count is usually elevated (15–20,000/mm^3).

A. After **acute ingestion** there may be initial mild nausea and vomiting, but systemic signs of intoxication are minimal and usually are delayed for several hours while lithium distributes into tissues. Initially high serum levels drop rapidly with tissue equilibration.

B. In contrast, patients with **chronic intoxication** usually have more serious systemic manifestations on admission and toxicity may be severe with levels only slightly above therapeutic. Typically, patients with chronic intoxication have elevated BUN and creatinine levels and other evidence of dehydration.

IV. **Diagnosis.** Lithium intoxication should be suspected in any patient with a known psychiatric history who is confused, ataxic, or tremulous.

A. **Specific levels.** The diagnosis is supported by an elevated **lithium** level.

1. Most hospital clinical laboratories can perform a stat **serum lithium** concentration. However, the serum lithium level is not an accurate predictor of toxicity.

a. With chronic poisoning, toxicity may be associated with levels only slightly above the therapeutic range.

b. On the other hand, patients with acute ingestion may have levels as high as 9.3 meq/L without signs of intoxication, owing to measurement before final tissue distribution.

2. If cerebrospinal fluid is available, a CSF **lithium** level may provide more information about brain levels: CSF lithium levels higher than 0.4 meq/L were associated in one case report with central nervous system toxicity.

3. *Note:* Specimens obtained in a green-top tube (lithium heparin) will give a markedly false elevation of the serum lithium level.

B. **Other useful laboratory studies.** CBC, electrolytes, glucose, BUN, creatinine, ECG.

V. **Treatment**

A. **Emergency and supportive measures**

1. In obtunded patients, maintain the airway and assist ventilation if necessary (see p 2).

   2. Treat coma (p 17), seizures (p 21), and hyperthermia (p 19) if they occur.
   3. In dehydrated patients, replace fluid deficits with intravenous crystalloid solutions. Initial treatment should include repletion of sodium and water with 1–2 L of normal saline (children: 10–20 mL/kg). Once fluid deficits are replaced, give hypotonic (eg, half-normal saline) solutions because continued administration of normal saline may lead to hypernatremia in patients with nephrogenic diabetes insipidus.
B. Specific drugs and antidotes. There is no specific antidote.
C. Decontamination. Decontamination measures are appropriate after acute ingestion but not chronic intoxication.
   1. Induce emesis or perform gastric lavage (see p 42).
   2. Activated charcoal (p 45) does not adsorb lithium but may be useful if other drug ingestion is suspected.
   3. Cathartics (p 45) or even whole gut lavage (p 46) may enhance gut decontamination, especially in cases involving sustained-release preparations that do not dissolve readily during the lavage procedure.
D. Enhanced elimination. Lithium is excreted exclusively by the kidney. The clearance is about 25% of the glomerular filtration rate and is reduced by sodium depletion or dehydration.
   1. Hemodialysis removes lithium effectively and is indicated for intoxicated patients with seriously abnormal mental status and for patients unable to excrete lithium renally (ie, anephric or anuric patients). The clearance with dialysis (50–100 mL/min) is only marginally better than that achieved with normal renal elimination (25–30 mL/min). Repeated and prolonged dialysis may be necessary because of slow movement of lithium out of the central nervous system.
   2. Forced diuresis only slightly increases lithium excretion compared with normal hydration and is not recommended.
   3. Hemoperfusion and repeat-dose charcoal are not effective.

Reference

Hansen HE, Amdisen A: Lithium intoxication: Report of 23 cases and review of 100 cases from the literature. *Q J Med* 1978;**47**:123.

LOMOTIL
Ilene B. Anderson, PharmD

ANTIDOTE   IPECAC   LAVAGE   CHARCOAL

Lomotil is a combination product containing diphenoxylate and atropine that is commonly prescribed for symptomatic treatment of diarrhea. Children are especially sensitive to small doses of Lomotil and may develop delayed toxicity after accidental ingestion.

   I. Mechanism of toxicity
      A. Diphenoxylate is an opioid analogue of meperidine. It is metabolized to difenoxin, which has 5 times the antidiarrheal activity of diphenoxylate. Both agents have opioid effects (see p 223) in overdose.
      B. Atropine is an anticholinergic agent (see p 71) that may contribute to lethargy and coma. It also slows drug absorption and may delay the onset of symptoms.

II. **Toxic dose.** The toxic dose of Lomotil is difficult to predict because of wide individual variability in response to drug effects and promptness of treatment. The lethal dose is unknown, but death in children has been reported after ingestion of **fewer than 5 tablets.**

III. **Clinical presentation.** Depending on the individual and the time since ingestion, manifestations may be of primarily anticholinergic or opioid intoxication.

A. Initial evaluation may reveal lethargy or agitation, flushed face, dry mucous membranes, ileus, hyperpyrexia, and tachycardia resulting from the anticholinergic effects of atropine. The pupils may be large.

B. Signs of serious opioid intoxication, such as small pupils, coma, and respiratory arrest, are often delayed for several hours after ingestion.

IV. **Diagnosis.** Diagnosis is based on the history and signs of anticholinergic or opioid intoxication.

A. **Specific levels.** Specific serum levels are not available.

B. **Other useful laboratory studies.** CBC, electrolytes, glucose, arterial blood gases (if respiratory insufficiency is suspected).

V. **Treatment**

A. **Emergency and supportive measures**
1. Maintain the airway and assist ventilation if necessary (see p 2).
2. Treat coma (p 17) and hypotension (p 14) if they occur.
3. Because of the danger of abrupt respiratory arrest, observe all children with Lomotil ingestion in an intensive care unit for 18–24 hours.

B. **Specific drugs and antidotes**
1. Administer **naloxone**, 1–2 mg IV (see p 325), to patients with lethargy, apnea, or coma. Repeated doses of naloxone may be required, because its duration of effect (2–3 hours) is much shorter than that of Lomotil.
2. There is no evidence that physostigmine (see p 336) is beneficial for this overdose, although theoretically it may reverse signs of anticholinergic poisoning.

C. **Decontamination**
1. Induce emesis or perform gastric lavage (see p 42).
2. Administer activated charcoal and cathartic (see p 45).
3. Gut emptying is probably not necessary following a very small ingestion if activated charcoal is given promptly.

D. **Enhanced elimination.** There is no role for these procedures.

Reference

Curtis JA, Goel KM: Lomotil poisoning in children. *Arch Dis Child* 1979;**54**:222.

**LYSERGIC ACID
DIETHYLAMIDE (LSD) AND
OTHER HALLUCINOGENS**
Howard E. McKinney, PharmD

ANTIDOTE   IPECAC   LAVAGE   CHARCOAL

Patients seeking medical care after self-administering mind-altering substances may have used any of a large variety of chemicals. Several of these agents are discussed elsewhere in this manual (eg, amphetamines [p 62], cocaine [p 127], phencyclidine [p 233], toluene [p 281]). The drugs discussed in this section, LSD and other hallucinogens, have recently become known as **entactogens** ("to touch within"), and several have been widely used for personal experimentation as well as clinically to facilitate psychotherapeutic interviews. Table II-29 lists some of the more common entactogens.

I. **Mechanism of toxicity.** Despite many intriguing theories and much current research, the biochemical mechanism of entactogenesis is not known. LSD and many other agents are thought to alter the activity of serotonin and dopamine in the brain. Central and peripheral sympathetic stimulation may account for some of the side effects such as anxiety, psychosis, dilated pupils, and hyperthermia.

II. **Toxic dose.** The toxic dose is highly variable depending on the agent and the circumstances (Table II-29). In general, entactogenic effects do not appear to be dose-related; therefore, increasing the dose does not intensify the desired effects. Likewise, paranoia or panic attacks may occur with any dose and depend on the surroundings and the patient's current emotional state. On the other hand, hallucinations, visual illusions, and sympathomimetic side effects are dose-related. The toxic dose may be only slightly greater than the therapeutic dose.

III. **Clinical presentation**
   A. **Mild to moderate intoxication**
      1. The person experiencing a "bad trip" is conscious, coherent, and oriented but is anxious and fearful and may display paranoid or bizarre reasoning. The patient may also be tearful, combative, or self-destructive. Delayed intermittent "flashbacks" may occur after the acute effects have worn off and are usually precipitated by use of another mind-altering drug.
      2. The person with dose-related sympathomimetic side effects may also exhibit tachycardia, mydriasis (dilated pupils), diaphoresis, bruxism, short attention span, tremor, hyperreflexia, hypertension, and fever.
   B. **Life-threatening toxicity**
      1. This is due to intense sympathomimetic stimulation and includes seizures, severe hyperthermia, hypertension, and cardiac arrhythmias. Hyperthermic patients are usually obtunded, agitated or thrashing about, diaphoretic, and hyperreflexic. Untreated, hyperthermia may result in hypotension, coagulopathy, rhabdomyolysis, and multiple organ failure (see p 19). Hyperthermia has been associated with LSD, MDA, MDMA, and PMA.
      2. Use of 2,5-dimethoxy-4-bromoamphetamine (DOB) has resulted in ergotlike vascular spasm, circulatory insufficiency, and gangrene (see pp 62 and 146).

IV. **Diagnosis.** Diagnosis is based on a history of use and the presence of signs of sympathetic stimulation. Diagnosis of hyperthermia requires a high level of suspicion and use of a thermometer that accurately measures core temperature (rectal, tympanic membrane, or esophageal probe).
   A. **Specific levels.** Serum drug levels are neither widely available nor clinically useful in emergency management. Most of the agents, including LSD, are not identified by a routine toxicology screen.
   B. **Other useful laboratory studies.** CBC, electrolytes, glucose, BUN, creatinine. In hyperthermic patients, obtain prothrombin time, creatine phosphokinase (CPK), urine for myoglobin.

V. **Treatment**
   A. **Emergency and supportive measures**
      1. For the patient with a "bad trip" or panic reaction, provide gentle reassurance and relaxation techniques in a quiet environment. Treat agitation (see p 22) or severe anxiety states with diazepam (p 302) or midazolam (p 323). Avoid use of antipsychotic agents, which may cause hypotension, lower the seizure threshold, and produce dystonic reactions.

TABLE II-29. EXAMPLES OF HALLUCINOGENS AND ENTACTOGENS

Drug or Compound	Common Name	Comments
5-Hydroxy-N,N-dimethyltryptamine	Bufotenine	From skin secretions of the toad *Bufo vulgaris*.
N,N-dimethyltryptamine	DMT	"Businessman's trip"; short duration (30–60 minutes).
2,5-Dimethoxy-4-bromo-amphetamine[a]	DOB	Potent ergotlike vascular spasm may result in ischemia, gangrene.
2,5-Dimethoxy-4-methyl-amphetamine[a]	DOM, STP	Potent sympathomimetic.
4,9-Dihydro-7-methoxy-1-methyl-3-pyrido(3,4)-indole	Harmaline	South American drink yage or ayahuasca.
Lysergic acid diethylamide	LSD, acid	Potent hallucinogen. Average dose 50–150 mcg.
n-Methyl-1-(1,3-benzodioxol-5-yl)-2-butanamine	MBDB	Nearly pure entactogen without hallucinosis or sympathomimetic stimulation.
3,4-Methylenedioxy-amphetamine[a]	MDA	Potent sympathomimetic. Several hyperthermic deaths reported.
3-4-Methylenedioxy-methamphetamine[a]	MDMA, ecstasy, Adam	Sympathomimetic; hyperthermia reported.
3,4-Methylenedioxy-n-ethylamphetamine[a]	MDE, Eve	
3,4,5-Trimethoxyphenethylamine	Mescaline	Derived from peyote cactus.
3-Methoxy-4,5-methylene-dioxyallylbenzene	Myristicin, nutmeg	
p-Methoxyamphetamine[a]	PMA	
4-Phosphoryloxy-N-N-dimethyltryptamine	Psilocybin	From *Psilocybe* mushrooms.

[a]Amphetamine derivatives. See also p 62.

2. Treat seizures (p 21), hyperthermia (p 19), rhabdomyolysis (p 24), hypertension (p 16), and cardiac arrhythmias (p 9) if they occur.

B. Specific drugs and antidotes. There are no specific antidotes. Sedating doses of **diazepam** (2–10 mg) may alleviate anxiety, and hypnotic doses (10–20 mg) can induce sleep for the duration of the "trip" (usually 4–10 hours).

C. Decontamination. Most entactogens are taken orally in small doses.
  1. Do *not* induce emesis, because it is relatively ineffective and is likely to aggravate psychologic distress. Gastric lavage should be performed *only* if a significant quantity (eg, massive intentional overdose) has been ingested within the last 30–60 minutes.
  2. Administer activated charcoal (see p 45) to bind remaining drug in the gut.

D. Enhanced elimination. These procedures are not useful. Although urinary acidification may increase the urine concentration of some agents, it does not significantly enhance total body elimination and it may aggravate myoglobinuric renal failure.

Reference

Strassman RJ: Adverse reactions to psychedelic drugs: A review of the literature. *J Nerv Ment Dis* 1984;**172**:577.

MAGNESIUM
James F. Buchanan, PharmD

ANTIDOTE   IPECAC   LAVAGE   CHARCOAL

Magnesium (Mg) is a divalent cation required for a variety of enzymatic reactions involving protein synthesis and carbohydrate metabolism. It is also an essential ion for proper neuromuscular functioning.

I. Mechanism of toxicity. Elevated serum magnesium concentrations impair neuromuscular electrical function; the exact mechanism is unknown. Large amounts of orally administered magnesium cause diarrhea that can result in major fluid and electrolyte losses. Excess magnesium is usually rapidly excreted by the kidneys; therefore, intoxication usually occurs only in patients with preexisting renal insufficiency.

II. Toxic dose. Although magnesium is usually poorly absorbed (50%) and any excess absorbed magnesium is rapidly excreted, acute ingestion of very large amounts, especially by patients with renal insufficiency, may cause significant elevation of the serum level.

III. Clinical presentation. Lethargy, weakness, and decreased deep tendon reflexes occur with levels higher than 4 meq/L. With levels higher than 10 meq/L, complete loss of deep tendon reflexes, hypotension, bradycardia, conduction abnormalities, and respiratory arrest may occur. The serum osmolality and osmolar gap may be elevated.

IV. Diagnosis. Because magnesium intoxication occurs mainly in patients with renal insufficiency who are receiving magnesium-containing cathartics or antacids, clinicians should be alert to development of weakness or hyporeflexia in such patients.

  A. Specific levels. Serum magnesium concentration is usually rapidly available. The normal range is 1.5–2.2 meq/L.

  B. Other useful laboratory studies. CBC, electrolytes, BUN, creatinine, serum osmolality and osmolar gap, calcium, ECG.

V. Treatment

  A. Emergency and supportive measures

    1. Maintain the airway and assist ventilation if necessary (see p 2).
    2. Replace fluid and electrolyte losses caused by excessive catharsis.
    3. Treat hypotension with intravenous fluids and dopamine (see p 14).
  B. Specific drugs and antidotes. There is no specific antidote. Administration of intravenous **calcium** (see p 298) may temporarily alleviate respiratory depression.
  C. Decontamination
    1. After acute massive ingestion, induce emesis or perform gastric lavage.
    2. Do *not* administer activated charcoal or cathartic.
  D. Enhanced elimination
    1. Hemodialysis rapidly removes magnesium and is the only route of elimination in anuric patients.
    2. Hemoperfusion and repeat-dose charcoal are not effective.

Reference

Ferdinandus J, Pederson JA, Whang R: Hypermagnesemia as a cause of refractory hypotension, respiratory depression, and coma. *Arch Intern Med* 1981;**141**:669.

MANGANESE
Paul D. Blanc, MD

ANTIDOTE   IPECAC   LAVAGE   CHARCOAL

Manganese (Mn) intoxication is generally due to chronic rather than acute exposure. Sources of exposure are almost universally industrial—mining, metal working, foundries, and welding.

  I. Mechanism of toxicity. The precise mechanism is not known. The central nervous system is the target organ, and enzymatic inhibition leading to neurotransmitter imbalance is suspected.
  II. Toxic dose. The primary route of exposure is inhalation; manganese is poorly absorbed from the gastrointestinal tract. The OSHA workplace permissible exposure limit (PEL) for manganese dusts is 5 mg/m^3. The air level considered to be immediately dangerous to life or health (IDLH) is 10,000 ppm.
  III. Clinical presentation. Acute high-level manganese inhalation can produce an irritant-type pneumonitis (see p 163). More typically, toxicity occurs after chronic exposure to low levels over months or years. The patient usually presents with an affective psychiatric disorder, frequently misdiagnosed as schizophrenia or atypical psychosis. Organic signs of neurologic toxicity, such as parkinsonism or other extrapyramidal movement disorders, usually appear later, some time after a primarily psychiatric presentation.
  IV. Diagnosis. Diagnosis depends on a thorough occupational and psychiatric history.
    A. Specific levels. Testing of whole blood, serum, or urine may be performed, but the results should be interpreted with caution, as they may not correlate with clinical effects.
      1. Elevated urine manganese concentrations (> 25 mcg/L) may confirm recent acute exposure. Chelation challenge does not have a role in diagnosis.
      2. Hair and nail levels are not useful.
    B. Other useful laboratory studies. Arterial blood gases, chest x-ray (after inhalation exposure).

V. Treatment

A. Emergency and supportive measures

1. **Acute inhalation.** Administer supplemental oxygen. Treat broncho-spasm (see p 8) and noncardiogenic pulmonary edema (see p 7) if they occur.

2. **Chronic intoxication.** Psychiatric and neurologic effects are treated with the usual psychiatric and antiparkinsonian drugs.

B. Specific drugs and antidotes. EDTA and other chelators have **not** been proved effective after chronic neurologic damage has occurred. The efficacy of chelators early after acute exposure has not been studied.

C. Decontamination

1. **Acute inhalation.** Remove victim from exposure and give supplemental oxygen, if available.

2. **Ingestion.** Because manganese is so poorly absorbed from the gastrointestinal tract, gut decontamination is probably not necessary. Give activated charcoal (see p 45) for large overdoses.

D. Enhanced elimination. There is no role for dialysis or hemoperfusion.

Reference

Chandra SV: Psychiatric illness due to manganese poisoning. *Acta Psychiatr Scand (Suppl)* 1983;**303**:49.

MARIJUANA
Neal L. Benowitz, MD

ANTIDOTE   IPECAC   LAVAGE   CHARCOAL

Marijuana consists of the leaves and flowering parts of the plant cannabis sativa and is usually smoked in cigarettes ("joints" or "reefers") or pipes or added to food (usually cookies or brownies). Resin from the plant may be dried and compressed into blocks called hashish. Marijuana contains a number of cannabinoids; the primary psychoactive one is delta-9-tetrahydrocannabinol (THC). THC is also available in capsule form as an experimental treatment for emesis associated with cancer chemotherapy and for glaucoma.

I. Mechanism of toxicity. THC may have stimulant, sedative, or hallucinogenic actions depending on the dose and time after consumption. Both catecholamine release (resulting in tachycardia) and inhibition of sympathetic reflexes (resulting in orthostatic hypotension) may be observed.

II. Toxic dose. Typical marijuana cigarettes contain 1–3% THC, but more potent varieties may contain up to 15% THC. Hashish contains 3–6% and hashish oil 30–50% THC. Toxicity is dose-related, but there is much individual variability, influenced in part by prior experience and degree of tolerance.

III. Clinical presentation

A. Subjective effects after smoking a marijuana cigarette include euphoria, palpitations, heightened sensory awareness, and altered time perception followed after about 30 minutes by sedation. More severe intoxication may result in impaired short-term memory, depersonalization, visual hallucinations, and acute paranoid psychosis. Occasionally, even with low doses of THC, subjective effects may precipitate a panic reaction.

B. Physical findings may include tachycardia, orthostatic hypotension, conjunctival injection, incoordination, slurred speech, and ataxia. Stupor with pallor, conjunctival injection, fine tremor, and ataxia have been observed in children after eating marijuana cookies.

C. **Other health problems** include salmonellosis and pulmonary aspergillosis from use of contaminated marijuana. Marijuana may be contaminated by paraquat, but the latter is destroyed by pyrolysis and there is no evidence of paraquat toxicity from smoking marijuana.

D. **Intravenous use** of marijuana extract or hash oil may cause dyspnea, abdominal pain, fever, shock, disseminated intravascular coagulation, acute renal failure, and death.

IV. **Diagnosis.** Diagnosis is usually based on the history and typical findings such as tachycardia and conjunctival injection combined with evidence of altered mood or cognitive function.

A. **Specific levels.** Blood levels are not commonly available. Cannabinoids may be measured in the urine by enzyme immunoassay, which detects the major metabolites. These metabolites may be present in the urine for several days after single acute exposure or weeks after chronic THC exposure. Urine levels do not correlate with degree of intoxication or functional impairment.

B. **Other useful laboratory studies.** CBC, electrolytes, glucose, electrocardiographic monitor.

V. **Treatment**

A. **Emergency and supportive measures**
1. Most psychologic disturbances may be managed by simple reassurance, possibly with adjunctive use of diazepam (see p 302) or midazolam (p 323).
2. Sinus tachycardia usually does not require treatment but if necessary may be controlled with beta blockers such as propranolol (p 338).
3. Orthostatic hypotension responds to head-down position and intravenous fluids.

B. **Specific drugs and antidotes.** There is no specific antidote.

C. **Decontamination**
1. For significant ingestions, perform gastric lavage (see p 43). Ipecac is recommended for children seen to ingest marijuana-containing food or cigarettes. However, because of the antiemetic action of THC, ipecac may be ineffective.
2. Administer activated charcoal and cathartic (see p 45).

D. **Enhanced elimination.** These procedures are not effective owing to the large volume of distribution of cannabinoids.

References

Brandenburg D, Wernick R: Intravenous marijuana syndrome. *West J Med* 1986;**145**:94.
Jones RT: Cannabis and health. *Annu Rev Med* 1983;**34**:247.

MERCURY
*Margaret Atterbury, MD, and
Kent R. Olson, MD*

ANTIDOTE   IPECAC   LAVAGE   CHARCOAL

Mercury exists in several forms: metallic (elemental) mercury, mercury salts, and organic mercury. **Metallic mercury** is used in the extraction of gold and silver from ore, in dental amalgams, and in a variety of technical equipment. **Mercuric salts** are used in some antiseptics and stool fixatives and formerly were used as diuretics. **Organomercurials** have been used as fungicides and antiseptics; methyl mercury and other organomercurials may accumulate in sea life after environmental contamination.

I. **Mechanism of toxicity.** Mercury reacts with sulfhydryl (SH) groups, binding to proteins and inactivating enzymes. The nervous system is particularly sensitive. **Metallic mercury vapor** is well absorbed by the central nervous system and is also a pulmonary irritant. **Inorganic mercuric salts** are highly corrosive to the skin, eyes, and gastrointestinal tract and are also nephrotoxic. **Organomercurial compounds** are toxic to the central nervous system, and methyl mercury is teratogenic.

II. **Toxic dose.** Acute toxicity depends largely on the form and the route of exposure (inhalation, ingestion, or percutaneous). Chronic exposure to any form may result in toxicity. See Table II-30 for a summary of absorption and toxicity.

   A. **Metallic mercury,** a liquid at room temperature, is poorly absorbed and essentially nontoxic if ingested unless abnormal gut motility delays fecal elimination. However, the vapor is well absorbed by inhalation if mercury is heated or otherwise vaporized. The OSHA workplace permissible exposure limit (PEL) is 0.05 mg/m^3 as an 8-hour time-weighted average; the air level considered immediately dangerous to life or health (IDLH) is 28 mg/m^3.

   B. **Inorganic mercuric salts.** The acute lethal oral dose of mercuric chloride is approximately 1 g. Severe toxicity and death have been reported after use of peritoneal lavage solutions containing mercuric chloride concentrations of 0.2–0.8%.

   C. **Organic mercury** compounds have variable absorption; medicinal organomercurial antiseptics (Mercurochrome, thimerosal [Merthiolate], acetomeroctol, and merbromin) are not well absorbed from the gut or skin and release very little mercury. Chronic methyl mercury consumption can lead to neurologic and fetal toxicity; the daily "safe" limit for ingestion of methyl mercury-contaminated fish is 0.03 mg.

III. **Clinical presentation**

   A. **Acute inhalation of high concentrations of metallic mercury vapor** may cause severe chemical pneumonitis and noncardiogenic pulmonary edema.

   B. **Acute ingestion of inorganic mercuric salts** causes vomiting, diarrhea (often bloody), and shock. Renal failure occurs within 24 hours, heralded by proteinuria and hematuria. Hepatitis may occur.

   C. **Chronic inorganic mercury poisoning** (by exposure to vapor or salts) causes permanent central nervous system toxicity, including irritability, memory loss, shyness, depression, insomnia, and tremor ("erythism"). Gingivitis, stomatitis, and salivation are also common.

TABLE II-30. SUMMARY OF ABSORPTION AND TOXICITY OF MERCURY COMPOUNDS

Form	Absorption		Toxicity	
	Oral	Inhalation	Neurologic	Renal
Metallic mercury				
Hg^0 liquid	Poor	NA	Rare	Rare
Hg^0 vapor	...	Good	Likely	Likely
Mercury salts				
Hg$^+$	Poor	Not volatile	Rare	Rare
Hg^{2+}	Good	Not volatile	Rare	Likely
Organomercurials				
RHg$^+$	Good	Rare but possible	Likely	Possible
R$_2$Hg medicinal	Poor	Not inhaled	Rare	Possible

D. Acute **organic mercury poisoning** may cause paresthesias, ataxia, dysarthria, and visual and hearing disturbances. Chronic organomercurial poisoning can cause severe permanent central nervous system toxicity. Methyl mercury is a potent teratogen.

IV. Diagnosis. Diagnosis depends on an accurate history of the exposure and the form of mercury.

A. With acute metallic mercury inhalation (eg, after heating liquid mercury), symptoms of pneumonitis may be delayed for a few hours; chest x-ray and arterial blood gases may reveal early signs of toxicity.

B. After ingestion of inorganic mercuric salts, pronounced vomiting and diarrhea are so common that the absence of severe gastroenteritis makes serious intoxication unlikely.

C. Specific levels. Obtain blood and urine for mercury levels. Collection of 24-hour urine mercury is useful in determining body burden. In acute situations a spot collection may be diagnostic. Normal whole blood mercury levels are usually below 10 mcg/dL; normal urine levels are below 50 mcg/L.

1. With acute **mercuric salt** exposure, toxic blood levels of 25–50 mcg/dL are associated with serious toxicity, including acute renal failure. Urine levels may lag after acute ingestion but are often elevated despite normal blood levels in patients with chronic poisoning.

2. **Organic mercury** is usually excreted through the biliary system, and urine levels are not useful, although blood levels may be elevated. Hair levels may also be helpful in confirming past organomercury exposure.

D. Other useful laboratory studies. CBC, electrolytes, glucose, BUN, creatinine, liver function tests, urinalysis.

V. Treatment

A. Emergency and supportive measures

1. After **inhalation of metallic mercury vapor,** give supplemental oxygen and observe closely for several hours for development of acute pneumonitis and pulmonary edema (see p 7).

2. After **mercuric salt ingestion,** anticipate severe gastroenteritis and treat shock aggressively with intravenous fluid replacement (see p 14). Treat renal failure supportively; it is usually reversible, but hemodialysis may be required for 1–2 weeks.

3. Provide symptomatic supportive care after **organic mercury ingestion.**

B. Specific drugs and antidotes. For serious systemic intoxication, especially in patients with inorganic mercuric salt ingestion, administer **dimercaprol** (BAL; see p 294), 3–5 mg/kg IM every 6 hours. Oral **penicillamine** (see p 332) is also an effective chelator. Follow blood and urine mercury levels, and stop chelation when urine mercury levels are below 50 mcg/L. Unfortunately, chelation therapy is of no apparent benfit for established neurologic toxicity.

C. Decontamination

1. **Inhalation**

a. Immediately remove victim from exposure and give supplemental oxygen, if available.

b. After spill of metallic mercury, carefully clean up all liquid and discard contaminated carpeting or porous tile, or arrange for professional toxic cleanup with self-contained vacuum system. Do *not* vacuum with home vacuum cleaner; this may disperse liquid mercury, increasing its airborne concentration.

2. **Ingestion of liquid mercury.** Because liquid mercury usually passes through the system without being absorbed, there is no need for gut decontamination. With extremely large ingestions, especially in patients with multiple blind loops of bowel or intestinal perforation,

there is a risk of chronic intoxication. Multiple-dose cathartics, whole gut lavage (see p 46), or even surgical removal may be necessary depending on x-ray evidence of large pockets of mercury.

3. Ingestion of inorganic mercuric salts
- **a.** Perform gastric lavage (see p 43). Do **not** induce emesis because of the risk of serious corrosive injury.
- **b.** Administer activated charcoal (see p 45), although it is of uncertain benefit.
- **c.** Arrange for endoscopic examination if corrosive injury is suspected. Do **not** administer activated charcoal if endoscopy is planned, because it may obscure the view.

4. Ingestion of organic mercury. Immediately discontinue exposure and stop breast feeding. Consider therapeutic abortion if the patient is pregnant.

D. Enhanced elimination. There is no role for dialysis, hemoperfusion, or repeat-dose charcoal in removing mercury. However, dialysis may be required for supportive treatment of renal failure, and it may slightly enhance removal of the mercury-chelator complex in patients with renal failure (hemodialysis clearance of the mercury-BAL complex is about 5 mL/min).

References

Elhassani SB: The many faces of methylmercury poisoning. *J Toxicol Clin Toxicol* 1982;**19**:875.

Rosenman KD et al: Sensitive indicators of inorganic mercury toxicity. *Arch Environ Health* 1986;**41**:208.

METALDEHYDE
Chris Dutra, MD

ANTIDOTE   IPECAC   LAVAGE   CHARCOAL

Metaldehyde is widely used in the USA as a snail and slug poison. In Europe, it is also used as a solid fuel for small heaters. The pellets are often mistaken for cereal or candy.

I. Mechanism of toxicity. The mechanism of toxicity is not well understood. Metaldehyde, like paraldehyde, is a polymer of acetaldehyde, and depolymerization to form acetaldehyde may account for some of its toxic effects.

II. Toxic dose. Ingestion of 100–150 mg/kg may cause myoclonus and convulsions, and ingestion of more than 400 mg/kg is potentially lethal. Death occurred in a child after ingestion of 3 g.

III. Clinical presentation. Symptoms usually begin within 1–3 hours after ingestion.
- **A. Small ingestions** (5–10 mg/kg) cause salivation, facial flushing, abdominal cramps, diarrhea, and fever.
- **B. Larger doses** may produce irritability, ataxia, drowsiness, myoclonus, opisthotonus, convulsions, and coma. Rhabdomyolysis and hyperthermia may result from seizures or excessive muscle activity. Liver and kidney damage have been reported.

IV. Diagnosis. Diagnosis is based on a history of ingestion and clinical presentation. Ask about containers in the garage or planting shed; metaldehyde is frequently packaged in brightly colored cardboard boxes similar to cereal containers.
- **A. Specific levels.** Serum levels are not generally available.

B. **Other useful laboratory studies.** CBC, electrolytes, glucose, BUN, creatinine, liver function tests, creatine phosphokinase (CPK), urinalysis.

V. **Treatment**

A. **Emergency and supportive measures**

1. Maintain the airway and assist ventilation if necessary (see p 2).
2. Treat coma (p 17) and seizures (p 21) if they occur. Paraldehyde should *not* be used to treat seizures because of its chemical similarity to metaldehyde.
3. Treat fluid loss from vomiting or diarrhea with intravenous crystalloid fluids (p 14).
4. Monitor asymptomatic patients for at least 4–6 hours after ingestion.

B. **Specific drugs and antidotes.** There is no specific antidote.

C. **Decontamination**

1. Perform gastric lavage (see p 43). Do *not* induce emesis because of the risk of abrupt onset of seizures.
2. Administer activated charcoal and a cathartic (see p 45).
3. Gut emptying is probably not necessary following a small ingestion if activated charcoal is given promptly.

D. **Enhanced elimination.** There is no apparent benefit from dialysis, hemoperfusion, or forced diuresis. Repeat-dose charcoal has not been studied.

Reference

Longstreth WT Jr, Pierson DJ: Metaldehyde poisoning from slug bait ingestion. *West J Med* 1982;**137**:134.

METAL FUME FEVER
Donna E. Foliart, MD, MPH

ANTIDOTE   IPECAC   LAVAGE   CHARCOAL

Metal fume fever is an acute febrile illness associated with the inhalation of freshly formed respirable particles of metal oxides. Although most commonly identified with the inhalation of zinc oxide, metal fume fever may also result from exposure to oxides of copper, magnesium, cadmium, iron, manganese, nickel, selenium, tin, and antimony. Metal fume fever occurs in workplace settings involving welding, melting, smelting, and galvanizing.

I. **Mechanism of toxicity.** Animal and human data suggest that particles of metal oxides in the range of 0.02–0.25μ in diameter are most pathogenic. As there is no latent period for sensitization, metal fume fever does not appear to have an immunologic basis.

II. **Toxic dose.** The toxic dose is variable. Resistance to the condition develops after a few days of exposure but wears off rapidly when exposure ceases. The OSHA workplace permissible exposure limit (PEL) for zinc oxide fumes is 5 mg/m^3 as an 8-hour time-weighted average, which is calculated to prevent metal fume fever in most exposed workers.

III. **Clinical presentation.** Symptoms begin 4–8 hours after exposure, when the victim develops a metallic, sweet taste, followed by fever, malaise, myalgias, and headache. Over the next 2–4 hours, the symptoms may progress to profuse sweating, back pain, cough, and substernal chest pain. There is fever, tachycardia, and sometimes localized rales on chest examination. The white blood cell count may be elevated (12,000–16,000). The chest x-ray is usually normal. Typically, all symptoms resolve spontaneously within 24–36 hours.

IV. Diagnosis. A history of welding, especially with galvanized metal, and typical symptoms and signs are sufficient to make the diagnosis.
  A. Specific levels. There are no specific tests to diagnose or exclude metal fume fever. Urine determinations of the metals are not useful, because the oxides are poorly absorbed and background excretion of endogenous metals (zinc, copper, manganese) is variable.
  B. Other useful laboratory studies. CBC, arterial blood gases, chest x-ray.
V. Treatment
  A. Emergency and supportive measures
    1. Administer supplemental oxygen, and give bronchodilators if there is wheezing (see p 8).
    2. Provide other symptomatic care (eg, acetaminophen) as needed; symptoms are self-limited and rarely severe.
  B. Specific drugs and antidotes. There is no specific antidote.
  C. Decontamination. Decontamination is not necessary; by the time symptoms develop, the exposure has usually been over for several hours.
  D. Enhanced elimination. There is no role for these procedures.

Reference

Mueller EJ, Seger DL: Metal fume fever: A review. *J Emerg Med* 1985;2:271.

METHANOL
Ilene B. Anderson, PharmD

ANTIDOTE   IPECAC   LAVAGE   CHARCOAL

Methanol (wood alcohol) is a common ingredient in many solvents, windshield-washing solutions, duplicating fluids, and paint removers. It is sometimes used as an ethanol substitute by alcoholics. Although methanol itself produces mainly inebriation, its metabolic products may cause metabolic acidosis, blindness, and death after a characteristic latent period of 6–30 hours.

I. Mechanism of toxicity. Methanol is slowly metabolized by alcohol dehydrogenase to formaldehyde and subsequently by aldehyde dehydrogenase to formic acid (formate). Systemic acidosis is caused by the formic acid as well as by lactic acid, while blindness is due primarily to formate. Both ethanol and methanol compete for the enzyme alcohol dehydrogenase; the preference of this enzyme for metabolizing ethanol forms the basis for ethanol therapy in methanol poisonings.
II. Toxic dose. The fatal oral dose of methanol is estimated to be 30–240 mL (20–150 g). The minimum toxic dose is approximately 100 mg/kg. The OSHA workplace permissible exposure limit (PEL) for inhalation is 200 ppm as an 8-hour time-weighted average, and the level considered immediately dangerous to life or health (IDLH) is 25,000 ppm.
III. Clinical presentation
  A. In the first few hours after ingestion, methanol-intoxicated patients present with inebriation and gastritis. Acidosis is not usually present because metabolism to toxic products has not yet occurred. There may be a noticeable elevation in the osmolar gap (see p 29); an osmolar gap of as little as 10 mosm/L is consistent with toxic concentrations of methanol.
  B. After a latency period of up to 30 hours, severe anion gap metabolic acidosis, visual disturbances, blindness, seizures, coma, and death may occur. Patients describe the visual disturbance as haziness or "like standing in a snowfield." The latent period is longer when ethanol has been ingested concurrently with methanol.
IV. Diagnosis. Diagnosis is usually based on the history, symptoms, and labo-

ratory findings because stat methanol levels are rarely available. Calculation of the osmolar (see p 29) and anion gaps (see p 30) can be used to
estimate the methanol level and to predict the severity of the ingestion.

A. Specific levels
1. **Serum methanol** levels higher than 20 mg/dL should be considered
   toxic, and levels higher than 40 mg/dL should be considered very
   serious. Following the latency period, a methanol level of zero does
   not rule out a serious intoxication in a symptomatic patient because
   all the methanol may already have been metabolized to formate.
2. Elevated **serum formate** concentrations may confirm the diagnosis
   and are a better measure of toxicity, but formate levels are not yet
   widely available.

B. Other useful laboratory studies. CBC, electrolytes, glucose, BUN, creatinine, serum osmolality and osmolar gap, arterial blood gases, ethanol
level.

V. Treatment
A. Emergency and supportive measures
1. Maintain the airway and assist ventilation if necessary (see p 2).
2. Treat coma (p 17) and seizures (p 21) if they occur.
3. Treat metabolic acidosis with intravenous sodium bicarbonate
   (p 296). Correction of acidosis should be guided by arterial blood
   gases.

B. Specific drugs and antidotes
1. **Ethanol.** Start an oral or intravenous infusion of ethanol (see p 312) to
   saturate the enzyme alcohol dehydrogenase and prevent the formation of methanol's toxic metabolites. Ethanol therapy is indicated in
   patients with the following:
   a. A history of a significant methanol ingestion, when methanol
      serum levels are not immediately available and the osmolar gap is
      greater than 5 mosm/L.
   b. Metabolic acidosis and an osmolar gap greater than 5–10 mosm/L
      not accounted for by ethanol.
   c. Methanol blood concentration greater than 20 mg/dL.
2. **Folic acid** (see p 314) may enhance the conversion of formate to
   carbon dioxide and water. A reasonable dose is 50 mg IV every 4
   hours.
3. An experimental drug, 4-methylpyrazole, inhibits alcohol dehydrogenase and prevents methanol metabolism but is not yet available in
   the USA.

C. Decontamination
1. Induce emesis or perform gastric lavage (see p 42). Because methanol is rapidly absorbed, gastric lavage is preferred over emesis if the
   patient is in the hospital. Ipecac is used mainly for initial home or
   prehospital treatment.
2. Activated charcoal has not been shown to efficiently adsorb methanol. In addition, charcoal may delay the absorption of orally administered ethanol.

D. Enhanced elimination. Hemodialysis rapidly removes both methanol
and formate. The indications for dialysis are suspected methanol poisoning with significant metabolic acidosis, an osmolar gap greater than
10 mosm/L, or a measured serum methanol concentration greater than
40 mg/dL. Dialysis should be continued until the methanol concentration is less than 20 mg/dL. *Note:* The ethanol infusion must be increased
during dialysis (see p 312).

Reference

Jacobsen D, McMartin KE: Methanol and ethylene glycol poisonings: Mechanism of toxicity, clinical course, diagnosis and treatment. *Med Toxicol* 1986;1:309.

METHEMOGLOBINEMIA
Paul D. Blanc, MD

ANTIDOTE   IPECAC   LAVAGE   CHARCOAL

Methemoglobin is an oxidized form of hemoglobin. Many oxidant chemicals and drugs are capable of inducing methemoglobinemia: nitrites and nitrates, bromates and chlorates, aniline derivatives, antimalarial agents, dapsone, sulfonamides, local anesthetics, and numerous others (Table II–31). Occupational risk groups include chemical and munitions workers. An important environmental source for methemoglobinemia in infants is nitrate-contaminated well water. Amyl and butyl nitrite are often abused for their alleged sexual enhancement properties. Oxides of nitrogen and other oxidant combustion products make smoke inhalation an important potential cause of methemoglobinemia.

I. **Mechanism of toxicity.** Methemoglobin inducers act by oxidizing ferrous (Fe^{2+}) to ferric (Fe^{3+}) hemoglobin. This abnormal hemoglobin is incapable of carrying oxygen, inducing a functional anemia. In addition, the shape of the oxygen-hemoglobin dissociation curve is altered, aggravating cellular hypoxia. Methemoglobinemia does not cause hemolysis; however, many oxidizing agents that induce methemoglobinemia may also cause hemolysis.

II. **Toxic dose.** The ingested dose or inhaled air level of toxin required to induce methemoglobinemia is highly variable. Neonates and persons with congenital methemoglobin reductase deficiency or glucose-6-phosphate dehydrogenase (G6PD) deficiency have an impaired ability to regenerate normal hemoglobin and are therefore more likely to accumulate methemoglobin after oxidant exposure.

III. **Clinical presentation.** The severity of symptoms usually correlates with measured methemoglobin level (Table II–32). Symptoms and signs are due to decreased blood oxygen content and cellular hypoxia and are nonspecific: headache, dizziness, and nausea, progressing to dyspnea, confusion, seizures, and coma. Even at low levels, skin discoloration ("chocolate cyanosis"), especially of the nails, lips, and ears, is striking.

IV. **Diagnosis.** The patient with mild to moderate methemoglobinemia appears markedly cyanotic yet may be relatively asymptomatic. The diagnosis is suggested by the finding of "chocolate brown" blood (put a drop of blood on filter paper and compare with normal blood), which is apparent when the methemoglobin level exceeds 15%. Differential diagnosis includes other causes of cellular hypoxia (eg, carbon monoxide, cyanide, hydrogen sulfide) and sulfhemoglobinemia.

    A. **Specific levels.** The co-oximeter type of arterial blood gas analyzer will directly measure oxygen saturation and methemoglobin saturation. Sulfhemoglobin and the antidote methylene blue both produce erron-

TABLE II–31. COMMON AGENTS CAPABLE OF INDUCING METHEMOGLOBINEMIA

Local anesthetics	Analgesics	Miscellaneous
Benzocaine	Phenazopyridine	Aniline dyes
Lidocaine	Phenacetin	Chlorates
Antimicrobials	**Nitrites and nitrates**	Nitrobenzene
Dapsone	Amyl nitrite	Aminophenol
Sulfanilamide	Butyl nitrite	
Sulfathiazole	Isobutyl nitrite	
	Sodium nitrite	
	Nitroglycerin	

TABLE II-32. CORRELATION OF SYMPTOMS WITH METHEMOGLOBIN LEVELS

Methemoglobin Level	Typical Symptoms
< 15%	Usually asymptomatic
15–20%	Cyanosis, mild symptoms
20–45%	Marked cyanosis, moderate symptoms
45–70%	Severe cyanosis, severe symptoms
> 70%	Usually lethal

eously high results on the co-oximeter. The cross-positive result due to sulfhemoglobin is about 10% of the sulfhemoglobin level; a dose of 2 mL/kg methylene blue gives a false-positive methemoglobin of approximately 15%.

1. Note that the routine arterial blood gas machine measures the serum P_{O2} (which is normal) and calculates a falsely normal oxygen saturation.
2. Pulse oximetry may give a falsely normal oxygen saturation.

B. **Other useful laboratory studies.** CBC, electrolytes, glucose, BUN, creatinine, arterial blood gases, chest x-ray.

V. Treatment

A. **Emergency and supportive measures**
   1. Maintain the airway and assist ventilation if necessary (see p 2). Administer supplemental oxygen.
   2. Usually, mild methemoglobinemia (< 20%) will resolve spontaneously without intervention.

B. **Specific drugs and antidotes. Methylene blue** (see p 322) is indicated in the symptomatic patient with methemoglobin levels higher than 15% or when even minimal compromise of oxygen-carrying capacity is potentially harmful (eg, preexisting anemia, congestive heart failure, angina pectoris, etc). Give methylene blue, 1–2 mg/kg (0.1–0.2 mL/kg of 1% solution) over several minutes. *Caution:* Methylene blue can slightly worsen methemoglobinemia when given in excessive amounts; in patients with G6PD deficiency, it may cause hemolysis. Ascorbic acid, which can reverse methemoglobin by an alternate metabolic pathway, is of minimal use acutely because of its slow action.

C. **Decontamination**
   1. **Inhalation.** Remove victim from exposure and give supplemental oxygen, if available.
   2. **Skin.** Remove contaminated clothing, and wash exposed skin with soap and water.
   3. **Ingestion**
      a. Induce emesis or perform gastric lavage (see p 42).
      b. Administer activated charcoal and cathartic (see p 45).
      c. Gut emptying is probably not necessary following a small ingestion if activated charcoal is given promptly.

D. **Enhanced elimination.** In patients with severe intoxication, if methylene blue is contraindicated (eg, G6PD deficiency) or has not been effective, exchange transfusion may be necessary. Hyperbaric oxygen is theoretically capable of supplying all oxygen needs without hemoglobin and may be useful in extremely serious cases that do not respond rapidly to antidotal treatment.

Reference

Hall AH, Kulig KW, Rumack BH: Drug- and chemical-induced methaemoglobinemia: Clinical features and management. *Med Toxicol* 1986;**1**:253.

METHYL BROMIDE
Gary Pasternak, MD

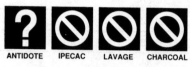

ANTIDOTE   IPECAC   LAVAGE   CHARCOAL

Methyl bromide is a gas used as an insecticidal fumigant, a fire extinguisher ingredient, and a chemical intermediate in the synthesis of chemicals and dyes. It is an odorless and colorless gas with poor warning properties. The nervous system is the primary target of methyl bromide toxicity, with the respiratory tract, skin, and cardiovascular system also affected. A delayed onset of symptoms is typical, and serious symptoms can develop within a few minutes to as long as 48 hours postexposure.

I. **Mechanism of toxicity.** Proposed mechanisms include inhibition of sulfhydryl enzymes, methylation of other proteins, and a direct toxic effect of methyl bromide on cells. Methyl bromide likely acts as an alkylating agent, a major target being tissue-reduced glutathione. NIOSH considers methyl bromide a potential occupational carcinogen.

II. **Toxic dose**
   A. **Inhalation.** The OSHA workplace permissible exposure limit (PEL) in air is 5 ppm as an 8-hour time-weighted average. Toxic effects are generally noted after inhalation at levels of 200 ppm. The air level considered immediately dangerous to life or health (IDLH) is 2000 ppm.
   B. **Skin.** Dermal penetration is very efficient, and methyl bromide easily penetrates clothing and protective gear. Retention of the gas in clothing and rubber boots can be a source of prolonged percutaneous exposure.

III. **Clinical presentation**
   A. **Irritant effects.** Methyl bromide is irritating to the eyes, skin, and mucous membranes of the upper respiratory tract. Lung irritation may result in noncardiogenic pulmonary edema, which may be immediate or delayed. However, because of its poor warning properties, significant exposure can occur before the onset of symptoms. Moderate skin exposure can result in dermatitis and, in severe cases, chemical burns.
   B. **Acute systemic effects.** With significant acute exposure, systemic toxicity may occur, including malaise, visual disturbances, headache, nausea, vomiting, vertigo, tremor, seizures, and coma. Death is due to pulmonary or circulatory failure.
   C. **Chronic neurologic sequelae** such as dementia, psychosis, and extrapyramidal symptoms have been described.

IV. **Diagnosis.** Diagnosis is based primarily on a history of exposure to the compound and typical symptoms. Some patients may describe the acute irritant effects of chlorpicrin or other irritant agents that are often added to commercial methyl bromide to provide warning properties.
   A. **Specific levels. Serum bromide** levels may be useful if intake of inorganic bromide can be excluded (endogenous serum bromide does not usually exceed 0.1 meq/L, and therapeutic bromide concentrations are usually < 1 meq/L). Because bromide remains in the body longer than methyl bromide and bromide itself is less toxic, elevated bromide concentrations may indicate exposure but do not necessarily correlate with the toxic effect of methyl bromide.

   B. **Other useful laboratory studies.** CBC, electrolytes (falsely elevated chloride is seen with some methods: 1 meq bromide = 1.5 meq chloride), glucose, BUN, creatinine, arterial blood gases, chest x-ray.
V. **Treatment**
   A. **Emergency and supportive measures**
      1. Administer supplemental oxygen, and treat bronchospasm (see p 8), pulmonary edema (p 7), seizures (p 21), and coma (p 17) if they occur.
      2. Monitor patients for a minimum of 6–12 hours to detect development of delayed symptoms, especially pulmonary edema.
   B. **Specific drugs and antidotes.** Methyl bromide reduction of tissue glutathione provides the rationale for the use of dimercaprol (BAL) and acetylcysteine, but these agents have not been critically tested in controlled studies.
   C. **Decontamination**
      1. Remove victim from exposure and administer supplemental oxygen, if available.
      2. Remove all contaminated clothing and wash affected skin with soap and water. Irrigate exposed eyes with copious water or saline.
   D. **Enhanced elimination.** There is no role for these procedures.

Reference

Behrens RH, Dukes DC: Fatal methyl bromide poisoning. *Br J Ind Med* 1986;**43**:561.

METHYLENE CHLORIDE
Peter Wald, MD

| ANTIDOTE | IPECAC | LAVAGE | CHARCOAL |

Methylene chloride is widely used in paint and varnish removers and as a solvent in degreasing operations; it is found in some Christmas tree lights and magic trick sets. It is metabolized to carbon monoxide in vivo, and it may produce phosgene, chlorine, or hydrogen chloride upon combustion. It was considered to be the least toxic of all the chlorinated hydrocarbon solvents prior to its implication as a suspected human carcinogen.

   I. **Mechanism of toxicity.** Like other chlorinated hydrocarbon solvents, methylene chloride is an irritant to mucous membranes and defats the skin epithelium; it is a direct central nervous system depressant and may sensitize the myocardium to arrhythmogenic effects of catecholamines. In addition:
      A. **Carbon monoxide** is generated in vivo during metabolism by the mixed-function oxidases in the liver. The contribution of carbon monoxide to methylene chloride intoxication is unknown.
      B. Methylene chloride is a **suspected human carcinogen.**
  II. **Toxic dose.** Toxicity may occur after inhalation or ingestion.
      A. **Inhalation.** OSHA considers methylene chloride a potential human carcinogen and has no established permissible exposure limit (PEL). The ACGIH workplace exposure threshold limit value (TLV) is 50 ppm for an 8-hour shift, which may result in a carboxyhemoglobin level of 3–4%. The air level considered immediately dangerous to life or health (IDLH) is 5000 ppm.
      B. **Ingestion.** The acute oral toxic dose is approximately 0.5–5 mL/kg.
 III. **Clinical presentation**
      A. **Inhalation** is the most common route of exposure and results in mucous

membrane and skin irritation, nausea, vomiting, and headache. Severe exposures may lead to pulmonary edema, cardiac arrhythmias, and central nervous system depression with respiratory arrest.

B. **Ingestion** can cause corrosive injury and systemic intoxication.

C. Extensive **skin exposure** can cause significant burns and systemic symptoms due to skin absorption.

D. **Chronic exposure** can cause bone marrow, hepatic, and renal toxicity.

IV. Diagnosis. Diagnosis is based on a history of exposure and clinical presentation.

    A. Specific levels

        1. Carboxyhemoglobin blood levels should be obtained, although they may not correlate with the severity of the exposure.

        2. Expired air and blood levels of **methylene chloride** may be obtained but are not useful in clinical management.

    B. Other useful laboratory studies. CBC, electrolytes, glucose, BUN, creatinine, liver enzymes, arterial blood gases.

V. Treatment

    A. Emergency and supportive measures

        1. Maintain the airway and assist ventilation if necessary (see p 2).

        2. Administer supplemental oxygen, and treat coma (p 17) and pulmonary edema (p 7) if they occur.

        3. Monitor the ECG for at least 4–6 hours, and treat arrhythmias (p 9) if they occur. Avoid the use of epinephrine, which may potentiate cardiac arrhythmias.

        4. If corrosive injury is suspected after ingestion, consult a gastroenterologist regarding possible endoscopy.

    B. Specific drugs and antidotes. Administer 100% **oxygen** by tight-fitting mask or endotracheal tube if the carboxyhemoglobin level is elevated.

    C. Decontamination

        1. Inhalation. Remove the victim from exposure and give supplemental oxygen, if available.

        2. Skin and eyes. Remove contaminated clothing, and wash exposed skin with soap and water. Irrigate exposed eyes with copious saline or tap water.

        3. Ingestion

            a. Do *not* induce emesis because of the risk of rapid central nervous system depression. Perform gastric lavage (see p 43) if the patient presents within 30–60 minutes or has ingested a large overdose.

            b. Administer activated charcoal and a cathartic (see p 45), orally or by gastric tube. The effectiveness of activated charcoal is not known.

    D. Enhanced elimination. There is no documented efficacy for repeat-dose activated charcoal, hemodialysis, hemoperfusion, or hyperbaric oxygen.

Reference

Stewart RD, Hake CL: Paint-remover hazard. *JAMA* 1976;235:398.

MONOAMINE OXIDASE INHIBITORS
Neal L. Benowitz, MD

ANTIDOTE   IPECAC   LAVAGE   CHARCOAL

Most monoamine oxidase (MAO) inhibitors are used in treating severe depression; procarbazine is a cancer chemotherapeutic drug. Available drugs in this class include furazolidone (Furoxone), isocarboxazid (Marplan), nialamide

(Niamid), pargyline (Eutonyl), phenelzine (Nardil), procarbazine (Matulane), and tranylcypromine (Parnate). Serious toxicity from MAO inhibitors occurs either with overdose or owing to interactions with certain other drugs or foods (Table II–33).

I. **Mechanism of toxicity.** MAO inhibitors irreversibly inactivate MAO, an enzyme responsible for degradation of catecholamines within neurons in the central nervous system. MAO is also found in the liver and the intestinal wall, where it metabolizes tyramine and therefore limits its absorption by the systemic circulation.

   A. Toxicity results from release of excessive neuronal stores of vasoactive amines, inhibition of metabolism of catecholamines or interacting drugs, or absorption of large amounts of dietary tyramine (which in turn releases catecholamines from neurons).

   B. In addition, severe rigidity and hyperthermia may occur when patients receiving MAO inhibitors use therapeutic doses of meperidine (Demerol), dextromethorphan, and possibly fluoxetine (Prozac); the mechanism is unknown but may be related to inhibition of serotonin metabolism in the central nervous system.

II. **Toxic dose.** MAO inhibitors have a low therapeutic index. Acute ingestion of 2–3 mg/kg or more should be considered potentially life-threatening. Serious drug or food interactions may occur in patients receiving therapeutic doses of MAO inhibitors.

III. **Clinical presentation.** Symptoms may be delayed 6–24 hours after acute overdose but occur rapidly following ingestion of interacting drugs or foods. Because of irreversible inactivation of MAO, toxic effects (and the potential for drug or food interactions) may persist for several days.

   A. Anxiety, flushing, headache, tremor, sweating, tachypnea, tachycardia, and hypertension are common with mild intoxication.

   B. Severe intoxication may result in severe hypertension (which may be complicated by intracranial hemorrhage), delirium, hyperthermia, and eventually cardiovascular collapse and multisystem failure.

IV. **Diagnosis.** Diagnosis is based on clinical features of sympathomimetic drug intoxication with a history of MAO use, particularly with use of drugs or foods known to interact.

   A. **Specific levels.** Specific drug levels are not available.

   B. **Other useful laboratory studies.** CBC, electrolyes, glucose, BUN, creatinine, creatine phosphokinase (CPK), ECG and electrocardiographic monitoring. Obtain a CT head scan if intracranial hemorrhage is suspected.

V. **Treatment**

   A. **Emergency and supportive measures**

      1. Maintain the airway and assist ventilation if necessary (see p 2). Administer supplemental oxygen.

TABLE II-33. INTERACTIONS WITH MONOAMINE OXIDASE INHIBITORS[a]

Drugs		Foods
Amphetamine	Metaraminol	Beer
Buspirone	Methyldopa	Broad beans
Dextromethorphan	Phenylephrine	Cheese (natural or aged)
Ephedrine	Phenylpropanolamine	Chicken liver
Fluoxetine	Reserpine	Pickled herring
Guanethidine	Trazodone	Snails
L-Dopa	Tryptophan	Wine (red)
LSD (lysergic acid diethylamide)		Yeast (dietary supplement)
Meperidine (Demerol)		

[a]Possible interactions, based on case reports or pharmacologic considerations.

2. Treat hypertension (p 16), hypotension (p 14), coma (p 17), seizures (p 21), and hyperthermia (p 19) if they occur.
3. Continuously monitor temperature, other vital signs, and ECG for a minimum of 6 hours in asymptomatic patients, and admit all symptomatic patients for continuous monitoring for 24 hours.

B. Specific drugs and antidotes. There is no specific antidote.

C. Decontamination
1. Do **not** induce emesis because of the risk of seizures and of aggravating hypertension. Perform gastric lavage (see p 43).
2. Administer activated charcoal and cathartic (see p 45).
3. Gut emptying is probably not necessary following a very small ingestion if activated charcoal is given promptly.

D. Enhanced elimination. Dialysis and hemoperfusion are not effective. Repeat-dose activated charcoal has not been studied.

Reference

Linden CH, Rumack BH, Strehlke C: Monoamine oxidase inhibitor overdose. *Ann Emerg Med* 1984;**13**:1137.

MUSHROOMS
Kent R. Olson, MD

ANTIDOTE   IPECAC   LAVAGE   CHARCOAL

There are more than 5000 varieties of mushrooms in the USA, about 100 of which are potentially toxic. The majority of toxic mushrooms cause mild to moderate self-limited gastroenteritis. A few species may cause severe or even fatal reactions. The 7 major types of poisonous mushroom varieties are described in Table II–34. *Amanita phalloides* and other amatoxin-containing mushrooms are discussed on p 212.

I. **Mechanism of toxicity.** The various mechanisms thought responsible for poisoning are listed in Table II–34. The majority of toxic incidents are due to gastrointestinal irritants that cause vomiting and diarrhea shortly after ingestion.
II. **Toxic dose.** This is not known. The amount of toxin varies considerably between members of the same species, depending on local geography and weather conditions. In most cases, the exact amount of toxic mushroom ingested is unknown because the victim has unwittingly added a toxic species to a meal of edible fungi.
III. **Clinical presentation.** The various clinical presentations are described in Table II–34. In most cases, the onset of vomiting and diarrhea is rapid. When the onset is delayed more than 6–12 hours, this suggests amatoxin or monomethylhydrazine poisoning. However, if a meal containing a mixture of toxic mushrooms has been ingested, early onset of symptoms does not rule out amatoxin poisoning.
IV. **Diagnosis.** The diagnosis may be difficult because the victim may not realize that the illness has been caused by mushrooms, especially if symptoms are delayed 12 or more hours after ingestion. If leftover mushrooms are available, obtain assistance from a mycologist through a local university or mycologic society. However, note that the mushrooms brought for identification may not be the same ones that were eaten.
A. **Specific levels.** Specific toxin levels are not available.
B. **Other useful laboratory studies.** CBC, electrolytes, glucose, BUN, creatinine, liver enzymes, and prothrombin time (PT).
V. **Treatment**

TABLE II-34. CLASSIFICATION OF MUSHROOM TOXICITY[a]

Toxins	Mushrooms	Onset	Symptoms and Signs
Amatoxins	*Amanita phalloides, A ocreata, A verna, A virosa,* some *Lepiota* and *Galerina* species.	6–12 h	Vomiting, diarrhea, abdominal cramps, hepatic failure.
Monomethylhydrazine	*Gyrometra (Helvella) esculenta,* others.	6–12 h	Vomiting, diarrhea, weakness, seizures, hemolysis, hepatitis, methemoglobinemia.
Muscarine	*Clitocybe dealbata, C cerusata, Inocybe, Omphalotus olearius.*	0.5–2 h	Salivation, sweating, vomiting, diarrhea, miosis.
Coprine	*Coprinus armamentarius, Clitocybe clavipes.*	30 min	Disulfiramlike reaction with alcohol may occur up to 5 days after ingesting fungi.
Ibotenic acid, muscimol	*Amanita muscaria, A pantherina,* others.	0.5–2 h	Muscular jerking, anticholinergic syndrome, hallucinations.
Psilocybin	*Psilocybe cubensis,* others.	0.5–1 h	Hallucinations.
Gastrointestinal irritants	Many species.	0.5–2 h	Vomiting, diarrhea.

[a] Modified and reproduced, with permission, from Becker CE et al: Diagnosis and treatment of *Amanita phalloides*-type mushroom poisoning: Use of thioctic acid. *West J Med* 1976;**125**:100.

A. Emergency and supportive measures
  1. Treat hypotension due to gastroenteritis with intravenous crystalloid solutions (see p 14) and supine positioning.
  2. Monitor patients for 12–24 hours for delayed-onset gastroenteritis associated with amatoxin and monomethylhydrazine poisoning.
B. Specific drugs and antidotes
  1. For **monomethylhydrazine** poisoning, give **pyridoxine,** 20–30 mg/kg IV (see p 339) for seizures; treat methemoglobinemia with **methylene blue,** 1 mg/kg IV (p 322).
  2. For **muscarine** intoxication, **atropine,** 0.01–0.03 mg/kg IV (p 293), may alleviate cholinergic symptoms.
  3. **Ibotenic acid-induced** or **muscimol-induced** anticholinergic symptoms may improve with **physostigmine** (p 336).
  4. Treat **amatoxin-type** poisoning as described below.
C. Decontamination
  1. If the patient presents shortly after any wild mushroom ingestion, induce emesis or perform gastric lavage (see p 42). Emesis is preferred because the gastric tube may not remove larger mushroom segments.
  2. Administer activated charcoal and cathartic (see p 45), orally or by gastric tube.
D. Enhanced elimination. There is no accepted role for enhanced removal procedures. Repeat-dose charcoal is often given to patients with amatoxin poisoning (see p 49 and p 299) in the hope of interrupting the enterohepatic recirculation, but this is of uncertain value.

Reference

Lincoff G, Mitchel DH: *Toxic and Hallucinogenic Mushroom Poisoning: A Handbook for Physicians and Mushroom Hunters.* Van Nostrand Reinhold, 1977.

MUSHROOMS, AMATOXIN-TYPE
Kent R. Olson, MD

ANTIDOTE   IPECAC   LAVAGE   CHARCOAL

Amatoxins are a group of highly toxic peptides found in several species of mushrooms, including *Amanita phalloides, Amanita virosa, Amanita ocreata, Amanita verna, Galerina autumnalis, Galerina marginata,* and some species of *Lepiota.* These mushrooms are often picked and eaten by amateur foragers who have misidentified them as an edible species.

I. **Mechanism of toxicity.** Amatoxins are highly stable and resistant to heat and are not removed by any form of cooking. They are thought to act by inhibiting cellular protein synthesis by interfering with RNA polymerase. Absorption by intestinal cells causes cell death and sloughing after a delay of 8–12 hours. Absorption by the liver results in severe hepatic necrosis.

   Death occurring within the first 1–2 days is usually due to massive fluid loss from gastroenteritis, while death occurring later is usually due to hepatic failure.

II. **Toxic dose.** Amatoxins are among the most potent toxins known; the minimum lethal dose is about 0.1 mg/kg. One *Amanita* cap may contain 10–15 mg. In contrast, *Galerina* species contain far less toxin; 15–20 caps would be a fatal dose for an adult.

III. **Clinical presentation.** The onset of symptoms is characteristically delayed 8–12 hours or more after ingestion.
   A. **Gastroenteritis.** Initially, vomiting is accompanied by severe abdominal cramps and explosive watery diarrhea. Severe fluid losses can occur rapidly, and some patients die of shock within 24 hours.
   B. **Hepatic failure.** Those who survive the gastroenteritis phase may appear to improve for 1–2 days before the onset of hepatic failure. Hepatic transaminase levels often exceed 10,000 units, and the bilirubin and prothrombin time steadily rise. Hepatic encephalopathy is a grave prognostic sign and usually predicts a fatal outcome.

IV. **Diagnosis.** Diagnosis is usually based on a history of wild mushroom ingestion and the characteristic delay of 8–12 hours before onset of severe gastroenteritis (see also monomethylhydrazine-type mushrooms, p 210). However, if a variety of mushrooms has been eaten, stomach upset may occur much earlier owing to a different toxic species, making diagnosis of amatoxin poisoning more difficult.

   Any available mushroom specimens that may have been ingested should be examined by a mycologist. Pieces of mushroom retrieved from the emesis or even mushroom spores found on microscopic examination may provide clues to the ingested species.

   A **qualitative test (the Meixner test)** may determine the presence of amatoxins in mushroom specimens. A single drop of concentrated hydrochloric acid is added to dried juice from the mushroom cap that has been dripped onto newspaper or other unrefined paper; a blue color suggests the presence of amatoxins. *Caution:* This test should not be used to determine edibility of mushroom specimens!
   A. **Specific levels.** A radioimmunoassay for amatoxins exists but is not widely available. The toxin is rapidly bound in the body within the first several hours after ingestion, and amatoxins are generally not detectable in the serum or urine more than 24 hours after exposure.
   B. **Other useful laboratory studies.** CBC, electrolytes, glucose, BUN, creatinine, liver transaminases, bilirubin, prothrombin time.

V. Treatment. The mortality rate may be higher than 60% if the patient is not treated but is probably less than 10–15% with intensive supportive care.

A. Emergency and supportive measures

1. Maintain the airway and assist ventilation if necessary (see p 2).
2. Treat fluid and electrolytes losses aggressively, because massive fluid losses may cause circulatory collapse. Administer normal saline or other crystalloid solution, 10- to 20-mL/kg boluses, with monitoring of central venous pressure or even pulmonary artery pressure (p 14) to guide fluid therapy.
3. Provide vigorous supportive care for hepatic failure (p 34); **liver transplant** may be lifesaving in patients who develop encephalopathy.

B. Specific drugs and antidotes. There is no proved effective antidote for amatoxin poisoning, although many popular therapies have been promoted and are still widely used. Animal studies suggest that early treatment with penicillin, silibinin, or cimetidine may partially protect against hepatic injury. Consult a medical toxicologist or a regional poison control center (see Table I-41, p 51) for further information.

C. Decontamination

1. If recent ingestion (< 1–2 hours) is suspected, induce emesis (unless the patient is already vomiting). Gastric lavage may not remove mushroom pieces.
2. Administer activated charcoal and cathartic (see p 45), orally or by gastric tube.

D. Enhanced elimination

1. **Repeat-dose activated charcoal** may trap small quantities of amatoxin undergoing enterohepatic recirculation.
2. Cannulation of the bile duct and removal of bile have been effective in dog studies.
3. There is no proved role for forced diuresis, hemoperfusion, or hemodialysis in the removal of amatoxins.

Reference

Pond SM et al: Amatoxin poisoning in northern California, 1982–1983. *West J Med* 1986;**145**:204.

NAPHTHALENE AND PARADICHLOROBENZENE
James F. Buchanan, PharmD

ANTIDOTE   IPECAC   LAVAGE   CHARCOAL

Naphthalene and paradichlorobenzene are common ingredients in mothballs and toilet bowl deodorizers. Both compounds have a similar pungent odor and are difficult to distinguish visually. Naphthalene is no longer commonly used because it has been largely replaced by the far less toxic paradichlorobenzene.

I. Mechanism of toxicity. Both compounds cause gastrointestinal upset, and both may cause central nervous system stimulation. In addition, naphthalene may produce hemolysis, especially in patients with glucose-6-phosphate dehydrogenase (G6PD) deficiency.

II. Toxic dose

A. Naphthalene. As little as one mothball containing naphthalene (250–500 mg) may produce hemolysis in a patient with G6PD deficiency. The amount necessary to produce lethargy or seizures is not known but may be as little as 1–2 g (4–8 mothballs).

B. Paradichlorobenzene is much less toxic than naphthalene; up to 20-g ingestions have been well-tolerated in adults. The oral LD_{50} for paradichlorobenzene in rats is 2.5–3.2 g/kg.

III. Clinical presentation. Acute ingestion usually causes prompt nausea and vomiting.

A. Naphthalene. Agitation, lethargy, and seizures may occur with naphthalene ingestion. In patients with G6PD deficiency, naphthalene ingestion may cause acute hemolysis.

B. Paradichlorobenzene ingestions are virtually always innocuous. Serious poisoning in animals is reported to cause tremors and hepatic necrosis.

IV. Diagnosis. Diagnosis is usually based on a history of ingestion and the characteristic "mothball" smell around the mouth and in the vomitus. Differentiation between naphthalene and paradichlorobenzene by odor or color is difficult. Paradichlorobenzene is reportedly more rapidly soluble in turpentine.

A. Specific levels. Serum levels are not available.

B. Other useful laboratory studies. CBC. If hemolysis is suspected, obtain haptoglobin, free hemoglobin, and urine hemoglobin.

V. Treatment

A. Emergency and supportive measures

1. Maintain the airway and assist ventilation if necessary (see p 2).
2. Treat coma (p 17) and seizures (p 21) if they occur.
3. Treat hemolysis and resulting hemoglobinuria, if they occur, by intravenous hydration and urinary alkalinization (see rhabdomyolysis, p 24).

B. Specific drugs and antidotes. There is no specific antidote.

C. Decontamination

1. Naphthalene
   a. Induce emesis or perform gastric lavage (see p 42). Gastric lavage is preferred over emesis because of the risk of seizures.
   b. Administer activated charcoal and cathartic (see p 45).
   c. Gut emptying is probably not necessary following a small ingestion if activated charcoal is given promptly.

2. Paradichlorobenzene
   a. Gut emptying is probably not needed unless a massive overdose has been ingested.
   b. Administer charcoal and cathartic (see p 45) orally.

D. Enhanced elimination. There is no role for these procedures.

Reference

Siegel E, Wason S: Mothball toxicity. *Pediatr Clin North Am* 1986;**33**:369.

NICOTINE
Neal L. Benowitz, MD

ANTIDOTE   IPECAC   LAVAGE   CHARCOAL

Nicotine poisoning may occur in children after they ingest tobacco or drink saliva expectorated by a tobacco chewer (which is often collected in a can or other containers); in adults after suicidal ingestion of nicotine-containing pesticides (such as Black Leaf 40, which contains 40% nicotine sulfate); and occasionally after cutaneous exposure to nicotine, such as in tobacco harvesters. Nicotine chewing gum (Nicorette) has been recently marketed, but owing to its slow absorption and high degree of presystemic metabolism, nicotine intoxication from this product is uncommon.

I. **Mechanism of toxicity.** Nicotine binds to nicotinic cholinergic receptors resulting initially, via actions on ganglia, in predominantly sympathetic nervous stimulation. With higher doses, parasympathetic stimulation and then ganglionic and neuromuscular blockade may occur. Direct effects on the brain may also result in vomiting and seizures.

II. **Toxic dose.** Cigarette tobacco contains about 1.5% nicotine, or 10–15 mg of nicotine per cigarette. Moist snuff is also about 1.5% nicotine; most containers hold 30 g of tobacco. Chewing tobacco contains 2.5–8% nicotine; nicotine gum contains 2 mg per piece (in the USA) and 2 mg or 4 mg in Canada and Europe. Owing to presystemic metabolism and spontaneous vomiting, which limit absorption, the bioavailability of nicotine that is swallowed is about 30–40%.
   A. Rapid absorption of 2–5 mg can cause nausea and vomiting, particularly in a person who does not habitually use tobacco. Absorption of 40–60 mg in an adult is said to be lethal, although this dose spread throughout the day is not unusual in a cigarette smoker.
   B. In a child, ingestion of 1 cigarette or 3 butts should be considered potentially toxic, although serious poisoning from ingestion of cigarettes is very uncommon.

III. **Clinical presentation.** Nicotine intoxication commonly causes dizziness, nausea, vomiting, pallor, and diaphoresis. Abdominal pain, salivation, lacrimation, and diarrhea may be noted. Pupils may be dilated or constricted. Confusion, agitation, lethargy, and convulsions are seen with severe poisonings. Initial tachycardia and hypertension may be followed by bradycardia and hypotension. Respiratory muscle weakness with respiratory arrest is the most likely cause of death.
   Symptoms usually begin within 15 minutes after exposure and resolve in 1 or 2 hours, although more prolonged symptoms may be seen with higher doses or cutaneous exposure, the latter due to continued absorption from the skin.

IV. **Diagnosis.** Vomiting, pallor, and diaphoresis are suggestive of nicotine poisoning but are nonspecific. The diagnosis is usually made by a history of tobacco or insecticide exposure. Nicotine poisoning should be considered in a small child with unexplained vomiting whose parents consume tobacco.
   A. **Specific levels.** Nicotine is detected in urine screens, but because it is so commonly present, it will not be reported unless specifically requested. Serum levels can be performed but are not useful in acute management.
   B. **Other useful laboratory studies.** CBC, electrolytes, glucose, arterial blood gases.

V. **Treatment**
   A. **Emergency and supportive measures**
      1. Maintain the airway and assist ventilation if necessary (see p 2).
      2. Treat seizures (p 21), coma (p 17), hypotension (p 14), hypertension (p 16), and arrhythmias (p 9) if they occur.
      3. Observe for at least 4–6 hours to rule out delayed toxicity, especially after skin exposure.
   B. **Specific drugs and antidotes**
      1. **Mecamylamine (Inversine)** is a specific antagonist of nicotine actions; however, it is available only in tablets, a form not suitable for a patient who is vomiting, convulsive, or hypotensive.
      2. Signs of parasympathetic stimulation (bradycardia, salivation, wheezing, etc), if they occur, may respond to **atropine** (see p 293).

C. Decontamination

1. Skin and eyes. Remove all contaminated clothing and wash exposed skin with copious soap and water. Irrigate exposed eyes with copious saline or water.

2. Ingestion

   a. Do **not** induce emesis because of the risk of seizures. Perform gastric lavage (see p 43).

   b. Administer activated charcoal and cathartic (see p 45).

   c. Gut emptying is probably not necessary following a very small ingestion if activated charcoal is given promptly.

D. Enhanced elimination. Hemoperfusion is not likely to be useful because the endogenous clearance of nicotine is high, its half-life is relatively short (2 hours), and the volume of distribution is large.

References

Benowitz NL et al: Prolonged absorption with development of tolerance to toxic effects after cutaneous exposure to nicotine. *Clin Pharmacol Ther* 1987;**42**:119.

Saxena K, Scheman A: Suicide plan by nicotine poisoning: A review of nicotine toxicity. *Vet Hum Toxicol* 1985;**27**:495.

NITRATES AND NITRITES
Neal L. Benowitz, MD

ANTIDOTE   IPECAC   LAVAGE   CHARCOAL

Organic nitrates (eg, nitroglycerin, isosorbide dinitrate) are widely used as vasodilators for the treatment of ischemic heart disease and heart failure. Organic nitrates such as nitroglycerin are also used in explosives. Bismuth subnitrate, ammonium nitrate, and silver nitrate are used in antidiarrheal, diuretic, and topical burn medications, respectively. Sodium and potassium nitrate and nitrite are used in preserving cured foods and may also occur in high concentrations in some well water. Butyl, amyl, ethyl, and isobutyl nitrite are often sold as "room deodorizers" or "liquid incense" and are inhaled for abuse purposes.

I. Mechanism of toxicity. Nitrates and nitrites both cause vasodilation, which can result in hypotension.

   A. Nitrates relax veins at lower doses and arteries at higher doses. Nitrates may be converted into nitrites in the gastrointestinal tract, especially in infants.

   B. Nitrites are potent oxidizing agents. Oxidation of hemoglobin by nitrites may result in methemoglobinemia (see p 204), which hinders oxygen-carrying capacity and oxygen delivery. Many organic nitrites (eg, amyl nitrite, butyl nitrite) are volatile and may be inhaled.

II. Toxic dose. In the quantities found in food, nitrates and nitrites are generally not toxic; however, infants may develop methemoglobinemia after ingestion of sausages or well water because they readily convert nitrate to nitrite and because their hemoglobin is more susceptible to oxidation compared with that of adults.

   A. Nitrates. The estimated adult lethal oral dose of nitroglycerin is between 200–1200 mg. Hypotension occurs at low doses, but massive doses are required to produce methemoglobinemia.

   B. Nitrites. Ingestion of as little as 15 mL of butyl nitrite produced 40% methemoglobinemia in an adult. The estimated adult lethal oral dose of sodium nitrite is 1 g.

III. Clinical presentation. Headache, skin flushing, and orthostatic hypotension with reflex tachycardia are the most common adverse effects of nitrates and nitrites and occur commonly even with therapeutic doses of organic nitrates.

  A. **Hypotension** may aggravate or produce symptoms of cardiac ischemia or cerebrovascular disease and may even cause seizures. However, fatalities due to hypotension are rare.

  B. Workers or patients regularly exposed to nitrates may develop tolerance and may suffer **angina** or **myocardial infarction** due to rebound coronary vasoconstriction upon sudden withdrawal of the drug.

  C. **Methemoglobinemia** (see p 204) is most common after nitrite exposure; the skin is cyanotic, even at levels low enough to be asymptomatic (eg, 15%).

IV. Diagnosis. Hypotension with reflex tachycardia and headache are suggestive of intoxication. Methemoglobinemia of 15% or more (see p 204) may be diagnosed by noting a chocolate brown coloration of the blood when it is dripped onto filter paper.

  A. **Specific levels.** Tests for serum levels are not commercially available. With the use of a nitrite dipstick (normally used to detect bacteria in urine), nitrite can be detected in the serum of patients intoxicated by butyl nitrite.

  B. **Other useful laboratory studies.** CBC, arterial blood gases, methemoglobin concentration, ECG and electrocardiographic monitoring.

V. Treatment

  A. **Emergency and supportive measures**

    1. Maintain the airway and assist ventilation if necessary (see p 2). Administer supplemental oxygen.

    2. Treat hypotension with supine positioning, intravenous crystalloid fluids, and low-dose pressors if needed (see p 14).

    3. Monitor vital signs and ECG for 4–6 hours.

  B. **Specific drugs and antidotes.** Symptomatic methemoglobinemia may be treated with **methylene blue** (see p 322). Treat myocardial ischemia caused by nitrate withdrawal with nitrates.

  C. **Decontamination**

    1. **Inhalation.** Remove victim from exposure and administer supplemental oxygen, if available.

    2. **Skin and eyes.** Remove contaminated clothing and wash with copious soap and water. Irrigate exposed eyes with water or saline.

    3. **Ingestion**

      a. Induce emesis or perform gastric lavage (see p 42).

      b. Administer activated charcoal and a cathartic (see p 45).

      c. Gut emptying is probably not necessary following a small ingestion if activated charcoal is given promptly.

  D. **Enhanced elimination.** Hemodialysis and hemoperfusion are not effective. Severe methemoglobinemia in infants not responsive to methylene blue therapy may require **exchange transfusion.**

Reference

Wason S et al: Isobutyl nitrite toxicity by ingestion. *Ann Intern Med* 1980;**92**:637.

NITROGEN OXIDES
Kent R. Olson, MD

ANTIDOTE   IPECAC   LAVAGE   CHARCOAL

Nitrogen oxides (nitric oxide, nitrogen dioxide) are dangerous chemical gases commonly released from nitrous or nitric acid, from reactions between nitric acid and organic materials, and from burning of nitrocellulose and many other products. Exposure to nitrogen oxides occurs in electric arc welding, electroplating, and engraving. They are found in engine exhaust, and they are produced when stored grain with a high nitrite content ferments in storage silos.

I. **Mechanism of toxicity.** Nitrogen oxides are irritant gases with relatively low water solubility. Slow accumulation and hydration to nitric acid in the alveoli result in delayed onset of chemical pneumonitis. In addition, nitrogen oxides can oxidize hemoglobin to methemoglobin.

II. **Toxic dose.** The OSHA Permissible Exposure Limit (PEL) for nitric oxide is 25 ppm as an 8-hour time-weighted average. There is no PEL for nitrogen dioxide, but the 15-minute Short-Term Exposure Limit (STEL) is 1 ppm. The air levels considered immediately dangerous to life or health (IDLH) are 100 ppm and 50 ppm, respectively.

III. **Clinical presentation.** Because of the poor water solubility of nitrogen oxides, there is very little upper respiratory irritation at low levels (< 10 ppm nitrogen dioxide) and prolonged exposure may occur with only a mild cough or nausea. With more concentrated exposures, upper respiratory symptoms such as burning eyes, sore throat, and painful brassy cough may occur.

   A. After a delay of up to 24 hours, chemical pneumonia may develop, with progressive cough, tachypnea, hypoxemia, and pulmonary edema. The onset may be more rapid after exposure to higher concentrations.

   B. Following recovery from acute chemical pneumonia and after chronic low-level exposure to nitrogen oxides, permanent restrictive and obstructive lung disease from bronchiolar damage may become evident.

   C. Methemoglobinemia has been described in victims exposed to nitrogen oxides in smoke during major structural fires.

IV. **Diagnosis.** Diagnosis is based on a history of exposure, if known. Because of the potential for delayed effects, all patients with significant smoke inhalation should be observed for several hours.

   A. **Specific levels.** There are no specific blood levels.

   B. **Other useful laboratory studies.** CBC, electrolytes, arterial blood gases, methemoglobin level, chest x-ray, pulmonary function tests.

V. **Treatment**

   A. **Emergency and supportive measures**

      1. Observe closely for signs of upper airway obstruction, and intubate the trachea and assist ventilation if necessary (see p 4). Administer humidified supplemental oxygen.

      2. Observe symptomatic victims for a minimum of 24 hours after exposure and treat chemical pneumonia and noncardiogenic pulmonary edema (see p 7) if they occur.

   B. **Specific drugs and antidotes**

      1. Administration of corticosteroids is favored by many toxicologists, but there is no convincing evidence that they can improve nitrogen oxide-induced chemical pneumonia or pulmonary edema or prevent chronic bronchitis.

      2. Treat methemoglobinemia (see p 204) with **methylene blue** (see p 322).

   C. **Decontamination**

      1. **Inhalation.** Remove victim from exposure immediately and give supplemental oxygen, if available.

      2. **Skin and eyes.** Remove contaminated clothing and flush exposed skin with water. Irrigate exposed eyes with copious water or saline.

   D. **Enhanced elimination.** There is no role for enhanced elimination procedures.

Reference

Yockey CC, Eden BM, Byrd RB: The McConnell missile accident: Clinical spectrum of nitrogen dioxide exposure. *JAMA* 1980;**244**:1221.

NITROPRUSSIDE
Neal L. Benowitz, MD

ANTIDOTE   IPECAC   LAVAGE   CHARCOAL

Sodium nitroprusside is a short-acting parenterally administered vasodilator used to treat severe hypertension and cardiac failure. It is also used to induce hypotension for certain surgical procedures. Toxicity may occur with acute high-dose nitroprusside treatment or with prolonged infusions.

I. **Mechanism of toxicity.** Nitroprusside is rapidly hydrolyzed and releases free cyanide, which is normally quickly converted to thiocyanate by rhodanase enzymes in the liver and blood vessels.
   A. **Acute cyanide poisoning** may occur with short-term high-dose nitroprusside infusions.
   B. **Thiocyanate** is eliminated by the kidney and may accumulate in patients with renal insufficiency, especially after prolonged infusions.

II. **Toxic dose.** The toxic dose depends on renal function and the **rate** of infusion.
   A. **Cyanide** poisoning is uncommon at nitroprusside infusion rates of less than 8–10 mcg/kg/min but has been reported after infusion of 4 mcg/kg/min for 3 hours.
   B. **Thiocyanate** toxicity does not occur with acute brief use in persons with normal renal function but may result from prolonged infusions.

III. **Clinical presentation.** The most common adverse effect of nitroprusside is hypotension, which is often accompanied by reflex tachycardia.
   A. **Cyanide** poisoning is accompanied by headache, hyperventilation, anxiety, agitation, seizures, and metabolic acidosis. The ECG may reveal ischemic patterns.
   B. **Thiocyanate** poisoning causes somnolence, confusion, delirium, tremor, and hyperreflexia. Seizures and coma may rarely occur with severe toxicity.
   C. **Methemoglobinemia** occurs rarely and is usually mild.

IV. **Diagnosis.** Lactic acidosis, coma, or seizures after short-term high-dose nitoprusside infusion should suggest cyanide poisoning, while confusion or delirium developing gradually after several days of continuous use should suggest thiocyanate poisoning.
   A. **Specific levels. Cyanide** and **thiocyanate** serum levels may be obtained but are not usually available rapidly enough to guide treatment when cyanide poisoning is suspected. Cyanide levels may not accurately reflect toxicity because of simultaneous production of methemoglobin, which binds some of the cyanide. Thiocyanate levels higher than 50–100 mg/L may cause delirium and somnolence.
   B. **Other useful laboratory studies.** CBC, electrolytes, glucose, BUN, creatinine, serum lactate, ECG, arterial blood gases and measured arterial and venous oxygen saturation (see Cyanide, p 134), methemoglobin level.

V. **Treatment**
   A. **Emergency and supportive measures**
      1. Maintain the airway and assist ventilation if necessary (see p 2). Administer supplemental oxygen.
      2. For hypotension, stop the infusion immediately and administer intravenous fluids or pressors if necessary (p 14).
   B. **Specific drugs and antidotes.** If cyanide poisoning is suspected, administer **sodium thiosulfate** (see p 340). **Sodium nitrite** treatment may aggravate hypotension and should not be used. Hydroxocobalamin (p 316) is a cyanide antidote available in some European countries.

C. **Decontamination.** These procedures are not relevant because the drug is administered only parenterally.
D. **Enhanced elimination.** Nitroprusside and cyanide are both metabolized rapidly, so there is no need to consider enhanced elimination for these. **Hemodialysis** may accelerate **thiocyanate** elimination and is especially useful in patients with renal failure.

Reference

Cottrell JE et al: Prevention of nitroprusside-induced cyanide toxicity with hydroxocobalamin. *N Engl J Med* 1978;**298**:809.

NITROUS OXIDE
Margaret Atterbury, MD

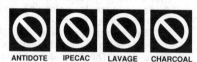

ANTIDOTE   IPECAC   LAVAGE   CHARCOAL

Nitrous oxide, or laughing gas, is used as a general anesthetic agent and as a propellant in many commercial products such as whipped cream or cooking oil spray. Abuse of nitrous oxide is not uncommon in the medical and dental professions.

I. **Mechanism of toxicity**
   A. **Acute toxicity** following exposure to nitrous oxide is mainly due to asphyxia if adequate oxygen is not supplied with the gas.
   B. **Chronic toxicity** to the hematologic and nervous systems is believed to be secondary to the selective inactivation of vitamin B_{12}.
II. **Toxic dose.** The toxic dose is not established. Chronic occupational exposure to 2000 ppm nitrous oxide produced asymptomatic but measurable depression of vitamin B_{12} in dentists.
III. **Clinical presentation**
   A. Signs of **acute toxicity** are related to **asphyxia.** These include headache, dizziness, confusion, syncope, seizures, and cardiac arrhythmias. Interstitial emphysema and pneumomediastinum have been reported following forceful inhalation from a pressurized whipped cream dispenser.
   B. **Chronic nitrous oxide abuse** may produce megaloblastic anemia, thrombocytopenia, leukopenia, peripheral neuropathy, and myelopathy, similar to effects of vitamin B_{12} deficiency.
IV. **Diagnosis.** Diagnosis is based on a history of exposure and clinical presentation with evidence of asphyxia and an empty can or tank or with manifestations of chronic vitamin B_{12} deficiency but with normal vitamin B_{12} levels.
   A. **Specific levels.** Specific levels are not generally available and are unreliable owing to off-gassing. Case reports of 5 fatalities from nitrous oxide abuse reported postmortem blood concentrations of 46–180 mL/L.
   B. **Other useful laboratory studies.** CBC, platelet count, arterial blood gas, vitamin B_{12}.
V. **Treatment**
   A. **Emergency and supportive measures**
      1. Maintain the airway and assist ventilation if necessary (see p 2). Administer high-flow supplemental oxygen.
      2. After significant asphyxia, anticipate and treat coma (p 17), seizures (p 21), and cardiac arrhythmias (pp 9–13).
   B. **Specific levels.** There is no specific antidote. Chronic effects should resolve over 2–3 months after discontinuing exposure.

C. **Decontamination.** Remove victim from exposure and give supplemental oxygen, if available.
D. **Enhanced elimination.** These procedures are not effective.

Reference

Sweeney B et al: Toxicity of bone marrow in dentists exposed to nitrous oxide. *Br Med J* 1985;**291**:567.

NONSTEROIDAL ANTI-INFLAMMATORY AGENTS
Kathryn H. Keller, PharmD

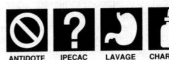

ANTIDOTE   IPECAC   LAVAGE   CHARCOAL

The nonsteroidal anti-inflammatory drugs (NSAIDs) are a chemically diverse group of agents that share similar pharmacologic properties and are widely used for control of pain and inflammation (Table II–35). Overdose by most of the agents in this group usually produces only mild gastrointestinal upset. However, toxicity may be severe following overdose with **oxyphenbutazone, phenylbutazone, mefenamic acid, piroxicam,** or **diflunisal.**

TABLE II–35. COMMON NSAIDs

Drug	Maximum Daily Adult Dose (mg)	Half-Life (h)	Comments
Carboxylic acids			
Diclofenac	195	2	
Fenoprofen	3200	3	Acute renal failure
Ibuprofen	3200	2.5	Massive overdose may cause coma, renal failure, metabolic acidosis, and cardiorespiratory depression.
Indomethacin	200	3–11	
Ketoprofen	300	2–4	
Meclofenamate	400	3	
Mefenamic acid	750	3	Seizures, twitching
Naproxen	1500	10–20	
Sulindac	400	7	
Suprofen	800	2–4	
Tolmetin	2000	5–6	
Enolic acids			
Oxyphenbutazone	600	27–64	Seizures, acidosis
Phenylbutazone	600	75	Seizures, acidosis
Piroxicam	20	45–50	Seizures, coma

I. Mechanism of toxicity. NSAIDs produce their pharmacologic and most toxicologic effects by inhibiting the enzyme cyclooxygenase; this results in decreased production of prostaglandins and decreased pain and inflammation. Central nervous system, hemodynamic, pulmonary, and hepatic dysfunction also occur with some agents, but the relationship to prostaglandin production remains uncertain. Prostaglandins are also involved in maintaining the integrity of the gastric mucosa and regulating renal blood flow; thus, acute or chronic intoxication may affect these organs.

II. Toxic dose. Human data are insufficient to establish a reliable correlation between amount ingested, plasma concentrations, and clinical toxic effects. Generally, significant symptoms occur after ingestion of more than 5–10 times the usual therapeutic dose.

III. Clinical presentation. In general, patients with NSAID overdose are asymptomatic or have mild gastrointestinal upset (nausea, vomiting, abdominal pain, sometimes hematemesis). Occasionally patients exhibit drowsiness, lethargy, ataxia, nystagmus, tinnitus, and disorientation.

  A. With the more toxic agents **oxyphenbutazone, phenylbutazone, mefenamic acid,** or **piroxicam** and with massive **ibuprofen** overdose, seizures, coma, renal failure, and cardiorespiratory arrest may occur. Hepatic dysfunction, hypoprothrombinemia, and metabolic acidosis are also commonly reported.

  B. Diflunisal overdose produces toxicity resembling salicylate poisoning (see p 261).

IV. Diagnosis. Diagnosis is usually based primarily on a history of ingestion of NSAIDs, because symptoms are mild and nonspecific and quantitative levels are not usually available.

  A. Specific levels. Specific serum levels are not usually readily available and do not contribute to clinical management.

  B. Other useful laboratory studies. CBC, electrolytes, glucose, BUN, creatinine, liver function tests, prothrombin time (PT), urinalysis.

V. Treatment

  A. Emergency and supportive measures

  1. Maintain the airway and assist ventilation if necessary (see p 2). Administer supplemental oxygen.
  2. Treat seizures (p 21), coma (p 17), and hypotension (p 14) if they occur.
  3. Antacids may be used for mild gastrointestinal upset. Replace fluid losses with intravenous crystalloid solutions (p 14).

  B. Specific drugs and antidotes. There is no antidote. Vitamin K (see p 341) may be used for patients with elevated prothrombin time (PT) caused by hypoprothrombinemia.

  C. Decontamination

  1. Induce emesis or perform gastric lavage (see p 42). The latter is preferable for the more toxic agents because of the risk of seizures.
  2. Administer activated charcoal and cathartic (see p 45).
  3. Gut emptying is probably not necessary following small ingestions if activated charcoal is given promptly.

  D. Enhanced elimination. NSAIDs are highly protein-bound and extensively metabolized. Thus, hemodialysis, peritoneal dialysis, and forced diuresis are not likely to be effective.

  1. **Charcoal hemoperfusion** may be effective for **phenylbutazone** overdose, although there are limited clinical data to support its use.
  2. There are no data on the use of repeat-dose activated charcoal therapy.

Reference

Vale JA, Meredith TJ: Acute poisoning due to nonsteroidal anti-inflammatory drugs: Clinical features and management. *Med Toxicol* 1986;1:12.

OPIATES AND OPIOIDS
Kent R. Olson, MD

ANTIDOTE   IPECAC   LAVAGE   CHARCOAL

Opiates are a group of naturally occurring compounds derived from the juice of the poppy *Papaver somniferum*. Morphine is the classic opiate derivative used widely in medicine; heroin (diacetylmorphine) is a well-known, highly addictive street narcotic. The term **opioids** refers to these and other derivatives of naturally occurring opium (eg, morphine, heroin, codeine, hydrocodone) as well as new, totally synthetic opiate analogues (eg, fentanyl, butorphanol, meperidine, methadone; Table II–36). A wide variety of prescription medications contain opioids, often in combination with aspirin or acetaminophen.

Dextromethorphan (see p 141) is an opioid with potent antitussive but no analgesic or addictive properties. Diphenoxylate is an opioid that is combined with atropine (see Lomotil, p 190) as a treatment for diarrhea.

I. **Mechanism of toxicity.** In general, the opioids share the ability to stimulate a number of specific opiate receptors in the central nervous system, causing sedation and respiratory depression. Death is due to respiratory failure, usually as a result of apnea or pulmonary aspiration of gastric contents. In addition, acute noncardiogenic pulmonary edema may occur by unknown mechanisms.

II. **Toxic dose.** The toxic dose varies widely depending on the specific compound, the route and rate of administration, and tolerance to the effects of

TABLE II-36. COMMON OPIATES AND OPOIDS[a]

Drug	Type of Activity	Usual Dose[a] (mg)	Elimination Half-Life (h)	Duration of Analgesia (h)
Morphine	Agonist	10	3	4–5
Hydromorphone	Agonist	1.5	2.5	4–5
Methadone	Agonist	10	35	4–6
Heroin	Agonist	4	(b)	3–4
Meperidine	Agonist	100	3	2–4
Fentanyl	Agonist	0.2	4	1–2
Codeine	Agonist	60	3	3–4
Oxycodone	Agonist	4.5	4	3–4
Propoxyphene	Agonist	100	15	4–5
Pentazocine	Mixed	50	3	3–4
Nalbuphine	Mixed	10	3.5	3–6
Butorphanol	Mixed	2	3	3–4
Naloxone	Antagonist	1–2	1	NA

[a] Usual dose: Dose equivalent to 10 mg of morphine.
[b] Rapidly hydrolyzed to morphine.

the drug. Some newer fentanyl derivatives have a potency up to 2000 times that of morphine. The duration of effect and elimination half-lives of the opioids also vary greatly (Table II–36).

III. **Clinical presentation**

A. **With mild or moderate overdose,** lethargy is common. The pupils are usually small, often "pinpoint" size. Blood pressure and pulse rate are decreased, bowel sounds are diminished, and the muscles are usually flaccid.

B. **With higher doses,** coma is accompanied by respiratory depression and apnea often results in rapid death. Noncardiogenic pulmonary edema may occur, often *after* resuscitation and administration of the opiate antagonist naloxone.

C. **Seizures** are not common after acute opioid overdose but occur occasionally with certain compounds (eg, meperidine, propoxyphene, dextromethorphan). Seizures may occur in renally compromised patients receiving repeated doses of meperidine.

D. Some newer synthetic opioids have mixed agonist and antagonist effects with unpredictable results in overdose.

IV. **Diagnosis.** Diagnosis is easy when typical manifestations of opiate intoxication are present (pinpoint pupils, respiratory and CNS depression), and the patient quickly awakens after administration of naloxone. Signs of intravenous drug abuse (eg, needle track marks) are often present. When opioids are combined with other drugs or signs of intravenous drug abuse are absent, then diagnosis is based on the history, the response to naloxone, and results of toxicologic screening.

A. **Specific levels.** Specific serum levels are not usually performed because of poor correlation of levels with clinical effects. Qualitative screening of the urine is an effective way to confirm recent use. Fentanyl derivatives and some other synthetic opioids are not detected by routine toxicologic screens.

B. **Other useful laboratory studies.** CBC, electrolytes, glucose, arterial blood gases, chest x-ray, stat serum acetaminophen or salicylate levels (if ingested overdose was a combination product).

V. **Treatment**

A. **Emergency and supportive measures**

1. Maintain the airway and assist ventilation if necessary (see p 2). Administer supplemental oxygen.

2. Treat coma (p 17), seizures (p 21), and hypotension (p 14) if they occur.

B. **Specific drugs and antidotes. Naloxone** (p 325) is a specific opioid antagonist with no agonist properties of its own; huge doses may be given safely.

1. Administer naloxone, 0.4–2 mg IV. Repeat dose every 2–3 minutes if there is no response, up to a total dose of 10–20 mg if opioid overdose is strongly suspected.

2. *Caution:* The duration of effect of naloxone (2–3 hours) is shorter than that of many opioids. Therefore, do not release the patient who has awakened after naloxone treatment until at least 3–4 hours have passed since the last dose of naloxone. In general, if naloxone was required to reverse opioid-induced coma, it is safer to admit the patient for at least 6–12 hours of observation.

C. **Decontamination**

1. Induce emesis or perform gastric lavage (see p 42).

2. Administer activated charcoal and cathartic (see p 45).

3. Gut emptying is probably not necessary following small ingestions if activated charcoal is given promptly.

4. *Caution:* Because of the risk of rapid onset of coma and respiratory depression, do not induce vomiting or give oral activated charcoal unless the patient has received naloxone and is wide awake.

    D. Enhanced elimination. Because of the very large volumes of distribution of the opioids, there is no role for enhanced elimination procedures.

Reference

Goldfrank L et al: A dosing nomogram for continuous infusion intravenous naloxone. *Ann Emerg Med* 1986;**15**:566.

ORGANOPHOSPHATES
Olga F. Woo, PharmD

ANTIDOTE   IPECAC   LAVAGE   CHARCOAL

Organophosphates are widely used pesticides that may cause acute or chronic poisonings after accidental or suicidal exposure. Poisonings are particularly common in rural areas and third-world countries where organophosphates are widely available. Organophosphates usually contain solvents such as toluene or xylene that may be listed as inert ingredients but can produce toxic effects in an overdose.

  I. Mechanism of toxicity. Organophosphates are rapidly absorbed by inhalation and ingestion and through the skin. Organophosphates and their potent sulfoxidation ("-oxon") derivatives inhibit the enzyme acetylcholinesterase, allowing the accumulation of excessive acetylcholine at muscarinic receptors (cholinergic effector cells), at nicotinic receptors (skeletal neuromuscular junctions and autonomic ganglia), and in the central nervous system.

  II. Toxic dose. A substantial proportion of the acetylcholinesterase enzyme activity must be inhibited before characteristic signs and symptoms of intoxication occur. The degree of intoxication is also affected by the rate of exposure (acute versus chronic), by the ongoing metabolic degradation and elimination of the organophosphate, and by the rate of metabolism to its more toxic "-oxon" derivative.

    There is a wide spectrum of relative potency of organophosphates (Table II–37). Some organophosphates are highly lipophilic, are stored in fat tissue (eg, fenthion), and may cause persistent toxicity for several days after exposure.

  III. Clinical presentation. Signs and symptoms of acute organophosphate poisoning usually occur within 1–2 hours of exposure but may be delayed up to several hours, especially after skin exposure. Clinical manfestations may be classified into muscarinic, nicotinic, or central nervous system. In addition, hypdrocarbon pneumonitis (see p 165) may occur if the product is aspirated into the lungs.

    A. Muscarinic (parasympathetic) manifestations include vomiting, diarrhea, abdominal cramping, bronchospasm, miosis, bradycardia, and excessive salivation and sweating.

    B. Nicotinic (ganglionic) manifestations include muscle fasciculations, tremor, and weakness. Death is usually caused by respiratory muscle paralysis. Blood pressure and pulse rate may be increased because of nicotinic effects or decreased because of muscarinic effects.

    C. Central nervous system poisoning causes agitation, seizures, and coma.

    D. Some organophosphates may cause a delayed, often permanent peripheral neuropathy.

  IV. Diagnosis. Diagnosis is based on the history of exposure and the presence of characteristic muscarinic, nicotinic, and CNS manifestations. There is

TABLE II-37. RELATIVE TOXICITIES OF ORGANOPHOSPHATES

Low toxicity (LD_{50} > 1000 mg/kg)[a]

Acephate	Phoxim
Bromophos	Pirimiphos-methyl
Etrimfos	Propylthiopyrophosphate
Iodofenphos	Temephos
Malathion	Tetrachlorvinphos
Merphos	

Moderate toxicity (LD_{50} > 500 mg/kg)[a]

Bromophos-ethyl	Heptenophos
Chlorpyrifos	Isoxathion
Coumaphos	Leptophos
Cythioate	Naled
DEF	Phencapton
Demeton-methyl	Phenthoate
Diazinon	Phosalone
Dichlofenthion	Phosmet
Dichlorovos	Profenofos
Dimethoate	Propetamphos
Dioxathion	Pyrazophos
EPBP	Pyridaphenthion
Ethion	Quinalphos
Ethoprop	Sulprofos
Fenitrothion	Thiometon
Fenthion	Triazophos
Formothion	Trichlorfon

High toxicity (LD_{50} < 50 mg/kg)[a]

Azinphos-methyl	Isophenfos
Bomyl	Isoflurophate
Carbophenothion	Methamidophos
Chlorfenvinphos	Methidathion
Chlormephos	Mevinphos
Chlorthiophos	Monocrotophos
Cyanofenphos	Parathion
Demeton	Phorate
Dialifor	Phosfolan
Dicrotophos	Phosphamidon
Disulfoton	Prothoate
EPN	Schradan
Famphur	Sulfotepp
Fenamiphos	Terbufos
Fenophosphon	Tetraethylpyrophosphate
Fensulfothion	Triorthocresylphosphate
Fonofos	

[a] Based on oral LD_{50} values in the rat.

frequently a solvent odor, and some describe a garliclike odor of the organophosphate.
   A. **Specific levels.** Laboratory confirmation may be obtained by measuring decreases in the plasma pseudocholinesterase (PChE) and red blood cell acetylcholinesterase (AChE) activities. *Note:* Because of wide interindividual variability, significant depression of enzyme activity may occur but still fall within the "normal" range.
      1. The AChE activity provides a more reliable measure of the toxic effect; a 25% or greater depression in activity from baseline generally indicates true exposure.
      2. PChE activity is a very sensitive indicator of exposure but is not as reliable as AChE activity (PChE may be depressed owing to genetic

deficiency, medical illness, or chronic organophosphate exposure). PChE activity usually recovers within weeks after exposure, whereas AChE recovery may take several months.

  B. Other useful laboratory studies. CBC, electrolytes, glucose, BUN, creatinine, liver enzymes, arterial blood gases, ECG, chest x-ray.

V. Treatment

  A. Emergency and supportive measures

  1. Maintain the airway and assist ventilation if necessary (see p 2). Pay careful attention to respiratory muscle weakness; sudden respiratory arrest may occur. Administer supplemental oxygen.

  2. Treat hydrocarbon pneumonitis (p 165), seizures (p 21), and coma (p 17) if they occur.

  3. Observe patients for at least 6–8 hours to rule out delayed-onset symptoms resulting from skin absorption or fat storage.

  B. Specific drugs and antidotes. Specific treatment includes the antimuscarinic agent **atropine** and the enzyme reactivator **pralidoxime.**

  1. Give **atropine,** 0.5–2 mg IV initially (see p 293), repeated frequently as needed. Large cumulative doses of atropine (up to 100 mg or more) may occasionally be required in severe cases. The most clinically important indication for continued atropine administration is persistent wheezing or bronchorrhea. Atropine will reverse muscarinic but not nicotinic effects.

  2. **Pralidoxime** (2-PAM, Protopam; see p 337) is a specific antidote that acts to regenerate the enzyme activity at all affected sites (muscarinic, nicotinic, and probably CNS). It should be given immediately (adults: 1–2 g IV; children: 25–50 mg/kg IV, maximum 1 g) and repeated every 6–8 hours to control muscular weakness and fasciculations. Pralidoxime is most effective if started within the first 24 hours of the exposure prior to irreversible phosphorylation of the enzyme.

  C. Decontamination

  1. Remove all contaminated clothing and wash exposed areas with soap and water, including the hair and under the nails. Irrigate exposed eyes with copious tepid water or saline.

  2. Do **not** induce emesis because of the danger of abrupt respiratory arrest and seizures. Perform gastric lavage (see p 43), protecting the airway with a cuffed endotracheal tube if patient is obtunded. Gut emptying is probably of no benefit if started more than 60 minutes after ingestion and is not necessary for small ingestions.

  3. Administer activated charcoal (see p 45) orally or by gastric tube. Cathartics are not necessary if the patient already has diarrhea.

  D. Enhanced elimination. Dialysis and hemoperfusion are not indicated because of the large volume of distribution of organophosphates and the effectiveness of the specific therapy described above.

Reference

Namba T et al: Poisoning due to organophosphate insecticides: Acute and chronic manifestations. *Am J Med* 1971;**50:**475.

OXALIC ACID
Kent R. Olson, MD

ANTIDOTE   IPECAC   LAVAGE   CHARCOAL

Oxalic acid and oxalates are used as bleaches, metal cleaners, and rust removers and in chemical synthesis and leather tanning. Soluble and insoluble oxalate salts are found in several species of plants.

I. **Mechanism of toxicity.** Oxalic acid solutions are highly irritating and corrosive. Ingestion and absorption of oxalate cause acute hypocalcemia resulting from precipitation of the insoluble calcium oxalate salt. Calcium oxalate crystals may deposit in the brain, heart, kidneys, and other sites, causing serious systemic damage.

   The insoluble calcium oxalate salt found in dieffenbachia and similar plants is not absorbed but causes local mucous membrane irritation (see p 245).

II. **Toxic dose.** Ingestion of 5–15 g of oxalic acid has caused death. The OSHA workplace permissible exposure limit (PEL) for oxalic acid vapor is 1 mg/m^3.

III. **Clinical presentation.** Toxicity may occur as a result of skin or eye contact, inhalation, or ingestion.

   A. **Acute skin or eye contact** causes irritation and burning, which may lead to serious corrosive injury if the exposure and concentration are high.

   B. **Inhalation** may cause sore throat, cough, and wheezing. Large exposures may lead to chemical pneumonitis or pulmonary edema.

   C. **Ingestion** of soluble oxalates may result in weakness, tetany, convulsions, and cardiac arrest due to profound hypocalcemia. The QT interval may be prolonged, and variable conduction defects may occur. Oxalate crystals may be found on urinalysis.

IV. **Diagnosis.** The diagnosis is based on a history of exposure and evidence of local or systemic effects described, along with severe hypocalcemia or oxalate crystalluria.

   A. **Specific levels.** Serum oxalate levels are not available.

   B. **Other useful laboratory studies.** CBC, electrolytes, glucose, BUN, creatinine, calcium, ECG and electrocardiographic monitoring, urinalysis.

V. **Treatment**

   A. **Emergency and supportive measures**
      1. Protect the airway (see p 1), which may become acutely swollen and obstructed after ingestion or inhalation. Administer supplemental oxygen, and assist ventilation if necessary (p 2).
      2. Treat coma (p 17), seizures (p 21), and arrhythmias (pp 9–13) if they occur.
      3. Monitor the ECG and vital signs for at least 6 hours after exposure, and admit symptomatic patients to an intensive care unit.

   B. **Specific drugs and antidotes.** Administer 10% **calcium solution** (see p 298) to counteract symptomatic hypocalcemia.

   C. **Decontamination**
      1. **Emesis** (see p 42) is appropriate after ingestion of plants containing soluble oxalates; but with oxalic acid, strong commercial oxalate salts, or plants containing insoluble oxalate crystals, do **not** induce emesis because of the risk of aggravating corrosive injury. Alternatively, perform gastric lavage (see p 43).
      2. **Gut emptying** is not necessary following small ingestions of low-concentration oxalate.
      3. Precipitate ingested oxalate in the stomach by administering calcium (chloride, gluconate, or lactate) orally or via gastric tube.
      4. The effectiveness of activated charcoal is unknown.

   D. **Enhanced elimination.** Maintain **high-volume urine flow** (3–5 mL/kg/h) to help prevent calcium oxalate precipitation in the tubules. Oxalate is removed by hemodialysis, but the indications for this treatment are not established.

Reference

Stauffer M: Oxalosis: Report of a case with a review of the literature and discussion of the pathogenesis. *N Engl J Med* 1960;263:386.

PARALDEHYDE
Timothy McCarthy, PharmD

ANTIDOTE   IPECAC   LAVAGE   CHARCOAL

Paraldehyde is a cyclic trimer of acetaldehyde. Although it has been largely replaced by newer agents, paraldehyde was widely used in the past as an anticonvulsant, a sedative-hypnotic, and an anesthetic. It has a characteristic penetrating odor and a disagreeable taste. It is incompatible with plastic and must be stored and administered in glass containers only. It rapidly decomposes to acetaldehyde and acetic acid upon exposure to light and air.

I. **Mechanism of toxicity.** Paraldehyde is a potent CNS depressant. It is a strong irritant to intestinal mucosa, especially if it has partially decomposed to acetic acid. If the product has developed a brown discoloration or the pungent smell of acetic acid, it should *not* be used.

II. **Toxic dose.** The typical therapeutic dose of paraldehyde for control of seizures or alcohol withdrawal is 5–10 mL IM or PO or 0.1–0.2 mL/kg IV every 4–6 hours. Deaths have been reported after a rectal dose of only 12 mL (undecomposed paraldehyde) and an oral dose of 25 mL. However, survival has been reported after ingestion of 125 mL. Coingestion of alcohol or other depressant drugs increases the risk of serious toxicity.

III. **Clinical presentation.** Peak effects are usually seen within 30–60 minutes after ingestion but may be delayed up to 2–3 hours after rectal administration. Lethargy, stupor, and coma are common. Gastritis, often hemorrhagic, may occur. Metabolic acidosis with an elevated anion gap may be due to acetic acid or may be a manifestation of starvation-type ketoacidosis in a patient with paraldehyde-induced gastritis. Severe leukocytosis (> 30,000), hypercoagulability, tachycardia, hypotension, tachypnea, right ventricular failure, and pulmonary edema have been reported.

IV. **Diagnosis.** The diagnosis is based on a history of exposure and is suggested by the typical pungent odor on the breath, metabolic acidosis, and altered mental status.

   A. **Specific levels.** Serum levels are not routinely available. The anticonvulsant therapeutic level is approximately 200 mg/L; serum levels higher than 500 mg/L are often associated with death.

   B. **Other useful laboratory studies.** CBC, electrolytes, glucose, arterial blood gases.

V. **Treatment**

   A. **Emergency and supportive measures**
   1. Maintain the airway and assist ventilation if necessary (see p 2). Administer supplemental oxygen.
   2. Treat coma (p 17), hypotension (p 14), metabolic acidosis (p 30), and pulmonary edema (p 7) if they occur.

   B. **Specific drugs and antidotes.** There is no specific antidote.

   C. **Decontamination**
   1. Do *not* induce emesis because paraldehyde is mildly corrosive and because of the risk of abrupt decline in mental status. Perform gastric lavage (see p 43). Gut emptying is not necessary after small ingestions (< 10–20 mL).
   2. Administer activated charcoal and a cathartic (see p 45) orally or by gastric tube.

   D. **Enhanced elimination.** The volume of distribution is 0.9 L/kg, making paradehyde accessible to enhanced elimination procedures. However, there are few data to support use of extracorporeal methods of enhanced elimination.

Reference

DiMaio VJ, Garriott JC: A fatal overdose of paraldehyde during treatment of a case of delirium tremens. *J Forensic Sci* 1974;**18**:755.

PARAQUAT AND DIQUAT
Kent R. Olson, MD

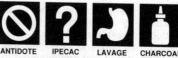

ANTIDOTE   IPECAC   LAVAGE   CHARCOAL

Paraquat and diquat are dipyridyl herbicides used primarily for weed control. Paraquat has also been used for large-scale control of illegal marijuana growing. Solutions available for home use are generally extremely dilute (0.2%), whereas commercial preparations may contain up to 21% paraquat. Weedol is a granular formulation containing a 2.5% mixture of paraquat and diquat salts.

I. **Mechanism of toxicity**
   A. **Paraquat** is a strong cation in aqueous solution, and concentrated solutions (20–24%) may cause corrosive injury when applied to the skin or ingested. After absorption, paraquat is selectively taken up and concentrated by pulmonary alveolar cells over several days. Lipid peroxidation then results in cell necrosis and proliferation of fibrous connective tissue, leading to pulmonary fibrosis. Although paraquat is poorly absorbed through intact skin, it is absorbed across abraded skin and fatalities have been reported following skin application.
   B. **Diquat** is also corrosive in concentrated solutions. Unlike paraquat, diquat does not cause pulmonary fibrosis. Instead, it causes gastrointestinal fluid sequestration, renal failure, and cerebral and brain stem hemorrhagic infarctions.
II. **Toxic dose.** Paraquat and diquat are both extremely toxic, although diquat is less toxic than paraquat.
   A. **Paraquat.** Ingestion of as little as 2–4 g, or 10–20 mL of concentrated 20% paraquat solution, has resulted in death. With ingestion of 60 mL or more, the onset of toxicity and death is more rapid. If food is present in the stomach, it may bind paraquat, preventing its absorption and reducing its toxicity.
      Once applied to plants or soil, paraquat is rapidly bound and is not likely to be toxic. When burned, it is combusted and does not produce poisoning.
   B. **Diquat.** The animal LD_{50} is approximately 400 mg/kg. Survival has been reported after ingestion of 60 g (300 mL of a 20% solution) of diquat.
III. **Clinical presentation**
   A. **Paraquat.** After ingestion of concentrated solutions, there is pain and swelling in the mouth and throat and oral ulcerations may be visible. Nausea, vomiting, and abdominal pain are common. Renal failure develops over 3–5 days, and progressive pulmonary fibrosis occurs over 10–15 days, with death from irreversible pulmonary fibrosis. With ingestion of more than 60 mL of concentrated solution, death may occur within 24 hours owing to massive gastroenteritis, corrosive esophageal injury, pulmonary edema, and cardiogenic shock.
   B. **Diquat.** Corrosive injury may also occur. Severe gastroenteritis may cause massive fluid and electrolyte loss and renal failure. Pulmonary toxicity has not been reported, but cerebral and brain stem hemorrhagic infarctions may occur.
IV. **Diagnosis.** Diagnosis is based on a history of ingestion and the presence of gastroenteritis and oral burns. The oral mucosal burns may have the appearance of a pseudomembrane on the soft palate, sometimes confused with diphtheria.
   A. **Specific levels.** Prognosis may be correlated with specific paraquat

serum levels. These may be obtained free of charge 24 hours a day from ICI Americas, Inc; telephone 1-(800)-327-8633.

  1. Paraquat levels associated with a high likelihood of death are 2 mg/L at 4 hours, 0.9 mg/L at 6 hours, and 0.1 mg/L at 24 hours after ingestion.

  2. A qualitative test for paraquat in the urine may confirm large exposure. Alkalinize 3–5 mL of urine with sodium bicarbonate, then add a few milligrams of sodium dithionite. An intense blue-green color suggests the presence of paraquat. Note, however, that severe toxicity may occur even when this test is negative.

  B. Other useful laboratory studies. CBC, electrolytes, glucose, BUN, creatinine, liver function tests, urinalysis, arterial blood gases, chest x-ray.

V. Treatment

  A. Emergency and supportive measures. Contact ICI Americas, Inc, 24 hours a day at 1-(800)-327-8633 for assistance with treatment.

    1. Maintain the airway and assist ventilation if necessary (see p 2).

    2. **Avoid excessive oxygen** administration, as this may aggravate lipid peroxidation reactions in the lungs. Treat significant hypoxemia with supplemental oxygen, but use only the lowest oxygen concentration necessary to achieve a P_{O2} of 60 mm or more.

    3. Treat fluid and electrolyte imbalance caused by gastroenteritis with intravenous crystalloid solutions (see p 14).

  B. Specific levels. There is no specific antidote.

  C. Decontamination

    1. **Skin and eyes.** Remove all contaminated clothing, and wash exposed skin with soap and water. Irrigate exposed eyes with copious saline or water.

    2. **Ingestion.**

      a. If lavage or charcoal is not immediately available (eg, at home, work, or in the ambulance), induce vomiting with manual stimulation, soapy water, or ipecac (see p 42). Once in the hospital, immediately perform gastric lavage (see p 43).

      b. Administer activated charcoal as soon as the gastric tube is placed and again after lavage (see p 45). Various clays, such as bentonite and fuller's earth, adsorb paraquat and diquat but are no better than charcoal. Ingestion of any food or even plain dirt may afford some protection if other adsorbents are not immediately available. Give a cathartic along with the adsorbent (see p 45).

  D. Enhanced elimination. Although the volume of distribution of paraquat is relatively large (2.8 L/kg) and little paraquat is actually removed, some recommend repeated and prolonged hemoperfusion (every day for 8 hours) in an attempt to limit transfer of paraquat from tissues to the lung. Increased survival has been reported with this technique, although no controlled studies have been performed. Hemodialysis and forced diuresis are not effective.

Reference

Gaudreault P, Friedman PA, Lovejoy FH Jr: Efficacy of activated charcoal and magnesium citrate in the treatment of oral paraquat intoxication. *Ann Emerg Med* 1985;**14**:123.

PENTACHLOROPHENOL AND DINITROPHENOL
Michael T. Kelly, MD

ANTIDOTE   IPECAC   LAVAGE   CHARCOAL

Pentachlorophenol is a chlorinated aromatic hydrocarbon widely used as an herbicide, fungicide, and defoliant. It is applied to wood, leather, burlap, twine, and rope to prevent fungal rot and decay. Eighty percent of all pentachlorophenol produced is used as a wood preservative. Sodium pentachlorophenol is even an ingredient in some paints. Common synonyms for pentachlorophenol are: chlorophen, PCP, penchlorol, Penta, pentachlorofenol, pentanol, and pentachlorophenate. **Dinitrophenol** is an herbicide, fungicide, insecticide, and chemical intermediary and is used in some explosives; it has also been used as a weight-reducing agent but is banned for this use. Its structure and toxicity are similar to those of pentachlorophenol.

I. **Mechanism of toxicity.** Pentachlorophenol and dinitrophenol, like salicylate, uncouple oxidative phosphorylation in the mitochondria. This results in a generalized increase in metabolic activity and inefficient production of adenosine triphosphate (ATP), resulting in excessive generation of lactic acid and heat.
   A. Pentachlorophenol is fetotoxic in rats when given in the first trimester.
   B. Dinitrophenol may oxidize hemoglobin to methemoglobin (see p 204).
II. **Toxic dose.** These agents are readily absorbed through the skin, lungs, and gastrointestinal tract. Most cases of accidental poisoning involve skin absorption.
   A. **Inhalation.** The air level of pentachlorophenol considered immediately dangerous to life or health (IDLH) is 150 mg/m^3. The OSHA permissible exposure limit (PEL) is 0.5 mg/m^3 as an 8-hour time-weighted average.
   B. **Skin.** An epidemic of moderate intoxication occurred in a neonatal nursery after diapers were inadvertently washed in 23% sodium pentachlorophenate.
   C. **Ingestion.** The minimum lethal oral dose of pentachlorophenol for humans is not known, but serious intoxication is reported after ingestion of 2 g. Ingestion of 1–3 g of dinitrophenol is considered lethal.
III. **Clinical presentation.** The toxic effects of pentachlorophenol and dinitrophenol are nearly identical.
   A. **Acute exposure** causes irritation of the skin, eyes, and upper respiratory tract. Systemic absorption results in headache, sweating, hyperthermia, vomiting, weakness, tachycardia, tachypnea, lethargy, convulsions, and coma. Pulmonary edema may occur. Dinitrophenol may induce methemoglobinemia. Death is usually due to cardiovascular collapse or hyperthermia.
   B. **Chronic exposure** to pentachlorophenol may be associated with pancreatitis, hepatitis, and aplastic anemia.
IV. **Diagnosis.** The diagnosis should be suspected in patients with fever, metabolic acidosis, diaphoresis, and tachypnea.
   A. **Specific levels.** Blood levels are not readily available; levels higher than 1 mg/L indicate excessive exposure.
   B. **Other useful laboratory studies.** CBC, electrolytes, glucose, BUN, creatinine, creatine phosphokinase (CPK), liver enzymes, amylase, urinalysis, arterial blood gases, methemoglobin level, chest x-ray.
V. **Treatment**
   A. **Emergency and supportive measures**
      1. Maintain the airway and assist ventilation if necessary (see p 2).
      2. Treat coma (p 17), seizures (p 21), hypotension (p 14), and hyperthermia (p 19) if they occur.
      3. Monitor asymptomatic patients for at least 6 hours after exposure.
   B. **Specific drugs and antidotes.** There is no specific antidote. Treat methemoglobinemia with **methylene blue** (see p 322).
   C. **Decontamination**
      1. **Inhalation.** Remove victim from exposure and administer supplemental oxygen, if available.
      2. **Skin and eyes.** Remove contaminated clothing and store in a plastic bag; wash exposed areas thoroughly with soap and copious water.

Irrigate exposed eyes with copious saline or tepid water. Rescuers should wear protective gear and respirators to avoid exposure.

3. **Ingestion**
   a. Do *not* induce emesis because of the risk of seizures and coma. Perform gastric lavage (see p 43).
   b. Administer activated charcoal and a cathartic (see p 45), orally or by gastric tube. Activated charcoal may be given with the first gastric lavage aliquot to enhance adsorption of toxin.
D. **Enhanced elimination.** There is no evidence that enhanced elimination procedures are effective.

Reference

Wood S et al: Pentachlorophenol poisoning. *J Occup Med* 1983;**25:**527.

PHENCYCLIDINE (PCP)
Evan T. Wythe, MD

ANTIDOTE   IPECAC   LAVAGE   CHARCOAL

Phencyclidine (PCP) is a dissociative anesthetic agent with properties similar to those of ketamine. It was previously marketed for veterinary use, but it became popular as an inexpensive street drug in the late 1960s. PCP may be snorted, smoked, ingested, or injected, and it is frequently substituted for or added to other illicit psychoactive drugs such as THC (tetrahydrocannabinol, marijuana), mescaline, or LSD. PCP is known by a variety of street names, including "peace pill," "angel dust," "hog," and "krystal."

I. **Mechanism of toxicity.** PCP is a dissociative anesthetic that produces generalized loss of pain perception with little or no depression of airway reflexes or ventilation. It also has CNS-stimulant, anticholinergic, dopaminergic, opiate, and alpha-adrenergic activity.

II. **Toxic dose.** In tablet form the usual street dose is 1–6 mg, which results in hallucinations, euphoria, and disinhibition. Ingestion of 6–10 mg causes toxic psychosis and signs of sympathomimetic stimulation. Acute ingestion of 150–200 mg has resulted in death. Smoking PCP produces rapid onset of effects and thus may be an easier route for users to titrate to the desired level of intoxication.

III. **Clinical presentation**
   A. **Mild intoxication** causes lethargy, euphoria, hallucinations, and occasionally bizarre or violent behavior. Patients may rapidly swing between quiet catatonia and loud or agitated behavior. Vertical and horizontal nystagmus are prominent.
   B. **Severe intoxication** produces signs of adrenergic hyperactivity, including hypertension, rigidity, hyperthermia, tachycardia, diaphoresis, convulsions, and coma. The pupils are often paradoxically small. **Death** may occur as a result of self-destructive behavior or as a complication of hyperthermia (eg, rhabdomyolysis, renal failure, coagulopathy, brain damage).

IV. **Diagnosis.** The diagnosis is suggested by the presence of rapidly fluctuating behavior, vertical nystagmus, and signs of sympathomimetic excess.
   A. **Specific levels**
      1. Specific serum PCP levels are not readily available. Levels between 30–100 ng/mL have been associated with toxic psychosis.
      2. Qualitative urine screening for PCP is widely available. PCP ana-

logues may not appear on routine screening, although they can cross-react in some immunologic assays.

B. Other useful laboratory studies. CBC, electrolytes, glucose, BUN, creatinine, creatine phosphokinase (CPK), urinalysis for myoglobin.

V. Treatment

A. Emergency and supportive measures

1. Maintain the airway and assist ventilation if necessary (see p 2).
2. Treat coma (p 17), seizures (p 21), hypertension (p 16), hyperthermia (p 19), and rhabdomyolysis (p 24) if they occur.
3. Agitated behavior (p 22) may respond to limiting sensory stimulation but may require sedation.
4. Monitor temperature and other vital signs for a minimum of 6 hours, and admit all patients with hyperthermia or other evidence of significant intoxication.

B. Specific drugs and antidotes. There is no specific antidote.

C. Decontamination. No decontamination measures are necessary after smoking or injecting PCP.

1. For ingestions, do **not** induce emesis because of the risk of rapid onset of seizures and coma. Perform gastric lavage (see p 43).
2. Administer activated charcoal and a cathartic (see p 45) orally or by gastric tube.
3. Gut emptying is probably not necessary after small ingestions if activated charcoal is given promptly.

D. Enhanced elimination. Because of its large volume of distribution, PCP is not effectively removed by dialysis, hemoperfusion, or other enhanced removal procedures.

1. Repeat-dose activated charcoal has not been studied but might marginally increase elimination by adsorbing PCP partitioned into the acidic stomach fluid.
2. Although urinary acidification increases the urinary concentration of PCP, there is no evidence that this significantly enhances elimination; and it may be dangerous because urinary acidification may aggravate myoglobinuric renal failure.

Reference

Patel R et al: Myoglobinuric acute renal failure in phencyclidine overdose: Report of observation in eight cases. *Ann Emerg Med* 1980;**9**:549.

PHENOL AND RELATED COMPOUNDS
Olga F. Woo, PharmD

ANTIDOTE   IPECAC   LAVAGE   CHARCOAL

Phenol (carbolic acid) was introduced into household use as a potent germicidal agent but has limited use today because less toxic compounds have replaced it. **Hexachlorophene** is a chlorinated biphenol that was widely used as a topical antiseptic and preoperative scrub until recently, when its adverse neurologic effects were recognized. Other phenolic compounds include **creosote, creosol, hydroquinone, eugenol, dinitrophenol,** and **pentachlorophenol.** Pentachlorophenol and dinitrophenol toxicity is discussed on p 231.

I. Mechanism of toxicity. Phenol denatures protein and penetrates tissues well. It is a potent irritant that may cause corrosive injury to the eyes, skin, and respiratory tract. Systemic absorption causes central nervous system stimulation. The mechanism of CNS intoxication is not known. Some phe-

nolic compounds (eg, dinitrophenol and hydroquinone) may induce **methemoglobinemia** (see p 204).
II. **Toxic dose.** The minimum toxic and lethal doses have not been well established. Phenol is well absorbed by inhalation, skin application, and ingestion.
   A. **Inhalation.** The OSHA workplace permissible exposure limit (PEL) is 5 ppm as an 8-hour time-weighted average. The level considered immediately dangerous to life or health (IDLH) is 100 ppm.
   B. **Skin application.** Death has occurred in infants from repeated dermal applications of small doses (one infant died after a 2% solution of phenol was applied for 11 hours on the umbilicus under a closed bandage).
   C. **Ingestion.** Deaths have occurred after adult ingestions of 1–32 g of phenol; however, survival after ingestion of 45–65 g has been reported. As little as 50–500 mg has been reported as fatal in infants.
III. **Clinical presentation.** Toxicity may result from inhalation, skin or eye exposure, or ingestion.
   A. **Inhalation.** Vapors of phenol may cause respiratory tract irritation and chemical pneumonia. Smoking of clove cigarettes (clove oil contains the phenol derivative eugenol) may cause severe tracheobronchitis.
   B. **Skin and eyes.** Topical exposure to the skin may produce a deep white patch that turns red, then stains the skin brown. This lesion is often relatively painless. Eye irritation and severe corneal damage may occur if concentrated liquids are spilled into the eye.
   C. **Ingestion** usually causes vomiting and diarrhea, and diffuse corrosive gastrointestinal tract injury may occur. Systemic absorption may cause agitation, confusion, seizures, coma, hypotension, arrhythmias, and respiratory arrest.
IV. **Diagnosis.** Diagnosis is based on a history of exposure, the presence of a characteristic odor, and painless white skin burns.
   A. **Specific levels.** In the workplace, workers exposed to benzene have urine phenol levels monitored to determine if they are within the normal range (0.5–80 mg/L). Urine phenol levels may also be elevated after use of phenol-containing throat lozenges and mouthwashes.
   B. **Other useful laboratory studies.** CBC, electrolytes, glucose, BUN, creatinine, ECG. After hydroquinone exposure, obtain a methemoglobin level.
V. **Treatment**
   A. **Emergency and supportive measures**
      1. Maintain the airway and assist ventilation if necessary (see p 2).
      2. Treat coma (p 17), seizures (p 21), hypotension (p 14), and arrhythmias (p 13) if they occur.
      3. If corrosive injury to the gastrointestinal tract is suspected, consult a gastroenterologist for possible endoscopy.
   B. **Specific drugs and antidotes.** No specific antidotes are available. If methemoglobinemia occurs, administer **methylene blue** (see p 322).
   C. **Decontamination**
      1. **Inhalation.** Remove victim from exposure and administer supplemental oxygen, if available.
      2. **Skin and eyes.** Remove contaminated clothing and wash exposed skin with soapy water or, if available, mineral oil, olive oil, or petroleum jelly. Immediately flush exposed eyes with copious tepid water or saline.
      3. **Ingestion**
         a. Do *not* induce emesis, because phenol is corrosive and may induce seizures. Perform gastric lavage (see p 43).
         b. Administer activated charcoal and a cathartic (see p 45), orally or by gastric tube.

    c. Gut emptying is probably not necessary after small ingestions if activated charcoal is given promptly.

  D. Enhanced elimination. Enhanced removal methods are generally not effective because of the large volume of distribution of these lipid soluble compounds. Hexachlorophene is excreted in the bile, and repeat-dose activated charcoal may possibly be effective in increasing its clearance from the gut.

Reference

Soares ER, Tift JP: Phenol poisoning: Three fatal cases. *J Forensic Sci* 1982;**27**:729.

PHENOTHIAZINES AND RELATED DRUGS
Neal L. Benowitz, MD

ANTIDOTE   IPECAC   LAVAGE   CHARCOAL

Phenothiazines and butyrophenones are widely used to treat psychosis and agitated depression. In addition, some of these drugs (eg, prochlorperazine, promethazine, droperidol) are used as antiemetic agents. Suicidal overdose is common, but because of the high toxic-therapeutic ratio, acute overdose seldom results in death. Table II-38 describes available antipsychotic agents.

  I. Mechanism of toxicity. A variety of pharmacologic effects are responsible for toxicity involving primarily the cardiovascular and central nervous systems.

    A. Cardiovascular. Anticholinergic effects produce tachycardia. Alpha-adrenergic blockade causes orthostatic hypotension. With very high doses, quinidinelike membrane-depressant effects on the heart may occur.

    B. Central nervous system effects. Centrally mediated sedation and anticholinergic effects contribute to central nervous system depression. Extrapyramidal dystonic reactions are relatively common with therapeutic doses and are probably due to central dopamine receptor blockade. The seizure threshold may be lowered by unknown mechanisms. Temperature regulation is also disturbed, resulting in poikilothermy.

  II. Toxic dosage. Extrapyramidal reactions, anticholinergic side effects, and orthostatic hypotension are seen after therapeutic doses. Tolerance to the sedating effects of the antipsychotics is well-described, and patients on chronic therapy may tolerate much larger doses than other persons.

    A. Typically daily doses are given in Table II–38.

    B. The toxic dose after acute ingestion is highly variable. Serious central nervous system depression and hypotension may occur after ingestion of 200–1000 mg of chlorpromazine in children or 3–5 g in adults.

  III. Clinical presentation. Major toxicity is manifested in the cardiovascular and central nervous systems.

    A. Mild intoxication causes sedation, small pupils, and orthostatic hypotension. Anticholinergic manifestations include dry mouth, absence of sweating, tachycardia, and urinary retention.

    B. Severe intoxication may cause coma, seizures, and respiratory arrest. The ECG usually shows QT interval prolongation and occasionally QRS prolongation. Hypothermia or hyperthermia may occur.

    C. Extrapyramidal dystonic side effects of therapeutic doses include torticollis, jaw muscle spasm, oculogyric crisis, rigidity, bradykinesia, and pill-rolling tremor.

    D. Patients on chronic antipsychotic medication may develop the **neuro-**

TABLE II-38. COMMON PHENOTHIAZINES AND OTHER ANTIPSYCHOTIC DRUGS

Drug	Type[a]	Equivalent Dose (mg)	Usual Adult Daily Dose (mg)	Toxicity[b]
Chlorpromazine	P	100	200–2000	E, A, H
Chlorprothixene	T	100	75–200	E
Ethopropazine	P	50	50–400	A, H
Fluphenazine	P	2	2.5–20	E, A
Haloperidol	B	2	1–100	E
Loxapine	O	15	60–100	E
Mesoridazine	P	50	150–400	A, H
Molindone	O	10	50–225	E
Perphenazine	P	10	10–30	E
Prochlorperazine[c]	P	15	15–40	E
Promethazine[c]	P	25	25–200	A, E
Thioridazine	P	100	150–300	A, H
Thiothixene	T	5	5–60	E
Trifluoperazine	P	5	1–40	E
Trimethobenzamide[c]	O	250	600–1000	A, E

[a] P = Phenothiazine; T = Thiothixine; B = Butyrophenone; O = Other. [b] E = Extrapyramidal reactions; A = Anticholinergic effects; H = Hypotension;
[c] Used primarily as an antiemetic.

leptic malignant syndrome (see p 20) characterized by rigidity, hyperthermia, sweating, lactic acidosis, and rhabdomyolysis.

IV. **Diagnosis.** The diagnosis is based on a history of ingestion and is suggested by the findings of sedation, small pupils, hypotension, and QT interval prolongation. Dystonias in children should always suggest the possibility of antipsychotic exposure, possibly owing to intentional administration by parents.

   A. **Specific levels.** Quantitative blood levels are not routinely available and do not help in diagnosis or treatment. Qualitative screening may easily detect phenothiazines in urine or gastric juice, but butyrophenones such as haloperidol are usually not included in the screens (see Table I-28).

   B. **Other useful laboratory studies.** CBC, electrolytes, glucose, BUN, creatinine, creatine phosphokinase (CPK), arterial blood gases, abdominal x-ray (to look for radiopaque pills), chest x-ray.

V. **Treatment**

   A. **Emergency and supportive measures**

      1. Maintain the airway and assist ventilation if necessary (see p 2).
      2. Treat coma (p 17), seizures (p 21), hypotension (p 14), and hyperthermia (p 19) if they occur.
      3. Monitor vital signs and ECG for at least 6 hours, and admit the patient for at least 24 hours if there are signs of significant intoxication.

B. Specific drugs and antidotes. There is no specific antidote.
1. Treat **dystonic reactions** with **diphenhydramine,** 0.5–1 mg/kg IM or IV (see p 305), or **benztropine,** 1–2 mg IM or IV (p 295).
2. Treat quinidinelike cardiotoxic effects (eg, QRS interval widening) with **bicarbonate,** 1–2 meq/kg IV (see p 296).
3. Some authorities recommend **bromocriptine** for treatment of neuroleptic malignant syndrome, but other treatments for hyperthermia (p 19) are also effective.

C. Decontamination
1. Induce emesis or perform gastric lavage (see p 42) if the patient presents within 30–60 minutes or has ingested a large overdose. Gastric lavage is preferred because of the risk of seizures and coma. Gut emptying is not necessary following small ingestions.
2. Administer activated charcoal and a cathartic (see p 45) orally or by gastric tube.

D. Enhanced elimination. Owing to extensive tissue distribution and large volumes of distribution, these drugs are not effectively removed by dialysis or hemoperfusion. Repeat-dose activated charcoal has not been evaluated.

Reference

Black JL, Richelson E, Richardson JW: Antipsychotic agents: A clinical update. *Mayo Clin Proc* 1985;**60:**777.

PHENYLPROPANOLAMINE AND RELATED DECONGESTANTS
Neal L. Benowitz, MD

ANTIDOTE   IPECAC   LAVAGE   CHARCOAL

Phenylpropanolamine (PPA), phenylephrine (PHE), ephedrine (EPH), and pseudoephedrine (PEP) are sympathomimetic drugs widely available in nonprescription nasal decongestants and cold preparations. These remedies usually also contain antihistamines and cough suppressants. PPA is also widely used as an appetite suppressant. Combinations of nonprescription sympathomimetics and caffeine are often sold on the underground market as amphetamine or cocaine substitutes.

I. **Mechanism of toxicity.** All these agents stimulate the adrenergic system, with variable effects on alpha- and beta-adrenergic receptors depending on the compound.
   A. PPA and PHE are direct alpha-adrenergic agonists. In addition, PPA produces mild β_1-adrenergic stimulation and acts in part indirectly by enhancing norepinephrine release.
   B. EPH and PEP have both direct and indirect alpha- and beta-adrenergic activity but clinically produce more beta-adrenergic stimulation than PPA or PHE.

II. **Toxic dose.** Table II–39 lists the usual therapeutic doses of each agent. Patients developing autonomic insufficiency and those taking monoamine oxidase (MAO) inhibitors (see p 208) may be extraordinarily sensitive to these and other sympathomimetic drugs, developing severe hypertension after ingestion of even subtherapeutic doses.
   A. PPA, PHE, and EPH have low toxic:therapeutic ratios, with toxicity often occurring after ingestion of just 2–3 times the therapeutic dose.
   B. PEP is slightly less toxic, with symptoms occurring after 4–5 times the usual therapeutic dose.

TABLE II-39. COMMON OVER-THE-COUNTER SYMPATHOMIMETIC DRUGS

Drug	Major Effects[a]	Usual Daily Adult Dose (mg)	Usual Daily Pediatric Dose (mg/kg)
Ephedrine	β, α	100–200	2–3
Phenylephrine	α	40–60	0.5–1
Phenylpropanolamine	α	100–150	1–2
Pseudoephedrine	β, α	180–360	3–5

[a] α = alpha-adrenergic; β = beta-adrenergic.

III. **Clinical presentation.** The major toxic effect of these drugs is **hypertension,** which may be severe. Hypertensive complications include headache, confusion, seizures, and intracranial hemorrhage.
  A. **Intracranial hemorrhage** may occur in normal, healthy young persons after what might appear to be only modest elevation of the blood pressure (ie, 170/110 mm Hg) and is often associated with focal neurologic deficits, coma, or seizures.
  B. Hypertension caused by PPA and PHE is usually accompanied by reflex **sinus bradycardia** or even **atrioventricular (AV) block,** while EPH and PEP generally cause hypertension with tachycardia. The presence of other drugs such as antihistamines or caffeine prevents reflex bradycardia and may enhance hypertensive effects of PPA and PHE.
  C. PPA may also cause myocardial infarction or diffuse myocardial necrosis.
  D. The time course of intoxication by these drugs is usually brief, with resolution within 4–6 hours (unless sustained-release preparations are involved).
IV. **Diagnosis.** Diagnosis is usually based on a history of excessive ingestion of diet pills or decongestant medications and the presence of hypertension. Bradycardia or AV block suggests PPA or PHE. Severe headache, focal neurologic deficits, or coma should raise the possibility of intracerebral hemorrhage.
  A. **Specific levels.** Serum drug levels are not generally available and do not alter treatment. Urine toxicology screens may be reported as positive for amphetamine because of the presence of these drugs.
  B. **Other useful laboratory studies.** BUN, creatinine, creatine phosphokinase (CPK) with MB band fractions, ECG and electrocardiographic monitoring, CT head scan if intracranial hemorrhage is suspected.
V. **Treatment**
  A. **Emergency and supportive measures**
    1. Maintain the airway and assist ventilation if necessary (see p 2).
    2. Treat seizures (p 21), arrhythmias (pp 9–13) and hypertension (p 16 and **B,** below) if they occur.
    3. Monitor the vital signs and ECG for a minimum of 4–6 hours after exposure and longer if a sustained-release preparation has been ingested.
  B. **Specific drugs and antidotes.** There is no specific antidote.
    1. Treat **hypertension** if the diastolic pressure is higher than 100–105 mm Hg, especially in a patient with no prior history of hypertension. If there is CT or obvious clinical evidence of intracranial hemorrhage, consult a neurosurgeon before treating hypertension.
      a. Use a vasodilator such as **phentolamine** (see p 335) or **nitroprus-**

side (p 330). Nifedipine (p 328) may be effective for mild hypotension.

    b. *Caution:* Do *not* use beta blockers to treat hypertension without first giving a vasodilator; paradoxic worsening of the hypertension may result.

  2. **Arrhythmias**

    a. Tachyarrhythmias usually respond to low-dose **propranolol** (p 338) or **esmolol** (p 311).

    b. *Caution:* Do *not* treat AV block or sinus bradycardia associated with hypertension; this is a reflex (baroreceptor) response that serves to limit hypertension. Hypertension may be aggravated by use of atropine.

 C. **Decontamination**

  1. Do *not* induce emesis because of the risk of aggravating hypertension. Perform gastric lavage (see p 43) if the patient presents within 30–60 minutes or has ingested a large overdose.

  2. Administer activated charcoal and a cathartic (see p 45) orally or by gastric tube.

  3. Gut emptying is probably not necessary after small ingestions if activated charcoal is given promptly.

 D. **Enhanced elimination.** Dialysis and hemoperfusion are not effective. Urinary acidification may enhance elimination of PPA, EPH, and PEP but may also aggravate myoglobin deposition in the kidney in patients with rhabdomyolysis.

Reference

Pentel P: Toxicity of over-the-counter stimulants. *JAMA* 1984;**252**:1898.

PHENYTOIN
Kathryn H. Keller, PharmD

ANTIDOTE   IPECAC   LAVAGE   CHARCOAL

Phenytoin is used orally for the prevention of grand mal and psychomotor seizures. Intravenous phenytoin is used to treat status epilepticus and occasionally as an antiarrhythmic agent (see p 335). Oral formulations include suspensions, capsules, and tablet preparations. The brand Dilantin Kapseals exhibits delayed absorption characteristics not usually shared by generic products.

 I. **Mechanism of toxicity.** Toxicity may be caused by the phenytoin itself or by the propylene glycol diluent used in parenteral preparations.

  A. **Phenytoin** alters neuronal ion fluxes, increasing refractory periods and decreasing repetitive neuronal firing. Toxic levels usually cause central nervous system depression.

  B. The **propylene glycol** diluent in parenteral preparations may cause cardiac arrest when infused rapidly (> 40–50 mg/min [0.5–1 mg/kg/min]). The mechanism is not known.

 II. **Toxic dose.** The minimum acute toxic oral overdose is approximately 20 mg/kg. Because phenytoin exhibits dose-dependent elimination kinetics, accidental intoxication can easily occur in patients on chronic therapy owing to drug interactions or slight dosage adjustments.

 III. **Clinical presentation.** Toxicity due to phenytoin may be associated with acute oral overdose or chronic accidental overmedication. In addition, life-threatening adverse effects may occur after rapid intravenous administration.

  A. **Mild to moderate intoxication** commonly causes nystagmus, ataxia, and dysarthria. Nausea, vomiting, diplopia, hyperglycemia, agitation, irritability, and hallucinations have also been reported.

B. **At very high levels,** stupor, coma, and respiratory arrest may occur. Although seizures have been reported, the literature reports are unconvincing.

C. **Cardiac toxicity** observed with rapid intravenous injection does not occur with oral overdose.

IV. **Diagnosis.** Diagnosis is based on a history of ingestion or is suspected in any epileptic patient with altered mental status or ataxia. Nystagmus is such a common feature of phenytoin intoxication that its absence should suggest an alternative diagnosis.

A. **Specific levels.** Serum phenytoin levels are generally available in all hospital clinical laboratories. Obtain repeated blood samples because slow absorption may result in delayed peak levels. The therapeutic concentration range is 10–20 mg/L.

1. Above 20 mg/L, nystagmus is common. Above 30 mg/L, ataxia occurs, and with levels higher than 40 mg/L, lethargy is common. Survival has been reported in 2 patients with levels above 100 mg/L.

2. Because phenytoin is protein-bound, patients with renal failure or hypoalbuminemia may experience toxicity at lower serum levels.

B. **Other useful laboratory studies.** BUN, creatinine, serum albumin, electrocardiographic monitoring.

V. **Treatment**

A. **Emergency and supportive measures**

1. Maintain the airway and assist ventilation if necessary (see p 2). Administer supplemental oxygen.

2. Treat stupor and coma (p 17) if they occur. Protect the patient from self-injury caused by ataxia.

3. If seizures occur, consider an alternative diagnosis and treat with other usual anticonvulsants (p 21).

4. If hypotension occurs with intravenous phenytoin administration, immediately stop the infusion and administer intravenous fluids and pressors (p 14) if necessary.

B. **Specific drugs and antidotes.** There is no specific antidote.

C. **Decontamination**

1. Induce emesis or perform gastric lavage (see p 42).

2. Administer activated charcoal and a cathartic (see p 45) orally or by gastric tube.

3. Gut emptying is probably not necessary after small ingestions if activated charcoal is given promptly.

D. **Enhanced elimination.** Repeat-dose activated charcoal (see p 49 and p 299) may enhance phenytoin elimination. There is no role for diuresis, dialysis, or hemoperfusion.

Reference

Mauro LS et al: Enhancement of phenytoin elimination by multiple-dose activated charcoal. *Ann Emerg Med* 1987;**16**:1132.

PHOSGENE
Peter Wald, MD

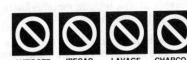

ANTIDOTE IPECAC LAVAGE CHARCOAL

Phosgene was originally manufactured as a war gas. It is now used in the manufacture of dyes, resins, and pesticides. It is also commonly produced when chlorinated compounds are burned, such as in a fire, or in the process of welding metal that has been cleaned with chlorinated solvents.

I. **Mechanism of toxicity.** Phosgene is an irritant. However, because it is poorly water-soluble, in lower concentrations it does not cause immediate upper airway or skin irritation. This allows the victim to inhale it deeply into the lungs for prolonged periods, where it is slowly hydrolyzed to hydrochloric acid in the alveoli. This results in necrosis and inflammation of the small airways and transudative (noncardiogenic) pulmonary edema.

II. **Toxic dose.** The OSHA workplace permissible exposure limit (PEL) is 0.1 ppm as an 8-hour time-weighted average. The level considered immediately dangerous to life or health (IDLH) is 2 ppm. Exposure to as little as 50 ppm may be rapidly fatal.

III. **Clinical presentation.** Exposure to moderate concentrations of phosgene causes mild cough and minimal mucous membrane irritation. After an asymptomatic interval of 30 minutes to 8 hours (depending on the duration and concentration of exposure), the victim develops dyspnea, hypoxemia, and pulmonary edema. Permanent pulmonary insufficiency may be a sequela of serious exposure.

IV. **Diagnosis.** Diagnosis is based on a history of exposure and the clinical presentation. Many other toxic gases may cause delayed-onset pulmonary edema (see p 163).

  A. **Specific level.** There are no specific blood or urine levels.

  B. **Other useful laboratory studies.** Chest x-ray, arterial blood gases.

V. **Treatment**

  A. **Emergency and supportive measures**

   1. Maintain the airway and assist ventilation if necessary (see p 2). Administer supplemental oxygen, and treat noncardiogenic pulmonary edema (see p 7) if it occurs.

   2. Monitor the patient for at least 12–24 hours after exposure because of the potential for delayed-onset pulmonary edema.

  B. **Specific drugs and antidotes.** There is no specific antidote.

  C. **Decontamination.** Remove the victim from exposure and give supplemental oxygen, if available. Rescuers should wear self-contained breathing apparatus.

  D. **Enhanced elimination.** These procedures are not effective.

Reference

Bradley BL, Unger KM: Phosgene inhalation: A case report. *Tex Med* (May) 1982;**78**:51.

PHOSPHINE
Gary Pasternak, MD

ANTIDOTE   IPECAC   LAVAGE   CHARCOAL

Phosphine is a colorless gas that is heavier than air with a characteristic fishy odor, frequently used for fumigation. Although poisoning has become rare, it is a serious potential hazard in operations producing metal phosphides where phosphine can be released in the chemical reaction of water and metal alloys. Workers at risk include metal refiners, acetylene workers, fire fighters, and pest-control operators.

I. **Mechanism of toxicity.** Phosphine is a highly toxic gas, especially to organs of high oxygen flow and demand such as the lungs, brain, kidneys, heart, and liver. The pathophysiologic action of phosphine is not clearly understood.

II. **Toxic dose.** The OSHA workplace permissible exposure limit (PEL) is 0.3 ppm, much lower than the minimal detectable (fishy odor) concentration of 1–3 ppm. Hence, the odor threshold does not provide sufficient warning of dangerous concentrations. A level of 200 ppm is considered immediately dangerous to life or health (IDLH).

Chronic exposure to sublethal concentrations for extended periods may produce toxic symptoms.

III. **Clinical presentation.** Toxicity occurs following inhalation exposure and is characterized by severe pulmonary irritation, cough, dyspnea, headache, dizziness, lethargy, and stupor. Seizures, gastroenteritis, and renal and hepatic toxicity may also occur. The onset of symptoms is usually rapid, although delayed onset of pulmonary edema may occur.

IV. **Diagnosis.** The diagnosis is based on a history of exposure to the agent. *Caution:* Pulmonary edema may have a delayed onset, and initial respiratory symptoms may be mild or absent.

   A. **Specific levels.** Plasma phosphine levels are not clinically useful. Chronic low-level exposure to phosphine may be identified through blood and urine phosphorus levels, although this procedure is not well established.

   B. **Other useful laboratory studies.** BUN, creatinine, liver enzymes, arterial blood gases, chest x-ray.

V. **Treatment**

   A. **Emergency and supportive measures**
      1. Maintain the airway and assist ventilation if necessary (see p 2). Administer supplemental oxygen, and treat noncardiogenic pulmonary edema (p 7) if it occurs.
      2. Treat seizures (p 21) and hypotension (p 14) if they occur.
      3. Patients with a history of significant phosphine inhalation should be admitted and observed for 48–72 hours for delayed onset of pulmonary edema.

   B. **Specific drugs and antidotes.** There is no specific antidote.

   C. **Decontamination.** Immediately remove the victim from exposure and administer supplemental oxygen, if available.

   D. **Enhanced elimination.** Dialysis and hemoperfusion have not been shown to be useful in hastening elimination of phosphine.

Reference

Finkel AJ (editor): Phosphine. Pages 117–118 in: *Hamilton and Hardy's Industrial Toxicology*, 4th ed. PSG, 1983.

PHOSPHORUS
Peter Wald, MD

ANTIDOTE   IPECAC   LAVAGE   CHARCOAL

There are 2 naturally occurring types of elemental phosphorus: red and white-yellow. **Red phosphorus** is not absorbed and is essentially nontoxic. In contrast, **white** or **yellow phosphorus** is a highly toxic cellular poison. Although no longer a component of matches, white phosphorus is still used in the manufacture of fireworks and fertilizer and as a rodenticide.

   I. **Mechanism of toxicity.** Phosphorus is highly corrosive and is also a general cellular poison. Cardiovascular collapse occurring after ingestion is probably due not only to fluid loss from vomiting and diarrhea but also to direct toxicity on the heart and vascular tone.

   White-yellow phosphorus spontaneously combusts in air to yield phosphorus oxide, a highly irritating fume.

II. Toxic dose

A. Ingestion. The fatal oral dose of white-yellow phosphorus is approximately 1 mg/kg. Deaths have been reported after ingestion of as little as 15 mg.

B. Inhalation. The OSHA workplace permissible exposure limit (PEL) for white-yellow phosphorus is 0.1 mg/m^3 as an 8-hour time-weighted average.

III. Clinical presentation

A. Acute inhalation may cause conjunctivitis, mucous membrane irritation, cough, wheezing, chemical pneumonia, and noncardiogenic pulmonary edema. **Chronic inhalation** of phosphorus (over at least 10 months) may result in mandibular necrosis ("phossy jaw").

B. Skin or eye contact may cause severe dermal or ocular burns.

C. Acute ingestion may cause gastrointestinal burns, severe vomiting, and diarrhea with "smoking" stools. Systemic effects include headache, confusion, seizures, coma, arrhythmias, and shock. Metabolic derangements may occur, including hypocalcemia, hyperphosphatemia, and hypophosphatemia. If the victim survives, hepatic or renal failure may occur after 4–8 days.

IV. Diagnosis.

Diagnosis is based on a history of exposure and the clinical presentation. Smoking stools caused by spontaneous combustion of elemental phosphorus suggests phosphorus ingestion.

A. Specific levels. Because serum phosphorus may be elevated, depressed, or normal, it is not a useful test for diagnosis or estimation of severity.

B. Other useful laboratory studies. BUN, creatinine, liver function tests, urinalysis, arterial blood gases, chest x-ray (after acute inhalation).

V. Treatment

A. Emergency and supportive measures

1. After inhalation, observe closely for signs of upper airway injury and perform endotracheal intubation and assist ventilation if necessary (see p 2). Administer supplemental oxygen. Treat bronchospasm (p 8) and pulmonary edema (p 7) if they occur.
2. Treat fluid losses from gastroenteritis with aggressive intravenous crystalloid fluid replacement (p 14).
3. Consider endoscopy if oral, esophageal, or gastric burns are suspected (p 114).

B. Specific drugs and antidotes. There is no specific antidote.

C. Decontamination

1. **Inhalation.** Remove the victim from exposure and give supplemental oxygen, if available.
2. **Skin and eyes.** Remove contaminated clothing and wash exposed areas with soap and water. Irrigate exposed eyes with copious tepid water or saline.
3. **Ingestion**
   a. Do **not** induce emesis because of the potential for corrosive injury. Perform careful gastric lavage (see p 43).
   b. Administer activated charcoal (even though there is no evidence that it adsorbs phosphorus) and a cathartic (see p 45).

D. Enhanced elimination. There is no effective method of enhanced elimination.

References

McCarron MM, Gaddis GP, Trotter AT: Acute yellow phosphorus poisoning from pesticide pastes. *Clin Toxicol* 1981;**18**:693.

Simon FA, Pickering LK: Acute yellow phosphorus poisoning: "Smoking stool syndrome." *JAMA* 1976;**235**:1343.

PLANTS AND HERBS
Olga F. Woo, PharmD

ANTIDOTE   IPECAC   LAVAGE   CHARCOAL

Plant ingestions are second only to drugs as the most common poisoning exposure in children. Fortunately, serious poisoning or death is extremely rare because the quantity of toxin ingested is small. During the past 2 decades, public interest in natural foods and traditional medical remedies and in "herbal highs" has resulted in increasing use of herbal products.

Unfortunately, there is little consumer awareness of the potential harm from some herbal preparations. Besides toxicity from natural products contained in some medicinal plants, "herbal" or "traditional" preparations may sometimes actually contain allopathic drugs such as phenylbutazone, corticosteroids, salicylates, or ephedrine or toxic metal salts such as mercury or lead.

I. **Mechanism of toxicity.** Table II–40 is a list of potentially toxic plants, categorized in groups 1, 2a, 2b, and 3.
   A. **Group 1** plants contain systemically active poisons that may cause serious intoxication.
   B. **Group 2a** plants contain insoluble calcium oxalate crystals that cause burning pain and swelling of the mucous membranes.
   C. **Group 2b** plants contain soluble oxalate salts (sodium or potassium) that can produce acute hypocalcemia, renal injury, and other organ damage secondary to precipitation of calcium oxalate crystals in various organs (see p 227). Mucous membrane irritation and gastroenteritis may also occur.
   D. **Group 3** plants contain various chemical agents that generally produce only mild to moderate gastrointestinal irritation after ingestion or dermatitis after skin contact.

II. **Toxic dose**
   A. **Plants.** The amount of toxin ingested is usually unknown. Concentrations of the toxic agent may vary depending on the plant part, the season, and soil conditions. In general, childhood ingestion of small amounts of even group 1 plants results in little or no toxicity because of the small amount of toxin absorbed.
   B. **Herbs.** Herbal teas and medications often contain only minute, "homeopathic" amounts of the toxin, in which case toxicity might occur only after chronic overuse or massive acute overdose.

III. **Clinical presentation**
   A. **Group 1.** The presentation depends upon the active toxic agent (Table II–40). In most cases, vomiting, abdominal pain, and diarrhea occur within 60–90 minutes of a significant ingestion. With some toxins (eg, ricin), severe gastroenteritis may result in massive fluid and electrolyte loss, shock, and death.
   B. **Group 2a.** Insoluble calcium oxalate crystals cause immediate burning prickly pain upon contact with mucous membranes. Swelling of the lips, tongue, and pharynx may occur, and in rare cases glottic edema may result in airway obstruction. Symptoms usually resolve within a few hours.
   C. **Group 2b.** Soluble oxalates may be absorbed into the circulation, where they precipitate with calcium, resulting in acute hypocalcemia and multiple-organ injury, including renal tubular necrosis.
   D. **Group 3.** Skin or mucous membrane irritation may occur, although it is less severe than with group 2 plants. Vomiting and diarrhea are com-

TABLE II-40. POISONOUS PLANTS AND HERBS

Common Name	Botanical Name	Toxic Group	Remarks
Acorn	*Quercus* spp	3	Tannin; irritant
Akee	*Blighia sapida*	1	Hypoglycemia and hepatotoxicity
Almond, bitter	*Prunus* spp	1	Cyanogenic glycosides (see p 134)
Aloe vera	*Aloe vera*	3	Hypersensitivity; skin irritant
Amaryllis	*Hippeastrum equestre*	3	
American bittersweet	*Celastrus scandens*	3	
American ivy	*Parthenocissus* spp	2b	Soluble oxalates (see p 227)
Angel's trumpet	*Brugmansia arborea*	1, 3	Anticholinergic alkaloids (see p 71)
Anthurium	*Anthurium* spp	2a	Calcium oxalate crystals (see text)
Apple (seeds)	*Malus domestica*	1	Cyanogenic glycosides (see p 134)
Apricot (chewed pits)	*Prunus* spp	1	Cyanogenic glycosides (see p 134)
Arrowhead vine	*Syngonium podophyllum*	2a	Calcium oxalate crystals (see text)
Asparagus fern	*Asparagus plumosus*	3	
Autumn crocus	*Colchicum autumnale*	1	Colchicine (see p 129)
Avocado (leaves)	*Avocado*	1	Unknown toxin
Azalea	*Azalea* spp	1	Andromedotoxin: hypotension, AV block, arrhythmias; lethargy
Azalea	*Rhododendron* genus	1	Andromedotoxin: hypotension, bradycardia, AV block; lethargy
Bahia	*Bahia oppositifolia*	1	Cyanogenic glycosides (see p 134)
Baneberry	*Actaea* spp	3	Irritant oil protoanemonin: severe gastroenteritis
Barbados nut; purging nut	*Jatropha* spp	1	Phytotoxins: severe gastroenteritis
Barberry	*Berberis* spp	3	
Beech	*Fagus sylvatica*	3	Saponins
Begonia	*Begonia rex*	2a	Calcium oxalate crystals (see text)
Belladonna	*Atropa belladonna*	1	Atropine (see p 71)
Bellyache bush	*Jatropha* spp	1	Phytotoxins: severe gastroenteritis
Be-still tree	*Thevetia peruviana*	1	Cardiac glycosides (see p 112)
Birch (bark, leaves)	*Betula* spp	1, 3	Methyl salicylate, irritant oils
Bird of paradise	*Poinciana gillesi*	3	
Black cohosh	*Cimicifuga* spp	3	
Black locust	*Robinia pseudoacacia*	1	Phytotoxins: severe gastroenteritis
Black nightshade	*Hyoscyamus* spp	1	Anticholinergic alkaloids (see p 71)
Black snakeroot	*Zigadenus* spp	1	Similar to veratramine: hypotension, bradycardia, lethargy
Bleeding heart	*Dicentra*	3	
Bloodroot	*Sanguinaria canadensis*	3	
Blue cohosh	*Caulophyllum thalictroides*	1, 3	Cytisine: similar to nicotine (see p 214)
Boston ivy	*Parthenocissus* spp	2b	Soluble oxalates (see p 227)
Boxwood; box plant	*Buxus* spp	3	
Broom; scotch broom	*Cytisus* spp	1	Cytisine: similar to nicotine (see p 214)
Buckeye	*Aesculus* spp	1, 3	Coumarin glycosides (see p 132)
Buckthorn; tullidora	*Karwinskia humboldtiana*	1	Chronic ingestion may cause ascending paralysis
Buckthorn	*Rhamnus* spp	3	Anthraquinone cathartic
Bunchberry	*Cornus canadensis*	3	
Burdock root	*Arctium minus*	1, 3	Anticholinergic alkaloids (see p 71)
Burning bush	*Euonymus* spp	3	
Buttercups	*Ranunculus* spp	3	Irritant oil protoanemonin
Cactus (thorn)	*Cactus*	3	Cellulitis, abscess may result
Caladium	*Caladium* spp	2a	Calcium oxalate crystals (see text)
Caladium	*Xanthosoma* spp	2a	Calcium oxalate crystals (see text)
California geranium	*Senecio* spp	1	Hepatotoxic pyrrolizidine alkaloids

continued

TABLE II-40. POISONOUS PLANTS AND HERBS (Continued)

Common Name	Botanical Name	Toxic Group	Remarks
California privet	*Ligustrum* spp	3	
Calla lily	*Zantedeschia* spp	2a	Calcium oxalate crystals (see text)
Cannabis	*Cannabis sativa*	1	Mild hallucinogen
Caraway	*Carum carvi*	3	When used as herbal medication
Cardinal flower	*Lobelia* spp	1	Lobeline: nicotinelike alkaloid (see p 214)
Carnation	*Dianthus caryophyllus*	3	
Carolina allspice	*Calycanthus* spp	1	Strychninelike alkaloid
Cascara	*Rhamnus* spp	3	Anthraquinone cathartic
Cassava	*Manihot esculenta*	1	Cyanogenic glycosides (see p 134)
Castor bean	*Ricinus communis*	1	Phytotoxins: severe gastroenteritis
Catnip	*Nepeta cataria*	1, 3	Mild hallucinogen
Century plant	*Agave americana*	3	Thorns can cause cellulitis
Chamomile	*Chamomilla recucita*	3	Highly antigenic
Cherry (chewed pits)	*Prunus* spp	1	Cyanogenic glycosides (see p 134)
Chili pepper	*Capsicum* spp	3	Irritant to skin, eyes, mucous membranes
Chinaberry	*Melia azedarach*	1, 3	Severe fatal gastroenteritis reported; contains convulsant
Christmas rose	*Helleborus niger*	1, 3	Similar to cardiac glycosides (see p 112)
Chrysanthemum; mum	*Chrysanthemum* spp	3	Pyrethrins (see p 254)
Coffeeberry	*Rhamnus* spp	3	Anthraquinone cathartic
Cola nut; gotu kola	*Cola* spp	1	Caffeine, theobromin
Comfrey	*Symphytum officinale*	1, 3	Irritant tannin and hepatotoxic pyrrolizidine alkaloids
Conquer root	*Exogonium purga*	3	
Coral bean	*Sophora secundiflora*	1	Cytisine: similar to nicotine (see p 214)
Coral berry	*Symphoricarpos* spp	3	
Coriaria	*Coriaria myrtifolia*	1	Contains convulsant agent
Cotoneaster	*Cotoneaster*	1, 3	Cyanogenic glycosides (see p 134)
Coyotillo	*Karwinskia humboldtiana*	1	Chronic ingestion may cause ascending paralysis
Creeping charlie	*Glecoma hederacea*	1, 3	Volatile oils; mild stimulant
Crown of thorns	*Euphorbia* spp	3	
Cyclamen	*Cyclamen*	3	
Daffodil (bulb)	*Narcissus* spp	3	
Daphne	*Daphne* spp	1, 3	Bark: coumarin glycosides (see p 132); berries: blisters
Deadly nightshade	*Atropa belladonna*	1	Atropine (see p 71)
Death camas	*Zigadenus* spp	1	Similar to veratramine: hypotension, bradycardia, lethargy
Devils ivy	*Scindapsus aureus*	2a	Calcium oxalate crystals (see text)
Dogbane	*Apocynum* spp	1	Cardiac glycosides (see p 112)
Dolls-eyes	*Actaea* spp	3	Irritant oil protoanemonin: severe gastroenteritis
Dragon root	*Arisaema* spp	2a	Calcium oxalate crystals (see text)
Dumbcane	*Dieffenbachia* spp	2a	Calcium oxalate crystals (see text)
Dusty miller	*Senecio* spp	1	Hepatotoxic pyrrolizidine alkaloids
Elderberry	*Sambucus*	1	Unripe berries contain cyanogenic glycosides (see p 134)
Elephant's ear; taro	*Alocasia* spp	2a	Calcium oxalate crystals (see text)
Elephant's ear	*Colocasia* spp	2a	Calcium oxalate crystals (see text)
Elephant's ear	*Philodendron* spp	2a	Calcium oxalate crystals (see text)
English ivy; heart ivy	*Hedera helix*	3	Saponins
English laurel	*Prunus laurocerasus*	1	Cyanogenic glycosides (see p 134)
Ergot	*Claviceps* spp	1	Ergot alkaloids (see p 146)
Eucalyptus	*Eucalyptus*	3	Irritant oils

continued

TABLE II-40. POISONOUS PLANTS AND HERBS (Continued)

Common Name	Botanical Name	Toxic Group	Remarks
False hellebore	*Veratrum* spp	1, 3	Veratramine: hypotension, AV block, arrhythmias; seizures
Fava bean	*Vicia faba*	1	Hemolytic anemia in G6PD-deficient persons
Ficus (sap)	*Ficus benjamina*	3	
Firethorn	*Pyracantha*	3	
Fool's parsley	*Conium maculatum*	1	Coniine: nicotinelike alkaloid (see p 214)
Four o'clock	*Mirabilis jalapa*	3	Seeds have hallucinogenic effects
Foxglove	*Digitalis purpurea*	1	Cardiac glycosides (see p 112)
Glacier ivy	*Hedera glacier*	3	Saponins
Glory pea	*Sesbania* spp	3	Saponins
Goldenrod; rayless	*Haplopappus heterophyllus*	1	Higher alcohol tremetol: CNS depression
Golden chain	*Laburnum anagyroides*	1	Cytisine: similar to nicotine (see p 214)
Golden seal	*Hydrastis* spp	1, 3	Fatalities reported after use as herbal tea
Gordolobo	*Senecio* spp	1	Hepatotoxic pyrrolizidine alkaloids
Grindelia	*Grindelia* spp	1	Balsamic resin: renal, cardiac toxicity
Groundsel	*Senecio* spp	1	Hepatotoxic pyrrolizidine alkaloids
Guaiac	*Guaiacum officinale*	3	
Harmaline	*Banisteriopsis* spp	1	Harmaline: hallucinogen (see p 191)
Harmel; Syrian rue	*Peganum harmala*	1	Harmaline: hallucinogen (see p 191)
Heart leaf	*Philodendron* spp	2a	Calcium oxalate crystals (see text)
Heath	*Ericaceae* family	1, 3	Andromedotoxin: hypotension, AV block, arrhythmias; lethargy
Heliotrope	*Heliotropium* spp	1	Pyrrolizidine alkaloids: hepatotoxicity
Hemlock; poison hemlock	*Conium maculatum*	1	Coniine: nicotinelike alkaloid (see p 214)
Henbane; black henbane	*Hyoscyamus* spp	1	Anticholinergic alkaloids (see p 71)
Holly (berry)	*Ilex aquifolium*	3	
Hops	*Humulus lupulus*	1	Sedative
Horse chestnut	*Aesculus* spp	1, 3	Coumarin glycosides (see p 132)
Hyacinth	*Hyacinthus*	3	
Hydrangea	*Hydrangea* spp	1, 3	Cyanogenic glycosides (see p 134)
Indian currant	*Symphoricarpos* spp	3	
Indian tobacco	*Lobelia* spp	1	Lobeline: nicotinelike alkaloid (see p 214)
Inkberry	*Phytolacca americana*	3	If absorbed may cause hemolysis; cooked berries edible
Iris	*Iris*	3	
Ivy bush; sheepkill	*Kalmia* spp	1	Andromedotoxin: hypotension, AV block, arrhythmias; lethargy
Jack-in-the-pulpit	*Arisaema* spp	2a	Calcium oxalate crystals (see text)
Jalap	*Exogonium purga*	3	
Jequirity bean	*Abrus precatorius*	1	Phytotoxin abrin: severe fatal gastroenteritis reported
Jerusalem cherry (unripe berry)	*Solanum pseudocapsicum*	1, 3	Solanine and anticholinergic alkaloids (see p 71)
Jessamine	*Gelsemium sempervirens*	1	Alkaloids similar to strychnine (see p 274)
Jessamine, Carolina	*Gelsemium sempervirens*	1	Alkaloids similar to strychnine (see p 274)
Jessamine, day or night	*Cestrum* spp	1, 3	Solanine and anticholinergic alkaloids (see p 71)
Jessamine, yellow	*Gelsemium sempervirens*	1	Alkaloids similar to strychnine (see p 274)

continued

TABLE II-40. POISONOUS PLANTS AND HERBS (Continued)

Common Name	Botanical Name	Toxic Group	Remarks
Jetbead	Rhodotypos scandens	1	Cyanogenic glycosides (see p 134)
Jetberry bush	Rhodotypos scandens	1	Cyanogenic glycosides (see p 134)
Jimmyweed	Haplopappus heterophyllus	1	Higher alcohol tremetol: CNS depression
Jimsonweed	Brugmansia arborea	1, 3	Anticholinergic alkaloids (see p 71)
Jimsonweed; thornapple	Datura stramonium	1	Anticholinergic alkaloids (see p 71)
Juniper	Juniperus macropoda	1, 3	Hallucinogen (see p 191)
Kava-kava	Piper methysticum	1	Mild hallucinogen (see p 191)
Kentucky coffee tree	Gymnocladus dioica	1	Cytisine: similar to nicotine (see p 214)
Khat; chat	Catha edulis	1	Mild hallucinogen and stimulant
Labrador tea	Ledum spp	1	Andromedotoxin: hypotension, AV block, arrhythmias; lethargy
Lantana	Lantana camara	1	Hepatotoxic in animals; ingestion of unripe berries may cause cardiovascular collapse and death
Larkspur	Delphinium	1	Cardiotoxic delphinine: arrhythmias, AV block
Licorice root	Glycyrrhiza lepidata	1, 3	Hypokalemia after chronic use
Lily of the Nile	Agapanthus	3	Burning sensation when ingested
Lily-of-the-valley	Convallaria majalis	1	Cardiac glycosides (see p 112)
Lily-of-the-valley shrub	Pieris japonica	1	Andromedotoxin: hypotension, AV block, arrhythmias; lethargy
Mandrake	Mandragora officinarum	1	Anticholinergic alkaloids (see p 71)
Mandrake	Podophyllum peltatum	1, 3	Oil is keratolytic, irritant; hypotension, seizures reported after ingestion of resin; ripe fruit nontoxic
Marble queen	Scindapsus aureus	2a	Calcium oxalate crystals (see text)
Marijuana	Cannabis sativa	1	Mild hallucinogen
Marsh marigold	Caltha palustris	3	Irritant oil protoanemonin
Mate	Ilex paraguayensis	1, 3	Irritant tannins; caffeine
Mayapple	Podophyllum peltatum	1, 3	Oil is keratolytic, irritant; hypotension, seizures reported
Meadow crocus	Colchicum autumnale	1	Colchicine (see p 129)
Mescal bean	Sophora secundiflora	1	Cytisine: similar to nicotine (see p 214)
Mescal button	Lophophora williamsii	1	Mescaline: hallucinogen (see p 191)
Mistletoe, American	Phoradendron flavescens	1, 3	Cardiotoxic phoratoxin: potential pressor effects
Mistletoe, European	Viscum album	1	Cardiotoxic viscotoxin; vasoconstrictor
Mock azalea	Menziesia ferruginea	1	Andromedotoxin: hypotension, AV block, arrhythmias; lethargy
Monkshood	Aconitum napellus	1	Aconitine: hypotension, AV block, arrhythmias; seizures
Moonseed	Menispermaceae	1	Contains convulsant agent
Mormon tea	Ephedra viridis	1	Sympathomimetic (see p 238)
Morning glory	Ipomoea violacea	1	Seeds are hallucinogenic (see p 191)
Mountain laurel	Kalmia spp	1	Andromedotoxin: hypotension, AV block, arrhythmias; lethargy
Nectarine (chewed pits)	Prunus spp	1	Cyanogenic glycosides (see p 134)
Nephthytis	Syngonium podophyllum	2a	Calcium oxalate crystals (see text)

continued

TABLE II-40. POISONOUS PLANTS AND HERBS (Continued)

Common Name	Botanical Name	Toxic Group	Remarks
Nightshade	*Solanum* spp	1, 3	Solanine and anticholinergic alkaloids (see p 71)
Nightshade, black	*Hyoscyamus* spp	1	Anticholinergic alkaloids (see p 71)
Nightshade, deadly	*Atropa belladonna*	1	Atropine (see p 71)
Nutmeg	*Myristica fragrans*	1	Hallucinogen (see p 191)
Oakleaf ivy	*Toxicodendron* spp	3	Urushiol oleoresin contact dermatitis (*Rhus* dermatitis)
Oleander	*Nerium oleander*	1	Cardiac glycosides (see p 112)
Oleander, yellow	*Thevetia peruviana*	1	Cardiac glycosides (see p 112)
Paraguay tea	*Ilex paraguayensis*	1, 3	Irritant tannins; caffeine
Peach (chewed pits)	*Prunus* spp	1	Cyanogenic glycosides (see p 134)
Pear (chewed seeds)	*Prunus* spp	1	Cyanogenic glycosides (see p 134)
Pennyroyal (oil)	*Mentha pulegium*	1	Hepatotoxic cyclic ketone; seizures reported
Periwinkle	*Vinca*	1	*Vinca* alkaloids
Periwinkle, rose	*Catharanthus roseus*	1	Hallucinogen (see p 191)
Peyote; mescal	*Lophophora williamsii*	1	Mescaline: hallucinogen (see p 191)
Pheasant's-eye	*Adonis* spp	1	Cardiac glycosides (see p 112)
Pigeonberry	*Duranta repens*	3	Saponins
Pigeonberry	*Phytolacca americana*	3	If absorbed may cause hemolysis; cooked berries edible
Plum (chewed pits)	*Prunus* spp	1	Cyanogenic glycosides (see p 134)
Poinsettia	*Euphorbia* spp	3	
Poison ivy	*Toxicodendron* spp	3	Urushiol oleoresin contact dermatitis (*Rhus* dermatitis)
Poison oak	*Toxicodendron* spp	3	Urushiol oleoresin contact dermatitis (*Rhus* dermatitis)
Poison sumac	*Toxicodendron* spp	3	Urushiol oleoresin contact dermatitis (*Rhus* dermatitis)
Poison vine	*Toxicodendron* spp	3	Urushiol oleoresin contact dermatitis (*Rhus* dermatitis)
Pokeweed (unripe berries)	*Phytolacca americana*	3	If absorbed may cause hemolysis; cooked berries edible
Potato (unripe)	*Solanum* spp	1, 3	Solanine and anticholinergic alkaloids (see p 71)
Pothos; yellow pothos	*Scindapsus aureus*	2a	Calcium oxalate crystals (see text)
Prickly poppy	*Argemone mexicana*	1	Narcotic-analgesic, smoked as euphoriant
Pride-of-Madeira	*Echium* spp	1	Pyrrolizidine alkaloids: hepatotoxicity
Privet; common privet	*Ligustrum* spp	3	
Purslane	*Portulaca oleracea*	2b	Soluble oxalates (see p 227)
Pyracantha	*Pyracantha*	3	
Ragwort, tansy	*Senecio* spp	1	Hepatotoxic pyrrolizidine alkaloids
Rattlebox	*Sesbania* spp	3	Saponins
Rattlebox; bush tea	*Crotalaria* spp	1	Pyrrolizidine alkaloids: hepatotoxicity
Rattlebox, purple	*Daubentonia* spp	3	
Rhododendron	*Rhododendron* genus	1	Andromedotoxin: hypotension, bradycardia, AV block; lethargy
Rhubarb	*Rheum rhaponticum*	2b	Soluble oxalates (see p 227)
Rosary pea; rosary bean	*Abrus precatorius*	1	Phytotoxin abrin: severe fatal gastroenteritis reported
Rose periwinkle	*Catharanthus roseus*	1	Hallucinogen (see p 191)
Rustyleaf	*Menziesia ferruginea*	1	Andromedotoxin: hypotension, AV block, arrhythmias; lethargy
Sassafras	*Sassafras albidium*	1	Hepatocarcinogenic
Shamrock	*Oxalis* spp	2b	Soluble oxalates (see p 227)
Skunk cabbage	*Symplocarpus foetidus*	2a	Calcium oxalate crystals (see text)

continued

TABLE II–40. POISONOUS PLANTS AND HERBS (Continued)

Common Name	Botanical Name	Toxic Group	Remarks
Skunk cabbage	*Veratrum* spp	1, 3	Veratramine: hypotension, AV block, arrhythmias; seizures
Sky-flower	*Duranta repens*	3	Saponins
Snakeroot	*Rauwolfia serpentina*	1	Antihypertensive reserpine tranquilizer
Snowberry	*Symphoricarpos* spp	3	
Sorrel; soursob	*Oxalis* spp	2b	Soluble oxalates (see p 227)
Spathiphyllum	*Spathiphyllum*	2a	Calcium oxalate crystals (see text)
Spindle tree	*Euonymus* spp	3	
Split leaf	*Philodendron* spp	2a	Calcium oxalate crystals (see text)
Sprengeri fern	*Asparagus densiflorus*	3	
Squill	*Scilla*	1	Cardiac glycosides (see p 112)
Squill	*Urginea maritima*	1	Cardiac glycosides (see p 112)
Star-of-Bethlehem	*Ornithogalum* spp	1	Cardiac glycosides (see p 112)
String of pearls/beads	*Senecio* spp	1	Hepatotoxic pyrrolizidine alkaloids
Strychnine	*Strychnos nux-vomica*	1	Strychnine (see p 274)
Sweet clover	*Melilotus* spp	1	Coumarin glycosides (see p 132)
Sweet pea	*Lathyrus odoratus*	1	Neuropathy (lathyrism) after chronic use
Swiss cheese plant	*Monstera friedrichsthali*	2a	Calcium oxalate crystals (see text)
Tobacco	*Nicotiana* spp	1	Nicotine (see p 214)
Tomato (leaves)	*Lycopersicon esculentum*	1	Solanine: sympathomimetic; bradycardia
Tonka bean	*Dipteryx odorata*	1	Coumarin glycosides (see p 132)
Toyon (leaves)	*Heteromeles arbutifolia*	1	Cyanogenic glycosides (see p 134)
Tulip (bulb)	*Tulipa*	3	
Tung tree; candle nut	*Aleurites* spp	1, 3	Phytotoxins, saponins
Turbina	*Turbina corymbosa*	1	Hallucinogen (see p 191)
T'u-san-chi	*Gynura segetum*	1	Hepatotoxic pyrrolizidine alkaloids
Umbrella plant	*Cyperus alternifolius*	1	See essential oils (p 104)
Valerian	*Valeriana officinalis*	1	Valerine alkaloids: used as mild tranquilizer
Walnut (green shells)	*Juglans*	1	Moldy parts contain convulsant mycotoxins
Water hemlock	*Cicuta maculata*	1	Cicutoxin: seizures; vomiting; diaphoresis, salivation
Wild calla	*Calla palustris*	2a	Calcium oxalate crystals (see text)
Wild onion	*Zigadenus* spp	1	Similar to veratramine: hypotension, bradycardia, lethargy
Windflower	*Anemone*	3	Irritant oil protoanemonin
Wisteria	*Wisteria*	3	
Woodruff	*Galium odoratum*	1	Coumarin glycosides (see p 132)
Wood rose	*Ipomoea violacea*	1	Seeds are hallucinogenic (see p 191)
Wood rose	*Merremia tuberosa*	1	Seeds are hallucinogenic
Wormwood	*Artemesia absinthium*	1	See essential oils (p 104); smoked as relaxant
Yarrow	*Achillea millefolium*	3	Prepared as a tea
Yellow oleander	*Thevetia peruviana*	1	Cardiac glycosides (see p 112)
Yew	*Taxus*	1	Taxine: similar to cardiac glycosides (see p 112); seizures
Yohimbine	*Corynanthe yohimbe*	1	Aphrodisiac; mild hallucinogen; α_2-blocker

mon and are usually mild and self-limited. Fluid and electrolyte imbalance caused by severe gastroenteritis is rare.

IV. Diagnosis. Diagnosis is usually based on a history of exposure and suspected when plant material is seen in vomitus. Identification of the plant is essential to proper treatment. Because common names sometimes refer to more than one plant, it is preferable to confirm the botanical name. If in doubt about the plant identification, take the specimen to a local nursery.

  A. Specific levels. Serum toxin levels are not available for most plant toxins. In selected cases, laboratory analyses for therapeutic drugs may be used (eg, digoxin assay for oleander glycosides).

  B. Other useful laboratory studies. For patients with gastroenteritis, obtain CBC, electrolytes, glucose, BUN, creatinine, and urinalysis. If hepatotoxicity is suspected, obtain liver enzymes and prothrombin time.

V. Treatment. Most ingestions cause no symptoms or only mild gastroenteritis, and patients recover quickly with supportive care.

  A. Emergency and supportive measures

  1. Maintain the airway and assist ventilation if necessary (see p 2).
  2. Treat coma (p 17), seizures (p 21), arrhythmias (pp 9–13), and hypotension (p 14) if they occur.
  3. Replace fluid losses caused by gastroenteritis with intravenous crystalloid solutions.

  B. Specific drugs and antidotes. There are few effective antidotes. See the "Remarks" column in Table II–40 for specific information or referral to additional discussion elsewhere in Section II.

  C. Decontamination

  1. **Group 1 and group 2b plants**
     a. Unless intense vomiting has already occurred, induce emesis or perform gastric lavage (see p 42). Gut emptying is not necessary following very small ingestions and is not very effective if started more than 60 minutes after ingestion.
     b. Administer activated charcoal and a cathartic (see p 45) orally or by gastric tube.
  2. **Group 2a and group 3 plants**
     a. Wash the affected areas with plain water and give water or milk to drink.
     b. Do **not** induce emesis because of potential aggravation of irritant effects. Gastric lavage and activated charcoal are not necessary.

  D. Enhanced elimination. These procedures are not generally effective.

References

Kingsbury JM: *Poisonous Plants of the United States and Canada.* Prentice-Hall, 1964.
Ridker PM: Toxic effects of herbal teas. *Arch Environ Health* 1987;**42**:133.

POLYCHLORINATED BIPHENYLS (PCBs)
Bruce Bernard, MD

ANTIDOTE   IPECAC   LAVAGE   CHARCOAL

Polychlorinated biphenyls (PCBs) are a group of chlorinated hydrocarbon compounds that are widely used as high-temperature insulators for transformers and other electric equipment and are also found in carbonless copy papers and some inks and paints. Most PCB poisonings are chronic occupational exposures, with delayed-onset symptoms being the first indication that an exposure has occurred. In 1977, the Environmental Protection Agency banned further manufacturing of PCBs because they are suspected carcinogens.

I. **Mechanism of toxicity.** PCBs are irritating to mucous membranes. When burned, PCBs may produce highly toxic polychlorinated dibenzodioxins (PCDDs) and polychlorinated dibenzofurans (PCDFs; see p 142). It is difficult to establish the specific effects of PCB intoxication because PCBs are nearly always contaminated with small amounts of these compounds. PCBs, and particularly the PCDD and PCDF contaminants, are mutagenic and teratogenic and are considered potential human carcinogens.

II. **Toxic dose.** PCBs are well absorbed by all routes (skin, inhalation, ingestion) and are widely distributed in fat; bioaccumulation occurs even with low-level exposure.
  A. **Inhalation.** PCBs are mildly irritating to the skin at airborne levels of 0.1 mg/m^3 and very irritating at 10 mg/m^3. The OSHA workplace permissible exposure limits (PEL) are 0.5 mg/m^3 (for PCBs with 54% chlorine) and 1 mg/m^3 (for PCBs with 42% chlorine) as an 8-hour time-weighted average. The air levels considered immediately dangerous to life or health (IDLH) are 5 mg/m^3 and 10 mg/m^3, respectively.
  B. **Ingestion.** Acute toxicity after ingestion is unlikely; the oral LD_{50} is 1–10 g/kg.

III. **Clinical presentation**
  A. **Acute PCB exposure** may cause skin, eye, nose, and throat irritation.
  B. **Chronic exposure** may cause **chloracne** (cystic acneiform lesions predominantly found on the posterior neck, axillas, and upper back); the onset is usually 6 weeks or longer after onset of exposure. Skin pigmentation and porphyria may occur. Elevation of hepatic transaminases may occur, although the significance is unclear.

IV. **Diagnosis.** Diagnosis is usually based on a history of exposure and the presence of chloracne or elevated hepatic transaminases.
  A. **Specific levels.** PCB serum and fat levels are poorly correlated with health effects. Serum PCB concentrations are usually less than 20 mcg/L; higher levels may indicate exposure but not necessarily toxicity.
  B. **Other useful laboratory studies.** BUN, creatinine, liver enzymes.

V. **Treatment**
  A. **Emergency and supportive measures**
    1. Treat bronchospasm (see p 8) if it occurs.
    2. Monitor for elevated hepatic enzymes; chloracne; and nonspecific eye, gastrointestinal, and neurologic symptoms.
  B. **Specific drugs and antidotes.** There is no specific antidote.
  C. **Decontamination**
    1. **Inhalation.** Remove the victim from exposure and give supplemental oxygen, if available.
    2. **Skin and eyes.** Remove contaminated clothing and wash exposed skin with soap and water. Irrigate exposed eyes with copious tepid water or saline.
    3. **Ingestion**
       a. Induce emesis or perform gastric lavage (see p 42).
       b. Administer activated charcoal and a cathartic (see p 45) orally or by gastric tube. Gut emptying is probably not necessary after small ingestions if activated charcoal is given promptly.
  D. **Enhanced elimination.** There is no role for dialysis, hemoperfusion, or repeat-dose charcoal. Lipid-clearing drugs (eg, clofibrate and resins) have been suggested, but insufficient data exist to recommend them.

Reference

Kimbrough RD: Laboratory and human studies on polychlorinated biphenyls (PCBs) and related compounds. *Environ Health Perspect* 1985;59:99.

PYRETHRINS
Olga F. Woo, PharmD

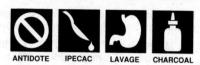

ANTIDOTE   IPECAC   LAVAGE   CHARCOAL

Pyrethrins are naturally occurring insecticides derived from the chrysanthemum plant. Pyrethroids (Table II-41) are synthetically derived compounds. Acute human poisoning from exposure to these insecticides is rare; however, inhalation frequently causes upper airway irritation and hypersensitivity reactions. Piperonyl butoxide is added to these compounds to prolong their activity by inhibiting mixed oxidase enzymes in the liver that metabolize the pyrethrins.

I. **Mechanism of toxicity.** In insects, pyrethrins and pyrethroids rapidly cause death by paralyzing the nervous system through disruption of the membrane ion transport system in nerve axons. Mammals are able to metabolize these compounds rapidly and thereby render them harmless.

II. **Toxic dose.** The toxic oral dose in mammals is greater than 100–1000 mg/kg. The potentially lethal acute oral dose is 10–100 g. Pyrethrins are not well absorbed across the skin or from the gastrointestinal tract. They have been used for many years as oral antihelmintic agents with minimum adverse effects other than mild gastrointestinal upset.

III. **Clinical presentation.** Toxicity to humans is primarily associated with hypersensitivity reactions and direct irritant effects rather than from any pharmacologic property.
   A. **Inhalation** of these compounds may precipitate wheezing in asthmatics. Inhalation or pulmonary aspiration may also cause a hypersensitivity pneumonitis.
   B. **Ingestion.** With massive oral doses, the central nervous system may be affected, resulting in seizures, coma, or respiratory arrest.
   C. **Anaphylactic** reactions including bronchospasm, oropharyngeal edema, and shock may occur in hypersensitive individuals.

IV. **Diagnosis.** Diagnosis is based on a history of exposure. There are no characteristic clinical symptoms or laboratory tests that are specific for identifying these compounds.
   A. **Specific levels.** These compounds are rapidly metabolized in the body, and methods for determining the parent compound are not routinely available.
   B. **Other useful laboratory studies.** Arterial blood gases, chest x-ray, pulmonary function tests.

V. **Treatment**
   A. **Emergency and supportive measures**
      1. Treat bronchospasm (see p 8) or anaphylaxis (see p 25) if they occur.
      2. Observe patients with massive ingestion for at least 4–6 hours for any signs of central nervous system depression or seizures.
   B. **Specific drugs and antidotes.** There is no specific antidote.
   C. **Decontamination**
      1. **Inhalation.** Remove victim from exposure and give supplemental oxygen, if available.

TABLE II-41. PYRETHROIDS

Allethrin	Decamethrin	Permethrin
Barthrin	Fenothrin	Phthalthrin
Bioresmethrin	Fenpropanate	Resmethrin
Cypermethrin	Fenvalerate	Tetramethrin

2. **Ingestion.** In the majority of cases, a subtoxic dose has been ingested and no decontamination is necessary. Following very large ingestions (> 100 mg/kg):

a. Induce emesis or perform gastric lavage (see p 42). Use caution because most commercial products contain a hydrocarbon solvent, which may cause a chemical pneumonitis if aspirated (p 165).

b. Administer activated charcoal and a cathartic (p 45) orally or by gastric tube.

c. Gut emptying is probably not necessary after small ingestions if activated charcoal is given promptly.

D. **Enhanced elimination.** These compounds are rapidly metabolized by the body, and extracorporeal methods of elimination would not be expected to enhance their elimination.

Reference

Newton JG, Breslin AB: Asthmatic reactions to a commonly used aerosol insect killer. *Med J Aust* 1983;1:378.

QUINIDINE AND OTHER TYPE Ia ANTIARRHYTHMIC DRUGS
Neal L. Benowitz, MD

| ANTIDOTE | IPECAC | LAVAGE | CHARCOAL |

Quinidine, procainamide (Pronestyl), and disopyramide (Norpace) are type Ia antiarrhythmic agents. Quinidine and procainamide are commonly used for suppression of acute and chronic supraventricular and ventricular arrhythmias. Disopyramide is used for ventricular arrhythmias. All 3 agents have a low toxic:therapeutic ratio and may produce fatal intoxication (Table II–42).

I. **Mechanism of toxicity.** Type Ia agents inhibit the fast sodium-dependent channel, slowing phase zero of the cardiac action potential. At high concentrations, this results in reduced myocardial contractility and excitability, and severe depression of cardiac conduction velocity. Repolarization is also delayed, resulting in a prolonged QT interval that may be associated with polymorphic ventricular tachycardia (torsade de pointes; see Fig I–5, p 13).

Quinidine and disopyramide also have anticholinergic activity; quinidine has alpha-adrenergic receptor-blocking activity, and procainamide has ganglionic- and neuromuscular-blocking activity.

TABLE II-42. TYPE Ia ANTIARRHYTHMIC DRUGS

Drug	Serum Half-Life (h)	Usual Adult Daily Dose (mg)	Therapeutic Serum Levels (mg/L)	Major Toxicity[a]
Quinidine	6	1000–2000	2–4	S, B, V, H
Disopyramide	7	400–800	2–4	B, V, H
Procainamide	4	1000–4000	4–10	B, V, H
NAPA	10	N/A	15–25	H

[a]S = seizures; B = bradycardia; V = ventricular tachycardia; H = hypotension.

II. **Toxic dose.** Acute ingestion of 1 g of quinidine, 5 g of procainamide, or 1 g of disopyramide in an adult should be considered potentially lethal.

III. **Clinical presentation.** The primary manifestations of toxicity involve the cardiovascular and central nervous systems.
   A. **Cardiotoxic effects** of the type Ia agents include sinus bradycardia; sinus node arrest or asystole; PR, QRS, or QT interval prolongation; sinus tachycardia (caused by anticholinergic effects); polymorphous ventricular tachycardia; and depressed myocardial contractility, which, along with alpha-adrenergic or ganglionic blockade, may result in hypotension and occasionally pulmonary edema.
   B. **Central nervous system toxicity.** Quinidine and disopyramide can cause anticholinergic effects such as dry mouth, dilated pupils, and delirium. All type Ia agents can produce seizures, coma, and respiratory arrest.
   C. **Other effects.** Quinidine commonly causes nausea, vomiting, and diarrhea after acute ingestion and, especially with chronic doses, cinchonism (tinnitus, vertigo, deafness, visual disturbances). Procainamide may cause gastrointestinal upset and, with chronic therapy, a lupuslike syndrome.

IV. **Diagnosis.** Diagnosis is based on a history of exposure and typical cardiotoxic features such as QRS and QT interval prolongation, AV block, or polymorphous ventricular tachycardia.
   A. **Specific levels.** Rapid serum levels are generally available for each agent. Serious toxicity with these drugs usually occurs only with levels above the therapeutic range; however, some complications, such as polymorphous ventricular tachycardia, may occur at therapeutic levels.
      1. Methods for detecting quinidine may vary in specificity, with some also measuring metabolites and contaminants.
      2. Procainamide has an active metabolite, N-acetylprocainamide (NAPA); with therapeutic procainamide dosing, NAPA levels can range up to 15 mg/L.
   B. **Other useful laboratory studies.** CBC, electrolytes, glucose, BUN, creatinine, arterial blood gases, ECG and electrocardiographic monitoring.

V. **Treatment**
   A. **Emergency and supportive measures**
      1. Maintain the airway and assist ventilation if necessary (see p 2).
      2. Treat hypotension (p 14), arrhythmias (pp 9–13), coma (p 17), and seizures (p 21) if they occur.
      3. Treat recurrent ventricular tachycardia with lidocaine, phenytoin, or overdrive pacing (p 13). Do **not** use other type Ia or type Ic agents, as they may worsen cardiac toxicity.
      4. Continuously monitor vital signs and ECG for a minimum of 6 hours, and admit symptomatic patients until the ECG returns to normal.
   B. **Specific drugs and antidotes.** Treat cardiotoxic effects such as wide QRS interval or hypotension with **hypertonic sodium bicarbonate** (see p 296), 1–2 meq/kg rapid IV bolus, repeated every 5–10 minutes and as needed. Markedly impaired conduction or high-degree atrioventricular block unresponsive to bicarbonate therapy is an indication for insertion of a cardiac pacemaker.
   C. **Decontamination**
      1. Do **not** induce emesis because of the risk of rapid onset of seizures or coma. Perform gastric lavage (see p 43).
      2. Administer activated charcoal and a cathartic (see p 45) orally or by gastric tube.
   D. **Enhanced elimination**
      1. **Quinidine** has a very large volume of distribution, and therefore it is not effectively removed by dialysis. Acidification of the urine may enhance excretion, but this is not recommended because it may aggravate cardiac toxicity.

    2. Disopyramide, procainamide, and *N*-acetylprocainamide (NAPA) have smaller volumes of distribution and are effectively removed by **hemoperfusion or dialysis.**

    3. The efficacy of repeat-dose activated charcoal has not been studied for the type Ia agents.

Reference

Shub C et al: The management of acute quinidine intoxication. *Chest* 1978;**73**:173.

QUININE
Neal L. Benowitz, MD

ANTIDOTE   IPECAC   LAVAGE   CHARCOAL

Quinine is an optical isomer of quinidine (see p 255). Quinine was once widely used for the treatment of malaria and is still occasionally used for chloroquine-resistant cases, but it is now prescribed primarily for the treatment of nocturnal muscle cramps. It has also been used as an abortifacient.

  I. Mechanism of toxicity. The mechanism of quinine toxicity is believed to be similar to that of quinidine (see p 255); however, quinine is a much less potent cardiotoxin. Quinine also has toxic effects on the retina that can result in blindness. At one time, vasoconstriction of retinal arterioles resulting in retinal ischemia was thought to be the cause of blindness; however, recent evidence indicates a direct toxic effect on photoreceptor and ganglion cells.

  II. Toxic dose. Quinine sulfate is available in capsules and tablets containing 130–325 mg. The minimum toxic dose is approximately 3–4 g in adults; 1 g has been fatal in a child.

 III. Clinical presentation. Toxic effects involve the cardiovascular and central nervous systems, the eyes, and other organ systems.

    A. Mild intoxication produces nausea, vomiting, and cinchonism (tinnitus, deafness, vertigo, headache, and visual disturbances).

    B. Severe intoxication may cause ataxia, obtundation, convulsions, coma, and respiratory arrest. With massive intoxication, quinidinelike cardiotoxicity (hypotension, QRS and QT interval prolongation, AV block, and ventricular arrhythmias) may be fatal.

    C. Retinal toxicity occurs 9–10 hours after ingestion and includes blurred vision, impaired color perception, constriction of visual fields, and blindness. Funduscopy may reveal retinal artery spasm, disk pallor, and macular edema. Although gradual recovery occurs, many patients are left with permanent visual impairment.

    D. Other toxic effects of quinine include hypokalemia, hypoglycemia, hemolysis (in patients with glucose-6-phosphate dehydrogenase [G6PD] deficiency), and congenital malformations when used in pregnancy.

 IV. Diagnosis. Diagnosis is based on a history of ingestion and the presence of cinchonism and visual disturbances. Quinidinelike cardiotoxic effects may or may not be present.

    A. Specific levels. Serum quinine levels can be measured by the same assay as for quinidine, as long as quinidine is not present. Plasma quinine levels above 10 mg/L have been associated with visual impairment; 87% of patients with levels above 20 mg/L reported blindness. Levels above 16 mg/L have been associated with cardiac toxicity.

    B. Other useful laboratory studies. CBC, electrolytes, glucose, BUN, creatinine, arterial blood gases, ECG and electrocardiographic monitoring.

V. Treatment
A. Emergency and supportive measures
1. Maintain the airway and assist ventilation if necessary (see p 2).
2. Treat coma (p 17), seizures (p 21), hypotension (p 14), and arrhythmias (pp 9–13) if they occur.
3. Avoid type Ia and type Ic antiarrhythmic drugs; they may worsen cardiotoxicity.
4. Continuously monitor vital signs and the ECG for at least 6 hours after ingestion, and admit symptomatic patients to an intensive care unit.

B. Specific drugs and antidotes
1. Treat cardiotoxicity with **hypertonic sodium bicarbonate** (see p 296), 1–2 meq/kg rapid IV bolus, as described for quinidine (see p 255).
2. Stellate ganglion block has previously been recommended for quinine-induced blindness, the rationale being to increase retinal blood flow. However, recent evidence indicates that this treatment is not effective and the procedure may have serious complications.

C. Decontamination
1. Do **not** induce emesis because of the risk of rapid onset of coma or seizures. Perform gastric lavage (see p 43).
2. Administer activated charcoal and a cathartic (see p 45) orally or by gastric tube.
3. Gut emptying is probably not necessary after very small ingestions if activated charcoal is given promptly.

D. Enhanced elimination.
Because of extensive tissue distribution (volume of distribution, 3 L/kg), dialysis and hemoperfusion procedures are ineffective. Acidification of the urine may slightly increase renal excretion but does not significantly alter the overall elimination rate and may aggravate cardiotoxicity.

Reference

Boland ME, Roper SM, Henry JA: Complications of quinine poisoning. *Lancet* 1985;1:384.

RADIATION
Evan T. Wythe, MD, and
Kent R. Olson, MD

ANTIDOTE   IPECAC   LAVAGE   CHARCOAL

Radiation poisoning is a rare but potentially catastrophic complication of the nuclear age. Poisoning may result from internal or external contamination and from particle-emitting solids, liquids, or gases, or electromagnetic sources. **Particle-emitting** radiation sources may produce beta and alpha particles, neutrons, protons, and positrons. **Electromagnetic** radiation includes gamma rays and x-rays.

I. **Mechanism of toxicity.** Radiation impairs biologic function by ionizing atoms and breaking chemical bonds, resulting in the intracellular formation of highly reactive free radicals that damage DNA and RNA. Cells with a high turnover rate (eg, skin, gastrointestinal tract, hematopoietic system) are affected first.
   A. **Particle-emitting dusts, liquids, or gases** may be highly contaminating to rescuers, transport vehicles, and attending health personnel.
   B. In contrast, **electromagnetic** radiation injures the victim but does not render the victim radioactive or dangerous to others. However, embedded electromagnetic radiation emitters may pose a danger.
II. **Toxic dose.** Various terms are used to describe radiation dose: R (roentgen), rad (radiation absorbed dose), and rem. Rad is the unit of radiation

dose commonly referred to in exposures. Exposure to 100–200 rads causes nausea and vomiting. Exposure to 200 rads is potentially lethal, and 600 rads is nearly 100% fatal. Brief exposure to 5000 rads or more usually causes death within minutes to hours.

III. **Clinical presentation.** The onset and character of radiation poisoning are determined largely by the dose.

    A. **Exposure to 100 rads** or more usually produces a prodrome within a few hours, characterized by nausea, vomiting, abdominal cramps, and diarrhea.

    B. With **exposure to 600 rads** or more, severe necrotic gastroenteritis may result in marked dehydration and death within a few days.

    C. With massive **exposures of several thousand rads,** confusion and lethargy may occur, followed within minutes to hours by ataxia, convulsions, coma, and cardiovascular collapse.

    D. **Bone marrow depression** usually follows exposure to at least 200–1000 rads. Leukopenia often contributes to death due to infections. Although thrombocytopenia and neutropenia are usually not evident for 2 weeks or more, the lymphocyte count is usually depressed within 48 hours of serious exposure; a count of less than 300–500 lymphocytes/mm^3 during this period indicates a poor prognosis, while 1200/mm^3 or more suggests likely survival.

    E. **Other complications** of radiation exposure include skin burns and hair loss.

IV. **Diagnosis.** Diagnosis depends on a history of exposure. Onset of symptoms within 2 hours usually indicates a dose of more than 400 rads, whereas if symptoms are delayed more than 6 hours, the exposure is often less than 50 rads.

    A. **Specific levels.** Serum radiation levels are neither available nor useful. Radiation-measuring instruments such as a Geiger counter may be used to measure particulate radiation contamination of the victim or hospital environment.

    B. **Other useful laboratory studies.** CBC, electrolytes, glucose, BUN, creatinine, urinalysis. Immediately draw lymphocytes for HLA typing in case bone marrow transplant is required later.

V. **Treatment**

    A. **Emergency and supportive measures.** Serious medical problems always take precedence over radiologic concerns.

        1. Maintain the airway and assist ventilation if necessary (see p 2).

        2. Treat coma (p 17) and seizures (p 21) if they occur.

        3. Replace fluid losses from gastroenteritis with intravenous crystalloid solutions (see p 14).

        4. Treat leukopenia and resulting infections as needed.

        5. For **expert assistance** in evaluation and treatment of victims and on-scene management, immediately contact the federally administered Oak Ridge Radiation Emergency Assistance Center & Training Site, 24 hours a day; telephone (615) 576-3131; or (615) 481-1000, ext 1502 or beeper 241. Also contact any local state agencies responsible for radiation safety.

    B. **Specific drugs and antidotes. Chelating agents or pharmacologic blocking drugs** may be useful in cases of ingestion or inhalation of certain biologically active radioactive particles, if they are given before or shortly after exposure (Table II–43). Contact the Oak Ridge Center (see above) for specific advice on use of these agents.

    C. **Decontamination**

        1. **Particulate exposure.** The victim is potentially highly contaminating to rescuers.

            a. Remove the victim from exposure and if condition permits, remove all clothing and wash the victim with soap and water.

TABLE II-43. CHELATING AND BLOCKING AGENTS FOR RADIATION EXPOSURE[a]

Radionuclide	Medication	Comments
Iodine	Potassium iodide	Blocks iodine uptake. Dose: 130 mg/d orally.
Rare earths, plutonium, transplutonics, yttrium	DTPA (pentetic acid)	Chelating agent. Dose: 1 g Ca-DTPA in D5W over 30–60 min. Wounds: Irrigate with 1 g DTPA in 250 mL of D5W.
Polonium, mercury, arsenic, bismuth, gold	BAL (dimercaprol)	Chelating agent (see p 294). Dose: 3–5 mg/kg IV every 4 hours for 3 days.
Uranium	Bicarbonate	Alkalinize urine, reduce risk of acute tubular necrosis.
Cesium, rubidium, thallium	Prussian blue (ferric hexacyanoferrate [II])	Not approved for use in USA. Dose: 1 g in 100–200 mL of water orally 3 times daily.
Radium	Calcium gluconate	Displaces radium. Dose: 10 mL once or twice daily.
Strontium	Ammonium chloride	Demineralizing agent. Dose: 3 g orally 3 times daily.
Tritium	Plain water	Isotopic dilution. Dose: 6–12 L/d of water orally.
Strontium, radium	Barium sulfate	Reduces absorption. Dose: 100 g BaSO$_4$ in 250 mL of water orally.
Calcium, barium	Sodium alginate	Inhibits absorption. Dose: 10 g in water orally.
Copper, polonium, lead, mercury, gold	Penicillamine	Chelating agent (see p 332). Dose: 1 g orally every 4–6 hours.

[a]Reference: Ricks RC: *Hospital Emergency Department Management of Radiation Accidents.* Oak Ridge Associated Univ, 1984.

      b. All clothing and cleansing water must be saved and properly disposed of.

      c. Rescuers should wear protective clothing and respiratory gear to avoid contamination. At the hospital, measures must be taken to prevent contamination of facilities and personnel.

      d. Induce emesis or perform gastric lavage (see p 42) if radioactive material has been ingested.

      e. The role of activated charcoal and cathartics (see p 45) is unknown.

   2. Electromagnetic radiation exposure. There is no need for decontamination once the patient has been removed from the source of exposure, unless electromagnetic radiation emitter fragments are embedded in body tissues. The patient is not radioactive and does not pose a contamination threat.

  D. Enhanced elimination. Chelating agents may be useful for certain exposures (Table II–43). There is no known role for dialysis or hemoperfusion.

Reference

Leonard RB, Ricks RC: Emergency department radiation accident protocol. *Ann Emerg Med* 1980;9:462.

SALICYLATES
Susan Kim, PharmD

      ANTIDOTE   IPECAC   LAVAGE   CHARCOAL

Salicylates are widely used for their analgesic and anti-inflammatory properties. They are found in a variety of prescription and over-the-counter analgesics, cold preparations, and topical keratolytic products. Before the introduction of child-resistant containers, salicylate overdose was one of the leading causes of accidental death in children. Two distinct syndromes of intoxication may occur, depending on whether the exposure is **acute** or **chronic**.

  I. Mechanism of toxicity. Salicylates have a variety of toxic effects.

   A. Central stimulation of the respiratory center results in hyperventilation, leading to respiratory alkalosis and compensatory metabolic acidosis and contributing to dehydration.

   B. Intracellular effects include uncoupling of oxidative phosphorylation and interruption of glucose and fatty acid metabolism.

   C. The mechanism by which cerebral and pulmonary edema occur is not known but may be related to alteration in capillary integrity.

   D. Salicylates alter platelet function and bleeding time and may also prolong the prothrombin time.

  II. Toxic dose. The average therapeutic single dose is 10 mg/kg, and the usual daily therapeutic dose is 40–60 mg/kg/d.

   A. Acute ingestion of 150–200 mg/kg will produce mild intoxication; severe intoxication is likely after acute ingestion of 300–500 mg/kg.

   B. Chronic intoxication may occur with ingestion of 100 mg/kg/d for 2 or more days.

  III. Clinical presentation. Patients may become intoxicated following acute accidental or suicidal overdose or as a result of chronic repeated overmedication for several days.

   A. Acute ingestion. Vomiting occurs shortly after ingestion, followed by hyperpnea, tinnitus, and lethargy. Respiratory alkalemia and metabolic acidosis are apparent when arterial blood gases are determined. With severe intoxication, coma, seizures, hypoglycemia, hyperthermia, and pulmonary edema may occur. Death is due to central nervous system failure and cardiovascular collapse.

B. Chronic intoxication. Victims are usually young children or confused elderly. The diagnosis is often overlooked because the presentation is nonspecific; confusion, dehydration, and metabolic acidosis are often attributed to sepsis, pneumonia, or gastroenteritis. However, morbidity and mortality rates are much higher than after acute overdose. Cerebral and pulmonary edema are more common than with acute intoxication, and severe poisoning occurs at lower salicylate levels.

IV. Diagnosis. Diagnosis is not difficult if there is a history of acute ingestion, accompanied by typical signs and symptoms. In the absence of a history of overdose, diagnosis is suggested by the characteristic arterial blood gases, which reveal a mixed respiratory alkalemia and metabolic acidosis.

A. Specific levels. Obtain a stat and serial serum salicylate concentrations.

1. **Acute ingestion.** Salicylate levels are plotted on the nomogram (Fig II–2) to determine expected toxicity. Single determinations are **not** sufficient because of the possibility of delayed absorption from sustained-release tablets or a tablet bezoar.

2. **Chronic intoxication.** The nomogram cannot be used to predict toxicity, and intoxication is poorly correlated with serum levels. Chronic therapeutic concentrations in arthritis patients range from 100 to 300 mg/L (10–30 mg/dL). Systemic acidemia increases brain salicylate concentration, worsening toxicity.

B. Other useful laboratory studies. CBC, electrolytes, anion gap calculation, glucose, BUN, creatinine, liver function tests, prothrombin time, arterial blood gases, chest x-ray. Abdominal x-ray may reveal radiopaque enteric-coated or sustained-release tablets.

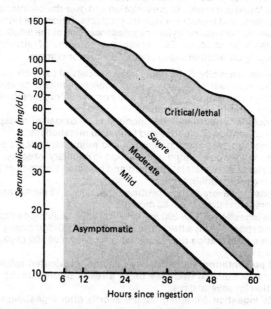

Figure II-2. Nomogram for determining severity of salicylate intoxication. Absorption kinetics assume acute (1-time) ingestion of non-enteric-coated preparation. (Redrawn and reproduced, with permission, from Done AK: Salicylate intoxication: Significance of measurement of salicylate in blood in cases of acute ingestion. *Pediatrics* 1960;26:800.)

V. Treatment
A. Emergency and supportive measures
1. Maintain the airway and assist ventilation if necessary (see p 2). Administer supplemental oxygen. Obtain serial arterial blood gases and chest x-rays to observe for pulmonary edema (more common with chronic intoxication).
2. Treat coma (p 17), seizures (p 21), pulmonary edema (p 7), and hyperthermia (p 19) if they occur.
3. Treat metabolic acidosis with intravenous sodium bicarbonate (do *not* allow the serum pH to fall below 7.4).
4. Replace fluid and electrolyte deficits caused by vomiting and hyperventilation with intravenous crystalloid solutions. Be cautious with fluid therapy, because excessive fluid administration may contribute to pulmonary edema.
5. Monitor asymptomatic patients for a minimum of 6 hours (longer if an enteric-coated preparation has been ingested or there is suspicion of a tablet bezoar). Admit symptomatic patients to an intensive care unit.
B. Specific drugs and antidotes.
There is no specific antidote for salicylate intoxication. **Sodium bicarbonate** is frequently given both to prevent acidemia and to promote salicylate elimination by the kidneys (see D, below).
C. Decontamination.
(Not necessary for patients with chronic intoxication.)
1. Induce emesis or perform gastric lavage (see p 42).
2. Administer activated charcoal and a cathartic (see p 45) orally or by gastric tube. *Note:* With very large ingestions of salicylate (eg, 30–60 g), very large doses of activated charcoal (300–600 g) are theoretically necessary to adsorb all the salicylate and prevent desorption. In these cases, the charcoal may be given in several 50- to 100-g doses at 3- to 5-hour intervals.
3. Gut emptying is probably not necessary after small ingestions (ie, < 200–300 mg/kg) if activated charcoal is given promptly.
D. Enhanced elimination
1. **Urinary alkalinization** is effective in enhancing urinary excretion of salicylate although difficult to achieve in critically ill patients.
   a. Add 100 meq of sodium bicarbonate (see p 296) to 1 L of 5% dextrose and infuse intravenously at 150–200 mL/h (2–3 mL/kg/h). If the patient is dehydrated, start with a bolus of 10–20 mL/kg. Fluid and bicarbonate administration is potentially dangerous in patients at high risk for pulmonary edema (eg, chronic intoxication).
   b. Unless renal failure is present, also add potassium, 30–40 meq, to each liter of intravenous fluids (potassium depletion inhibits alkalinization).
2. **Hemodialysis** is very effective in rapidly removing salicylate and correcting acid-base and fluid abnormalities. Indications for hemodialysis are as follows:
   a. Patients with acute ingestion and serum levels higher than 1200 mg/L (120 mg/dL) or with severe acidosis and other manifestations of intoxication.
   b. Patients with chronic intoxication with serum levels higher than 600 mg/L (60 mg/dL) and any confusion or lethargy.
   c. Any patient with severe manifestations of intoxication.
3. **Hemoperfusion** is also very effective but does not correct acid-base or fluid disturbances.
4. **Repeat-dose activated charcoal** therapy effectively reduces the serum salicylate half-life but may contribute to dehydration and electrolyte disturbances.

References

Hillman RJ, Prescott LF: Treatment of salicylate poisoning with repeated oral charcoal. *Br Med J* 1985;**291**:1472.
Prescott LF et al: Diuresis or urinary alkalinisation for salicylate poisoning? *Br Med J* 1982;**285**:1383.

SCORPIONS
Howard E. McKinney, PharmD

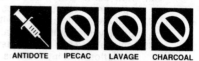

The order Scorpionida contains several families, genera, and species of scorpions. All have paired venom glands in a bulbous segment called the telson, located just anterior to a stinger on the end of the 6 terminal segments of the abdomen (often called a tail).

The only dangerous species in the USA is the *Centruroides exilicauda*. The most serious envenomations are usually reported in children under age 10 years. This scorpion is found primarily in the arid southwestern USA but has been found as a stowaway in cargo as far north as Michigan.

Other dangerous scorpions are found in Mexico (*Centruroides* species), Brazil (*Tityus* species), India (*Buthus* species), and north Africa and the eastern Mediterranean (*Leiurus* species).

I. **Mechanism of toxicity.** The scorpion grasps the skin with its anterior pincers, arches its pseudoabdomen, and stabs with the stinger. Stings also result from stepping on the stinger. The venom of *C exilicauda* contains numerous digestive enzymes (eg, hyaluronidase, phospholipase) and also several neurotoxins. Alteration in sodium channel flow results in excessive stimulation at neuromuscular junctions and the autonomic nervous system.

II. **Toxic dose.** Variable amounts of venom from none to the complete contents of the telson may be ejected through the stinger.

III. **Clinical presentation**
  A. **Common scorpion stings.** Most stings result only in local, immediate, excruciating, burning pain. Some local tissue inflammation and occasionally local paresthesias may occur. Symptoms usually resolve within several hours. This represents the typical scorpion sting seen in the USA.
  B. **Dangerous scorpion stings.** In some victims, especially children under age 10 years, systemic symptoms occur, including restlessness, diaphoresis, diplopia, nystagmus, hyperexcitability, muscle fasciculations, opisthotonus, salivation, hypertension, tachycardia, and, rarely, convulsions, paralysis, and respiratory arrest. Pulmonary edema, cardiovascular collapse, and death have been reported, as well as coagulopathies, disseminated intravascular coagulation, pancreatitis, and renal failure with hemoglobinuria and jaundice.

IV. **Diagnosis.** Either the patient saw the scorpion, or the clinician must recognize the symptoms. In the case of *Centruroides* stings, tapping on the site usually produces severe pain ("tap test").
  A. **Specific levels.** Serum toxin levels are not available.
  B. **Other useful laboratory studies.** None are needed for minor envenomations. For severe envenomations, obtain CBC, electrolytes, glucose, BUN, creatinine, creatine phosphokinase (CPK), coagulation profile, arterial blood gases.

V. **Treatment.** The majority of even *Centruroides* stings can be managed with symptomatic care at home.
  A. **Emergency and supportive measures**

1. For severe envenomations, maintain the airway and assist ventilation if necessary (see p 2). Administer supplemental oxygen.
2. Treat hypertension (p 16), tachycardia (p 12), and convulsions (p 21) if they occur.
3. Do **not** overtreat with excessive sedation.
4. Clean the wound and provide tetanus prophylaxis if indicated.
5. Do **not** immerse the injured extremity in ice or perform local incision or suction.

B. **Specific drugs and antidotes.** Some **antivenins** have been produced, but none are approved for human use. In selected cases, they can be located by a regional poison control center (see Table I–41, p 51).

C. **Decontamination.** These procedures are not applicable.

D. **Enhanced elimination.** These procedures are not applicable.

Reference

Curry SC et al: Envenomation by the scorpion *Centruroides sculpturatus*. *J Toxicol Clin Toxicol* 1983–84;**21**:417.

SEDATIVE-HYPNOTIC AGENTS
Evan T. Wythe, MD

| ANTIDOTE | IPECAC | LAVAGE | CHARCOAL |

Sedative-hypnotic agents are widely used for the treatment of anxiety and insomnia. As a group they are one of the most frequently prescribed medications. Barbiturates (see p 85), benzodiazepines (p 90), antihistamines (p 73), and anticholinergic agents (p 71) are discussed elsewhere in this book. In this section are listed some of the less commonly used hypnotic agents.

I. **Mechanism of toxicity.** The exact mechanism of action and the pharmacokinetics vary for each agent. The major toxic effect resulting in serious poisoning or death is central nervous system depression resulting in coma, respiratory arrest, and pulmonary aspiration of gastric contents.

II. **Toxic dose.** The toxic dose varies considerably between drugs and also depends largely on individual tolerance and the presence of other drugs such as alcohol (Table II–44). For most of these drugs, ingestion of 3–5 times the usual hypnotic dose results in coma. However, coingestion of alcohol may cause coma after smaller ingestions, while individuals chronically using large doses of these drugs may tolerate much larger doses.

III. **Clinical presentation.** Overdose with any of these drugs may cause drowsiness, ataxia, nystagmus, stupor, coma, and respiratory arrest. Deep coma may result in absent reflexes, fixed pupils, and depressed or absent electroencephalographic (EEG) activity. Hypothermia is common. Most agents also slow gastric motility and decrease muscle tone and may cause hypotension with very large overdose, primarily by depression of cardiac contractility.

A. **Chloral hydrate** is metabolized to trichloroethanol, which also has CNS-depressant activity. Trichloroethanol may also sensitize the myocardium to the effects of catecholamines, resulting in cardiac arrhythmias.

B. **Ethchlorvynol** has a pungent odor sometimes described as pearlike, and gastric fluid often has a pink or green color depending on the capsule form (200- and 500-mg are red; 750-mg is green).

C. **Glutethimide** often produces mydriasis (dilated pupils) and other anticholinergic side effects, and patients may exhibit prolonged and cyclic or fluctuating coma. It is sometimes taken in combination with codeine ("loads"), which may produce opioid effects.

D. **Meprobamate** has been reported to form tablet concretions in large

TABLE II-44. COMMON SEDATIVE-HYPNOTIC AGENTS[a]

Drug	Usual Adult Oral Hypnotic Dose (mg)	Approximate Lethal Dose (g)	Usual Half-Life[b] (h)
Chloral hydrate	500–1000	5–10	5–10
Ethchlorvynol	500–1000	5–10	10–20
Glutethimide	250–500	10–20	10–40
Meprobamate	600–1200	10–20	8–12
Methaqualone	150–250	3–8	10–40
Methyprylon	200–400	5–10	3–6

[a] See also benzodiazepines (p 90), barbiturates (p 85), paraldehyde (p 229), antihistamines (p 73), and anticholinergic agents (p 71).
[b] Half-life in overdose may be considerably longer.

overdose, occasionally requiring surgical removal. Hypotension is more common with this agent than with other sedative-hypnotics.
   E. **Methaqualone** is unusual among sedative-hypnotic agents in frequently causing muscular hypertonicity, clonus, and hyperreflexia.
IV. **Diagnosis.** Diagnosis is usually based on a history of ingestion, because clinical manifestations are fairly nonspecific. Hypothermia and deep coma may cause the patient to appear to be dead; thus, careful evaluation should precede the diagnosis of brain death.
   A. **Specific levels.** Serum drug levels and qualitative urine screening are usually available through commercial toxicology laboratories.
      1. Drug levels do not always correlate with severity of intoxication, especially in patients who have tolerance to the drug or who have also ingested other drugs or alcohol. In addition, early after ingestion blood levels may not reflect brain concentrations.
      2. Some agents (chloral hydrate, glutethimide) have active metabolites, levels of which may correlate better with the state of intoxication.
   B. **Other useful laboratory studies.** CBC, electrolytes, glucose, serum ethanol, BUN, creatinine, arterial blood gases, chest x-ray.
V. **Treatment**
   A. **Emergency and supportive measures**
      1. Maintain the airway and assist ventilation if necessary (see p 2). Admninister supplemental oxygen.
      2. Treat coma (p 17), hypothermia (p 18), hypotension (p 14), and pulmonary edema (p 7) if they occur.
      3. Monitor patients for at least 6 hours after ingestion, because delayed absorption may occur.
   B. **Specific drugs and antidotes.** Flumazenil (see p 313) is a specific antagonist of benzodiazepine receptors and is available in Europe. It is currently undergoing clinical trials in the USA.
   C. **Decontamination**
      1. Induce emesis or perform gastric lavage (see p 42).
      2. Administer activated charcoal and a cathartic (p 45) orally or by gastric tube.
      3. Gut emptying is probably not necessary after small ingestions if activated charcoal is given promptly.
      4. If a gastric concretion (bezoar) is suspected because of sustained coma or sustained high serum drug levels, obtain a plain abdominal x-ray or perform a contrast material swallow x-ray to attempt to

identify a mass. Repeat-dose charcoal (p 299), whole gut lavage (p 46), or even surgical removal may be necessary.

D. **Enhanced elimination.** Because of extensive tissue distribution, dialysis and hemoperfusion are not very effective for most of the drugs in this group.

1. **Repeat-dose charcoal** may enhance elimination of glutethimide (which undergoes enterohepatic recirculation) and meprobamate, although no studies have been performed to document this.

2. Meprobamate has a relatively small volume of distribution (0.75 L/kg), and **hemoperfusion** is indicated for deep coma complicated by intractable hypotension.

3. **Resin hemoperfusion** has been reported to be partially effective for ethchlorvynol overdose.

References

Bertino JS Jr, Reed MD: Barbiturate and nonbarbiturate sedative hypnotic intoxication in children. *Pediatr Clin North Am* 1986;**33**:703.

Bowyer K, Glasser SP: Chloral hydrate overdose and cardiac arrhythmias. *Chest* 1980;**77**:232.

SELENIUM
Mary Twieg, MD, and Kent R. Olson, MD

ANTIDOTE   IPECAC   LAVAGE   CHARCOAL

Selenium is a trace metal considered an essential element in the human diet, with multiple roles in metabolic chemistry. Excessive selenium absorption is well known to cause chronic toxicity. Selenium is used in the electronics industry in rectifiers, photoelectric cells, and solar batteries; in glass, rubber, steel, and ceramic manufacturing; and in some paints, varnishes, fungicides, and insecticides. **Selenious acid** is used in gun blueing solutions. Food sources of selenium include seafoods (especially shrimp), meat, milk products, and grains. Geographic concentration of selenium due to environmental factors has been reported.

I. **Mechanism of toxicity.** Elemental selenium is not well absorbed and poses no significant risk of toxicity. Other forms of selenium are well absorbed by the skin, lungs, or gastrointestinal tract.

A. **Hydrogen selenide** (selenium hydride) is a highly irritating gas produced by acid reaction with metal selenides.

B. **Selenious acid** is a caustic agent with systemic toxic effects.

C. **Selenium,** once absorbed, may have a variety of toxic effects, including inhibition of sulfhydryl enzymes and displacement of sulfur in certain tissues.

II. **Toxic dose**

A. **Ingestion.** Little is known about the oral toxic dose because there are few reports of poisoning. Coingestion of vitamin C may reduce selenite to elemental selenium and decrease its absorption.

1. **Acute overdose.** The oral mean lethal dose of selenite salts in the dog is about 4 mg/kg. Ingestion of as little as 20 mL of gun blueing solution (2% selenious acid) has been fatal.

2. **Chronic ingestion.** The recommended nutritional daily intake is 50–200 mcg/d. The drinking water standard is 10 mcg/L. Chronic ingestion of 3–6 mg/d has been associated with chronic intoxication.

B. **Inhalation.** The OSHA workplace permissible exposure limit (PEL) for hydrogen selenide is 0.05 ppm as an 8-hour time-weighted average; and

the level immediately dangerous to life or health (IDLH) is just 2 ppm (Table II–45).
III. **Clinical presentation**
   A. **Inhalation** of irritant selenium gases such as hydrogen selenide may cause burning eyes and throat, coughing, wheezing, chemical pneumonia, and pulmonary edema. Skin irritation is common after direct exposure.
   B. **Acute ingestion** may cause vomiting, hypersalivation, and garlicky odor on the breath. Hypotension, coma, and convulsions have been reported. Prolonged QT intervals and T-wave changes may occur. Death has occurred after small ingestions of selenious acid in gun blueing solutions.
   C. **Chronic intoxication** has been associated with discoloration and loss of hair and nails, polyneuritis, fatigue, garlicky breath, elevation of hepatic enzymes, dermatitis, and nausea and vomiting. Animal studies suggest that chronic excessive selenium exposure is embryotoxic and teratogenic, causes hepatic cirrhosis, and may be carcinogenic.
IV. **Diagnosis.** Diagnosis is difficult without a history of exposure but should be suspected in a patient with hair and nail loss or discoloration and other characteristic symptoms.
   A. **Specific levels.** Selenium can be measured in the blood, hair, or urine.
      1. On a normal diet, **whole blood** selenium levels range from 0.1 to 0.2 mg/L; in one patient with chronic intoxication after daily ingestion of 31 mg/d, whole blood selenium was 0.53 mg/L.
      2. Average **hair** levels are up to 0.5 ppm.
      3. Concentrations in **urine** reflect dietary intake. Excessive exposure should be considered when urine concentrations exceed 100 mcg/L.
   B. **Other useful laboratory studies.** CBC, electrolytes, glucose, BUN, creatinine, hepatic function tests, ECG. After inhalation exposure, obtain arterial blood gases and chest x-ray.
V. **Treatment**
   A. **Emergency and supportive measures**
      1. Maintain the airway and assist ventilation if necessary (see p 2). Administer supplemental oxygen.
      2. Treat coma (p 17), convulsions (p 21), bronchospasm (p 8), and pulmonary edema (p 7) if they occur.
      3. Observe for at least 6 hours after exposure.
      4. After ingestion of selenious acid, consider endoscopy to rule out esophageal or gastric corrosive injury.
   B. **Specific drugs and antidotes.** There is no established specific antidote. Although chelation with EDTA (see p 308) has been studied in animals, it is effective only if given within 15 minutes of the ingestion. High-dose vitamin C has produced equivocal results.
   C. **Decontamination**
      1. **Inhalation.** Immediately remove the victim from exposure and give supplemental oxygen, if available.
      2. **Skin and eyes.** Remove contaminated clothing and wash exposed

TABLE II–45. TOXIC LEVELS OF SELENIUM COMPOUNDS

Selenium Compound	Permissible Exposure Limit	Level Immediately Dangerous to Life or Health
Hydrogen selenide (selenium hydride)	0.05 ppm (0.2 mg/m^3)	2 ppm
Selenium compounds, general	(0.2 mg/m^3)	100 mg/m^3
Selenium hexafluoride	0.05 ppm (0.4 mg/m^3)	5 ppm

skin with soap and copious water. Irrigate exposed eyes with copious tepid water or saline.

3. **Ingestion**
   a. After **selenite** ingestion, induce emesis or perform gastric lavage (see p 42).
   b. Do **not** induce emesis after ingestion of **selenious acid;** instead, perform gastric lavage.
   c. Administer activated charcoal and a cathartic (see p 45) orally or by gastric tube.
   d. In vitro experiments indicate that vitamin C can reduce selenium salts to elemental selenium, which is poorly absorbed. Its use has not been studied in vivo, but oral or nasogastric administration of several grams of ascorbic acid is probably reasonable.

D. **Enhanced elimination.** There is no known role for any enhanced removal procedure.

Reference

Centers for Disease Control: Selenium intoxication: New York. *MMWR* 1984;**33**:157.

SNAKEBITE
Howard E. McKinney, PharmD

ANTIDOTE   IPECAC   LAVAGE   CHARCOAL

Of the 14 families of snakes, 5 are poisonous (Table II–46). Roughly 8000 envenomations resulting in 10–20 deaths occur yearly in the USA. Rattlesnake bite is the most common envenomation in the USA, and the victim is often a young, intoxicated male who was playing with the snake. Snakes strike accurately to about one-third their body length, with a maximum striking distance of a few feet.

TABLE II–46. EXAMPLES OF POISONOUS SNAKES

Family and Genera	Common Name	Comments
Colubridae		
Lampropeltis	King snake	Human envenomation difficult because of
Heterodon	Hognose	small mouth and small fixed fangs in the rear
Coluber	Racer	of mouth. May cause severe systemic coagu-
Dispholidus	Boomslang	lopathy.
Crotalidae		
Crotalus	Rattlesnake	Most common envenomation in USA. Long rotat-
Agkistrodon	Copperhead, cottonmouth	ing fangs in the front of the mouth. Heat-sensing
Bothrops	Fer-de-lance	facial pits (hence the name "pit vipers").
Elapidae		
Micrurus	Coral snake	Human envenomation difficult because of
Naja	Cobra	small mouth and small fixed fangs in rear
Bungarus	Krait	of mouth. Neurotoxicity usually predomi-
Dendroaspis	Mamba	nates.
Hydrophidae	Sea snakes	Also have small rear-located fangs.
Viperidae		
Bitis	Puff adder, gaboon viper	Long rotating fangs in the front of the
Cerastes	Cleopatra's asp	mouth but do not have heat-sensing facial
Echis	Saw-scaled viper	pits.

I. **Mechanism of toxicity.** Snake venoms are complex mixtures of 50 or more components that function to immobilize, kill, and predigest prey. The relative predominance of neurotoxic or digestive venom components depends on the species of the snake and geographic variables.

II. **Toxic dose.** The potency of the venom and the amount of venom injected vary considerably. About 20% of all snake strikes are "dry" bites in which there is no envenomation.

III. **Clinical presentation.** The most common snake envenomations in the USA are rattlesnake (Crotalidae) bites. Bites from common North American Elapidae (eg, coral snake) and Colubridae (eg, king snake) are also discussed here. For bites from other, exotic snakes, contact a regional poison center (see Table I–41, p 51) for specific consultation.

   A. **Crotalidae.** Fang marks may look like puncture wounds or shaving razor nicks. The fangs often penetrate only a few millimeters but occasionally enter deeper tissue spaces or veins.

      1. **Local effects.** Within minutes of envenomation, stinging, burning pain begins and progressive proximal swelling, erythema, petechiae, ecchymosis, and hemorrhagic blebs develop over the next several hours. The limb may swell to twice its normal size within the first few hours. Hypovolemic shock may occur secondary to fluid and blood sequestration in injured areas.

      2. **Systemic effects** may include nausea and vomiting, weakness, muscle fasciculations, diaphoresis, perioral and peripheral parasthesias, a rubbery or minty taste, thrombocytopenia, and coagulopathy. Circulating vasodilatory compounds may contribute to hypotension. Pulmonary edema has been reported.

      3. With *Crotalus scutulatus scutulatus* (Mojave rattlesnake) envenomation, there may be little or no swelling or evidence of tissue digestion; instead, delayed-onset (up to several hours) muscle weakness, ptosis, and respiratory arrest may occur. Facial and laryngeal edema have also been reported.

   B. **Elapidae.** Coral snake envenomation is rare because the snake's mouth is small, and it must hold on and "chew" the extremity for several seconds or more to work its rear fangs into the skin.

      1. **Local effects.** There is usually minimal swelling and inflammation around the fang marks. Local paresthesias may occur.

      2. **Systemic effects.** Nausea and vomiting, euphoria, and confusion may occur. After a delay of up to 12 hours or more, diplopia, dysarthria, muscle fasciculations, generalized muscle weakness, and respiratory arrest may occur.

   C. **Colubridae.** These small-mouthed rear-fanged snakes must also hang onto their victims and "chew" the venom into the skin.

      1. **Local effects.** There is usually little local reaction other than mild pain and paresthesias, although swelling of the extremity may occur.

      2. **Systemic effects.** The most serious effect of envenomation is systemic coagulopathy, which may be fatal.

IV. **Diagnosis.** Correct diagnosis and treatment depend on proper identification of the offending snake.

   A. Attempt to establish whether the bite was by an indigenous (wild) species or an exotic zoo animal or illegally imported pet. (The owner of an illegal pet snake may be reluctant to admit this for fear of fines or confiscation.) Envenomation occurring during the fall and winter months (October–March) when snakes usually hibernate is not likely to be caused by a wild species.

   B. If the snake is available, attempt to have it identified by a herpetologist. *Caution:* Be careful not to handle a "dead" snake; accidental envenomation may still occur up to several hours after death.

     C. Specific levels. These tests are not applicable.

     D. Other useful laboratory studies. CBC, platelet count, prothrombin time, fibrin split products, fibrinogen, blood type and screen, creatine phosphokinase (CPK), urine for myoglobin. If compromised respiratory function is suspected, obtain serial arterial blood gases.

V. Treatment

  A. Emergency and supportive measures. Regardless of the species, prepare for both systemic manifestations and local "digestive" effects. Monitor patients closely for at least 3–4 hours after typical Crotalid bite and for at least 12–24 hours after *C scutulatus scutulatus* or Elapid bites.

     1. Systemic effects

       a. Monitor for respiratory muscle weakness. Maintain the airway and assist ventilation if necessary (see p 2). Administer supplemental oxygen.

       b. Treat severe coagulopathy with fresh-frozen plasma (and antivenin; see below). Treat hypotension with intravenous crystalloid fluids (p 14) and rhabdomyolysis (p 24) with fluids and sodium bicarbonate.

     2. Local effects

       a. Monitor local swelling at least hourly with measurements of limb girth, the presence and extent of local ecchymosis, and assessment of circulation.

       b. Treat local wound complications with the assistance of an experienced surgeon; do *not* overzealously perform fasciotomy unless compartment syndrome is documented with compartment pressure monitoring.

       c. Provide tetanus prophylaxis if needed.

  B. Specific drugs and antidotes. For patients with documented envenomation, administer specific **antivenin.** Virtually all local and systemic manifestations of envenomation improve after antivenin adminstration.

     1. For **rattlesnake** and **Crotalidae** envenomations in general, the presence of fang marks, progressive swelling and ecchymosis, and pain at the bite site are considered minimal indications for **polyvalent Crotalidae antivenin** (see p 290). *Caution:* Life-threatening anaphylactic reactions may occur with antivenin administration, even after a negative skin test. For Mojave rattlesnake bite, the decision to administer antivenin is more difficult because there are few local signs of toxicity.

     2. For **coral snake** envenomation, consult a regional poison center (see Table I-41, p 51) or an experienced herpetologist to determine the advisability of *Micrurus fulvius* **antivenin** (see p 292). In general, if there is evidence of coagulopathy or neurologic toxicity, administer antivenin.

     3. For **Colubridae** envenomations, there are no antivenins available.

     4. For **other exotic snakes,** consult a regional poison center (see Table I-41, p 51) for asistance in diagnosis, location of specific antivenin, and indications for administration.

  C. Decontamination. First-aid measures are generally ineffective and may cause additional tissue damage.

     1. Remain calm, remove the victim to at least 20 feet from the snake, wash the area with soap and water, and remove any constricting clothing or jewelry. Do *not* apply ice to the site.

     2. Loosely splint and immobilize the extremity near heart level. *Do not apply a tourniquet.*

     3. Do *not* make cuts over the bite site. If performed within 15 minutes, **suction** over the fang marks (ie, with a Sawyer extractor) may remove some venom but this should not delay transport to a hospital.

D. Enhanced elimination. Dialysis, hemoperfusion, and charcoal administration are not applicable.

References

Kitchens CS, Van Mierop LH: Envenomation by the eastern coral snake *(Micrurus fulvius fulvius)*: A study of 39 victims. *JAMA* 1987;**258**:1615.

Wingert WA, Chan L: Rattlesnake bites in southern California and rationale for recommended treatment. *West J Med* 1988;**148**:37.

SPIDERS
Howard E. McKinney, PharmD

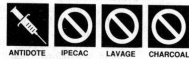

ANTIDOTE   IPECAC   LAVAGE   CHARCOAL

Most of the more than 50,000 species of spiders in the USA possess poison glands connected to fangs in the large, paired, jawlike structures known as chelicerae. However, only a very few spiders have fangs long and tough enough to pierce human skin. In the USA, these include *Latrodectus* (black widow), *Loxosceles* (brown spiders), *Phidippus* (jumping spider), and *Tarantulas* (a common name given to many large spiders). Most envenomations seem to occur when the spider's nest or young are disturbed, typically during gardening, moving firewood, or house repairs. **Tarantulas** rarely cause significant envenomation but produce a painful bite because of their large size. Spiders not common to North America are not discussed here.

I. **Mechanism of toxicity.** Spider venoms contain various protein and polypeptide toxins that are poorly characterized but appear to be designed to induce rapid paralysis of the insect victim and to aid in digestion.

   A. *Latrodectus* (black widow) toxin contains a highly potent neurotoxin that causes generalized release of neurotransmitters at muscle nerve endings.

   B. *Loxosceles* (brown spiders) and *Phidippus* (jumping spiders) toxins contain various digestive enzymes such as lipase, collagenase, and protease.

II. **Toxic dose.** Spider venoms are generally extremely potent toxins (far more potent than most snake venoms), but the delivered dose is extremely small.

III. **Clinical presentation.** Manifestations of envenomation are quite different depending on the species.

   A. *Latrodectus* (black widow) is a shiny black spider with a red hourglass marking on the abdomen.

      1. The black widow inflicts a bite that is often initially unnoticed but becomes painful within 30–120 minutes. By 3–4 hours, painful cramping and muscle fasciculations occur in the involved extremity. This cramping progresses toward the chest, back, or abdomen, producing boardlike rigidity, weakness, dyspnea, headache, and paresthesias. Black widow envenomation may mimic myocardial infarction or an acute surgical abdominal condition.

      2. Additional symptoms may include nausea, vomiting, diaphoresis, facial edema, ptosis, cardiac arrhythmias, fever, leukocytosis, restlessness, delirium, tachypnea, and tachycardia. Symptoms often persist for 18–36 hours.

      3. Rarely, hypertensive crisis or respiratory arrest may occur within 4–6 hours after severe envenomation, mainly in very young or very old victims.

   B. *Loxosceles* is brown, with a violin-shaped marking on its back. The

Loxosceles syndrome is often called "loxoscelism" or "necrotic arachnidism."

1. Envenomation usually produces a painful burning sensation at the bite site within 10 minutes. Over the next 1–12 hours, a "bull's-eye" lesion forms, consisting of a central vesicle (which may be hemorrhagic) surrounded by a blanched ring enclosed by a ring of ecchymosis. The entire lesion is about 1–5 cm in diameter.

2. Over the next 24–72 hours, an indolent necrotic ulcer develops that may persist for a month or more. This ulcer may be accompanied by a generalized pruritic morbilliform rash, fever, regional lymphadenopathy, nausea, vomiting, jaundice, hemolysis with resulting renal failure, and, rarely, disseminated intravascular coagulation and death.

C. *Phidippus.* Many necrotic spider bites in the USA are probably caused by *Phidippus* species, which inflicts a painful bite, resulting in localized wheals, rashes, ecchymosis, and pruritus that are occasionally complicated by arthralgias, myalgias, headache, fever, nausea, vomiting, and hypotension. The duration of effects is generally no more than 1–4 days, and death is very rare.

IV. **Diagnosis.** Bite marks of all spiders but the tarantulas are usually too small to be easily visualized, and victims often do not recall feeling the bite or seeing the spider.

Besides *Loxosceles* and *Phidippus,* many arthropods and insects may also produce small puncture wounds, pain, itching, redness, swelling, and even necrotic ulcers, so the offending animal often cannot be precisely identified unless it was captured or seen by the victim.

A. **Specific levels.** Serum toxin levels are not currently available. In the future, diagnostic serologic tests may be useful in diagnosing the specific responsible spider.

B. **Other useful laboratory studies.** CBC, electrolytes, glucose, BUN, creatinine, creatine phosphokinase (CPK), urinalysis, ECG.

V. **Treatment**

A. **Emergency and supportive measures**

1. **General**

a. Cleanse the wound and treat infection if it occurs.

b. Give tetanus prophylaxis if indicated.

2. *Latrodectus* **envenomation**

a. Monitor victims for at least 6–8 hours.

b. Maintain the airway and assist ventilation if necessary (see p 2).

c. Muscle cramping may be treated with **intravenous calcium** (p 298) or muscle relaxants such as **methocarbamol** (p 321). Pain may be treated with **morphine** (p 324).

3. *Loxosceles* **or** *Phidippus* **envenomation.** Provide local wound care and general supportive care. Monitor *Loxosceles* envenomations for hemolysis, renal failure, and other complications.

B. **Specific drugs and antidotes**

1. *Latrodectus.* Most patients can be effectively managed without using the equine-derived antivenin (**Antivenin** *Latrodectus mactans;* see p 291). It may still be indicated for elderly and pediatric patients who do not respond to conventional therapy for hypertension, muscle cramping, or respiratory distress and for pregnant victims threatening premature labor.

2. *Loxosceles.* Therapy for necrotic arachnidism has been difficult to evaluate because of the inherent difficulty of accurate diagnosis. There is as yet not enough evidence to recommend therapy with dapsone or colchicine, and there is not yet a commercially available antivenin.

C. **Decontamination.** These measures are not applicable. There is no proved value in the sometimes popular early excision of *Loxosceles* bites to prevent necrotic ulcer formation.

D. Enhanced elimination. These procedures are not applicable.

References

Banner W Jr: Bites and stings in the pediatric patient. *Curr Probl Pediatr* 1988;**18**:1.
Moss HS, Binder LS: A retrospective review of black widow spider envenomation. *Ann Emerg Med* 1987;**16**:188.

STRYCHNINE
Neal L. Benowitz, MD

| ANTIDOTE | IPECAC | LAVAGE | CHARCOAL |

Strychnine is an alkaloid derived from the seeds of a tree, *Strychnos nux-vomica*. At one time, strychnine was an ingredient in a variety of over-the-counter tonics and laxatives. Today, strychnine is no longer used in any pharmaceuticals. Instead, it is used primarily as a rodenticide and is sometimes found as an adulterant in illicit drugs such as cocaine or heroin.

I. **Mechanism of toxicity.** Strychnine competitively antagonizes glycine, an inhibitory neurotransmitter released by postsynaptic inhibitory neurons in the spinal cord. This causes increased neuronal excitability, which results in generalized seizurelike contraction of skeletal muscles. Simultaneous contraction of opposing flexor and extensor muscles causes severe muscle injury, with rhabdomyolysis, myoglobinuria, and, in some cases, acute renal failure.

II. **Toxic dose.** It is difficult to establish a toxic dose, although 16 mg was fatal in an adult in one case. Because life-threatening clinical manifestations can occur rapidly and because management decisions are based on clinical findings rather than on a history of ingested amount, any dose of strychnine should be considered life-threatening.

III. **Clinical presentation.** Symptoms and signs usually develop within 15–30 minutes of ingestion.

   A. Muscular stiffness and painful cramps precede generalized muscle contractions and opisthotonus. The face may be drawn into a forced smile ("sardonic grin" or "risus sardonicus"). Muscle contractions are intermittent and are easily triggered by emotional or physical stimuli. Repeated and prolonged muscle contractions often result in hyperthermia, rhabdomyolysis, myoglobinuria, and renal failure.

   B. The muscle contractions may resemble the tonic phase of a grand mal seizure, but strychnine does not cause true seizures and the patient is awake and painfully aware of the contractions.

   C. Death is usually due to respiratory arrest caused by intense contraction of the respiratory muscles. Death may also be secondary to hyperthermia or rhabdomyolysis and renal failure.

IV. **Diagnosis.** The diagnosis is based on a history of ingestion of rodenticide or recent intravenous drug abuse and the presence of seizurelike generalized muscle contractions, often accompanied by hyperthermia, lactic acidosis, and rhabdomyolysis (with myoglobinuria and elevated serum creatine phosphokinase [CPK]).

In the differential diagnosis, one should consider other causes of generalized muscle rigidity such as black widow spider bite (see p 272), neuroleptic malignant syndrome (p 20), or tetanus (see also Table I-15, p 23).

   A. **Specific levels.** Strychnine can be measured in the gastric fluid, urine, or blood. The toxic serum concentration is reported to be 1 mg/L, although in general, blood levels do not correlate with the severity of toxicity.

B. Other useful laboratory studies. CBC, electrolytes, BUN, creatinine, creatine phosphokinase (CPK), arterial blood gases, urine for myoglobin.

V. Treatment

A. Emergency and supportive measures

1. Maintain the airway and assist ventilation if necessary (see p 2).
2. Treat hyperthermia (p 19), metabolic acidosis (p 30), and rhabdomyolysis (p 24) if they occur.
3. Limit external stimuli such as noise, light, and touch.
4. **Treat muscle spasms** aggressively:
   a. Administer **diazepam** (see p 302), 0.1–0.2 mg/kg IV, or **midazolam** (p 323), 0.05–0.1 mg/kg IV, to patients with mild muscle contractions.
   b. In more severe cases, use **pancuronium** (p 326), 0.06–0.1 mg/kg IV, to produce complete neuromuscular paralysis. *Caution:* Neuromuscular paralysis will cause respiratory arrest; patients will need endotracheal intubation (p 4) and assisted ventilation (p 6).

B. Specific drugs and antidotes. There is no specific antidote.

C. Decontamination

1. Do *not* induce emesis because of the risk of inducing or aggravating muscle spasms. Perform gastric lavage (see p 43).
2. Administer activated charcoal and a cathartic (see p 45) orally or by gastric tube.

D. Enhanced elimination. Because strychnine is rapidly metabolized and symptoms abate within several hours, there is little to be gained from accelerated drug removal by dialysis or hemoperfusion. The use of repeat-dose activated charcoal has not been studied.

Reference

Boyd RE et al: Strychnine poisoning: Recovery from profound lactic acidosis, hyperthermia, and rhabdomyolysis. *Am J Med* 1983;**74**:507.

SULFUR DIOXIDE
Mary Twieg, MD

| ANTIDOTE | IPECAC | LAVAGE | CHARCOAL |

Sulfur dioxide is a colorless, nonflammable gas formed by the burning of materials that contain sulfur. It is a major air pollutant from automobiles, smelters, and plants burning soft coal or oils high in sulfur content. It is soluble in water to form caustic sulfurous acid, which may be oxidized to sulfuric acid; both are components of acid rain. Occupational exposures to sulfur dioxide occur in ore and metal refining, chemical manufacturing, and wood pulp treatment and in its use as a disinfectant, refrigerant, and dried food preservative.

I. **Mechanism of toxicity.** Sulfur dioxide is an irritant because it rapidly forms sulfurous acid on contact with moist mucous membranes. Most effects occur in the upper respiratory tract because 90% of inhaled sulfur dioxide is rapidly deposited there, but with very large exposures sufficient gas reaches the lower airways to cause chemical pneumonitis and pulmonary edema.

II. **Toxic dose.** The sharp odor or taste of sulfur dioxide is noticed at 3–5 ppm. Throat and conjunctival irritation begin at 8–12 ppm and are severe at 50 ppm. The OSHA workplace permissible exposure limit (PEL) is 2 ppm as an 8-hour time-weighted average, and the air level considered immediately dangerous to life or health (IDLH) is 100 ppm.

III. Clinical presentation

A. **Acute exposure** causes burning eyes, nose, and throat; lacrimation; and cough. Laryngospasm may occur. Wheezing may be seen in normal subjects as well as asthmatics (who are especially sensitive). With a very high-level exposure, chemical pneumonia and noncardiogenic pulmonary edema may occur.

B. **Chronic asthma and bronchitis** may be exacerbated.

C. **Sulfhemoglobinemia** has been reported owing to absorption of sulfur.

D. **Frostbite** injury to the skin may occur from exposure to liquid sulfur dioxide.

IV. Diagnosis. Diagnosis is based on a history of exposure and the presence of upper airway and mucous membrane irritation. Symptoms usually occur rapidly following exposure, and delay in onset of pulmonary edema is uncommon.

A. **Specific levels.** Blood levels are not available. Urinary sulfate excretion holds future promise as an indicator of exposure.

B. **Other useful laboratory studies.** Arterial blood gases, chest x-ray, pulmonary function tests.

V. Treatment

A. **Emergency and supportive measures**

1. Remain alert for progressive upper airway edema or obstruction, and be prepared to intubate the trachea and assist ventilation if necessary (see p 2).

2. Administer humidified oxygen, treat wheezing with bronchodilators (p 8), and observe for at least 4–6 hours for development of pulmonary edema (p 7).

B. **Specific drugs and antidotes.** There is no specific antidote.

C. **Decontamination**

1. **Inhalation.** Remove victim from exposure and give supplemental oxygen, if available.

2. **Skin and eyes.** Wash exposed skin and eyes with copious tepid water or saline. Treat frostbite injury as for thermal burns.

D. **Enhanced elimination.** There is no role for these procedures.

Reference

Smith LH, Martin DW, Naughton JL: Asthma, sulfur dioxide and the Clean Air Act. *West J Med* 1982;**136**:129.

THALLIUM
Mary Twieg, MD

ANTIDOTE IPECAC LAVAGE CHARCOAL

Thallium is a soft metal that quickly oxidizes upon exposure to air. It is a minor constituent in a variety of ores and is commonly found in flue dusts. The metal itself finds little use, but thallium salts are widely used in industry and chemical analysis; example of uses include the manufacture of optical lenses, photoelectric cells, and costume jewelry. It is no longer used in the USA as a depilatory or a rodenticide because of its high human toxicity.

I. **Mechanism of toxicity.** The mechanism of thallium toxicity is not entirely known. It appears to affect the mitochondria and a variety of enzyme systems, resulting in generalized cellular poisoning. Thallium metabolism has some similarities to that of potassium, and it may inhibit potassium flux across membranes. Some thallium salts are well absorbed across intact skin.

II. **Toxic dose.** The minimum lethal dose of thallium salts is probably 12–15 mg/kg, although toxicity varies widely depending on the compound, and there are reports of death after adult ingestion of as little as 200 mg. The more water-soluble salts (eg, thallous acetate, thallic chloride) are slightly more toxic than the less soluble forms (thallic oxide, thallous iodide).

III. **Clinical presentation.** Symptoms do not occur immediately but usually within 12–14 hours after ingestion.

   A. **Acute effects** include abdominal pain, vomiting, and diarrhea (with hemorrhage). Shock may be due to massive fluid or blood loss. Within 2–3 days, delirium, seizures and coma may occur.

   B. **Chronic effects.** Chronic neurologic toxicity includes muscle weakness and atrophy, chorea, and peripheral neuropathy. Hair loss and nail dystrophy (Mees' lines) may appear after 2–4 weeks.

IV. **Diagnosis.** Diagnosis may be made from a history of acute exposure and the presence of severe gastroenteritis, but in chronic exposures toxicity may not be suspected until alopecia or nail dystrophy occurs.

   A. **Specific levels.** Urinary thallium is normally less than 1.5 mcg/L. Concentrations greater than 100 mcg/L are considered toxic. Blood and hair thallium levels are not reliable measures of exposure.

   B. **Other useful laboratory studies.** CBC, electrolytes, glucose, BUN, creatinine, hepatic function tests.

V. **Treatment**

   A. **Emergency and supportive measures**

      1. Maintain the airway and assist ventilation if necessary (see p 2).

      2. Treat seizures (p 21) and coma (p 17) if they occur.

      3. Treat gastroenteritis with aggressive intravenous replacement of fluids (and blood, if needed). Use pressors only if shock does not respond to fluid therapy (p 14).

   B. **Specific drugs and antidotes.** There is currently no recommended specific treatment in the USA.

      1. **Prussian blue** (ferric ferrocyanide) is believed to enhance removal of thallium from tissues and increase renal and fecal elimination; however, it is not available for use in the USA, and charcoal is probably equally effective at enhancing fecal elimination.

      2. BAL and other chelators have been tried with varying success.

   C. **Decontamination**

      1. Induce emesis or perform gastric lavage (see p 42).

      2. Administer activated charcoal and a cathartic (see p 45) orally or by gastric tube.

   D. **Enhanced elimination. Repeat-dose activated charcoal** may enhance fecal elimination by binding thallium secreted into the gut lumen or via the biliary system, interrupting enterohepatic or enteroenteric recirculation. Forced diuresis, dialysis, and hemoperfusion are of no proved benefit.

Reference

Lehmann PA, Favari L: Acute thallium intoxication: Kinetic study of the relative efficacy of several antidotal treatments in rats. *Arch Toxicol* 1985;**57**:56.

THEOPHYLLINE
Kent R. Olson, MD

ANTIDOTE   IPECAC   LAVAGE   CHARCOAL

Theophylline is a methylxanthine widely used for the treatment of asthma. Intravenous infusions of aminophylline, the ethylenediamine salt of theophylline, are used to treat bronchospasm, congestive heart failure, and neonatal apnea. Theophylline is most commonly used orally in sustained-release preparations (eg, Theo-Dur, Slo-Phyllin, Theobid).

I. **Mechanism of toxicity.** The exact mechanism of toxicity is not known. Theophylline is known to inhibit phosphodiesterase at high levels, increasing intracellular cyclic adenosine monophosphate (cAMP). It also is known to release endogenous catecholamines at therapeutic concentrations and may itself stimulate beta-adrenergic receptors. It also is an antagonist of adenosine receptors.

The normal elimination half-life is 4–6 hours; this may be doubled by illnesses or interacting drugs that slow hepatic metabolism, such as congestive heart failure, influenza, erythromycin, or cimetidine, and may increase to as much as 20 hours after overdose.

II. **Toxic dose.** An acute single dose of 8–10 mg/kg will produce a therapeutic level of 15–20 mg/L. Acute overdose of more than 50 mg/kg is expected to result in a level above 100 mg/L and significant toxicity.

III. **Clinical presentation.** Two distinct syndromes of intoxication may occur, depending on whether the exposure is **acute** or **chronic.**

A. **Acute single overdose** is usually a result of a suicide attempt or accidental childhood ingestion but may also be caused by accidental or iatrogenic misuse (therapeutic overdose).

1. Usual manifestations include vomiting (sometimes with hematemesis), tremor, anxiety, and tachycardia. Metabolic effects include pronounced hypokalemia, hypophosphatemia, hyperglycemia, and metabolic acidosis.

2. With serum levels above 100 mg/L, hypotension, ventricular arrhythmias, and seizures are common; status epilepticus is frequently resistant to anticonvulsant drugs.

3. Seizures and other manifestations of severe toxicity may be delayed 12–16 hours or more after ingestion, in part because of delayed absorption of drug from sustained-release preparations.

B. **Chronic intoxication** occurs when excessive doses are administered repeatedly over 24 hours or longer, or when intercurrent illness or an interacting drug interferes with hepatic metabolism of theophylline. The usual victims are very young infants or elderly patients.

1. Vomiting may occur but is not as common as in acute overdose. Tachycardia is common, but hypotension is rare. Metabolic effects such as hypokalemia and hyperglycemia do **not** occur.

2. Seizures often occur with levels of 40–60 mg/L.

IV. **Diagnosis.** Diagnosis is based on a history of ingestion or the presence of tremor, tachycardia, and other manifestations in a patient known to be on theophylline. Hypokalemia strongly suggests acute overdose rather than chronic intoxication.

A. **Specific levels.** Serum theophylline levels are essential for diagnosis and determination of emergency treatment. After acute oral overdose, obtain repeated levels every 2–4 hours; single determinations are not sufficient, because continued absorption from sustained-release preparations may result in peak levels 12–16 hours or longer after ingestion.

1. Levels between 20–90 mg/L after acute overdose are not usually associated with severe symptoms such as seizures or ventricular arrhythmias.

2. However, with chronic intoxication severe toxicity commonly occurs with levels of 40–60 mg/L.

Note: Acute caffeine overdose (see p 100) will cause a similar clinical picture and will produce falsely elevated theophylline concentrations with most commercial immunoassays.

B. **Other useful laboratory studies.** CBC, electrolytes, glucose, BUN, creatinine, hepatic function tests, electrocardiographic monitoring.

V. **Treatment**

A. **Emergency and supportive measures**
1. Maintain the airway and assist ventilation if necessary (see p 2).
2. Treat seizures (p 21), arrhythmias (pp 12–13), and hypotension (p 14) if they occur.
3. Hypokalemia is caused by intracellular movement of potassium and does not reflect significant total body deficit; it usually resolves spontaneously without aggressive treatment.
4. Monitor vital signs, ECG, and serial theophylline levels for at least 12–16 hours after a significant oral overdose.

B. **Specific drugs and antidotes.** Hypotension, tachycardia, and ventricular arrhythmias are due primarily to excessive beta-adrenergic stimulation. Treat with **propranolol** (see p 338), 0.01–0.03 mg/kg IV, or low-dose **esmolol** (see p 311), 25–50 mcg/kg/min. Use beta blockers cautiously in patients with a prior history of asthma or wheezing.

C. **Decontamination**
1. Induce emesis or perform gastric lavage (see p 42). Ipecac may be more effective than gastric lavage for removal of sustained-release tablets.
2. Administer activated charcoal and a cathartic (p 45) orally or by gastric tube.
3. Undissolved sustained-release tablets may not be removed with even the largest (40F) gastric tube. For significant ingestions, consider the following special techniques:
   a. Administer repeat doses of activated charcoal and cathartic (p 49 and p 299).
   b. Administer whole gut lavage solution (p 46).

D. **Enhanced elimination.** Theophylline has a small volume of distribution (0.5 L/kg) and is efficiently removed by charcoal hemoperfusion or repeat-dose activated charcoal.
1. **Hemoperfusion** (see p 48) should be performed if the patient is in status epilepticus or if the serum theophylline concentration is greater than 100 mg/L. Hemodialysis is not as effective but may be used if hemoperfusion is not readily available.
2. **Repeat-dose activated charcoal** (see p 49 and p 299) is not as effective as hemoperfusion but may be used for patients with levels below 100 mg/L.

Reference

Olson KR et al: Theophylline overdose: Acute single ingestion versus chronic repeated overmedication. *Am J Emerg Med* 1985;3:386.

THYROID HORMONE
Belle L. Lee, PharmD

ANTIDOTE   IPECAC   LAVAGE   CHARCOAL

Thyroid hormone is available as synthetic triiodothyronine (T_3, liothyronine), synthetic tetraiodothyronine (T_4, levothyroxine), or natural desiccated animal thyroid (containing both T_3 and T_4; Table II–47). Despite concern over the potentially life-threatening manifestations of thyrotoxicosis, serious toxicity rarely occurs after acute thyroid hormone ingestion.

I. **Mechanism of toxicity.** Thyroid hormone stimulates the cardiovascular, gastrointestinal, and neurologic systems, presumably by potentiating adrenergic activity. The effects of T_3 overdose are manifested within the first 6 hours following an ingestion. In contrast, symptoms of T_4 overdose may

TABLE II-47. DOSAGE EQUIVALENTS OF THYROID HORMONE

Thyroid USP	65 mg (1 gr)
l-Thyroxine (T$_4$)	0.1 mg (100 mcg)
1-Triiodothyronine (T$_3$)	0.025 mg (25 mcg)

be delayed 2–5 days after ingestion while metabolic conversion to T$_3$ occurs.

II. Toxic dose

A. An acute ingestion of more than 3 mg of **levothyroxine** or 0.75 mg of **triiodothyronine** is considered toxic. An adult has survived an ingestion of 48 g of unspecified thyroid tablets; a 15-month-old child had moderate symptoms after ingesting 1.5 g of desiccated thyroid.

B. Euthyroid persons and children appear to have a high tolerance to the effects of an acute overdose. Patients with preexisting cardiac disease and those with chronic overmedication have a lower threshold of toxicity. Sudden deaths have been reported following chronic thyroid hormone abuse in healthy adults.

III. Clinical presentation.
The effects of an acute T$_4$ overdose may not be evident for several days because of delayed metabolism to more active T$_3$.

A. Mild to moderate intoxication may cause sinus tachycardia, elevated temperature, diarrhea, vomiting, headache, anxiety, agitation, psychosis, and confusion.

B. Severe toxicity. Supraventricular tachycardia, hyperthermia, and hypotension indicate serious toxicity. There is one case report of a seizure following acute overdose.

IV. Diagnosis.
Diagnosis is based on a history of ingestion and signs and symptoms of increased sympathetic activity.

A. Specific levels. Thyroid function tests (total serum T$_3$ and T$_4$ levels [T$_3$RIA and T$_4$RIA]) and **T$_3$ resin uptake** (T$_3$RU) should be obtained 2–6 hours after an ingestion and repeated over the following 5–7 days. However, there is relatively poor correlation between laboratory results and the clinical state in patients with thyroid overdose.

B. Other useful laboratory studies. CBC, electrolytes, glucose, BUN, creatinine, ECG and electrocardiographic monitoring.

V. Treatment

A. Emergency and supportive measures

1. Maintain the airway and assist ventilation if necessary (see p 2).
2. Treat seizures (p 21), hyperthermia (p 19), hypotension (p 14), and arrhythmias (pp 12–13) if they occur.
3. Repeated examinations over several days are necessary after T$_4$ or combined ingestions, because serious symptoms may be delayed.
4. Most patients will suffer no serious toxicity or will recover with simple supportive care.

B. Specific drugs and antidotes

1. Treat serious tachyarrhythmias with **propranolol** (see p 338), 0.01–0.1 mg/kg IV repeated every 2–5 minutes to desired effect, or **esmolol** (see p 311), 25–100 mcg/kg/min IV. Simple sinus tachycardia may be treated with oral propranolol, 0.1–0.5 mg/kg every 4–6 hours.
2. Peripheral metabolic conversion of T$_4$ to T$_3$ can be partially inhibited by **propylthiouracil**, 6–10 mg/kg/d (maximum 1 g) divided into 3 oral doses, for 5–7 days.

C. Decontamination

1. Induce emesis or perform gastric lavage (see p 42).
2. Administer activated charcoal and a cathartic (see p 45) orally or by gastric tube.

3. Gut emptying is not necessary following small ingestions if activated charcoal is given promptly.

D. Enhanced elimination. Diuresis and hemodialysis are not useful because thyroid hormones are extensively protein-bound. Charcoal hemoperfusion may be effective, but limited data are available. Exchange transfusion has been performed in children and adults, but data on its efficacy are limited.

Reference

Litovitz TL, White JD: Levothyroxine ingestions in children: An analysis of 78 cases. *Am J Emerg Med* 1985;**3**:297.

TOLUENE AND XYLENE
Mary Twieg, MD, and
Kent R. Olson, MD

ANTIDOTE   IPECAC   LAVAGE   CHARCOAL

Toluene (methylbenzene) and xylene (dimethylbenzene, xylol) are very common aromatic solvents widely used in glues, inks, dyes, lacquers, varnishes, paints, paint removers, pesticides, cleaners, and degreasers. Exposures often occur in occupational settings, but toluene is best known as a commonly abused agent that is intentionally inhaled to induce a "sniffer's high."

I. **Mechanism of toxicity.** Toluene and xylene cause generalized central nervous system depression, which may cause ataxia, coma, and respiratory arrest. Like other aromatic hydrocarbons, they may sensitize the myocardium to the arrhythmogenic effects of catecholamines. They are mild mucous membrane irritants affecting the eyes and respiratory and gastrointestinal tracts. Pulmonary aspiration can cause a hydrocarbon pneumonia (see p 165). Chronic abuse of toluene can cause renal tubular damage and myopathy.

II. **Toxic dose**
   A. **Ingestion.** There is little information concerning the toxic dose by ingestion, although as little as 15–20 mL of toluene is reported to cause serious toxicity. Whether this reflects the risk for aspiration chemical pneumonia rather than true systemic toxicity is not known.
   B. **Inhalation.** The OSHA workplace permissible exposure limit (PEL) is 100 ppm for toluene and 100 ppm for xylene. The air level considered immediately dangerous to life or health (IDLH) is 2000 ppm for toluene and 10,000 ppm for xylene.

III. **Clinical presentation.** Toxicity may be a result of ingestion, pulmonary aspiration, or inhalation.
   A. **Ingestion** of toluene or xylene may cause vomiting and diarrhea, and if pulmonary aspiration occurs, chemical pneumonia (see p 165) may result. Systemic absorption may result in central nervous system depression.
   B. **Inhalation** produces euphoria, dizziness, headache, nausea, and weakness. Exposure to high concentrations may rapidly cause coma, pulmonary edema, respiratory arrest, and death. Arrhythmias may occur owing to cardiac sensitization.
   C. **Chronic exposure** to toluene may cause myopathy, hypokalemia, renal tubular acidosis, and neuropathy.

IV. **Diagnosis.** Diagnosis is based on a history of exposure and typical manifestations of CNS effects such as euphoria or drunkenness. After acute ingestion, pulmonary aspiration is suggested if there is coughing, choking, tachypnea, or wheezing and is confirmed by chest x-ray.

A. Specific levels. In acute symptomatic exposures, toluene or xylene may be detectable in blood drawn with a gas-tight syringe but usually only for a few hours. The metabolites hippuric acid (toluene) and methyl-hippuric acid (xylene) are excreted in the urine and can be used to document exposure, but urine levels do not correlate with systemic effects.

B. Other useful laboratory studies. CBC, electrolytes, glucose, BUN, creatinine, liver function tests, creatine phosphokinase (CPK), urinalysis.

V. Treatment

A. Emergency and supportive measures

1. Maintain the airway and assist ventilation if necessary (see p 2). Administer supplemental oxygen, and monitor arterial blood gases and chest x-rays.

   a. If the patient is coughing or dyspneic, aspiration chemical pneumonia is likely. Treat as for hydrocarbon pneumonia (see p 165).

   b. If the patient remains asymptomatic after a 6-hour observation period, chemical pneumonia is unlikely and further observation or chest x-ray is not needed.

2. Treat coma (see p 17), arrhythmias (pp 12–13), and bronchospasm (p 8) if they occur. *Caution:* Avoid the use of epinephrine and other sympathomimetic amines because of the risk of aggravating arrhythmias. Tachyarrhythmias may be treated with propranolol (p 338), 1–2 mg IV, or esmolol (p 311), 25–100 mcg/kg/min IV.

B. Specific drugs and antidotes. There is no specific antidote.

C. Decontamination

1. **Inhalation.** Remove the victim from exposure and give supplemental oxygen, if available.

2. **Skin and eyes.** Remove contaminated clothes and wash exposed skin with soap and water. Irrigate exposed eyes with copious tepid water or saline.

3. **Ingestion**

   a. Do *not* induce emesis unless the ingestion is recent (5 minutes) and the emergency facility is more than 30 minutes away, because toluene and xylene are rapidly absorbed. Perform gastric lavage (see p 43) if the patient presents within 30–60 minutes or has ingested a large overdose (> 1–2 oz).

   b. Administer activated charcoal and a cathartic (see p 45) orally or by gastric tube. For small ingestions (< 30–60 mL), oral activated charcoal alone without gut emptying may be sufficient if the patient will ingest it voluntarily.

D. Enhanced elimination. There is no role for enhanced elimination.

Reference

Streicher HZ et al: Syndromes of toluene sniffing in adults. *Ann Intern Med* 1981;**94:**758.

TRICHLOROETHANE AND TRICHLOROETHYLENE
Gary Pasternak, MD

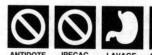

ANTIDOTE   IPECAC   LAVAGE   CHARCOAL

Trichloroethane and trichloroethylene are widely used solvents found as ingredients in many products including typewriter correction fluid ("white-out"), color film cleaners, insecticides, spot removers, fabric cleaning solutions, adhesives, and paint removers. They are used extensively in industry as degreasers. Trichloroethane is available in 2 isomeric forms, 1,1,2- and 1,1,1-, with the latter being the most common.

I. **Mechanism of toxicity**
   A. Trichloroethane and trichloroethylene act as respiratory and central nervous system depressants and skin and mucous membrane irritants. They have rapid anesthetic action, and both were used for this purpose medically until the advent of safer agents.
   B. Trichloroethane, trichloroethylene, and their metabolite trichloroethanol may sensitize the myocardium to the arrhythmogenic effects of catecholamines.
   C. Trichloroethylene or a metabolite may act to inhibit acetaldehyde dehydrogenase, blocking the metabolism of ethanol and causing "degreaser's flush."
   D. NIOSH considers 1,1,2-trichloroethane and trichloroethylene possible carcinogens.

II. **Toxic dose**
   A. **Trichloroethane.** The acute lethal oral dose to humans is reportedly between 0.5–5 mL/kg. The OSHA workplace permissible exposure limits (PEL) in air for the 1,1,1- and 1,1,2- isomers are 350 and 10 ppm, respectively, and the air levels considered immediately dangerous to life or health (IDLH) are 1000 and 500 ppm, respectively. Anesthetic levels are in the range of 10,000–26,000 ppm. The odor is dectable by a majority of people at 500 ppm, but olfactory fatigue commonly occurs.
   B. **Trichloroethylene.** The acute lethal oral dose is reported to be approximately 3–5 mL/kg. The OSHA permissible exposure limit (PEL) is 50 ppm, and the air level considered immediately dangerous to life or health (IDLH) is 1000 ppm.

III. **Clinical presentation.** Toxicity may be a result of inhalation, skin contact, or ingestion.
   A. **Inhalation or gastrointestinal absorption.** The symptoms of acute inhalation or ingestion overdose may include nausea, euphoria, ataxia, dizziness, agitation, and lethargy and, with significant intoxication, respiratory arrest, seizures, and coma. Hypotension and cardiac arrhythmias may occur. After severe overdose, renal and hepatic injury may be apparent 1–2 days after exposure.
   B. **Local effects** of exposure to liquid or vapors include irritation of the eyes, nose, and throat. Prolonged skin contact can cause defatting and dermatitis.
   C. **Ingestion.** Aspiration into the tracheobronchial tree may result in hydrocarbon pneumonia (see p 165).
   D. **Degreaser's flush.** Workers exposed to these vapors may have acute flushing and orthostatic hypotension if they ingest alcohol, owing to a disulfiramlike effect.

IV. **Diagnosis.** Diagnosis is based on the history of exposure and typical symptoms. Addictive inhalational abuse of typewriter correction fluid suggests trichloroethylene poisoning.
   A. **Specific levels**
      1. Although trichloroethane can be measured in expired air, blood, and urine, levels are not routinely rapidly available and are not needed for evaluation or treatment. Confirmation of overdose is possible by detecting the metabolite trichloroethanol in the blood or urine. Hospital laboratories are not generally sensitive to these amounts.
      2. Breath analysis is becoming more widely used for workplace exposure control, and serial measurements may allow for estimation of the amount absorbed. Expired air is collected in a plastic bag and analyzed by infrared or gas chromatography.
   B. **Other useful laboratory studies.** CBC, electrolytes, glucose, BUN, creat-

inine, liver function tests, arterial blood gases, chest x-ray, ECG and electrocardiographic monitoring.

V. Treatment

A. Emergency and supportive measures

1. Maintain the airway and assist ventilation if necessary (see p 2). Administer supplemental oxygen, and treat hydrocarbon aspiration pneumonitis (p 165) if it occurs.
2. Treat seizures (p 21), coma (p 17), and arrhythmias (pp 12–13) if they occur. *Caution:* Avoid the use of epinephrine or other sympathomimetic amines because of the risk of inducing or aggravating cardiac arrhythmias.
3. Monitor for a minimum of 4–6 hours after significant exposure.

B. Specific drugs and antidotes.
There is no specific antidote. Tachyarrhythmias caused by myocardial sensitization may be treated with **propranolol** (see p 338), 1–2 mg IV, or **esmolol** (see p 311), 25–100 mcg/kg/min IV.

C. Decontamination

1. **Inhalation.** Remove the victim from exposure and administer supplemental oxygen, if available.
2. **Skin and eyes.** Remove contaminated clothing and wash exposed skin with soap and water. Irrigate exposed eyes with copious tepid water or saline.
3. **Ingestion**
   a. Do **not** induce emesis because of the danger of rapid absorption and abrupt onset of seizures or coma. Perform gastric lavage (see p 43) if the patient presents within 30–60 minutes or has ingested a large overdose (> 1 mL/kg).
   b. Administer activated charcoal and a cathartic (see p 45) orally or by gastric tube. For small ingestions (< 30 mL), oral activated charcoal alone without gut emptying may be sufficient if the patient will ingest it voluntarily.

D. Enhanced elimination.
These procedures are not effective or necessary.

Reference

Gerace RV: Near-fatal intoxication by 1,1,1-trichloroethane. *Ann Emerg Med* 1981;**10**:533.

VACOR (PNU)
Neal L. Benowitz, MD

ANTIDOTE   IPECAC   LAVAGE   CHARCOAL

Vacor rat killer (2% N-3-pyridylmethyl-N'-*p*-nitrophenylurea; PNU) is a unique rodenticide that causes irreversible insulin-dependent diabetes and autonomic nervous system injury. It was removed from general sale in the USA in 1979 but is still available in some homes and for use by licensed exterminators. The product was sold in 39-g packets of cornmeallike material containing 2% PNU.

I. **Mechanism of toxicity.** PNU is believed to antagonize the actions of nicotinamide and, in a manner similar to that of alloxan and streptozocin, injure pancreatic beta cells. The mechanisms of autonomic neuropathy and central nervous system effects are unknown. Adrenergic neurons acting on blood vessels but not the heart are affected. As a result, orthostatic hypotension associated with an intact reflex tachycardia is the usual picture.

II. **Toxic dose.** Acute toxicity has usually occurred after ingestion of one 39-g packet of Vacor (approximately 8 g of PNU). The smallest dose reported to cause toxicity was 390 mg.

III. Clinical presentation. Initial symptoms include nausea and vomiting. Occasionally, confusion, stupor, and coma occur after several hours. After a delay of several hours to days, irreversible autonomic neuropathy and diabetes may occur.

- **A. Autonomic dysfunction.** Dizziness or syncope or both due to severe orthostatic hypotension occur with an onset from 6 hours to 2 days following ingestion. Orthostatic hypotension is usually accompanied by intact reflex tachycardia. Other manifestations of autonomic neuropathy include dysphagia and constipation.
- **B. Insulin-dependent diabetes mellitus,** with polyuria, polydipsia, hyperglycemia, and ketoacidosis, occurs after a few days. Hypoglycemia, resulting from insulin release, occasionally precedes hyperglycemia.

IV. Diagnosis. Sudden onset of orthostatic hypotension or diabetes mellitus should suggest the possibility of Vacor ingestion. A careful investigation should be performed to determine what rat-killing chemicals may be present in the home.

- **A. Specific levels.** PNU levels are not available.
- **B. Other useful laboratory studies.** CBC, electrolytes, glucose, BUN, creatinine, ECG.

V. Treatment

- **A. Emergency and supportive measures**
  1. Maintain the airway and assist ventilation if necessary (see p 2).
  2. Treat coma (see p 17) if it occurs.
  3. Orthostatic hypotension usually responds to supine positioning and intravenous fluids. Chronic therapy includes a high-salt diet and fludrocortisone (0.1–1 mg/d).
  4. Treat diabetes in the usual manner with fluids and insulin.
- **B. Specific drugs and antidotes.** Immediately administer **nicotinamide** (see p 327). Although its efficacy in humans is not proved, nicotinamide can prevent PNU-induced diabetes in rats.
- **C. Decontamination**
  1. Induce emesis or perform gastric lavage (see p 42).
  2. Administer activated charcoal and a cathartic (see p 45) orally or by gastric tube.
  3. Gut emptying is probably not necessary following small ingestions if activated charcoal is given promptly.
- **D. Enhanced elimination.** Forced diuresis, dialysis, and hemoperfusion are not effective. Repeat-dose charcoal treatment has not been studied.

Reference

LeWitt PA: The neurotoxicity of the rat poison Vacor: A clinical study of 12 cases. *N Engl J Med* 1980;**302**:73.

VASODILATORS
Olga F. Woo, PharmD

ANTIDOTE   IPECAC   LAVAGE   CHARCOAL

A variety of vasodilators and alpha-receptor blockers are used in clinical medicine. Hydralazine, diazoxide, and minoxidil are vasodilators commonly used for the treatment of hypertension. Alpha-adrenergic blocking agents (eg, phenoxybenzamine, phentolamine, tolazoline) have been used in clinical practice since the 1940s. The first selective α_1 inhibitor, prazosin, was introduced in the early 1970s; terazosin and trimazosin are newer α_1-selective agents. Serious acute overdoses of these agents seldom occur. Nitroprusside (see p 219) and nitrates (see p 216) are discussed elsewhere.

I. **Mechanism of toxicity.** All these drugs dilate peripheral arterioles to lower blood pressure. A reflex sympathetic response results in tachycardia and occasionally cardiac arrhythmias. Prazosin and other α_1 specific agents are associated with little or no reflex tachycardia.

II. **Toxic dose.** The minimum toxic or lethal doses of these drugs have not been established. An adult male developed priapism following an overdose of 150 mg of prazosin. No fatalities have been reported except with excessive intravenous doses of phentolamine and indoramin (available only in Europe).

III. **Clinical presentation.** Acute overdose may cause headache, nausea, dizziness, weakness, syncope, orthostatic hypotension, warm flushed skin, and palpitations. Lethargy and ataxia may occur in children. Severe hypotension may result in cerebral and myocardial ischemia and acute renal failure.

IV. **Diagnosis.** Diagnosis is based on a history of exposure and the presence of orthostatic hypotension, which may or may not be accompanied by reflex tachycardia.
   A. **Specific levels.** Blood levels of these drugs are not routinely available or clinically useful.
   B. **Other useful laboratory studies.** CBC, electrolytes, glucose, BUN, creatinine, ECG and electrocardiographic monitoring.

V. **Treatment**
   A. **Emergency and supportive measures**
      1. Maintain the airway and assist ventilation if necessary (see p 2).
      2. Hypotension (see p 14) usually responds to supine positioning and intravenous crystalloid fluids. Occasionally, pressor therapy is needed.
   B. **Specific drugs and antidotes.** There are no specific antidotes.
   C. **Decontamination**
      1. Induce emesis or perform gastric lavage (see p 42).
      2. Administer activated charcoal and a cathartic (see p 45) orally or by gastric tube.
      3. Gut emptying is probably not necessary following small ingestions if activated charcoal is given promptly.
   D. **Enhanced elimination.** There is no clinical experience with extracorporeal drug removal for these agents. Terazosin is long-acting and eliminated 60% in feces; thus, repeat-dose activated charcoal may enhance its elimination.

References

Isles C et al: Accidental overdosage of minoxidil in a child. (Letter.) *Lancet* 1981;**1**:97.
Robbins DN, Crawford ED, Lackner LH: Priapism secondary to prazosin overdose. *J Urol* 1983;**130**:975.

VITAMINS
James F. Buchanan, PharmD

ANTIDOTE   IPECAC   LAVAGE   CHARCOAL

Acute toxicity is unlikely following ingestion of vitamin products that do not contain iron (when iron is present, see p 177). Vitamins A and D may cause toxicity but usually only after chronic excessive use.

   I. **Mechanism of toxicity**
      A. **Vitamin A.** The mechanism by which excessive amounts of vitamin A produce increased intracranial pressure is not known.

    B. Vitamin D. Chronic ingestion of excessive amounts of vitamin D enhances calcium absorption and produces hypercalcemia.

    C. Niacin. Histamine release results in cutaneous flushing and pruritus.

    D. Pyridoxine. Chronic overdose may alter neuronal conduction, resulting in paresthesias and muscular incoordination.

II. Toxic dose

    A. Vitamin A. Acute ingestion of more than 12,000 IU/kg is considered toxic. Chronic ingestion of more than 25,000 IU/d for 2–3 weeks may produce toxicity.

    B. Vitamin D. Acute ingestion is highly unlikely to produce toxicity. Chronic ingestion in children of more than 5000 IU/d for several weeks (adults > 25,000 IU/d) may result in toxicity.

    C. Niacin. Acute ingestion of more than 100 mg may cause dermal flushing reaction.

    D. Pyridoxine. Chronic ingestion of 2–5 g/d for several months has resulted in neuropathy.

III. Clinical presentation. Most acute overdoses of multivitamins are associated with nausea, vomiting, and diarrhea.

    A. Chronic **vitamin A** toxicity is characterized by dry, peeling skin and signs of increased intracranial pressure (headache, altered mental status, blurred vision). Bulging fontanelles have been described in infants.

    B. Chronic excessive use of **vitamin D** is associated with hypercalcemia, producing weakness, altered mental status, gastrointestinal upset, renal tubular injury, and occasionally cardiac arrhythmias.

    C. Acute ingestion of **niacin** but not niacinamide (nicotinamide) may produce unpleasant cutaneous flushing and pruritus.

    D. Chronic excessive **pyridoxine** use may result in peripheral neuropathy.

    E. Large doses of **B vitamins** may intensify the yellow color of urine, and **riboflavin** may produce yellow perspiration.

IV. Diagnosis. The diagnosis of vitamin overdose is usually based on a history of ingestion. Cutaneous flushing and pruritus suggest a niacin reaction but may be caused by other histaminergic agents.

    A. Specific levels. Serum vitamin A (retinol) or carotenoid assays may assist in the diagnosis of hypervitaminosis A. Other serum vitamin concentration measurements are not useful in overdose.

    B. Other useful laboratory studies. CBC, electrolytes, glucose, BUN, creatinine, liver function tests.

V. Treatment

    A. Emergency and supportive measures

        1. Treat fluid losses caused by gastroenteritis with intravenous crystalloid solutions (see p 14).

        2. Treat vitamin A-induced elevated intracranial pressure and vitamin D-induced hypercalcemia if they occur.

        3. Antihistamines may alleviate niacin-induced histamine release.

    B. Specific drugs and antidotes. There are no specific antidotes.

    C. Decontamination. Usually, gut decontamination is unnecessary unless a toxic dose of vitamin A or D has been ingested, or if the product contains a toxic amount of iron (see p 177).

        1. Induce emesis or perform gastric lavage (p 42).

        2. Administer activated charcoal and a cathartic (p 45) orally or by gastric tube.

    D. Enhanced elimination. Forced diuresis, dialysis, and hemoperfusion are of no clinical benefit.

Reference

Feldman MH, Schlezinger NS: Benign intracranial hypertension associated with hypervitaminosis A. *Arch Neurol* 1970;**22**:1.

Section III. Therapeutic Drugs and Antidotes

ACETYLCYSTEINE (*N*-ACETYLCYSTEINE, NAC)

Kent R. Olson, MD

I. **Pharmacology.** Acetylcysteine (*N*-acetylcysteine, NAC) is a mucolytic agent that acts as a sulfhydryl group donor, substituting for the liver's usual sulfhydryl donor glutathione. It rapidly binds (detoxifies) the highly reactive intermediates of metabolism. It is very effective in preventing acetaminophen-induced liver injury but only when given early in the course of intoxication. It may be used empirically when the severity of ingestion is unknown or serum concentrations of the ingested drug are not immediately available.

II. **Indications**
   A. Acetaminophen overdose.
   B. Carbon tetrachloride poisoning (unproved).
   C. Chloroform poisoning (unproved).

III. **Contraindications.** Known hypersensitivity to the drug.

IV. **Adverse effects**
   A. Acetylcysteine typically causes nausea and vomiting when given **orally**. If the dose is vomited, it should be repeated. Use of a gastric tube and an antiemetic agent (eg, metoclopramide or prochlorperazine) may be necessary.
   B. Rapid **intravenous** administration can cause flushing and hypotension. One death was reported in a small child rapidly receiving a large dose intravenously.

V. **Drug interactions.** Activated charcoal adsorbs acetylcysteine and may interfere with its systemic absorption when both are given orally together; data suggest that peak acetylcysteine levels are decreased by about 30% and that the time to reach peak level may be delayed. However, the clinical importance of this incomplete adsorption is not established.

VI. **Dosage and method of administration**
   A. **Oral loading dose.** Give 140 mg/kg of the 10% (1.4 mL/kg) or 20% (0.7 mL/kg) solution diluted to 5% in juice or soda.
   B. **Maintenance oral dose.** Give 70 mg/kg every 4 hours for 17 doses (or until acetaminophen level is zero).
   C. If oral charcoal is administered, it may be removed by gastric suctioning before acetylcysteine is administered or the loading dose of acetylcysteine may be increased by approximately 30%.
   D. **Intravenous administration** is *not* approved in the USA. Contact a medical toxicologist or regional poison center (see p 51) for advice. In the UK, the dosing regimen is 150 mg/kg in 200 mL of 5% dextrose in water (D5W) over 15 minutes, followed by 50 mg/kg in 500 mL of D5W over 4 hours, and then 100 mg/kg in 1000 mL of D5W over 16 hours.

VII. **Formulations**
   A. The usual formulation is as a 10% (100 mg/mL) or 20% (200 mg/mL) solution, supplied as an inhaled mucolytic agent (Mucomyst). This form is available through most hospital pharmacies or respiratory therapy departments. This preparation is *not* approved for parenteral use. In rare circumstances when intravenous administration of this preparation is required, a micropore filter should be used.
   B. In the USA, the investigational intravenous formulation is available only at medical centers participating in an approved study.

ANTIVENIN, CROTALIDAE (RATTLESNAKE)

Howard E. McKinney, PharmD

I. **Pharmacology.** To produce the antivenin, horses are hyperimmunized with the pooled venoms of *Crotalus adamanteus* (eastern diamondback rattlesnake), *Crotalus atrox* (western diamondback), *Crotalus durissus terrificus* (tropical rattlesnake, cascabel), and *Bothrops atrox* (fer-de-lance). The lyophilized protein product from pooled equine sera is a combination of several antibodies against venom constituents and also contains residual serum components. After intravenous administration, the antivenin is distributed widely throughout the body where it binds to venom.

II. **Indications.** Antivenin is used for treatment of significant envenomation by Crotalidae species.

III. **Contraindications.** Known hypersensitivity to the antivenin or to horse serum is a relative contraindication; antivenin may still be indicated for severe envenomation despite allergic history.

IV. **Adverse effects**
- A. Immediate hypersensitivity reactions (including life-threatening anaphylaxis) may occur, even in patients with no history of horse serum sensitivity and negative skin test results.
- B. Mild flushing and wheezing often occur within the first 30 minutes of intravenous administration and may be terminated by slowing the rate of infusion.
- C. Delayed hypersensitivity (serum sickness) occurs in over 75% of patients receiving more than 4 vials of antivenin and in virtually all patients who receive more than 12 vials. The onset is 5–14 days.

V. **Drug interactions.** There are no known drug interactions.

VI. **Dosage and method of administration.** The initial dose is based on severity of symptoms, not on body weight (Table III-1). Children may require doses as large as or larger than those for adults. The end point of antivenin therapy is the reversal of systemic manifestations (eg, shock, coagulopathy, paresthesias) and the halting of progressive edema and pain. Antivenin may be effective up to 3 days or more following envenomation. If envenomation by the Mojave rattlesnake *(Crotalus scutulatus scutulatus)* is suspected, especially if there is an increased serum CPK (creatinine phosphokinase) level, administer 10 vials of antivenin even if there is minimal swelling or local pain.
- A. Treat all patients in an intensive care setting.
- B. Before skin test or antivenin administration, insert at least one and preferably 2 secure intravenous lines.
- C. Perform skin test for horse serum sensitivity (included in antivenin kit) according to package instructions. Do **not** perform the skin test unless signs of envenomation are present and imminent antivenin therapy is anticipated. If the skin test is positive, reconsider the need for antivenin as opposed to supportive care, but do not abandon antivenin therapy if it is needed. Even if the skin test is negative, anaphylaxis may still occur.

TABLE III-1. INITIAL DOSE OF CROTALIDAE ANTIVENIN

Severity of Envenomation	Initial Dose (vials)
None or minimal	None
Mild (local pain and swelling)	5
Moderate (proximal progression of swelling, ecchymosis, mild systemic symptoms)	10
Severe (hypotension, rapidly progressive swelling and ecchymosis, coagulopathy)	15

    D. If antivenin is used in a patient with a positive skin test, pretreat with intravenous diphenhydramine hydrochloride (see p 305), 1 mg/kg slowly, and have ready at the bedside a preloaded syringe containing epinephrine (1:10,000 for intravenous use) in case of anaphylaxis (p 309). Dilute the antivenin 1:10 to 1:1000 before administration.

    E. Reconstitute the lyophilized product with the 10 mL of diluent provided and gently swirl for 10–30 minutes to solubilize the material. Avoid shaking, which destroys the immunoglobulins (indicated by foam formation). Further dilution with 50–200 mL of saline may facilitate solubilization.

    F. Administer the diluted antivenin slowly (10–15 min/vial) by the intravenous route only.

VII. Formulation. Antivenin (Crotalidae) Polyvalent (equine). Supplies can be located by a regional poison center (see Table I–41).

ANTIVENIN, LATRODECTUS MACTANS (BLACK WIDOW SPIDER)

Howard E. McKinney, PharmD

  I. Pharmacology. To produce the antivenin, horses are hyperimmunized with *Latrodectus mactans* (black widow spider) venom. The lyophilized protein product from pooled equine sera contains antibody specific to certain venom fractions, as well as residual serum proteins such as albumin and globulins. After intravenous administration, the antivenin distributes widely throughout the body where it binds to venom.

  II. Indications

    A. Severe hypertension is not alleviated by analgesics or sedation.

    B. Black widow envenomation in a pregnant woman may cause abdominal muscle spasm severe enough to threaten spontaneous abortion or early onset of labor.

  III. Contraindications. Known hypersensitivity to horse serum is a contraindication.

  IV. Adverse effects

    A. Immediate hypersensitivity may occur, including life-threatening anaphylaxis.

    B. Delayed-onset serum sickness may occur after 10–14 days.

  V. Drug interactions. There are no known drug interactions.

  VI. Dosage and method of administration. Generally, one vial of antivenin is sufficient to treat black widow envenomation in adults or children.

    A. Treat all patients in an intensive care setting.

    B. Before skin test or antivenin administration, insert at least one and preferably 2 secure intravenous lines.

    C. Perform skin test for horse serum sensitivity (included in antivenin kit) according to the package instructions. If the skin test is positive, reconsider need for antivenin versus supportive care. Even if the skin test is negative, anaphylaxis may still occur.

    D. If antivenin is used in a patient with horse serum sensitivity, pretreat with intravenous diphenhydramine hydrochloride (see p 305), 1 mg/kg slowly, and have ready at the bedside a preloaded syringe containing epinephrine (1:10,000, for intravenous use) in case of anaphylaxis (p 309). Dilute the antivenin (1:10 to 1:1000) and give very slowly.

    E. Reconstitute the lyophilized product to 2.5 mL with the supplied diluent, using gentle swirling for 15–30 minutes to avoid shaking and destroying the immunoglobulins (indicated by the formation of foam).

    F. Dilute this solution to a total volume of 10–50 mL with normal saline.

    G. Administer the diluted antivenin slowly over 15–30 minutes.

  VII. Formulation. Lyophilized Antivenin *(Latrodectus mactans)*, 6000 units.

ANTIVENIN, MICRURUS FULVIUS (CORAL SNAKE)

Howard E. McKinney, PharmD

I. **Pharmacology.** To produce the antivenin, horses are hyperimmunized with venom from *Micrurus fulvius,* the eastern coral snake. The lyophilized protein preparation from pooled equine sera contains antibody to venom fractions as well as residual serum proteins. Administered intravenously, the antibody distributes widely throughout the body where it binds the target venom.

II. **Indications**
   A. Envenomation by the eastern coral snake *(M fulvius)* or the Texas coral snake *(Micrurus fulvius tenere).*
   B. **Not** effective for envenomation by the Arizona or Sonora coral snake *(Micrurus euryxanthus).*

III. **Contraindications.** Known hypersensitivity to the antivenin or to horse serum is a relative contraindication; if a patient with significant envenomation needs the antivenin, it should be given with caution.

IV. **Adverse effects**
   A. Immediate hypersensitivity, including life-threatening anaphylaxis, may occur even after a negative skin test for horse serum sensitivity.
   B. Delayed hypersensitivity (serum sickness) may occur 1–3 weeks after antivenin administration.

V. **Drug interactions.** There are no known drug interactions.

VI. **Dosage and method of administration.** Generally, the recommended dose is 4–10 vials, depending on the severity of symptoms and signs and not on body weight. Children may require doses as large as or even larger than those for adults.
   A. Treat all patients in an intensive care unit setting.
   B. Before skin test or antivenin administration, insert at least one and preferably 2 secure intravenous lines.
   C. Perform skin test for horse serum sensitivity (included in antivenin kit) according to the package instructions. Do **not** perform the skin test unless signs of envenomation are present and imminent antivenin therapy is anticipated. If the skin test is positive, reconsider need for antivenin versus supportive care, but do not abandon antivenin therapy if it is needed. Even if the skin test is negative, anaphylaxis may still occur.
   D. If antivenin is used in a patient with a positive skin test, pretreat with intravenous diphenhydramine hydrochloride (see p 305), 1 mg/kg slowly, and have ready at the bedside a preloaded syringe containing epinephrine (1:10,000, for intravenous use) in case of anaphylaxis (p 309). Dilute the antivenin (1:10 to 1:1000) and administer very slowly.
   E. Reconstitute the lyophilized material with the 10 mL of the diluent supplied, gently swirling for 10–30 minutes. Avoid shaking the preparation because this may destroy the immunoglobulins (indicated by the formation of foam). Dilution with 50–200 mL of saline may aid solubilization.
   F. Administer the antivenin intravenously over 15–30 minutes.

VII. **Formulation.** Antivenin *(Micrurus fulvius).*

APOMORPHINE

James F. Buchanan, PharmD

I. **Pharmacology.** Apomorphine is an alkaloid salt derived from morphine that has minimal analgesic properties but marked emetic efficacy. Vomiting is produced by direct stimulation of the medullary chemoreceptor trigger zone. Following subcutaneous administration, emesis occurs within an average time period of 5 minutes; oral administration is **not** recommended because of erratic absorption.

II. **Indications.** Apomorphine has been used for induction of emesis in the acute management of oral poisoning. Currently, apomorphine is rarely used in childhood or adult poisoning because of its potential for respiratory depression and its inconvenient formulation (see **VI**, below). It remains popular in veterinary practice.

III. **Contraindications**
   A. Unconscious patients or those with poor or absent gag reflex.
   B. Ingestion of hydrocarbons, caustics, or convulsant agents.
   C. Geriatric patients or those with significant cardiac disease.
   D. Known hypersensitivity to opiates.

IV. **Adverse effects**
   A. Respiratory depression and hypotension are the most common adverse effects.
   B. Excessive vomiting.
   C. Bradycardia.
   D. Central nervous system depression or stimulation, seizures. (**Note:** Protracted vomiting and central nervous system and respiratory depression may be reversed by naloxone, but this reversal is inconsistent.)

V. **Drug interactions.** Apomorphine may precipitate seizures in patients who have been poisoned by convulsant drugs or toxins.

VI. **Dosage and method of administration**
   A. **Adult.** Give 6 mg (range 2–10 mg) as a single subcutaneous dose. A 6-mg tablet is dissolved in 1–2 mL of sodium chloride solution or sterile water and filtered through a $0.22 - \mu m$ filter prior to administration.
   B. **Child.** Give 0.07–0.1 mg/kg or 3 mg/m^2 as a single subcutaneous dose. **Note:** Additional doses are not recommended even if emesis does not occur.

VII. **Formulation.** Parenteral: Apomorphine hydrochloride; soluble tablets, 6 mg.

ATROPINE

James F. Buchanan, PharmD

I. **Pharmacology.** Atropine is a parasympatholytic agent that blocks the action of acetylcholine at muscarinic receptors. Desired therapeutic effects for treating poisoning include decreased secretions from salivary and other glands, decreased bronchorrhea and wheezing, decreased intestinal peristalsis, increased heart rate, and enhanced atrioventricular conduction.

II. **Indications**
   A. Correction of bronchorrhea and excessive salivation associated with organophosphate and carbamate insecticide intoxication.
   B. Acceleration of the rate of sinus node firing and atrioventricular nodal conduction velocity in the presence of drug-induced atrioventricular conduction impairment (eg, digitalis, beta blockers, organophosphate or carbamate insecticides).

III. **Contraindications**
   A. Angle-closure glaucoma in which pupillary dilation may increase intraocular pressure.
   B. Patients with hypertension, tachyarrhythmias, congestive heart failure, and coronary artery disease who might not tolerate a rapid heart rate.
   C. Partial or complete obstructive uropathy.
   D. Myasthenia gravis.

IV. **Adverse effects**
   A. Some adverse effects include dry mouth, blurred vision, cycloplegia, mydriasis, urinary retention, tachycardia, aggravation of angina, and constipation.
   B. Doses less than 0.5 mg (in adults) and those administered by very slow intravenous push may result in paradoxic slowing of heart rate.

V. **Drug interactions**
   A. Atropinization may occur more rapidly if atropine and pralidoxime are given concurrently to patients with organophosphate or carbamate insecticide poisoning.
   B. Atropine has an additive effect with other antimuscarinic and antihistaminic compounds.
   C. Slowing of gastrointestinal motility may delay absorption of orally ingested materials.
VI. **Dosage and method of administration**
   A. **Organophosphate or carbamate insecticide poisoning.** For adults, give 1–5 mg IV; for a child, give 0.05 mg/kg IV; repeat every 5–10 minutes until satisfactory atropinization is achieved. The goal of therapy is drying of bronchial secretions and reversal of wheezing and significant bradycardia. In severe poisonings, several grams of atropine may be required.
   B. **Drug-induced bradycardia.** For adults, give 0.5–1 mg IV; for a child, give 0.01–0.05 mg/kg up to a maximum dose of 0.5 mg IV. Repeat as needed. Note that 3 mg is a fully vagolytic dose in adults. If response is not achieved by 3 mg, the patient is unlikely to benefit from further treatment unless bradycardia is caused by excessive cholinergic input (eg, organophosphate overdose).
VII. **Formulation.** Parenteral: Atropine sulfate injection, 0.05, 0.1, 0.3, 0.4, 0.5, 0.6, 0.8, 1, and 1.2 mg/mL solutions. Use preservative-free formulations when huge doses are required.

BAL (DIMERCAPROL)

James F. Buchanan, PharmD

I. **Pharmacology.** BAL (British antilewisite) is a dithiol chelating agent used in the treatment of poisoning by the heavy metals arsenic, mercury, lead, and gold. It is of no value for the treatment of poisoning by selenium, iron, or cadmium; in fact, it is contraindicated in these poisonings because the BAL-metal (mercaptide) complex may be more toxic than the metal alone. Adequate doses of BAL must be given to ensure an excess of free BAL. An insufficient concentration of BAL may allow dissociation of the BAL-metal complex. This chelate dissociates more rapidly in an acid urine; adequate renal function must exist to allow elimination of the mercaptide complex.
II. **Indications**
   A. Arsenic poisoning (except arsine, for which BAL is ineffective).
   B. Mercury poisoning (except monoalkyl mercury). BAL is most effective in preventing renal damage if administered within 2 hours after ingestion; it is not effective in reversing neurologic damage caused by chronic mercury poisoning.
   C. Lead poisoning (except alkyl lead compounds). EDTA and penicillamine are the preferred chelating agents, but BAL is indicated as adjunctive therapy in patients with acute lead encephalopathy (see EDTA [p 308], penicillamine [p 332], and DMSA [p 306]).
   D. Gold poisoning.
   E. Poisoning due to antimony, bismuth, chromium, copper, nickel, tungsten, or zinc.
III. **Contraindications**
   A. Heavy metal poisoning due to iron, cadmium, selenium, or uranium (BAL-metal complex is more toxic than the metal alone).
   B. Poisoning due to thallium, tellurium, or vanadium (BAL is ineffective).
   C. Glucose-6-phosphate dehydrogenase deficiency. BAL may cause hemolysis; use only in life-threatening situations.
   D. Hepatic impairment (except arsenic-induced jaundice).
   E. Renal impairment. Avoid BAL or use only with extreme caution.
   F. Pregnancy. Safety of BAL is not established. BAL is embryotoxic in mice. Use in pregnancy only for life-threatening acute intoxication.

IV. **Adverse effects**
  A. Local pain at injection site, sterile abscess formation.
  B. Dose-related hypertension, with or without tachycardia. Onset 15–30 minutes, duration 2 hours. Use with caution in hypertensive patients.
  C. Nephrotoxicity. Urine should be kept alkaline to protect renal function and to prevent dissociation of metal-BAL complex.
  D. Nausea, vomiting, headache, lacrimation, rhinorrhea, salivation, urticaria, myalgias, paresthesias, dysuria, fever (particularly in children), central nervous system depression, seizures.

V. **Drug interactions**
  A. BAL forms toxic complexes with iron, cadmium, selenium, and uranium. Avoid concurrent iron replacement therapy.
  B. BAL may abruptly terminate gold therapy-induced remission of rheumatoid arthritis.
  C. BAL interferes with iodine accumulation by the thyroid.

VI. **Dosage and method of administration (adults and children)**
  A. **Arsenic, mercury, and gold poisoning.** Give BAL, 3 mg/kg deep IM every 4 hours for 2 days, then every 12 hours for 7–10 days or until recovery.
  B. **Lead** (in conjunction with calcium EDTA therapy [see p 308])
    1. Symptomatic acute encephalopathy or blood lead greater than 100 µg/dL: give BAL, 4–5 mg/kg deep IM every 4 hours for 5 days.
    2. Symptomatic without encephalopathy or blood lead greater than 70 µg/dL: give BAL, 3 mg/kg deep IM every 4 hours for 5 days. May discontinue BAL if blood lead is less than 50 µg/dL after 3 days.

VII. **Formulation.** Parenteral (for deep IM injection only): BAL in oil, 100 mg/mL.

BENZTROPINE

James F. Buchanan, PharmD

I. **Pharmacology.** Benztropine is an antimuscarinic agent with pharmacologic activity similar to that of atropine. The drug also exhibits antihistaminic properties. Benztropine is used for the treatment of parkinsonism and for the control of extrapyramidal side effects associated with neuroleptic use.

II. **Indications.** Benztropine is an alternative in adults to diphenhydramine (the drug of choice for children) for the treatment of acute dystonic reactions associated with neuroleptic use.

III. **Contraindications**
  A. Angle-closure glaucoma.
  B. Obstructive uropathy (prostatic hypertrophy).
  C. Myasthenia gravis.

IV. **Adverse effects.** Adverse effects include sedation, blurred vision, tachycardia, urinary hesitancy or retention, and dry mouth. Adverse effects are minimal following single doses.

V. **Drug interactions**
  A. Benztropine has additive effects with other drugs exhibiting antimuscarinic properties (eg, antihistamines, phenothiazines, cyclic antidepressants, disopyramide).
  B. Slowing of gastrointestinal motility may delay or inhibit absorption of certain drugs.

VI. **Dosage and method of administration**
  A. **Parenteral.** Give 1–2 mg IV (children > 3 years old, 0.02 mg/kg, 1 mg maximum).
  B. **Oral.** Give 1–2 mg PO every 12 hours (children > 3 years old, 0.02 mg/kg, 1 mg maximum) to prevent recurrence of symptoms.

VII. **Formulations**
  A. **Parenteral.** Benztropine mesylate (Cogentin), 1 mg/mL.
  B. **Oral.** Benztropine mesylate (Cogentin), 0.5-, 1-, 2-mg tablets.

BICARBONATE, SODIUM

James F. Buchanan, PharmD

I. **Pharmacology**
A. Sodium bicarbonate is a buffering agent that reacts with hydrogen ions to correct acidemia and produce alkalemia. In addition, urinary alkalinization from renally excreted bicarbonate ion enhances the renal elimination of certain acidic drugs (eg, salicylate, phenobarbital) and helps prevent renal tubular myoglobin deposition in patients with rhabdomyolysis.
B. The sodium ion load and alkalemia produced by hypertonic sodium bicarbonate reverse sodium channel-dependent membrane-depressant effects of several drugs (eg, the cyclic antidepressants, type Ia and type Ic antiarrhythmic agents).
C. Sodium bicarbonate given orally or by gastric lavage forms an insoluble salt with iron and may prevent absorption of ingested iron tablets.

II. **Indications**
A. Severe metabolic acidosis resulting from intoxication by methanol, ethylene glycol, or salicylates or from excessive lactic acid production (eg, due to status epilepticus or shock).
B. To produce urinary alkalinization, to enhance elimination of salicylate or phenobarbital, or to prevent renal deposition of myoglobin after severe rhabdomyolysis.
C. Cardiotoxicity due to the cyclic antidepressants and type Ia or type Ic antiarrhythmic drugs.
D. In lavage fluid for excessive iron ingestion.

III. **Contraindications**
A. Significant metabolic or respiratory alkalemia or hypernatremia.
B. Pulmonary edema.

IV. **Adverse effects**
A. Excessive alkalemia: impaired oxygen release from hemoglobin, hypocalcemic tetany, paradoxic intracellular acidosis (from elevated P_{CO2} concentrations), hypokalemia.
B. Hypernatremia, hyperosmolality.
C. Aggravation of congestive heart failure and pulmonary edema.

V. **Drug interactions.** Do not mix with other parenteral drugs because of the possibility of drug inactivation or precipitation.

VI. **Dosage and method of administration (adults and children)**
A. **Metabolic acidemia.** Give 0.5–1 meq/kg IV bolus; repeat as needed to correct serum pH to at least 7.2. For salicylates, methanol, and ethylene glycol, bring the pH to 7.4–7.5.
B. **Urinary alkalinization.** Give 100 meq in 1 L of 5% dextrose at 2–3 mL/kg/h. Check urine pH frequently and adjust flow rate to maintain urine pH level at 6–7.
Note: Hypokalemia and fluid depletion prevent effective urinary alkalinization. Add 30 meq of potassium to each liter of IV fluids, unless renal failure is present.
C. **Cyclic antidepressant or related cardiotoxic drug intoxication.** Give 0.5–1 meq/kg IV bolus; repeat as needed to improve cardiotoxic manifestations and to maintain serum pH at 7.45–7.5.
D. **Gastric iron complexation.** Make a 1–2% solution by diluting sodium bicarbonate with normal saline, and use 4–5 mL/kg as a gastric lavage solution.

VII. **Formulations.** Several products are available, ranging from 4.2% (0.5 meq/mL) to 8.4% (1 meq/mL) in volumes of 10–500 mL. The most commonly used formulation available in most emergency "crash carts" is 8.4% ("hypertonic") sodium bicarbonate, 1 meq/mL, in 50-mL ampules or syringes.

BOTULIN ANTITOXIN

James F. Buchanan, PharmD

I. **Pharmacology.** Botulin antitoxin contains concentrated equine-derived antibodies directed against the toxins produced by the various strains of *Clostridium botulinum* (A, B, and E). The trivalent form (A, B, E) provides the greatest degree of coverage and is preferred over the older bivalent (A, B) type. The antibodies bind and inactivate freely circulating botulin toxins but do **not** remove toxin that is already bound to nerve terminals. Because antitoxin will not reverse established paralysis once it occurs, it must be administered before paralysis sets in. Treatment within 24 hours of the onset of symptoms may shorten the course of intoxication and may prevent progression to total paralysis.

II. **Indications.** Botulin antitoxin is used to treat clinical botulism to prevent progression of neurologic manifestations. It is generally not recommended for treatment of infant botulism.

III. **Contraindications.** There are no absolute contraindications. Known hypersensitivity to botulin antitoxin or horse serum requires extreme caution if this product is given.

IV. **Adverse effects**
   A. Immediate hypersensitivity reactions (anaphylaxis) due to the equine source of antibodies.
   B. Delayed Arthus' reaction (serum sickness) 1–2 weeks after antitoxin administration.

V. **Drug interactions.** There are no known drug interactions.

VI. **Dosage and method of administration**
   A. For established clinical botulism, give 1–2 vials IV every 4 hours for 4–5 doses. Duration of therapy depends on clinical response. Intramuscular administration is not recommended.
   B. Perform skin testing prior to administration (see package insert). Should the patient have known sensitivity to horse serum or demonstrate a positive skin test, provide desensitization as indicated in the package insert. In addition, pretreat the patient with diphenhydramine hydrochloride (see p 305), 1–2 mg/kg IV, and have epinephrine (see p 308) ready in case anaphylaxis occurs.

VII. **Formulation.** Parenteral: Trivalent botulin antitoxin (7500 IU type A, 5500 IU type B, 8500 IU type E); available from the Centers for Disease Control, 8 am to 4:30 pm (eastern standard time). Telephone (404) 639-3670; nights, weekends, and holidays, (404) 639-2888 (emergencies only).

BRETYLIUM

James F. Buchanan, PharmD

I. **Pharmacology.** Bretylium is a quaternary ammonium compound that is an effective antifibrillatory drug and also suppresses ventricular ectopic activity. It increases the threshold for ventricular fibrillation and reduces the disparity in action potential duration between normal and ischemic tissue, which is believed to abolish boundary currents responsible for reentrant arrhythmias. Its pharmacologic actions are complex. Initially, norepinephrine is released from sympathetic neurons; this is followed by a block of further norepinephrine release. In addition, norepinephrine uptake is inhibited at adrenergic neurons. The result is a transient increase in heart rate, blood pressure, and cardiac output that may last from a few minutes to 1 hour. Subsequent adrenergic blockade produces vasodilation, which may result in hypotension.

II. **Indications**
   A. Prophylaxis and treatment of ventricular fibrillation. May be particularly effective in hypothermic patients.

    B. Ventricular tachycardia resistant to other antiarrhythmic agents.

III. Contraindications

    A. Use with extreme caution in patients with digitalis intoxication, because the initial release of catecholamines may aggravate arrhythmias.

    B. Use with extreme caution in patients with arrhythmias due to intoxication with cyclic antidepressants or group Ia or group Ic antiarrhythmic agents because of additive cardiac depression.

    C. Use with extreme caution in patients with severe pulmonary hypertension or aortic stenosis.

IV. Adverse effects

    A. Hypotension (both supine and orthostatic).

    B. Nausea and vomiting from rapid intravenous administration.

    C. Initial catecholamine release may cause transient hypertension and worsening of arrhythmias.

V. Drug interactions

    A. The pressor effect of sympathomimetic amines may be enhanced.

    B. Cardiac-depressant effects may be additive with other antiarrhythmic drugs, particularly type Ia and type Ic drugs.

VI. Dosage and method of administration

    A. For ventricular fibrillation, give 5 mg/kg IV over 1 minute. If not effective, may repeat with 10 mg/kg (and defibrillation as necessary).

    B. For ventricular tachycardia, give adults and children older than 12 years 5–10 mg/kg IV over 8–10 minutes or IM, repeated as necessary at 15-minute intervals to a maximum of 30 mg/kg; repeat every 6 hours as needed.

    C. The continuous infusion rate following the loading dose is 1–2 mg/min (children > 12 years old, 20–30 μg/kg/min).

VII. Formulation. Parenteral: Bretylium tosylate (Bretylol, others), 50 mg/mL.

CALCIUM

James F. Buchanan, PharmD, and Kent R. Olson, MD

  I. Pharmacology

    A. Calcium is a cation necessary for the normal functioning of a variety of enzymes and organ systems, including muscle and nervous tissue. Hypocalcemia, or a blockade of calcium's effects, causes muscle cramps, tetany, and ventricular fibrillation. Antagonism of calcium-dependent channels results in hypotension, bradycardia, and atrioventricular block.

    B. Calcium ion rapidly binds to fluoride ion, abolishing its toxic effects.

    C. The neuromuscular effects of black widow spider venom can be antagonized to some degree by the administration of calcium, through a mechanism not fully understood.

    D. Calcium can reverse the negative inotropic effects of calcium antagonists; however, depressed automaticity and atrioventricular nodal conduction velocity and vasodilation may not respond to calcium administration.

    E. Calcium is directly antagonistic to the cardiotoxic effects of hyperkalemia.

  II. Indications

    A. Symptomatic hypocalcemia due to intoxication by fluoride, oxalate, phosphate, or the intravenous anticoagulant citrate.

    B. Reversal of corrosive effects of topical hydrofluoric acid exposure.

    C. Black widow spider envenomation with muscle cramping or rigidity.

    D. Calcium antagonist overdose with hypotension.

    E. Severe hyperkalemia with cardiotoxic manifestations.

  III. Contraindications

A. Hypercalcemia.

B. Digitalis intoxication (may aggravate digitalis-induced ventricular tachyarrhythmias).

IV. Adverse effects

A. Tissue irritation, particularly with calcium chloride; extravasation may cause local cellulitis or necrosis.

B. Hypercalcemia, especially in patients with diminished renal function.

C. Hypotension, bradycardia, syncope, and cardiac arrhythmias caused by rapid intravenous administration.

D. Constipation caused by orally administered calcium salts.

V. Drug interactions

A. Inotropic and arrhythmogenic effects of digitalis are potentiated by calcium.

B. A precipitate will form with solutions containing soluble salts of carbonates, phosphates, or sulfates and with various antibiotics.

VI. Dosage and method of administration

A. Oral fluoride or oxalate ingestion. Administer calcium-containing antacid (calcium carbonate) 2–3 g orally to complex fluoride or oxalate ion.

B. Symptomatic hypocalcemia, hyperkalemia, black widow spider envenomation, or calcium antagonist poisoning. Give 10% calcium gluconate, 10–20 mL (children, 0.2–0.3 mL/kg), or 10% calcium chloride, 5–10 mL (children, 0.1–0.2 mL/kg), slowly IV. Repeat as needed. *Note:* Calcium chloride contains nearly 3 times the milliequivalents of Ca^{2+} per milliliter of 10% solution compared with calcium gluconate.

C. Dermal hydrofluoric acid exposure. For any exposures involving the hand or fingers, obtain immediate consultation from an experienced hand surgeon.

1. For topical application of calcium gel, prepare gel by combining the proportion of 1 g of calcium gluconate or calcium carbonate per 30 g (approximately 30 mL) of water-soluble base material (Surgilube, K-Y Jelly). Apply liberally to exposed areas. For finger burns, place in a loose-fitting latex glove for sustained topical effect.

2. For subcutaneous injection, inject calcium gluconate 0.5–1 mL/cm^2 of affected skin, using a 27-gauge or smaller needle. May repeat 2–3 times at 1- to 2-hour intervals if pain is not relieved.

3. For intra-arterial injection, administer 10 mL of 10% calcium gluconate in 40 mL saline infused via the radial or brachial artery over 3–4 hours.

VII. Formulations

A. Oral. Calcium carbonate; suspension, tablets, chewable tablets, 300–800 mg.

B. Parenteral. Calcium gluconate 10%, 10 mL (4.5–4.8 meq, 1 g); calcium chloride 10%, 10 mL (13.6 meq, 1g).

CHARCOAL, ACTIVATED

James F. Buchanan, PharmD

I. Pharmacology. Activated charcoal, by virtue of its large surface area, adsorbs many drugs and toxins (see Section I, p 45). Small or highly ionic salts (eg, iron, lithium, or cyanide) or small molecules (eg, alcohols) are poorly adsorbed. Repeated oral doses of activated charcoal can increase the rate of elimination of drugs that have a small volume of distribution (V_d) and that undergo enterohepatic recirculation (eg, digitoxin) or diffuse into the gastrointestinal lumen from the intestinal circulation (eg, phenobarbital, theophylline). See also discussion in Section I, p 49.

II. Indications

A. Activated charcoal is used after any ingestion to limit drug or toxin

absorption. It is usually administered after the stomach has been emptied by ipecac-induced emesis or gastric lavage, although recent studies suggest that it is effective when used alone for most ingestions.
  B. Repeated doses of activated charcoal are indicated to enhance elimination of drugs or toxins when serum levels are high and their half-lives are long, if (1) more rapid elimination will benefit the patient, and (2) more aggressive means of removal (eg, hemodialysis or hemoperfusion) are not immediately indicated.
III. **Contraindications**
  A. Gastrointestinal ileus or obstruction.
  B. Acid or alkali ingestions, unless other drugs have also been ingested (charcoal makes endoscopic evaluation more difficult).
IV. **Adverse effects**
  A. Constipation (may be prevented by coadministration of a cathartic).
  B. Distention of the stomach, with potential risk of aspiration.
  C. Diarrhea, dehydration, and hypernatremia due to coadministered cathartics, especially with repeated doses.
  D. Intestinal bezoar with obstruction.
V. **Drug interactions**
  A. Activated charcoal may reduce, prevent, or delay the absorption of orally administered antidotes (eg, acetylcysteine [see p 289]).
  B. The adsorptive capacity of activated charcoal may be diminished by the concurrent ingestion of ice cream, milk, or sugar syrup.
VI. **Dosage and method of administration**
  A. **Initial dose.** Activated charcoal, 1 g/kg orally or via gastric tube, is administered or, if the quantity of toxin ingested is known, 10 times the amount of ingested toxin by weight is given.
  B. **Repeat dose.** Activated charcoal, 15–20 g every 4–8 hours is given orally or by gastric tube. Administer a small dose of cathartic with every second or third charcoal dose. Do *not* use cathartic with every activated charcoal dose.
VII. **Formulations.** There are a variety of formulations and a large number of brands and types of charcoal with various affinities and capacities for adsorption of toxins. Highly activated charcoal (Superchar) is reported to have a larger capacity than other types of charcoal. Activated charcoal is available as a powder, a liquid aqueous suspension, or a liquid suspension in sorbitol or propylene glycol.

CYANIDE ANTIDOTE KIT

See Nitrite (p 328) and Thiosulfate (p 340).

DANTROLENE

James F. Buchanan, PharmD

  I. **Pharmacology.** Dantrolene relaxes skeletal muscle by inhibiting the release of calcium from the sarcoplasmic reticulum, thereby reducing actin-myosin contractile activity. Dantrolene can help control hyperthermia that results from excessive muscle hyperactivity, particularly when hyperthermia is caused by a defect within the muscle cell (eg, malignant hyperthermia). Dantrolene is not a substitute for other temperature-controlling measures (eg, sponging and fanning).
 II. **Indications**
  A. The primary indication for dantrolene is malignant hyperthermia caused by reaction to anesthetic agents.
  B. Dantrolene may also be useful in treating hyperthermia and rhabdomyolysis caused by drug-induced muscular hyperactivity not controlled by usual cooling measures or neuromuscular paralysis.

III. **Contraindications.** No absolute contraindications exist. Patients with muscular weakness or respiratory impairment must be observed closely for possible respiratory arrest.

IV. **Adverse effects**
   A. Muscle weakness, which may aggravate respiratory depression.
   B. Drowsiness, diarrhea.
   C. Hypersensitivity hepatitis, occasionally fatal, reported after chronic therapy.

V. **Drug interactions.** Dantrolene may have additive central nervous system-depressant effects with sedative and hypnotic drugs.

VI. **Dosage and method of administration (adults and children)**
   A. **Parenteral.** Give 1–2 mg/kg rapidly IV; may be repeated as needed every 5–10 minutes, to a total dose of 10 mg/kg. Satisfactory response is usually achieved with 2–5 mg/kg.
   B. **Oral.** To prevent recurrence of hyperthermia, administer 1–2 mg/kg IV or PO (up to 100 mg maximum) 4 times a day for 2–3 days.

VII. **Formulations**
   A. **Parenteral.** Dantrolene sodium (Dantrium), 20 mg of lyophilized powder for reconstitution (after reconstitution, protect from light and use within 6 hours to ensure maximal activity).
   B. **Oral.** Dantrolene sodium (Dantrium), 25-, 50-, 100-mg capsules.

DEFEROXAMINE

James F. Buchanan, PharmD

I. **Pharmacology.** Deferoxamine is a specific chelating agent for iron. It binds free iron and, to some extent, loosely bound iron (eg, from ferritin or hemosiderin). Iron bound to hemoglobin, transferrin, cytochrome enzymes, and all other sites is unaffected. The red iron-deferoxamine (ferrioxamine) complex is water-soluble and is excreted renally, where it imparts an orange-pink or "vin rosé" color to the urine. One hundred milligrams of deferoxamine is capable of binding 8.5 mg of elemental iron.

II. **Indications**
   A. Deferoxamine is used to treat iron intoxication when the serum iron is greater than 450–500 μg/dL or when clinical signs of significant iron intoxication exist (e.g., shock, acidosis, severe gastroenteritis, leukocytosis, hyperglycemia).
   B. Deferoxamine is sometimes used as a "test dose" to determine the presence of free iron by observing for the characteristic "vin rosé" color in the urine.

III. **Contraindications**
   A. There are no absolute contraindications to deferoxamine use in patients with serious iron poisoning. The drug should be used with caution in patients with known sensitivity to deferoxamine.
   B. Effects on pregnancy are not known, but deferoxamine use in pregnant patients should be reserved for serious intoxications.

IV. **Adverse effects**
   A. Hypotension or an anaphylactoid reaction may occur from rapid intravenous bolus administration; this may be avoided by limiting the rate of administration to 15 mg/kg/h.
   B. Local pain, induration, and sterile abscess formation may occur at intramuscular injection sites. Large intramuscular injections may also cause hypotension.
   C. The ferrioxamine complex may itself cause hypotension and may accumulate in patients with renal impairment; hemodialysis may be necessary to remove the ferrioxamine complex.

V. **Drug interactions.** There are no known drug interactions.

VI. **Dosage and method of administration**

A. The intravenous route is preferred in all cases. In children or adults, give at an infusion rate generally not to exceed 15 mg/kg/h (rates up to 40–50 mg/kg/h have been given in massive iron intoxication). The maximum cumulative daily dose should generally not exceed 6 g. The end points of therapy are loss of "vin rosé"-colored urine; serum iron level less than 350 μg/dL; or resolution of clinical signs of intoxication.

B. Oral complexation is **not** recommended.

C. "Test dose" intramuscular injection is **not** recommended. If the patient is symptomatic, use the intravenous route. If the patient is not symptomatic but serious toxicity is expected, then intravenous access is essential and intravenous dosing provides more reliable administration.

VII. **Formulation.** Parenteral: Deferoxamine mesylate (Desferal), 500 mg of lyophilized powder.

DIAZEPAM

James F. Buchanan, PharmD, and Kent R. Olson, MD

I. **Pharmacology**

A. Diazepam and other benzodiazepines potentiate inhibitory gamma-aminobutyric acid (GABA) neuronal activity in the central nervous system. Pharmacologic effects include reduction of anxiety, suppression of seizure activity, central nervous system depression (possible respiratory arrest when given rapidly intravenously), and inhibition of spinal afferent pathways to produce skeletal muscle relaxation. In addition, diazepam has been reported to antagonize the cardiotoxic effect of chloroquine, although the mechanism is unknown.

B. Diazepam generally has little effect on the autonomic nervous system or cardiovascular system.

C. Diazepam is well absorbed orally but not intramuscularly. It is eliminated entirely by hepatic metabolism, with a serum half-life of approximately 40 hours. Active metabolites further extend the duration of effect.

II. **Indications**

A. **Anxiety.** Diazepam is used for the treatment of anxiety or agitation (eg, caused by sympathomimetic or hallucinogenic drug intoxication).

B. **Convulsions.** Diazepam is used for the treatment of acute seizure activity or status epilepticus due to idiopathic epilepsy or convulsant drug overdose. It is **not** effective for seizure prophylaxis or chronic treatment.

C. **Muscle relaxant.** Diazepam is used for relaxation of excessive muscle rigidity and contractions (eg, caused by strychnine poisoning or black widow spider envenomation).

D. **Chloroquine poisoning.** Diazepam may antagonize cardiotoxicity.

III. **Contraindications.** Do not use diazepam in patients with a known sensitivity to benzodiazepines.

IV. **Adverse effects**

A. Central nervous system-depressant effects may interfere with evaluation of neurologic function.

B. Excessive or rapid intravenous administration may cause respiratory arrest due to drug effect or cardiorespiratory depression caused by the diluent.

V. **Drug interactions**

A. Diazepam will potentiate central nervous system-depressant effects of opioids, ethanol, and other sedative-hypnotic and depressant drugs.

B. Diazepam may produce a false-negative reaction for glucose in the urine with Clinistix and Diastix test strips.

VI. **Dosage and method of administration**

    A. **Anxiety or agitation.** Give 0.1–0.2 mg/kg IV initially, depending on sever-
        ity; may repeat every 1–4 hours as needed. Oral dose is 0.1–0.3 mg/kg.
        Do *not* give intramuscularly (absorbed erratically by this route).
    B. **Convulsions.** Give 0.1–0.2 mg/kg IV every 10–15 minutes to a total of 30
        mg (adults) or 5 mg (young children) to 10 mg (older children). If convul-
        sions persist, use an alternative anticonvulsant (Phenytoin [see p 335],
        Phenobarbital [p 334], or Pentobarbital [p 333]). Do *not* give diazepam
        orally or intramuscularly. Rectal administration of 5 mg has been report-
        edly effective in children with status epilepticus when there is no intra-
        venous access.
    C. **Muscle relaxation.** Give 0.1–0.2 mg/kg IV initially; may repeat every 1–4
        hours as needed.
    D. **Chloroquine intoxication.** There is reported improvement of cardiotoxic-
        ity with administration of 1 mg/kg IV.
        Caution: This will likely cause apnea; the patient must be intubated, and
        ventilation must be controlled.
VII. Formulation. Parenteral: Diazepam (Valium, others), 5 g/mL solution.

DIAZOXIDE

James F. Buchanan, PharmD

  I. Pharmacology
    A. Diazoxide, a nondiuretic thiazide, is a direct arterial vasodilator used to
       treat severe hypertension. Heart rate and cardiac output increase owing
       to a reflex response to decreased peripheral vascular resistance. The
       duration of the hypotensive effect ranges from 3 to 12 hours, although
       the elimination half-life is 20–40 hours.
    B. Diazoxide is used in the treatment of oral hypoglycemic overdose be-
       cause it increases serum glucose by inhibiting insulin secretion, dimin-
       ishing peripheral glucose utilization, and enhancing hepatic glucose
       release.
  II. Indications
    A. Acute management of hypertensive crisis, although other antihyperten-
       sive agents generally are preferred (see Nifedipine [p 328], Phentol-
       amine [p 335], Nitroprusside [p 330], and Labetalol [p 319]).
    B. Oral hypoglycemic overdose, when serum glucose concentrations can-
       not be adequately maintained by intravenous glucose infusions.
  III. Contraindications
    A. Hypertension associated with aortic stenosis, aortic coarctation, hy-
       pertrophic cardiomyopathy, or arteriovenous shunt.
    B. Known hypersensivity to thiazides.
    C. Diazoxide is teratogenic in animals and is not approved for use in
       pregnancy.
  IV. Adverse effects
    A. Hypotension or excessive blood pressure reduction must be avoided in
       patients with compromised cerebral or cardiac circulation.
    B. Fluid retention from prolonged therapy may compromise patients with
       congestive heart failure.
    C. Hyperglycemia may occur, particularly in patients with diabetes or he-
       patic dysfunction.
  V. Drug interactions
    A. The hypotensive effect is potentiated by concomitant therapy with di-
       uretics or β-adrenergic blockers.
    B. Diazoxide displaces warfarin from protein-binding sites and may tran-
       siently potentiate its anticoagulant effects.
  VI. Dosage and method of administration (adults and children)

A. For hypertensive crisis, give 1–3 mg/kg IV (150 mg maximum) every 5–15 minutes as needed. *Note:* The use of a 300-mg rapid bolus is no longer recommended.

B. For oral hypoglycemic-induced hypoglycemia, give 0.1–2 mg/kg/h infusion; initiate at lower infusion rate and titrate up as needed. Hypotension is minimized by keeping the patient supine and increasing the infusion rate slowly.

VII. Formulation. Parenteral: Diazoxide (Hyperstat), 15 mg/mL.

DIGOXIN-SPECIFIC ANTIBODIES

James F. Buchanan, PharmD

I. **Pharmacology.** Digoxin-specific antibodies are produced in immunized sheep and have a high binding affinity for digoxin and (to a lesser extent) digitoxin and other cardiac glycosides. The Fab fragments used to treat poisoning are derived by cleaving the whole antibodies. Once the digoxin-Fab complex is formed, the digoxin molecule is no longer pharmacologically active. The complex enters the circulation, is renally eliminated, and has a half-life of 16–20 hours. Reversal of signs of digitalis intoxication occurs within 30–60 minutes of administration, with complete reversal by 3 hours.

II. **Indications.** Digoxin-specific antibodies are used for life-threatening arrhythmias or hyperkalemia due to cardiac glycoside intoxication (see p 112).

III. **Contraindications.** No contraindications are known. Caution is warranted in patients with known sensitivity to ovine (sheep) products or in those who have been previously treated with digoxin-Fab fragments. The safety of digoxin-Fab fragments in pregnancy is not established.

IV. **Adverse effects**

A. Monitor the patient for potential hypersensitivity reactions and serum sickness.

B. In patients with renal insufficiency and impaired clearance of the digitalis-Fab complex, the complex may potentially degrade, releasing active glycoside.

C. Removal of the inotropic effect of digitalis may exacerbate preexisting heart failure.

TABLE III–2. APPROXIMATE DIGOXIN-FAB DOSE IF AMOUNT INGESTED IS KNOWN

Tablets Ingested (0.25 mg)	Approximate Dose Absorbed (mg)	Recommended Dose Fab (mg)	Vials
5	1	68	1.7
10	2	136	3.4
25	5	340	8.5
50	10	680	17
75	15	1000	25
100	20	1360	34
150	30	2000	50

TABLE III-3. APPROXIMATE DIGOXIN-FAB DOSE BASED ON SERUM CONCENTRATION (SC) AT STEADY STATE (AFTER EQUILIBRATION)

$$\text{Dose of digoxin-Fab: No. of vials} = \frac{\text{Body load (mg)}}{0.6}$$

$$\text{Digoxin: Body load in mg} = \frac{\text{SC (ng/mL)} \times 5.6 \times \text{weight in kg}}{1000}$$

$$\text{Digitoxin: Body load in mg} = \frac{\text{SC (ng/mL)} \times 0.56 \times \text{weight in kg}}{1000}$$

    D. With removal of digitalis effect, patients with preexisting atrial fibrillation may develop accelerated ventricular response.

V. Drug interactions
    A. Digoxin-specific Fab fragments will cross-react with other cardiac glycosides including digitoxin, ouabain, and (potentially) glycosides in oleander, lily of the Nile, and strophanthus.
    B. The digoxin-Fab complex cross-reacts with the antibody utilized in quantitative immunoassay techniques. This results in falsely high serum concentrations of digoxin owing to measurement of the inactive Fab complex.

VI. Dosage and method of administration
    A. Each vial (40 mg) of digoxin-immune Fab binds 0.6 mg of digoxin.
    B. Estimation of the dose of Fab is based on the body burden of digitalis. This may be calculated if the approximate amount ingested is known (Table III-2) or if the "steady-state" (postdistributional) serum drug concentration is known (Table III-3). (Postdistributional serum drug concentration should be determined at least 12–16 hours after the last dose.)

VII. Formulation. Parenteral: Digibind, 40 mg of lyophilized digoxin-specific Fab fragments.

DIPHENHYDRAMINE

James F. Buchanan, PharmD

    I. Pharmacology. Diphenhydramine is an antihistamine with anticholinergic and antiemetic properties. The antihistaminic property affords relief from itching and minor irritation caused by plant-induced dermatitis and insect bites and, when used as pretreatment, provides partial protection against anaphylaxis caused by horse serum-derived antivenins or antitoxins. Drug-induced extrapyramidal symptoms respond to the anticholinergic effect of diphenhydramine. The effects are maximal 1 hour after intravenous injection and last up to 7 hours. The drug is eliminated by hepatic metabolism, with a serum half-life of 3–7 hours.

    II. Indications
    A. Pruritis caused by poison oak, poison ivy, or minor insect bites.
    B. Pretreatment before administration of horse serum-derived antivenins or antitoxins, especially in patients with a history of hypersensitivity or with a positive skin test.

    C. Drug-induced extrapyramidal symptoms.
III. Contraindications
    A. Angle-closure glaucoma.
    B. Prostatic hypertrophy with obstructive uropathy.
    C. Concurrent therapy with monoamine oxidase inhibitors.
IV. Adverse effects
    A. Sedation, drowsiness, and ataxia may occur.
    B. Paradoxic excitation is possible in small children.
    C. Excessive doses may cause flushing, tachycardia, blurred vision, delirium, toxic psychosis, urinary retention, and respiratory depression.
V. Drug interactions. Diphenhydramine has an additive sedative effect with opioids, ethanol, and other sedative or anticholinergic drugs.
VI. Dosage and method of administration
    A. Pruritis. Give 25–50 mg orally every 6–8 hours (children, 5 mg/kg/d in divided doses).
    B. Pretreatment before antivenin administration. Give 50 mg (children, 0.5–1 mg/kg) IV; if possible, it should be given at least 15–20 minutes before antivenin use.
    C. Drug-induced extrapyramidal symptoms. Give 50 mg (children, 0.5–1 mg/kg) IV. Provide oral maintenance therapy, 25–50 mg (children, 0.5–1 mg/kg) every 4–6 hours for 1–2 days to prevent recurrence.
VII. Formulations
    A. Oral. Diphenhydramine hydrochloride (Benadryl, others), 25- and 50-mg tablets and capsules; elixir, 12.5 mg/5 mL.
    B. Parenteral. Diphenhydramine hydrochloride (Benadryl, others), 10- and 50-mg/mL solutions.

DMSA

James F. Buchanan, PharmD

    I. Pharmacology. DMSA (2,3-dimercaptosuccinic acid) is a chelating agent currently being investigated for use in the treatment of heavy metal poisoning. The specificity of DMSA for certain heavy metals (lead, arsenic, mercury, and silver) appears greater than that of other chelating agents; the elimination of iron, calcium, and magnesium is unaffected. DMSA is rapidly absorbed after oral administration. It is eliminated primarily by renal excretion, with a half-life of approximately 2 days.
    II. Indications. DMSA is used for heavy metal poisoning caused by lead, mercury (particularly methyl mercury), and arsenic.
    III. Contraindications. There are no known contraindications. The teratogenic potential of DMSA in humans has not been determined.
    IV. Adverse effects
        A. Nausea and vomiting occasionally occur.
        B. Mild, transient increase in alanine aminotransferase has been noted in a minority of patients in one study.
        C. Urinary elimination of zinc and copper is minimally increased but is substantially less than that caused by calcium EDTA.
        D. Unidentified adverse human effects may exist owing to the limited experience with the drug. Animal studies report renal and pancreatic islet cell damage with high doses (150 mg/kg/d).
    V. Drug interactions. There are no known drug interactions.
    VI. Dosage and method of administration (adults and children)
        A. Oral. Give 30 mg/kg/d in 3 divided doses.
        B. Parenteral. Give 30 mg/kg/d in 3 divided doses.
    VII. Formulations (investigational)
        A. Oral. 2,3-Dimercaptosuccinic acid.
        B. Parenteral. Sodium 2,3-dimercaptosuccinate.
        C. Availability. For information on the availability and use of DMSA, con-

tact the Medical Department, Johnson & Johnson Baby Products Company, at (201) 874-1447 (weekdays, 8 am to 5 pm, eastern standard time) or (800) 526-3967 (24 hours toll-free).

DOPAMINE

Neal L. Benowitz, MD

I. **Pharmacology.** Dopamine is an endogenous catecholamine and the immediate metabolic precursor of norepinephrine. It stimulates α- and β-adrenergic receptors and, in addition, acts on specific dopaminergic receptors. Its relative activity at these various receptors is dose-related. At low infusion rates (1–5 μg/kg/min), dopamine stimulates β_1 activity (increased heart rate and contractility) and increases renal and mesenteric blood flow through dopaminergic agonist activity. At high infusion rates (>10–20 μg/kg/min), α-adrenergic stimulation predominates, resulting in increased peripheral vascular resistance. Dopamine is not effective orally. Following intravenous administration, its onset of action occurs within 5 minutes and the duration of effect is less than 10 minutes. The plasma half-life is about 2 minutes.

II. **Indications**
   A. Dopamine is used to increase blood pressure, cardiac output, and urine flow in patients with shock who have not responded to intravenous fluid challenge, correction of hypothermia, or reversal of acidosis.
   B. Low-dose infusion is most effective for hypotension caused by venodilation or reduced cardiac contractility; high-dose dopamine is indicated for shock resulting from decreased peripheral arterial resistance.

III. **Contraindications**
   A. Hypertension is a contraindication.
   B. High-dose infusion is relatively contraindicated in the presence of peripheral arterial occlusive disease with thrombosis or in patients with ergot poisoning.
   C. Use with extreme caution in patients intoxicated by halogenated or aromatic hydrocarbon solvents or anesthetics.
   D. Use with extreme caution in patients with known hypersensitivity to sulfite preservatives.

IV. **Adverse effects**
   A. Severe hypertension, which may result in intracranial hemorrhage, pulmonary edema, or myocardial necrosis.
   B. Aggravation of tissue ischemia, resulting in gangrene (with high-dose infusion).
   C. Ventricular arrhythmias, especially in patients intoxicated by halogenated or aromatic hydrocarbon solvents or anesthetics.
   D. Tissue necrosis after extravasation (p 308 for treatment of extravasation).
   E. Anaphylaxis induced by sulfite preservatives in sensitive patients.

V. **Drug interactions**
   A. Enhanced pressor response may occur in the presence of cocaine and cyclic antidepressants owing to inhibition of neuronal reuptake.
   B. Enhanced pressor response may occur in patients taking monoamine oxidase inhibitors, owing to inhibition of neuronal metabolic degradation.
   C. Cyclopropane and halogenated hydrocarbon anesthetics may enhance the arrhythmogenic effect of dopamine owing to sensitization of the myocardium to effects of catecholamines.
   D. Alpha- and beta-blocking agents antagonize the adrenergic effects of dopamine; haloperidol and other dopamine antagonists may antagonize the dopaminergic effects.

VI. **Dosage and method of administration (adults and children)**
   A. **Avoid extravasation.** *Caution:* The intravenous infusion must be free-flowing, and the infused vein should be observed frequently for signs of infiltration (pallor, coldness, induration). If extravasation occurs, immediately infiltrate the affected area with phentolamine (see p 335), 5–10 mg in 10–15 mL of normal saline (children, 0.1–0.2 mg/kg; maximum 10 mg total) via a fine (25- to 27-gauge) hypodermic needle; improvement is evidenced by hyperemia and return to normal temperature.
   B. As an initial infusion rate, for **predominantly inotropic effects,** begin with 1 μg/kg/min and increase infusion rate as needed to 5–10 μg/kg/min.
   C. For **predominantly vasopressor effect,** infuse 10–20 μg/kg/min and increase as needed. Doses above 50 μg/kg/min may result in severe peripheral vasoconstriction and gangrene.
VII. **Formulations**
   A. **Concentrate for admixture to intravenous infusion.** Dopamine hydrochloride (Intropin, others), 40, 80, and 160 mg/mL in 5-mL vials. All contain sodium bisulfite as a preservative.
   B. **Premixed parenteral for direct injection.** Dopamine hydrochloride (Intropin, others), 0.8, 1.6, and 3.2 mg/mL in 5% dextrose. All contain sodium bisulfite as a preservative.

EDTA, CALCIUM (CALCIUM DISODIUM EDTA, EDETATE CALCIUM DISODIUM)

James F. Buchanan, PharmD, and Kent R. Olson, MD

   I. **Pharmacology.** Calcium EDTA chelates a variety of polyvalent metals, particularly lead. The elimination of other metals such as zinc, cadmium, manganese, iron, copper, and heavy radioisotopes (eg, uranium, plutonium, and yttrium) is also enhanced by calcium EDTA to a lesser extent. Calcium EDTA should not be confused with sodium EDTA (edetate disodium), which is occasionally used to treat life-threatening severe hypercalcemia. Within 1 hour of intravenous administration, urinary excretion of the EDTA-metal complex begins, and symptoms of lead poisoning such as colic may improve within 2–3 hours. The plasma half-life of the drug is 20–60 minutes, and 50% of the injected dose is excreted in the urine within 1 hour.
   II. **Indications**
   A. Calcium EDTA is used for acute and chronic lead poisoning. When encephalopathy is present, concomitant administration of BAL (dimercaprol [p 294]) is recommended.
   B. Calcium EDTA may possibly be useful in poisoning caused by manganese, zinc, chromium, nickel, or heavy radioisotopes. It is ineffective for mercury, gold, or arsenic intoxication.
   III. **Contraindications**
   A. Anuria is a relative contraindication. Use with extreme caution in patients with renal dysfunction, because accumulation increases the nephrotoxicity of calcium EDTA.
   B. The safety of calcium EDTA in pregnancy has not been established.
   IV. **Adverse effects**
   A. Nephrotoxicity (proteinuria, hematuria, acute tubular necrosis) may be minimized by adequate hydration, establishment of adequate urine flow, avoidance of excessive doses, and intermittent therapy (minimum 2 days, preferably 2 weeks between treatments). Monitoring of renal function during treatment is essential. The limited volume of distribution and small molecular size suggest that the metal-EDTA complex could be readily removed by hemodialysis.
   B. Avoid rapid intravenous infusions in the presence of lead encephalopa-

III: THERAPEUTIC DRUGS AND ANTIDOTES

thy; worsening of intracranial hypertension may result. BAL (dimecaprol [see p 294]) should be the initial drug of choice in patients with lead encephalopathy.

C. Nausea, vomiting, myalgia, arthralgia, chills, fever, hypotension, and histamine release may occur.

D. Local pain may occur at the intramuscular injection site, and thrombophlebitis may occur with intravenous infusions (especially with concentrations > 0.5%).

E. Inadvertent use of sodium EDTA (EDTA disodium) may cause serious hypocalcemia.

F. Calcium EDTA may cause concurrent zinc depletion and loss of taste during therapy.

G. Rarely, hypercalcemia may occur owing to release of chelated calcium in exchange for lead.

V. **Drug interactions.** There are no known drug interactions.

VI. **Dosage and method of administration**

A. **Lead poisoning (adults and children)**

1. For lead poisoning with encephalopathy or blood lead level greater than 100 μg/dL, give calcium EDTA, 1500 mg/m^2/d (approximately 30 mg/kg) in 6 divided doses (every 4 hours) deep IM or as a continuous slow IV infusion (diluted to 2–4 mg/mL in saline) for 5 days (intramuscular route is preferred because of the large volume load with diluted intravenous preparation). Patients with encephalopathy should also receive BAL (dimercaprol [see p 294]) concomitant with calcium EDTA.

2. For lead poisoning that is symptomatic (but without encephalopathy) *or* blood lead level of 50–100 μg/dL *or* positive mobilization test (see **4**, below), give calcium EDTA, 1000 mg/m^2/d (approximately 20 mg/kg) continuous IV infusion or IM in 6 divided doses (every 4 hours) for 5 days.

3. Reevaluate blood lead concentration level at end of course of therapy for possible need of further calcium EDTA treatment.

4. A lead mobilization test (EDTA challenge test) may be given to assess lead burden. Give 500 mg/m^2 (approximately 10 mg/kg; 1 g maximum) IV over 1 hour, or IM. Collect urine in a lead-free container for 24 hours. If the number of micrograms of lead excreted is greater than the number of milligrams of EDTA given, the test is considered positive.

5. Oral EDTA therapy is **not** recommended for prevention or treatment; it may increase the absorption of lead from the gastrointestinal tract.

Note: The Federal Lead Standard requires removal from the workplace of any worker with blood lead level over 60 μg/dL; proper control measures must be undertaken before return to work. It is **not** appropriate to treat asymptomatic workers in order to lower their lead level below the standard. Consult the local or state health department or OSHA (see Table IV–15, p 501) for more detailed information.

B. **Other metals**

1. Consult with a regional poison center (see p 51).

2. Give calcium EDTA, 1000 mg (10 mg/kg; 1 g maximum) IV infusion over 5 hours daily for 3 days.

VII. **Formulation.** Parenteral: Calcium disodium edetate (Versenate), 200 mg/mL.

EPINEPHRINE

Neal L. Benowitz, MD

I. **Pharmacology.** Epinephrine is an endogenous catecholamine with α- and β-adrenergic agonist properties, used primarily in emergency situations to treat anaphylaxis or cardiac arrest. Beneficial effects include inhibition of mediator release from mast cells and basophils, bronchodilation, positive inotropic effects, and peripheral vasoconstriction. Epinephrine is not active after oral administration. Subcutaneous injection produces effects within 5–10 minutes, with peak effects at 20 minutes. Intravenous or inhalational administration produces even more rapid onset. Epinephrine is rapidly inactivated in the body, with an elimination half-life of 2 minutes.

II. **Indications**
  A. Anaphylaxis and anaphylactoid reactions.
  B. Occasionally used for hypotension due to overdose by beta blockers and other cardiac-depressant drugs.

III. **Contraindications**
  A. Hypertension is a contraindication.
  B. Use with extreme caution in patients intoxicated by halogenated and aromatic hydrocarbon solvents and anesthetics, because these may sensitize the myocardium to the arrhythmogenic effects of epinephrine.
  C. Digitalis intoxication may enhance arrhythmogenicity of epinephrine.
  D. Epinephrine is relatively contraindicated in patients with peripheral arterial occlusive vascular disease with thrombosis or in patients with ergot poisoning.
  E. Use with extreme caution in patients with known hypersensitivity to sulfite preservatives.

IV. **Adverse effects**
  A. Anxiety, restlessness, tremor, headache.
  B. Severe hypertension, which may result in intracranial hemorrhage, pulmonary edema, or myocardial necrosis or infarction.
  C. Ventricular arrhythmias.
  D. Tissue necrosis after extravasation.
  E. Aggravation of tissue ischemia, resulting in gangrene.
  F. Anaphylaxis, which may occur owing to the bisulfite preservative in patients with sulfite hypersensitivity.

V. **Drug interactions**
  A. Enhanced arrhythmogenic effect occurs when epinephrine is given with cyclopropane and halogenated general anesthetics or halogenated and aromatic hydrocarbon solvents.
  B. Propranolol and other nonselective beta blockers may produce a paradoxic increase in hypertension, owing to blockade of β_2-mediated vasodilation resulting in unopposed α-mediated vasoconstriction.
  C. Cocaine and cyclic antidepressants may enhance stimulant effects owing to inhibition of neuronal epinephrine reuptake.
  D. Monoamine oxidase inhibitors may enhance pressor effects because of decreased neuronal epinephrine metabolism.

VI. **Dosage and method of administration**
  A. **Avoid extravasation.** *Caution:* The intravenous infusion must be free-flowing, and the infused vein should be observed frequently for signs of infiltration (pallor, coldness, induration). If extravasation occurs, immediately infiltrate the affected area with phentolamine (see p 335), 5–10 mg in 10–15 mL of normal saline (children, 0.1–0.2 mg/kg; maximum 10 mg total) via a fine (25- to 27-gauge) hypodermic needle; improvement is evidenced by hyperemia and return to normal temperature.
  B. **Mild to moderate allergic reaction.** Give 0.3–0.5 mg SC or IM (children, 0.01 mg/kg of 1:1000 solution or 1:200 suspension; maximum 0.5 mg). May be repeated after 10–15 minutes if needed.
  C. **Severe anaphylaxis.** Give 0.05–0.1 mg IV (0.5–1 mL of a 1:10,000 solution) every 5–10 minutes (children, 0.01 mg/kg; maximum 0.1 mg), or an intravenous infusion at 1–4 μg/min. If intravenous access is not available, the endotracheal route may be used; give 0.5 mg (5 mL of a 1:10,000 solution) down the endotracheal tube.

   D. Hypotension. Infuse at 1 μg/min; titrate upward every 5 minutes as necessary.
VII. Formulation. Parenteral: Epinephrine hydrochloride (Adrenalin, others), 0.01 mg/mL (1:100,000), 0.1 mg/mL (1:10,000), 0.5 mg/mL (1:2000), and 1 mg/mL (1:1000). Most preparations contain sodium bisulfite or sodium metabisulfite as a preservative.

ESMOLOL

Kent R. Olson, MD

   I. Pharmacology. Esmolol is a short-acting, intravenous, cardioselective β_1-adrenergic blocker with no intrinsic sympathomimetic or membrane-depressant activity. In usual therapeutic doses, it causes little or no bronchospasm in patients with asthma. Esmolol produces peak effects within 6–10 minutes of administration of an intravenous bolus. It is rapidly hydrolyzed by red blood cell esterases, with an elimination half-life of 9 minutes; therapeutic and adverse effects disappear within 30 minutes after the infusion is discontinued.
  II. Indications
     A. Rapid control of supraventricular and ventricular tachyarrhythmias and hypertension, especially if caused by excessive sympathomimetic activity.
     B. Reversal of hypotension and tachycardia caused by excessive β-adrenergic activity resulting from theophylline overdose.
 III. Contraindications
     A. Contraindications include hypotension, bradycardia, or congestive heart failure secondary to intrinsic cardiac disease or cardiac-depressant effects of drugs and toxins (eg, cyclic antidepressants, barbiturates).
     B. Asthma and chronic obstructive pulmonary disease are considered relative contraindications because despite its cardioselectivity, esmolol may produce bronchospasm.
 IV. Adverse effects
     A. Hypotension and bradycardia may occur, especially in patients with intrinsic cardiac disease or cardiac-depressant drug overdose.
     B. Bronchospasm may occur, but it is less likely than with propranolol or other nonselective beta blockers and it is rapidly reversible after the infusion is discontinued.
     C. Esmolol may mask hypoglycemia-induced tachycardia and therefore should be used with caution in patients with diabetes.
  V. Drug interactions
     A. Esmolol may transiently increase the serum digoxin level by 10–20%, but the clinical significance of this is unknown.
     B. Recovery from succinylcholine-induced neuromuscular blockade may be slightly delayed (5–10 minutes).
     C. Esmolol is not compatible with sodium bicarbonate solutions.
 VI. Dosage and method of administration
     A. Esmolol must be diluted before intravenous injection to a final concentration of 10 mg/mL.
     B. Esmolol is given as an intravenous infusion, starting at 50 μg/kg/min and increasing as needed up to 100 μg/kg/min. Therapeutic effects will reach a new steady state approximately 30 minutes after each infusion adjustment. A loading dose of 500 μg/kg should be given if more rapid onset of clinical effects (5–10 minutes) is desired.
     C. Infusion rates greater than 200 μg/kg/min are likely to produce excessive hypotension.
VII. Formulation. Parenteral: Esmolol hydrochloride (Brevibloc), 2.5 g in 10-mL

ampules (250 mg/mL). Dilute to 10 mg/mL with 5% dextrose, lactated Ringer's injection, or saline solutions.

ETHANOL

James F. Buchanan, PharmD

I. **Pharmacology.** Ethanol (ethyl alcohol) acts as a competitive substrate for the enzyme alcohol dehydrogenase, preventing the metabolic formation of toxic metabolites from methanol or ethylene glycol. Blood ethanol concentrations of 100 mg/dL effectively saturate alcohol dehydrogenase and prevent further methanol and ethylene glycol metabolism. Ethanol is well absorbed from the gastrointestinal tract when given orally, but the onset is more rapid and predictable when it is given intravenously. The elimination of ethanol is zero order; the average rate of decline is 15 mg/dL/h; however, this is highly variable and will be influenced by prior chronic use of alcohol and concomitant use of hemodialysis (eg, to remove methanol or ethylene glycol).

II. **Indications**
   A. Methanol (methyl alcohol) poisoning with a reliable history of ingestion but when blood concentration measurements are not available; with metabolic acidosis and an unexplained elevated osmolar gap; or with a serum methanol concentration greater than 20 mg/dL, even in an asymptomatic patient.
   B. Ethylene glycol poisoning with a reliable history of ingestion; with metabolic acidosis and an unexplained elevated osmolar gap; or with an ethylene glycol level higher than 20 mg/dL.

III. **Contraindications**
   A. Ethanol is contraindicated in patients currently receiving (or having received within 2 weeks) disulfiram therapy. In such cases, hemodialysis is the recommended alternative to ethanol treatment.
   B. Use with caution in patients with head trauma or altered mental status or in those who have ingested other drugs with central nervous system-depressant properties.

IV. **Adverse effects**
   A. Nausea, vomiting, and gastritis may occur with oral administration.
   B. Inebriation, sedation, and hypoglycemia (particularly in children and malnourished adults) may occur.
   C. Vasodilation may result in postural hypotension.
   D. Intravenous use is sometimes associated with local phlebitis (especially with ethanol solutions > 10%).

V. **Drug interactions.** Ethanol potentiates the effect of central nervous system-depressant drugs.

VI. **Dosage and method of administration**
   A. Ethanol may be given orally or intravenously. The desired serum concentration is 100 mg/dL (20 mmol/L); this can be achieved by giving approximately 750 mg/kg (Table III–4) as a loading dose, followed by a

TABLE III-4. ETHANOL DOSING (ADULTS AND CHILDREN)

Dose	Intravenous 5%	10%	50% Oral
Loading	15 mL/kg	7.5 mL/kg	1.5 mL/kg
Maintenance	2–3 mL/kg/h	1–1.5 mL/kg/h	0.2–0.3 mL/kg/h
Maintenance during hemodialysis	3–5 mL/kg/h	1.5–2.5 mL/kg/h	0.3–0.5 mL/kg/h

maintenance infusion of approximately 100–150 mg/kg/h (give a larger dose to chronic alcoholics).

  B. Obtain serum ethanol levels after the loading dose and frequently during maintenance therapy to ensure a concentration of 100 mg/dL.
  C. Increase the infusion rate to 175–250 mg/kg/h (larger dose for chronic alcoholics) during hemodialysis to offset the increased rate of ethanol elimination.

VII. **Formulations**
  A. **Oral.** Pharmaceutical grade ethanol (96% USP). Commercial liquor may be used (for oral administration only) if pharmaceutical grade ethanol is not available; multiply the "proof" by 0.35 to convert to percent by weight.
  B. **Parenteral.** Ethanol, 5% in 5% dextrose solution; 10% in 5% dextrose solution.

FLUMAZENIL

Kent R. Olson, MD

  I. **Pharmacology**
  A. Flumazenil (Anexate, Ro 15-1788) is a highly selective competitive inhibitor of central nervous system benzodiazepine receptors. It has no demonstrable benzodiazepine agonist activity and no significant toxicity even in high doses. It has no effect on alcohol or opioid receptors.
  B. Flumazenil is effective orally or parenterally. After intravenous administration, the onset of benzodiazepine reversal occurs within 1–2 minutes and lasts for 2–5 hours, depending on the dose of flumazenil and the degree of preexisting benzodiazepine effect. It is eliminated by hepatic metabolism with a serum half-life of approximately 1 hour.

  II. **Indications**
  A. Rapid reversal of benzodiazepine-induced coma, both as a diagnostic aid and potential substitute for endotracheal intubation.
  B. Has been used for postoperative reversal of benzodiazepine sedation for surgical procedures and as an adjunct in weaning patients from ventilators.

  III. **Contraindications**
  A. Known hypersensitivity to the drug.
  B. Known history of withdrawal reactions to benzodiazepines or alcohol.
  C. Known seizure disorder.
  D. Increased intracranial pressure.
  E. Patients known or suspected to be physically dependent on benzodiazepines must be treated with extreme caution.

  IV. **Adverse effects**
  A. Anxiety, agitation, headache, dizziness, nausea, vomiting, tremor, and transient facial flushing.
  B. Rapid reversal of benzodiazepine effect in patients with benzodiazepine addiction or high tolerance may result in acute withdrawal state, including hyperexcitability, tachycardia, and seizures (rarely reported).

  V. **Drug interactions.** None known. Does not appear to alter kinetics of benzodiazepines or other drugs.

  VI. **Dosage and method of administration**
  A. Benzodiazepine overdose: Administer 0.2–3 mg IV (pediatric dose not established; start with 0.01–0.05 mg/kg). Administer at a rate not to exceed 0.5 mg/min. Repeat as needed to maintain desired level of consciousness. Because effects last only 2–5 hours, continue to monitor patient closely for at least 5–6 hours to prevent relapse.
  B. Reversal of conscious sedation or anesthetic doses of benzodiazepine: 0.2–1 mg IV is usually sufficient.

VII. Formulation. Flumazenil remains an investigational drug in the USA. It is available only to researchers participating in clinical trials.

FOLIC ACID

Kathryn H. Keller, PharmD

I. **Pharmacology.** Folic acid is a B-complex vitamin that is essential for protein synthesis and erythropoiesis. In addition, the administration of folate to patients with methanol (and possibly ethylene glycol) poisoning may enhance the elimination of the toxic metabolite formic acid.
II. **Indications**
   A. Adjunctive treatment for methanol poisoning.
   B. May also be administered in ethylene glycol poisoning.
III. **Contraindications.** There are no known contraindications.
IV. **Adverse effects.** Rare allergic reactions have been reported following intravenous administration.
V. **Drug interactions.** None known.
VI. **Dosage and method of administration.** The dose required for methanol or ethylene glycol poisoning is not established, although 50 mg IV (children, 1 mg/kg) every 4 hours has been recommended.
VII. **Formulation.** Parenteral: Sodium folate (Folvite), 5 mg/mL, 10-mL vials.

GLUCAGON

James F. Buchanan, PharmD

I. **Pharmacology.** Glucagon is a polypeptide hormone that stimulates the formation of adenyl cyclase, which in turn increases the intracellular concentration of cyclic adenosine monophosphate (cAMP). This results in enhanced glycogenolysis and elevated serum glucose concentration; vascular smooth muscle relaxation; and positive inotropic, chronotropic, and dromotropic effects. These effects occur independently of β-adrenergic stimulation. Glucagon is destroyed in the gastrointestinal tract and must be given parenterally. After intravenous administration, effects are seen within 1–2 minutes and persist for 10–20 minutes. The serum half-life is about 3–10 minutes.
II. **Indications**
   A. Hypotension, bradycardia, or conduction impairment caused by β-adrenergic blocker intoxication.
   B. Possibly effective for severe cardiac depression caused by intoxication with calcium antagonists, quinidine, or other type Ia and type Ic antiarrhythmic drugs.
   C. Persistent hypoglycemia due to intoxication with oral hypoglycemics (generally not recommended as first-line therapy, because hyperglycemic effect may not be sustained and treatment with intravenous dextrose is preferred).
III. **Contraindications.** There are no known contraindications.
IV. **Adverse effects**
   A. Hyperglycemia.
   B. Nausea and vomiting.
   C. Rare hypersensitivity reactions.
V. **Drug interactions.** Concurrent administration of epinephrine potentiates and prolongs the hyperglycemic and cardiovascular effects of glucagon.
VI. **Dosage and method of administration**
   A. **Beta-blocker overdose.** 5–10 mg IV, followed by 1–5 mg/h infusion (children, 0.15 mg/kg IV, followed by 0.05–0.1 mg/kg/h).
   B. **Hypoglycemia.** 0.5–1 mg SC, IM, or IV; may repeat in 5–20 minutes

(children, 0.025 mg/kg). The failure of glucagon to increase serum glucose suggests inadequate hepatic glycogen stores.

VII. Formulation. Parenteral: Glucagon for injection, 1 unit (approximately 1
mg), 10 units (approximately 10 mg).

GLUCOSE (D-Glucose, Dextrose)

James F. Buchanan, PharmD

I. **Pharmacology.** Glucose is an essential carbohydrate used as a substrate
for energy production within the body. Although many organs use fatty
acids as an alternative energy source, the brain is totally dependent on
glucose as its major energy source; thus, hypoglycemia may rapidly cause
serious brain injury.

II. **Indications**
   A. Hypoglycemia.
   B. Empirical therapy for patients with stupor, coma, or seizures who may
      have unsuspected hypoglycemia.
   C. Thiamine (see p 340) is routinely given along with glucose to alcoholic
      or malnourished patients, because administration of a large glucose
      load may precipitate acute Wernicke-Korsakoff syndrome in thiamine-
      depleted patients.

III. **Contraindications.** There are no absolute contraindications for the use of
glucose as empirical treatment of comatose patients with possible hypoglycemia. However, hyperglycemia and (possibly) recent ischemic brain
injury may be aggravated by excessive glucose administration.

IV. **Adverse effects**
   A. Hyperglycemia.
   B. Hyperosmolarity.
   C. Local phlebitis and cellulitis following extravasation (occurs with con-
      centrations > 10%) from the intravenous injection site.

V. **Drug interactions.** None known.

VI. **Dosage and method of administration**
   A. As empirical therapy for coma, give 50–100 mL of 50% dextrose via a
      secure intravenous line (children, 2–4 mL/kg of 25% dextrose; do **not**
      use 50% dextrose in children).
   B. Persistent hypoglycemia (eg, resulting from poisoning by hypoglycemic
      agent) requires repeated boluses of 25% (for children) or 50% dextrose
      and infusion of 5–10% dextrose, titrated as needed.

VII. **Formulation.** Parenteral: Dextrose injection, 50%, 50 mL; 25% dextrose, 20
mL; various solutions of 5–10% dextrose, some in combination with saline
or other crystalloids.

HALOPERIDOL

James F. Buchanan, PharmD

I. **Pharmacology.** Haloperidol is a butyrophenone neuroleptic drug useful for
the management of acutely agitated psychotic patients. It has strong central antidopaminergic activity and weak anticholinergic effects. Haloperidol is well absorbed from the gastrointestinal tract and by the
intramuscular route. Peak pharmacologic effects occur within 30–40 minutes of an intramuscular injection. The drug is metabolized and excreted
slowly in the urine and feces. Although the serum half-life is 12–24 hours,
the drug is detectable in the serum and urine for up to several weeks after
a single dose.

II. **Indications.** Haloperidol is used for the management of acute agitated
functional psychosis or extreme agitation induced by stimulants or phencyclidine. In general, drug-induced agitation is preferably managed by administration of diazepam (see p 302) or midazolam (see p 323).

dol is well absorbed from the gastrointestinal tract and by the intramuscular route. Peak pharmacologic effects occur within 30–40 minutes of an intramuscular injection. The drug is metabolized and excreted slowly in the urine and feces. Although the serum half-life is 12–24 hours, the drug is detectable in the serum and urine for up to several weeks after a single dose.

II. **Indications.** Haloperidol is used for the management of acute agitated functional psychosis or extreme agitation induced by stimulants or phencyclidine. In general, drug-induced agitation is preferably managed by administration of diazepam (see p 302) or midazolam (see p 323).

III. **Contraindications**
   A. Severe central nervous system depression in the absence of airway and ventilatory control.
   B. Severe parkinsonism.
   C. Known hypersensitivity to haloperidol.
   D. Teratogenic and fetotoxic in animals; safety in human pregnancy not established.

IV. **Adverse effects**
   A. Haloperidol produces less sedation and less hypotension than chlorpromazine but is associated with a higher incidence of extrapyramidal side effects.
   B. Rigidity, diaphoresis, and hyperpyrexia may also be a manifestation of neuroleptic malignant syndrome (see p 20) induced by haloperidol and other neuroleptic agents.
   C. Haloperidol should be used with caution in the presence of other central nervous system depressants (additive depressant effects).
   D. Haloperidol lowers the seizure threshold and should be used with caution in patients with known seizure disorder or who have ingested a convulsant drug.
   E. Anticholinergic effects (dry mouth, blurred vision, constipation, urinary retention) are less common than with phenothiazines.
   F. Transient hypotension and tachycardia are uncommon.
   G. Some oral haloperidol tablets contain tartrazine dye, which may precipitate allergic reactions in susceptible patients.

V. **Drug interactions**
   A. Haloperidol potentiates central nervous system-depressant effects of opioids, antidepressants, phenothiazines, ethanol, barbiturates, and other sedatives.
   B. Combined therapy with lithium may increase the risk of neuroleptic malignant syndrome (see p 20).

VI. **Dosage and method of administration**
   A. **Oral.** Give 2–5 mg of haloperidol orally; may repeat once if necessary; usual daily dose is 3–5 mg 2–3 times daily (children > 3 years old, 0.05–0.15 mg/kg/d or 0.5 mg/dose in 2–3 divided doses).
   B. **Parenteral.** Give 2–5 mg of haloperidol IM; may repeat once after 20–30 minutes and hourly if necessary (children > 3 years old, same as orally). Haloperidol is not approved for intravenous use in the USA, but that route has been widely used and is reportedly safe (however, do *not* administer the decanoate salt formulation IV).

VII. **Formulations**
   A. **Oral.** Haloperidol (Haldol), 0.5-, 1-, 2-, 5-, 10-, and 20-mg tablets.
   B. **Parenteral.** Haloperidol (Haldol), 5 mg/mL.

HYDROXOCOBALAMIN

Kathryn H. Keller, PharmD

I. **Pharmacology.** Hydroxocobalamin is a synthetic form of vitamin B_{12} used

    B. Allergic reactions have been reported.
  V. Drug interactions. No significant interactions have been reported with parenteral use for cyanide poisoning.
  VI. Dosage and method of administration
    A. Administer hydroxocobalamin intravenously in a dose equivalent to 50 times the amount of the cyanide exposure. If the amount of cyanide exposure is unknown, the recommended empirical dose is 4 g.
    B. *Note:* In the USA, only vials of 1 mg/mL are available, which prohibits its use owing to the impractical preparation time and the large volume of drug (4 L) that would need to be administered.
  VII. Formulations
    A. Parenteral (USA). Hydroxocobalamin, 1 mg/mL for intramuscular use.
    B. A preparation of 4 g of hydroxocobalamin in combination with 8 g of sodium thiosulfate is used in France for intravenous administration and is being prepared for investigational trials in the USA.

IPECAC SYRUP

James F. Buchanan, PharmD

  I. Pharmacology. Ipecac syrup is a mixture of plant-derived alkaloids, principally emetine and cephaeline, that produces emesis by direct irritation of the stomach and by stimulation of the central chemoreceptor trigger zone. Vomiting occurs in 90% of patients, usually within 20–30 minutes. Depending on the time after ingestion of the toxin, ipecac-induced emesis removes 30–50% of the stomach contents.
  II. Indications. Ipecac syrup is used for early, initial management of oral poisonings, particularly in the home immediately following ingestion or in health care facilities without the capacity to perform gastric lavage.
  III. Contraindications
    A. Comatose or obtunded mental state.
    B. Ingestion of a caustic or corrosive substance.
    C. Ingestion of a petroleum distillate or hydrocarbon.
    D. Ingestion of a drug or toxin likely to result in abrupt onset of seizures or coma (eg, cyclic antidepressants, strychnine, camphor, nicotine, cocaine, amphetamines, isoniazid).
    E. Severe hypertension.
  IV. Adverse effects
    A. Persistent gastrointestinal upset following emesis may significantly delay administration of activated charcoal or other oral antidotes.
    B. Mallory-Weiss tear or hemorrhagic gastritis may occur.
    C. Drowsiness occurs in about 20% and diarrhea in 25% of children.
    D. Single ingestions of therapeutic doses of ipecac syrup are not toxic, and failure to induce vomiting does not require removal of the ipecac. However, chronic repeated ingestion of ipecac (eg, in bulemics) may result in accumulation of cardiotoxic alkaloids and may lead to fatal cardiomyopathy and arrhythmias.
  V. Drug interactions
    A. Ipecac syrup potentiates nausea and vomiting associated with the ingestion of other gastric irritants.
    B. Ipecac syrup is adsorbed by activated charcoal; however, ipecac may still produce vomiting when given concurrently with charcoal.
  VI. Dosage and method of administration
    A. Children 6–12 months old. Give 5–10 mL. (*Note:* Not recommended for non-health care facility use.)
    B. Children 1–12 years old. Give 15 mL.
    C. Adults and children over 12 years old. Give 30 mL.
    D. Follow ipecac administration with 2–3 oz of water or clear liquid. If emesis does not occur within 30 minutes, repeat the dose of ipecac and

fluid. If emesis has not occurred within 30 minutes of the second dose, consider alternative gut-emptying procedure (eg, gastric lavage).

VII. **Formulation.** Ipecac syrup, 30 mL.

ISOPROTERENOL

James F. Buchanan, PharmD

I. **Pharmacology.** Isoproterenol is a catecholaminelike drug that stimulates β-adrenergic receptors (β_1 and β_2). Pharmacologic properties include positive inotropic and chronotropic cardiac effects, peripheral vasodilation, and bronchodilation. Isoproterenol is not absorbed orally and shows variable and erratic absorption from sublingual and rectal sites. The effects of the drug are rapidly terminated by tissue uptake and metabolism; effects persist only a few minutes after intravenous injection.

II. **Indications**
   A. Severe bradycardia or conduction block resulting in hemodynamically significant hypotension is an indication for use of isoproterenol. After beta-blocker overdose, exceedingly high doses may be required to overcome the pharmacologic blockade of β-receptors; alternative approaches, including emergency pacemaker insertion, may be required (see also Glucagon [p 314] and Atropine [p 293]).
   B. Isoproterenol is used to increase heart rate and normalize conduction to abolish polymorphous ventricular tachycardia (torsades de pointes) associated with QT interval prolongation (see p 13).

III. **Contraindications**
   A. Do not use isoproterenol for ventricular fibrillation or ventricular tachycardia (other than torsades de pointes).
   B. Use with extreme caution in the presence of halogenated or aromatic hydrocarbon solvents or anesthetics.

IV. **Adverse effects**
   A. Increased myocardial oxygen demand may result in angina pectoris or acute myocardial infarction.
   B. Peripheral β_2-mediated vasodilation may worsen hypotension.
   C. Isoproterenol may precipitate ventricular arrhythmias.
   D. Sulfite preservative in some parenteral preparations may cause hypersensitivity reactions.

V. **Drug interactions**
   A. Additive β-adrenergic stimulation occurs in the presence of other sympathomimetic drugs.
   B. Administration in the presence of cyclopropane, halogenated anesthetics, or other halogenated or aromatic hydrocarbons may enhance risk of ventricular arrhythmias because of sensitization of the myocardium to the arrhythmogenic effects of catecholamines.
   C. Digitalis-intoxicated patients are more prone to develop ventricular arrhythmias when isoproterenol is administered.
   D. Beta blockers may interfere with the action of isoproterenol at β-adrenergic receptors.

VI. **Dosage and method of administration**
   A. For intravenous infusion, begin with 0.5–1 μg/min infusion (children, 0.01–0.02 μg/kg/min) and increase as needed for desired effect.
   B. If dilute solution is not available, make a solution of 1:50,000 (20 μg/mL) by diluting 1 mL of the 1:5000 solution to a volume of 10 mL with normal saline.

VII. **Formulation.** Parenteral: Isoproterenol hydrochloride (Isuprel), 0.02 mg/mL (1:50,000) or 0.2 mg/mL (1:5000) (with sodium bisulfite or sodium metabisulfite).

LABETALOL

James F. Buchanan, PharmD

I. **Pharmacology.** Labetalol is a mixed β- and α-adrenergic antagonist; the nonselective β-antagonist properties are approximately 7 times greater than the α_1-antagonist activity. Hemodynamic effects generally include a decrease in heart rate, blood pressure, and systemic vascular resistance. Atrioventricular conduction velocity may be decreased. After intravenous injection, hypotensive effects are maximal within 10–15 minutes and persist about 2–4 hours. The drug is eliminated by hepatic metabolism and has a half-life of 5–6 hours.

II. **Indications.** Labetalol is used to treat hypertension and tachycardia associated with stimulant drug overdose (eg, cocaine, amphetamines).
Note: Hypertension with bradycardia suggests excessive α-mediated vasoconstriction; in this case, a pure alpha blocker such as phentolamine (p 335) is preferable, because the reversal of β_2-mediated vasodilation may worsen hypertension.

III. **Contraindications**
   A. Asthma.
   B. Congestive heart failure.
   C. Heart block.

IV. **Adverse effects**
   A. Paradoxic hypertension may theoretically result when labetalol is used in the presence of stimulant intoxicants possessing strong α-adrenergic agonist properties (eg, phenylpropanolamine) owing to the relatively weak α-antagonist properties of labetalol compared with its beta-blocking ability.
   B. Orthostatic hypotension may occur.
   C. Dyspnea and bronchospasm may result, particularly in asthmatics.
   D. Negative inotropic effects may occur.
   E. Nausea, abdominal pain, diarrhea, and lethargy may occur.

V. **Drug interactions**
   A. Additive blood pressure is lowered with other antihypertensive agents.
   B. Use with halothane potentiates hypotensive effect.
   C. Cimetidine increases oral bioavailability of labetalol.
   D. Labetalol is incompatible with 5% sodium bicarbonate injection (precipitates).

VI. **Dosage and method of administration**
   A. **Adult.** Give 20 mg slow IV bolus initially; may repeat with 40- to 80-mg doses at 10-minute intervals until blood pressure is controlled or a cumulative dose of 300 mg is achieved (most patients will respond to total doses of 50–200 mg). Alternatively, administer a constant infusion of 2 mg/min until blood pressure is controlled or a 300-mg cumulative dose is reached. After this, give oral labetalol starting at 100 mg twice daily.
   B. **Children older than 12 years.** Initial 0.25 mg/kg dose is given intravenously over 2 minutes.

VII. **Formulations**
   A. **Parenteral.** Labetalol hydrochloride (Normodyne, Trandate), 5 mg/mL.
   B. **Oral.** Labetalol hydrochloride (Normodyne, Trandate), 100-, 200-, 300-mg tablets.

LEUCOVORIN CALCIUM (FOLINIC ACID, CITROVORUM FACTOR)

Kathryn H. Keller, PharmD

I. **Pharmacology.** Leucovorin is a metabolically functional form of folic acid. Unlike folic acid, leucovorin does not require reduction by dihydrofolate reductase, and therefore it can participate directly in the one-carbon trans-

TABLE III-5. LEUCOVORIN DOSE DETERMINATION

Methotrexate Concentration (10^{-6} mol/L)	Hours After Methotrexate Exposure	Leucovorin Dose (Adults and Children)
0.1–1	24	10–15 mg/m^2 q6h for 12 doses
1–5	24	50 mg/m^2 q6h until serum level is $< 1 \times 10^{-7}$ mol/L
5–10	24	100 mg/m^2 q6h until serum level is $< 1 \times 10^{-7}$ mol/L

Reference: Methotrexate Management, in Rumack, B H et al (eds): *Poisindex*. Denver, CO. 1989.

fer reactions necessary for purine biosynthesis and cellular DNA and RNA production. In animal models of methanol intoxication, both leucovorin and folic acid reduce morbidity and mortality by catalyzing the oxidation of the highly toxic metabolite, formic acid, to nontoxic products.

II. Indications
  A. **Methotrexate poisoning.** Leucovorin treatment is essential because cells are incapable of utilizing folic acid owing to inhibition of dihydrofolate reductase.
  B. **Methanol poisoning.** Leucovorin is an alternative to folic acid.
III. Contraindications. There are no known contraindications.
IV. Adverse effects. Allergic reactions as a result of prior sensitization have been reported.
V. Drug interactions. Leucovorin antagonizes the antifolate effect of methotrexate.
VI. Dosage and method of administration
  A. **Methotrexate poisoning.** Administer intravenously a dose equal to or greater than the dose of methotrexate. If the dose is large but unknown, administer 75 mg within 12 hours (children, 10 mg/m^2/dose) and then 12 mg every 6 hours for 4 doses. Serum methotrexate levels can be used to guide leucovorin therapy (Table III-5). Do not use oral therapy.
  B. **Methanol poisoning.** For adults and children, give 1 mg/kg (up to 50–70 mg) IV every 4 hours for 1–2 doses. Oral folic acid is given thereafter at the same dosage every 4–6 hours until resolution of symptoms and adequate elimination of methanol from the body. Although leucovorin could be used safely for the entire course of treatment, its high cost does not justify such prolonged use in place of folic acid.
VII. Formulations
  A. **Parenteral.** Leucovorin calcium (Wellcovorin, others), 3 and 10 mg/mL in vials; 20, 25, 50, 100, 250 mg for reconstitution.
  B. **Oral.** Leucovorin calcium (Wellcovorin) , 5-, 10-, 15-, 25-mg tablets.

LIDOCAINE
James F. Buchanan, PharmD

I. Pharmacology
  A. Lidocaine is a type Ib antiarrhythmic agent used to treat ventricular arrhythmias. This drug inhibits the fast sodium channels, depresses automaticity within the His-Purkinje system and the ventricles, and prolongs the effective refractory period and action potential duration. Conduction within ischemic myocardial areas is depressed, abolishing reentrant circuits. Unlike quinidine and related drugs, lidocaine exerts minimal effect on the automaticity of the SA node and on conduction through the AV node and does not decrease myocardial contractility or blood pressure in usual doses.
  B. The oral bioavailability of lidocaine is poor owing to extensive first-pass

hepatic metabolism. After intravenous administration of a single dose, the onset of action is within 60–90 seconds and the duration of action is 10–20 minutes. The elimination half-life is approximately 1.5–2 hours; active metabolites have elimination half-lives of 2–10 hours and may accumulate in patients with congestive heart failure or liver or renal disease.

II. **Indications.** Lidocaine is used for the control of ventricular arrhythmias arising from poisoning by a variety of cardioactive drugs and toxins (eg, digoxin, cyclic antidepressants, stimulants, theophylline).

III. **Contraindications**
   A. The presence of nodal or ventricular rhythms in the setting of third-degree atrioventricular or intraventricular block. These are reflex escape rhythms that may provide lifesaving cardiac output, and abolishing them may result in asystole.
   B. Hypersensitivity to lidocaine or other amide-type local anesthetics.

IV. **Adverse effects**
   A. Excessive doses produce dizziness, confusion, agitation, and seizures.
   B. Conduction defects, bradycardia, and hypotension may occur with extremely high serum concentrations or in patients with underlying conduction disease.

V. **Drug interactions**
   A. Cimetidine and propranolol may decrease the hepatic clearance of lidocaine.
   B. Lidocaine may produce additive effects with other local anesthetics. In severe cocaine intoxication, lidocaine theoretically may cause additive neuronal depression.

VI. **Dosage and method of administration (adults and children).** Administer 1 mg/kg IV bolus (over 1 minute), followed by infusion of 1–4 mg/min (20–50 μg/kg/min) to maintain serum concentrations of 1–5 mg/L. If significant ectopy persists after the initial bolus, a repeat dose of 0.5 mg/kg IV can be given if needed at 10-minute intervals (to 3 mg/kg total loading dose).

VII. **Formulation.** Parenteral: Lidocaine hydrochloride (Xylocaine, others), 10 and 20 mg/mL for direct injection; 40, 100, 200 mg/mL for preparing infusion solution.

METHOCARBAMOL

Howard E. McKinney, PharmD

   I. **Pharmacology.** Methocarbamol is a centrally acting muscle relaxant. It does not directly relax skeletal muscle, and it does not depress neuromuscular transmission or muscle excitability; muscle relaxation is probably related to its sedative effects. After intravenous administration, the onset of action is nearly immediate. Elimination occurs by hepatic metabolism, with a serum half-life of 0.9–2.2 hours.

  II. **Indications**
   A. Control of painful muscle spasm caused by black widow spider envenomation.
   B. Management of muscle spasm caused by tetanus and strychnine poisoning.

 III. **Contraindications**
   A. Known hypersensitivity to the drug.
   B. History of epilepsy (intravenous methocarbamol may precipitate seizures).

 IV. **Adverse effects**
   A. Dizziness, drowsiness, nausea, flushing, and metallic taste may occur.
   B. Extravasation from intravenous site may cause phlebitis and sloughing.
   C. Hypotension, bradycardia, and syncope have occurred after intramuscular or intravenous administration.

     D. Urticaria and anaphylactic reactions have been reported.

     E. The urine may turn brown, black, or blue after standing.

  V. Drug interactions. Lidocaine produces additive sedation with alcohol and other central nervous system depressants.

 VI. Dosage and method of administration

     A. Parenteral. Administer 1 g (children, 15 mg/kg) IV over 5 minutes, followed by 0.5 g in 250 mL of 5% dextrose (children, 10 mg/kg in 5 mL of 5% dextrose) over 4 hours. The usual intramuscular dose is 500 mg every 8 hours for adults and 10 mg/kg every 8 hours for children.

     B. Oral. Give 0.5–1 g (children, 10–15 mg/kg) orally every 6 hours; maximum dose, 1.5 g every 6 hours.

VII. Formulations

     A. Parenteral. Methocarbamol (Robaxin), 100 mg/mL.

     B. Oral. Methocarbamol (Robaxin, others), 500-, 750-mg tablets.

METHYLENE BLUE

Kathryn H. Keller, PharmD

  I. Pharmacology. Methylene blue is a thiazine dye that reverses drug-induced methemoglobinemia by increasing the conversion of methemoglobin to hemoglobin. This requires the presence of adequate amounts of the enzyme methemoglobin reductase and glucose-6-phosphate dehydrogenase. Methylene blue is excreted in the urine and bile, which turn blue or green.

 II. Indications. Methylene blue is used to treat methemoglobinemia in which the patient has symptoms or signs of hypoxemia (eg, dyspnea, confusion, chest pain) or has a methemoglobin level greater than 25–30%.

III. Contraindications

     A. Glucose-6-phosphate dehydrogenase (G6PD) deficiency; treatment with methylene blue is ineffective and may cause hemolysis.

     B. Severe renal failure.

     C. Known hypersensitivity to methylene blue.

     D. Methemoglobin reductase deficiency.

 IV. Adverse effects

     A. Gastrointestinal upset, headache, and dizziness may occur.

     B. Excessive doses of methylene blue (> 7 mg/kg) can actually cause methemoglobinemia by directly oxidizing hemoglobin. Doses greater than 15 mg/kg are associated with hemolysis.

     C. Long-term administration may result in marked anemia.

     D. Extravasation may result in local tissue necrosis.

  V. Drug interactions. There are no interactions known, but the intravenous preparation should not be mixed with other drugs.

 VI. Dosage and method of administration (adults and children). Administer 1–2 mg/kg (0.1–0.2 mL/kg of 1% solution) slowly intravenous over several minutes. May be repeated in 30–60 minutes.

VII. Formulation. Parenteral: Methylene blue injection 1% (10 mg/mL).

METOCLOPRAMIDE

James F. Buchanan, PharmD

  I. Pharmacology. Metoclopramide, a dopamine antagonist, is an antiemetic that acts at the chemoreceptor trigger zone and may also increase gastrointestinal motility and facilitate gastric emptying. The onset of effect is 1–3 minutes after intravenous administration, and therapeutic effects persist for 1–2 hours after a single dose. The drug is excreted primarily by the kidney. The initial and terminal elimination half-lives are 5 minutes and 2.5–5 hours, respectively.

 II. Indications. Metoclopramide is used to control persistent nausea and vomiting, particularly when the ability to administer activated charcoal (eg, treatment of theophylline poisoning) or other oral antidotal therapy (eg, acetylcysteine for acetaminophen poisoning) is compromised.

III. **Contraindications**
   A. Pheochromocytoma (metoclopramide may cause hypertensive crisis).
   B. Obstruction or perforation of the gastrointestinal tract.
   C. Known hypersensitivity to the drug; possible cross-sensitivity with procainamide.

IV. **Adverse effects**
   A. Sedation, restlessness, fatigue, and diarrhea may occur.
   B. Extrapyramidal reactions may result, particularly with high-dose treatment. Pediatric patients appear to be more susceptible. These reactions may be prevented by pretreatment with diphenhydramine.
   C. The drug may increase the frequency and severity of seizures in patients with seizure disorders.
   D. Parenteral formulations that contain sulfite preservatives may precipitate bronchoconstriction in susceptible individuals.

V. **Drug interactions**
   A. Additive sedation occurs in the presence of other central nervous system depressants.
   B. Risk of extrapyramidal reactions may be increased in the presence of other dopamine antagonist agents (eg, haloperidol, phenothiazines).
   C. Hypotensive reactions may occur when the drug is administered with anesthetics having hypotensive properties.
   D. The drug may enhance the absorption of ingested drugs by promoting gastric emptying.

VI. **Dosage and method of administration**
   A. **Low dose.** Give 10–20 mg IM or slowly IV; this is reportedly effective for mild nausea (children, 0.1 mg/kg).
   B. **High dose.** For adults and children, give 1–2 mg/kg IV infusion over 15 minutes in dextrose or saline. May be repeated twice at 2- to 3-hour intervals. Pretreatment with 50 mg (children, 1 mg/kg) of diphenhydramine (see p 305) helps to prevent extrapyramidal reactions.

VII. **Formulation.** Parenteral: Metoclopramide hydrochloride (Reglan), 5 mg/mL.

MIDAZOLAM

Kent R. Olson, MD

I. **Pharmacology.** Midazolam is an ultrashort-acting parenteral benzodiazepine used for the acute management of agitation and anxiety. Intravenous injection causes rapid sedation owing to high transient brain levels. Midazolam is well absorbed by subcutaneous and intramuscular routes. The serum half-life is 2–4 hours, but because central nervous system effects are determined by the rate of redistribution from the brain, the usual duration of sedation is only 30 minutes to 2 hours after a single dose. However, sedation may persist for 10 hours or longer after a prolonged infusion.

II. **Indications**
   A. Acute anxiety or agitation secondary to hallucinogenic or stimulant drug intoxication, psychosis, or metabolic encephalopathy.
   B. Sedation and amnesia during neuromuscular paralysis for endotracheal intubation.
   C. Status epilepticus (may be given intramuscularly if intravenous access for other anticonvulsants such as diazepam is not established).

III. **Contraindications.** There are no absolute contraindications. Midazolam must be used with caution in patients with compromised respiratory status, especially if the equipment and experienced personnel to perform rapid intubation are not available.

IV. **Adverse effects.** Respiratory arrest may result, especially if the drug is given rapidly or in excessive doses or to patients already intoxicated by other depressant drugs.

  V. **Drug interactions.** Additive depressant effects with other sedative-hypnotic agents, ethanol, opiates.
 VI. **Dosage and method of administration**
     A. **Agitation or excessive muscle hyperactivity.** Give 0.05–0.1 mg/kg IV or 0.1–0.2 mg/kg IM; may repeat every 30–60 minutes as needed.
        Caution: There have been several reports of respiratory arrest after rapid intravenous administration of midazolam, especially when given in combination with intravenous opioids.
     B. **Status epilepticus with no IV access.** Give 0.1–0.2 mg/kg IM. May repeat 5–10 minutes.
VII. **Formulation.** Parenteral: Midazolam (Versed), 1 and 5 mg/mL solutions.

MORPHINE

Kent R. Olson, MD

  I. **Pharmacology.** Morphine is the principal alkaloid of opium and is a potent analgesic and sedative agent. In addition, it decreases venous tone and systemic vascular resistance, resulting in reduced preload and afterload. Morphine is variably absorbed from the gastrointestinal tract and is usually used parenterally. After intravenous injection, peak analgesia is attained within 20 minutes and usually lasts 3–5 hours. Morphine is eliminated by hepatic metabolism, with a serum half-life of about 3 hours; however, the clearance of morphine is slowed and duration of effect is prolonged in patients with renal failure.
 II. **Indications**
     A. Severe pain associated with black widow spider envenomation, rattlesnake envenomation, or other bites or stings.
     B. Pain due to corrosive injury to the eyes, skin, or gastrointestinal tract.
     C. Pulmonary edema due to congestive heart failure. Chemical-induced noncardiogenic pulmonary edema is *not* an indication for morphine therapy.
III. **Contraindications**
     A. Known hypersensitivity to morphine.
     B. Respiratory or central nervous system depression with impending respiratory failure, unless the patient is intubated or equipment and trained personnel are standing by to intervene if necessary.
 IV. **Adverse effects**
     A. Respiratory and central nervous system depression may result in respiratory arrest. Depressant effects may be prolonged in patients with liver disease and chronic renal failure.
     B. Hypotension may occur owing to decreased systemic vascular resistance and venous tone.
     C. Nausea, vomiting, and constipation may occur.
     D. Bradycardia, wheezing, flushing, pruritis, urticaria, and other histamine-like effects may occur.
  V. **Drug interactions**
     A. Morphine has additive depressant effects with other opioid agonists, ethanol and other sedative-hypnotic agents, tranquilizers, and antidepressants.
     B. Morphine is physically incompatible with solutions containing a variety of drugs, including aminophylline, phenytoin, phenobarbital, and sodium bicarbonate.
 VI. **Dosage and method of administration**
     A. Morphine may be injected subcutaneously, intramuscularly, or intravenously. The oral and rectal routes produce erratic absorption and are not recommended for use in acutely ill patients.

B. The usual initial dose is 5–10 mg IV or 10–15 mg SC or IM, with maintenance analgesic doses of 5–20 mg IM or IV every 4 hours. The pediatric dose is 0.1–0.2 mg/kg IM or IV every 4 hours.

VII. Formulation. Parenteral: morphine sulfate for injection; variety of available concentrations from 2 to 15 mg/mL.

NALOXONE

James F. Buchanan, PharmD

I. Pharmacology. Naloxone is a pure opioid antagonist that competitively blocks mu, kappa, and sigma opiate receptors within the central nervous system. Naloxone hydrochloride has no opioid agonist properties and can be given safely in large doses without producing respiratory or central nervous system depression. Naloxone is not effective orally but may be given subcutaneously, intramuscularly, or intravenously. After intravenous administration, opioid antagonism occurs within 1–2 minutes and persists for approximately 1–4 hours. The plasma half-life is about 60 minutes.

II. Indications

A. Use naloxone for reversal of acute opioid intoxication manifested by central nervous system and respiratory depression.

B. Use as empirical therapy for stupor or coma suspected to be caused by drug overdose.

C. Anecdotal reports indicate that high-dose naloxone may partially reverse the central nervous system and respiratory depression associated with clonidine and ethanol overdoses, although these effects are inconsistent.

III. Contraindication. Do not use in patients with a known hypersensitivity to naloxone.

IV. Adverse effects

A. Use in opiate-dependent patients may precipitate acute withdrawal syndrome.

B. Pulmonary edema or ventricular fibrillation has occurred shortly after naloxone administration in opioid-intoxicated patients.

C. Agitation, hypertension, and ventricular irritability may occur following opioid antagonism when other stimulants are present. Such reactions have been associated with postanesthetic use of naloxone when catecholamines and large fluid volumes have been administered.

V. Drug interactions. Naloxone antagonizes the analgesic effect of opioids.

VI. Dosage and method of administration. Avoid intramuscular route; absorption is erratic and incomplete.

A. Suspected opioid-induced coma

1. Administer 0.4–2 mg IV; may repeat at 2- to 3-minute intervals. If no response is achieved by a total dose of 10 mg, the diagnosis of opioid overdose should be questioned. The dose for children is the same as for adults.

2. Repeated doses of naloxone may be required to maintain reversal of the effects of opioids with prolonged elimination half-lives (eg, methadone, propoxyphene).

B. Infusion. Give 0.4–0.8 mg/h in 5% dextrose, titrated to clinical effect.

VII. Formulation. Parenteral: Naloxone hydrochloride (Narcan), 0.02, 0.4, 1 mg/mL.

NEUROMUSCULAR BLOCKERS

James F. Buchanan, PharmD

I. Pharmacology

A. Neuromuscular blocking agents produce skeletal muscle paralysis by inhibiting the action of acetylcholine at the neuromuscular junction.

Depolarizing agents (eg, succinylcholine; Table III–6) depolarize the motor end plate and block recovery; transient muscle fasciculations occur with the initial depolarization. Nondepolarizing agents (eg, pancuronium, vecuronium) competitively block the action of acetylcholine at the motor end plate; therefore, no initial muscle fasciculations occur.

B. The neuromuscular blockers produce complete muscle paralysis with no depression of central nervous system function. Thus, patients who are conscious will remain awake but unable to move and patients with status epilepticus may continue to have central nervous system seizure activity despite flaccid paralysis.

C. Succinylcholine produces the most rapid onset of effects, with total paralysis within 30–60 seconds after intravenous administration. It is rapidly hydrolyzed by plasma cholinesterases, and its effects dissipate in 10–20 minutes. Pancuronium produces paralysis within 2–3 minutes, and its effects subside after about 45 minutes. Vecuronium produces paralysis within about 1 minute, with recovery after about 15–20 minutes.

II. Indications
A. Neuromuscular blockers are used to abolish excessive muscular activity, rigidity, or peripheral seizure activity when continued hyperactivity may produce or aggravate rhabdomyolysis and hyperthermia. Examples include drug overdoses involving stimulants (amphetamines, cocaine, phencyclidine) or strychnine and status epilepticus with severe hyperthermia (preferred agent, pancuronium).

B. Neuromuscular blockers provide prompt flaccid paralysis to facilitate orotracheal intubation (preferred agents, succinylcholine or vecuronium).

III. Contraindications
A. Unpreparedness or inability to intubate the trachea and ventilate the patient after total paralysis ensues. Proper equipment and trained personnel must be assembled before the drug is given.

B. Known history of malignant hyperthermia. Succinylcholine use is associated with malignant hyperthermia in susceptible patients (incidence approximately 1 in 50,000).

IV. Adverse effects
A. Complete paralysis results in respiratory depression and apnea.

B. Succinylcholine can stimulate vagal nerves, resulting in sinus bradycardia and atrioventricular block. Children are particularly sensitive to vagotonic effects.

C. Muscle fasciculations may cause increased intraocular and intragastric pressure (the latter of which may result in emesis and aspiration of gastric contents). Rhabdomyolysis and myoglobinuria may be observed, especially in children.

D. Succinylcholine may produce hyperkalemia in patients with myopathy, recent severe burns, or spinal cord injury (this risk develops a few months after the injury).

E. Clinically significant histamine release with bronchospasm may occur with succinylcholine.

TABLE III-6. COMPARISON OF NEUROMUSCULAR BLOCKING AGENTS

Drug	Type	Onset	Duration
Succinylcholine	Depolarizing	30–60 s	2–3 min, dissipates over 10 min
Pancuronium	Nondepolarizing	2–3 min	Dose-dependent; at 0.06 mg/kg, duration of effect is 35–45 min
Vecuronium	Nondepolarizing	1–2 min	Dose-dependent; average, 25–40 min

   F. Neuromuscular blockade is potentiated by hypokalemia and hypocalcemia (nondepolarizing agents) and by hypermagnesemia (depolarizing and nondepolarizing agents).
   G. Prolonged effects may occur after succinylcholine use in patients with genetic deficiency of plasma cholinesterase.
V. Drug interactions
   A. Actions of the nondepolarizing agents are potentiated by ether, methoxyflurane, and enflurane and are inhibited or reversed by anticholinesterase agents (eg, neostigmine, physostigmine, carbamate and organophosphate insecticides).
   B. Organophosphate or carbamate insecticide intoxication may potentiate or prolong the effect of succinylcholine.
   C. Numerous drugs may potentiate neuromuscular blockade. These include calcium antagonists, aminoglycoside antibiotics, propranolol, and membrane-stabilizing drugs (eg, quinidine, propranolol).
VI. Dosage and method of administration
   A. Succinylcholine
      1. Give 0.6 mg/kg IV (infants, 2 mg/kg; children, 1 mg/kg) over 10–30 seconds; may repeat as needed.
      2. To prevent fasciculations, administer a small dose of a nondepolarizing agent (eg, pancuronium, 0.01 mg/kg) 2–3 minutes prior to the succinylcholine.
      3. Pretreat children with atropine (0.005–0.01 mg/kg) to prevent bradycardia or atrioventricular block.
   B. Pancuronium. For infants older than 1 month, children, and adults, give 0.06–0.1 mg/kg IV push, then 0.01–0.02 mg/kg every 20–40 minutes as needed.
   C. Vecuronium. For children older than 1 year and adults, give 0.08–0.1 mg/kg IV push, then 0.01–0.02 mg/kg every 10–20 minutes as needed.
VII. Formulations
   A. Succinylcholine chloride (Anectine, others), 20, 50, 100 mg/mL.
   B. Pancuronium bromide (Pavulon), 1, 2 mg/mL.
   C. Vecuronium bromide (Norcuron), 10 mg of lyophilized powder for reconstitution.

NICOTINAMIDE (NIACINAMIDE)

James F. Buchanan, PharmD

   I. Pharmacology. Nicotinamide (niacinamide), one of the B vitamins, is required for the functioning of the coenzymes nicotinamide adenine dinucleotide (NAD) and nicotinamide adenine dinucleotide phosphate (NADP). NAD and NADP are responsible for energy transfer reactions. Niacin deficiency, which results in pellagra, can be corrected with nicotinamide.
   II. Indications. Nicotinamide is used to prevent the neurologic and endocrinologic toxicity associated with the ingestion of Vacor (PNU), a rodenticide that is believed to act by antagonizing nicotinamide. Best results are achieved when nicotinamide therapy is instituted within 3 hours of ingestion.
   III. Contraindications. There are no contraindications.
   IV. Adverse effects
      A. Headache, dizziness.
      B. Hyperglycemia.
      C. Hepatotoxicity (reported after chronic use with daily dose > 3 g).
   V. Drug interactions. There are no known drug interactions.
   VI. Dosage and method of administration (adults and children). Give 500 mg IV initially, followed by 100–200 mg IV every 4 hours for 48 hours. Then give 100 mg PO 3–5 times daily for 2 weeks. If clinical deterioration from the Vacor progresses during initial therapy with nicotinamide, change dosing interval to every 2 hours. The maximum suggested daily dose is 3 g.

Note: Nicotinic acid (niacin) is *not* a substitute for nicotinamide in the treatment of Vacor ingestions.

VII. **Formulations**
   A. **Parenteral.** Niacinamide, 100 mg/mL.
   B. **Oral.** Niacinamide, 50-, 100-, 500-mg tablets.

NIFEDIPINE

James F. Buchanan, PharmD

I. **Pharmacology.** Nifedipine is a calcium antagonist that inhibits the influx of calcium ions through calcium channels. It acts primarily by dilating systemic and coronary arteries. Unlike some other calcium antagonists (eg, verapamil, diltiazem), nifedipine has minimal effects on cardiac conduction and contractility. Nifedipine is administered orally. The rapid onset of effect (15–30 minutes) following sublingual administration of the capsule contents appears to be due to swallowing of the liquid rather than actual buccal absorption. The drug is metabolized by the liver and has a serum half-life of 2–5 hours.

II. **Indications**
   A. Severe hypertension (eg, following overdose with vasoconstrictive substances such as phenylpropanolamine, cocaine, amphetamines, phencyclidine, or other stimulants).
   B. Adjunctive use as a vasodilator for treatment of peripheral or coronary arterial spasm (ie, ergot, cocaine poisoning).

III. **Contraindications**
   A. Known hypersensitivity to the drug.
   B. Volume depletion (relative contraindication).

IV. **Adverse effects**
   A. Hypotension may result, especially in volume-depleted patients.
   B. Tachycardia, headache, and flushing may occur.
   C. Cerebral perfusion may be compromised if blood pressure is lowered too rapidly in a patient with intracranial hypertension due to stroke or hypertensive encephalopathy.
   D. Use with extreme caution in patients with obstructive cardiomyopathy or aortic stenosis; increased gradient across the aortic valve may cause pulmonary edema and hypotension.

V. **Drug interactions.** Nifedipine has an additive blood pressure-lowering effect when given with other antihypertensives or beta blockers.

VI. **Dosage and method of administration.** The usual dose is a 10-mg capsule (punctured, chewed, and contents swallowed). It may be repeated as needed. Most hypertensive patients respond to 10–20 mg. For childhood hypertensive emergencies, give 0.25–0.5 mg/kg/dose.

VII. **Formulation.** Oral: Nifedipine (Procardia), 10- and 20-mg fluid-filled capsules.

NITRITE, SODIUM AND AMYL

Kathryn H. Keller, PharmD

I. **Pharmacology.** Sodium nitrite injectable solution and amyl nitrite crushable ampules for inhalation are components of the cyanide antidote package. Their value as an antidote to cyanide poisoning is 2-fold: nitrites oxidize hemoglobin to methemoglobin (methemoglobin binds free cyanide) and possibly enhance endothelial cyanide detoxification by producing vasodilation. Administration of a single therapeutic dose of intravenous sodium nitrite is anticipated to produce a methemoglobin concentration of about 20%.

II. **Indications**
   A. Cyanide poisoning.

  B. Possibly hydrogen sulfide poisoning.
III. Contraindications
  A. Profound hypotension is a contraindication.
  B. Significant preexisting methemoglobinemia (> 40%) is a contraindication.
  C. Administration to patients with concurrent carbon monoxide poisoning is a relative contraindication; it may further compromise oxygen transport to the tissues.
IV. Adverse effects
  A. Headache, facial flushing, dizziness, nausea, vomiting, tachycardia, and sweating may occur. These side effects may be masked by the symptoms of cyanide poisoning.
  B. Rapid intravenous administration may result in hypotension.
  C. Excessive methemoglobinemia may result.
V. Drug interactions
  A. Hypotension may be exacerbated by the concurrent presence of alcohol or other vasodilators.
  B. Methylene blue should never be administered to a cyanide-poisoned patient, because it may reverse nitrite-induced methemoglobinemia and result in release of free cyanide ion.
  C. Binding of methemoglobin to cyanide may lower the measured (free) methemoglobin level.
VI. Dosage and method of administration
  A. Amyl nitrite crushable ampules. Crush 1–2 ampules and place under the nose of the victim, who inhales them deeply.
  B. Sodium nitrite parenteral
   1. Administer 300 mg of sodium nitrite (10 mL of 3% solution) IV over 3–5 minutes (children, 0.33 mL/kg to a maximum of 10 mL; pediatric dosing should be based on the hemoglobin concentration, if known; Table III–7).
   2. Oxidation of hemoglobin to methemoglobin occurs within 30 minutes. If no response to treatment occurs within 30 minutes, an additional half-sized dose of intravenous sodium nitrite may be given.
VII. Formulations
  A. Amyl nitrite. Lilly Cyanide Antidote Package, 0.3 mL in crushable ampules.
  B. Sodium nitrite parenteral. Lilly Cyanide Antidote Package, 300 mg in 10 mL of sterile water (3%).

TABLE III-7. PEDIATRIC DOSING OF SODIUM NITRITE BASED ON HEMOGLOBIN CONCENTRATION

Hemoglobin (g/dL)	Initial Dose (mg/kg)	Initial Dose of 3% Sodium Nitrite (mL/kg)
7	5.8	0.19
8	6.6	0.22
9	7.5	0.25
10	8.3	0.27
11	9.1	0.3
12	10	0.33
13	10.8	0.36
14	11.6	0.39

NITROPRUSSIDE

James F. Buchanan, PharmD

 I. **Pharmacology.** Nitroprusside is an ultrashort-acting parenteral hypotensive agent that acts by directly relaxing vascular smooth muscle. Both arterial and venous dilation occur; the effect is more marked in patients with hypertension. A small increase in heart rate may be observed in hypertensive patients. Intravenous administration produces nearly immediate onset of action, with a duration of effect of 1–10 minutes. Nitroprusside is rapidly metabolized, with a serum half-life of about 1–2 minutes.

 II. **Indications.** Nitroprusside is used for rapid control of severe hypertension (eg, in patients with stimulant intoxication or monoamine oxidase inhibitor toxicity), and for peripheral arterial spasm caused by ergot derivatives.

III. **Contraindications**
   A. In patients with an intracranial mass lesion, systemic hypertension may be an appropriate reflex response to increased intracerebral pressure. In such cases, marked lowering of blood pressure may be harmful.
   B. The safety of nitroprusside during pregnancy has not been established.

IV. **Adverse effects**
   A. Nausea, vomiting, headache, and sweating may be due to excessively rapid lowering of the blood pressure.
   B. Cyanide toxicity, manifested by altered mental status and metabolic acidosis, may occur with rapid high-dose infusion (> 10–$15 \mu g/kg/min$).
   C. Thiocyanate intoxication, manifested by disorientation, delirium, muscle twitching, and psychosis, may occur with prolonged infusion therapy, particularly in patients with renal insufficiency.
   D. Rebound hypertension may be observed after sudden discontinuance.

 V. **Drug interactions.** Hypotensive effect is potentiated by other antihypertensive agents and inhalational anesthetics.

VI. **Dosage and method of administration**
   A. Use only in an intensive care setting with continuous blood pressure monitoring.
   B. Dissolve 50 mg of sodium nitroprusside in 3 mL of 5% dextrose; then dilute this solution in 250, 500, or 1000 mL of 5% dextrose to achieve a concentration of 200, 100, or 50 $\mu g/mL$, respectively. Protect the solution from light to avoid photodegradation by covering the bottle and tubing with paper or aluminum foil.
   C. The average dose by intravenous infusion is 3 $\mu g/kg/min$ in children and adults (range, 0.5–10 $\mu g/kg/min$), titrated to desired effect. The maximum rate should not exceed 10 $\mu g/kg/min$ to avoid risk of acute cyanide toxicity.

VII. **Formulation.** Parenteral: Nitroprusside sodium (Nipride, others), 50 mg of lyophilized powder for reconstitution.

NOREPINEPHRINE

Neal L. Benowitz, MD

 I. **Pharmacology.** Norepinephrine is an endogenous catecholamine that stimulates α-adrenergic receptors. It is used primarily as a vasopressor to increase systemic vascular resistance and venous return to the heart. Norepinephrine is also a weak β_1-adrenergic receptor agonist, and it may increase heart rate and cardiac contractility in patients with shock. Norepinephrine is not effective orally and is erratically absorbed after subcutaneous injection. After intravenous administration, the onset of action is nearly immediate, and the duration of effect is 1–2 minutes after the infusion is discontinued.

 II. **Indications.** Norepinephrine is used to increase blood pressure and cardiac output in patients with shock caused by venodilation or low systemic vascular resistance, or both. Hypovolemia, depressed myocardial contractility, hypothermia, and electrolyte imbalance should be corrected first or concurrently.

III. **Contraindications**
  A. Hypertension is a contraindication.
  B. Norepinephrine is relatively contraindicated in patients with peripheral arterial occlusive vascular disease with thrombosis or in those with ergot poisoning.
  C. Use with extreme caution in patients with known hypersensitivity to sulfite preservatives.
  D. Use with extreme caution in patients intoxicated by halogenated or aromatic hydrocarbon solvents or anesthetics.

IV. **Adverse effects**
  A. Severe hypertension, which may result in intracranial hemorrhage, pulmonary edema, or myocardial necrosis.
  B. Aggravation of tissue ischemia, resulting in gangrene.
  C. Tissue necrosis after extravasation.
  D. Anaphylaxis induced by sulfite preservatives in sensitive patients.

V. **Drug interactions**
  A. Enhanced pressor response may occur in the presence of cocaine and cyclic antidepressants, owing to inhibition of neuronal reuptake.
  B. Enhanced pressor response may occur in patients taking monoamine oxidase inhibitors owing to inhibition of neuronal metabolic degradation.
  C. Alpha- and beta-blocking agents may antagonize the adrenergic effects of norepinephrine.
  D. Anticholinergic drugs may block reflex bradycardia, which normally occurs in response to norepinephrine-induced hypertension, enhancing the hypertensive response.
  E. Cyclopropane and halogenated or aromatic hydrocarbon solvents and anesthetics may enhance myocardial sensitivity to arrhythmogenic effects of norepinephrine.

VI. **Dosage and method of administration**
  A. **Avoid extravasation.** *Caution:* The intravenous infusion must be free-flowing, and the infused vein should be observed frequently for signs of infiltration (pallor, coldness, induration). If extravasation occurs, immediately infiltrate the affected area with phentolamine (see p 335), 5–10 mg in 10–15 mL of normal saline (children, 0.1–0.2 mg/kg; maximum 10 mg) via a fine (25- to 27-gauge) hypodermic needle; improvement is evidenced by hyperemia and return to normal temperature.
  B. Norepinephrine bitartrate is rapidly oxidized on exposure to air; it must be kept in its airtight ampule until immediately before use. If the solution appears brown or contains a precipitate, do not use it. The stock solution must be diluted in 5% dextrose or 5% dextrose-saline for infusion; usually, a 4-mg ampule is added to 1 L of fluid to provide 4 μg/mL of solution.
  C. For intravenous infusion, begin at 4–8 μg/min (children, 1–2 μg/min or 0.1 μg/kg/min) and increase as needed every 5–10 minutes.

VII. **Formulation.** Parenteral: Norepinephrine bitartrate (Levophed), 1 mg/mL, 4-mL vial. Contains sodium bisulfite as a preservative.

OXYGEN

James F. Buchanan, PharmD

  I. **Pharmacology.** Oxygen is a necessary oxidant to drive biochemical reactions. Room air contains 21% oxygen.
  II. **Indications**
    A. Supplemental oxygen is indicated when normal oxygenation is impaired because of pulmonary injury, which may result from aspiration

(chemical pneumonitis) or inhalation of toxic gases. The arterial P_{O2} should be maintained at 70–80 mm Hg if possible.

B. Oxygen (100%) is indicated for carbon monoxide poisoning to increase the conversion of carboxyhemoglobin and carboxymyoglobin to hemoglobin and myoglobin and to increase oxygen saturation of the plasma and subsequent delivery to tissues.

C. Hyperbaric oxygen (100% oxygen is delivered to the patient in a pressurized chamber at 2–3 atm) is advocated by some clinicians for more rapid reversal of carbon monoxide poisoning.

III. Contraindications. In paraquat poisoning, oxygen may contribute to lung injury. Slightly hypoxic environments (10–12% oxygen) have been advocated to reduce the risk of pulmonary fibrosis from paraquat.

IV. Adverse effects

A. Prolonged, high concentrations of oxygen are associated with pulmonary alveolar tissue damage. In general, the FI_{O2} should not be maintained at greater than 80% for more than 24 hours.

B. Administration of high oxygen concentrations to patients with severe chronic obstructive pulmonary disease and chronic carbon dioxide retention who are dependent on hypoxemia to provide a drive to breathe may result in respiratory arrest.

Caution: Oxygen is extremely flammable.

V. Drug interactions. Oxygen potentiates toxic pulmonary effects associated with paraquat poisoning.

VI. Dosage and method of administration

A. Supplemental oxygen. Provide supplemental oxygen to maintain a P_{O2} of approximately 70–80 mm Hg. If a P_{O2} greater than 50 mm Hg cannot be maintained with an FI_{O2} of at least 60%, consider positive end-expiratory pressure or continuous positive airway pressure.

B. Carbon monoxide poisoning. Provide 100% oxygen by tight-fitting face mask with a good seal and oxygen reservoir. Consider hyperbaric oxygen if the patient does not respond rapidly and is stable enough for transport.

VII. Formulations

A. Nasal cannula. See Table III–8.

B. Ventimask. Provides variable inspired oxygen concentrations from 24% to 40%.

C. Nonrebreathing reservoir masks. Provide 60–90% inspired oxygen concentrations.

D. Hyperbaric oxygen. One hundred percent oxygen can be delivered at a pressure of 2–3 atm.

PENICILLAMINE

James F. Buchanan, PharmD

I. Pharmacology. Penicillamine is a derivative of penicillin that has no antimicrobial activity but effectively chelates heavy metals such as lead, mer-

TABLE III-8. AMOUNT OF OXYGEN PROVIDED BY NASAL CANNULA

Flow Rate (L/min)	Approximate Inspired Oxygen Concentration (%)
1	24
2	28
5	40

cury, arsenic, and copper. It is commonly used as adjunctive therapy following initial treatment with calcium EDTA (see p 308) or BAL (dimercaprol; p 294). Penicillamine is well absorbed orally, and the penicillamine-metal complex is eliminated in the urine. No parenteral form is available.
II. **Indications.** Penicillamine is used to treat heavy metal poisoning caused by lead (penicillamine may be used alone for minor intoxications or as adjunctive therapy after calcium EDTA or BAL in moderate to severe intoxications), mercury (after initial BAL therapy), copper, or arsenic (adjunctive therapy after initial BAL treatment).
III. **Contraindications**
   A. Penicillin allergy is a contraindication.
   B. Renal insufficiency is a relative contraindication because the complex is eliminated only through the urine.
   C. Concomitant administration with other hematopoietic-depressant drugs (eg, gold salts, immunosuppressants, antimalarial agents, phenylbutazone) is not recommended.
IV. **Adverse effects**
   A. Hypersensitivity reactions: rash, pruritus, drug fever, hematuria, and proteinuria.
   B. Leukopenia, thrombocytopenia, hemolytic anemia, agranulocytosis.
   C. Hepatitis, pancreatitis.
   D. Anorexia, nausea, vomiting, epigastric pain, impairment of taste.
V. **Drug interactions.** Penicillamine may potentiate hematopoietic-depressant effects of drugs such as gold salts, immunosuppressants, antimalarial agents, and phenylbutazone.
VI. **Dosage and method of administration**
   A. Penicillamine should be taken on an empty stomach, at least 1 hour before meals and at bedtime.
   B. Administer 250 mg orally 4 times daily (100 mg/kg/d for arsenic; 25–40 mg/kg/d for lead; in children, maximum 1 g/d) for 5 days. Reassess need for chelation therapy based on urinary levels of intoxicating metal.
VII. **Formulations.** Oral: Penicillamine (Cuprimine, Depen), 125-, 250-mg capsules, 250-mg tablets. (N-Acetylpenicillamine may demonstrate better central nervous system and peripheral nerve penetration, but it is not currently available in the USA.)

PENTOBARBITAL

James F. Buchanan, PharmD

I. **Pharmacology.** Pentobarbital is a short-acting barbiturate with anticonvulsant as well as sedative-hypnotic properties. It is used as a third-line drug in the treatment of status epilepticus. Following intravenous administration of a single dose, the onset of effect occurs within about 1 minute and lasts about 15 minutes. Pentobarbital demonstrates a biphasic elimination pattern; the half-life of the initial phase is 4 hours, and the terminal phase half-life is 35–50 hours. Effects are prolonged after termination of a continuous infusion.
II. **Indications.** Pentobarbital is used for the management of status epilepticus that is unresponsive to conventional anticonvulsant therapy (eg, diazepam, phenytoin, and phenobarbital). If the use of pentobarbital for seizure control is considered, consultation with a neurologist is recommended.
III. **Contraindications**
   A. Known sensitivity to the drug.
   B. Manifest or latent porphyria.
IV. **Adverse effects**
   A. Central nervous system depression, coma, and respiratory arrest may occur, especially with rapid bolus or excessive doses.

  B. Hypotension may result, especially with rapid intravenous infusion.
  C. Laryngospasm and bronchospasm have been reported after rapid intravenous injection, although the mechanism is unknown.
V. Drug interactions
  A. Pentobarbital has additive central nervous system and respiratory depression effects with other sedative drugs.
  B. Hepatic enzyme induction is generally not encountered with acute pentobarbital overdose, although it may occur within 24–48 hours.
VI. Dosage and method of administration
  A. Intermittent intravenous bolus. Give 100 mg IV slowly over at least 2 minutes; may repeat as needed at 2-minute intervals, to a maximum dose of 300–500 mg (children, 1 mg/kg IV, repeated as needed to a maximum of 5–6 mg/kg).
  B. Continuous intravenous infusion. Administer a loading dose of 5–6 mg/kg IV over 1 hour (not to exceed 50 mg/min; children, 1 mg/kg/min), followed by maintenance infusion of 0.5–3 mg/kg/h titrated to the desired effect. Electroencephalographic achievement of burst suppression correlates with serum pentobarbital concentration of 25–40 μg/mL.
VII. Formulation. Parenteral: Pentobarbital sodium (Nembutal, others), 50 mg/mL.

PHENOBARBITAL

James F. Buchanan, PharmD

  I. Pharmacology. Phenobarbital is a barbiturate commonly used as an anticonvulsant. Because of the delay in onset of the therapeutic effect of phenobarbital, diazepam (see p 302) is usually the initial agent for parenteral anticonvulsant therapy. After an oral dose of phenobarbital, peak brain concentrations are achieved within 10–15 hours. Onset of effect following intravenous administration is usually within 5 minutes, although peak effects may take up to 30 minutes. The plasma elimination half-life is 48–100 hours.
 II. Indications
  A. Control of tonic-clonic seizures and status epilepticus, generally as a second- or third-line agent after diazepam and phenytoin have been tried.
  B. Withdrawal from ethanol and other sedative-hypnotic drugs.
III. Contraindications
  A. Known sensitivity to barbiturates.
  B. Manifest or latent porphyria.
IV. Adverse effects
  A. Central nervous system depression, coma, and respiratory arrest may result, especially with rapid bolus or excessive doses.
  B. Hypotension may result from rapid intravenous administration. This can be prevented by limiting the rate of administration to less than 50 mg/min (children, 1 mg/kg/min).
 V. Drug interactions
  A. Phenobarbital has additive central nervous system and respiratory depression effects with other sedative drugs.
  B. Hepatic enzyme induction is *not* encountered with acute phenobarbital dosing.
VI. Dosage and method of administration
  A. For parenteral phenobarbital, administer slowly intravenously (rate < 50 mg/min; children, < 1 mg/kg/min) until seizures are controlled or the loading dose of 10–15 mg/kg is achieved. Slow the infusion rate if hypotension develops. Intermittent infusions of 2 mg/kg every 5–15 minutes may diminish the risk of respiratory depression or hypotension.
  B. If intravenous access is not immediately available, phenobarbital may

be given intramuscularly; the initial dose in adults and children is 3–5 mg/kg IM.
VII. Formulation. Parenteral: Phenobarbital sodium (Luminal, others), 30, 60, 65, 130 mg/mL.

PHENTOLAMINE
James F. Buchanan, PharmD

I. **Pharmacology.** Phentolamine is a presynaptic and postsynaptic α-adrenergic receptor blocker that produces peripheral vasodilation. By acting on both venous and arterial vessels, it decreases total peripheral resistance and venous return. Phentolamine has a rapid onset of action (usually 2 minutes) and short duration of effect (approximately 15–20 minutes).

II. **Indications**
   A. Hypertensive crisis associated with phenylpropanolamine or stimulant drug overdose (eg, amphetamine, cocaine, ephedrine, etc).
   B. Hypertensive crisis due to interaction between monoamine oxidase inhibitors and tyramine or other sympathomimetic amines.
   C. Hypertensive crisis associated with sudden withdrawal of sympatholytic antihypertensive drugs such as clonidine.
   D. Extravasation of vasoconstrictive agents such as epinephrine, norepinephrine, and dopamine.

III. **Contraindications.** Use with extreme caution in patients with intracranial hemorrhage or ischemic stroke; any lowering of blood pressure may aggravate brain injury.

IV. **Adverse effects**
   A. Hypotension and reflex tachycardia may occur from excessive doses.
   B. Anginal chest pain and cardiac arrhythmias may occur.
   C. Slow intravenous infusion (< 0.3 mg/min) may result in transient increased blood pressure caused by stimulation of β-adrenergic receptors.

V. **Drug interactions.** Additive or synergistic effects may occur with other antihypertensive agents, especially other α-adrenergic antagonists (eg, prazosin, terazosin, and yohimbine).

VI. **Dosage and method of administration**
   A. **Parenteral.** Give 1–5 mg IV (children, 0.02–0.1 mg/kg) as a bolus; may repeat at 5- to 10-minute intervals (or constant infusion of 0.1–2 mg/min) as needed to lower blood pressure to a desired level (usually < 100–110 mm Hg diastolic in adults, 80 mm Hg diastolic in children, but may vary depending on the clinical situation).
   B. **Catecholamine extravasation.** Infiltrate 5–10 mg in 10–15 mL of normal saline (children, 0.1–0.2 mg/kg; maximum 10 mg) into affected area with a fine (25- to 27-gauge) hypodermic needle; improvement is evidenced by hyperemia and return to normal temperature.

VII. **Formulation.** Parenteral: Phentolamine mesylate (Regitine), 5 mg.

PHENYTOIN
Kathyrn H. Keller, PharmD

I. **Pharmacology.** The neuronal membrane-stabilizing actions of phenytoin make this the primary drug for sustained control of acute and chronic seizure disorders and a useful drug for certain cardiac arrhythmias. Because of the relatively slow onset of anticonvulsant action, phenytoin is usually administered after diazepam. At serum concentrations considered therapeutic for seizure control, phenytoin acts similarly to lidocaine to reduce ventricular premature depolarizations and suppress ventricular tachycardia. After intravenous administration, peak therapeutic effects are attained within 1 hour. The therapeutic serum concentration for seizure control is 10–20 mg/L. Elimination is nonlinear, with an apparent half-life averaging 22 hours.

II. **Indications**
   A. Control of generalized tonic-clonic seizures or status epilepticus caused by various drugs and poisons.
   B. Control of cardiac arrhythmias associated with digitalis intoxication.
   C. Treating cardiac arrhythmias caused by cyclic antidepressant intoxication (controversial).

III. **Contraindications.** Do not use if the patient has a known hypersensitivity to phenytoin or other hydantoins.

IV. **Adverse effects**
   A. Rapid intravenous administration (> 50 mg/min in adults or 1 mg/kg/min in children) may produce hypotension, atrioventricular block, and cardiovascular collapse, probably owing to the propylene glycol diluent.
   B. Extravasation may result in local tissue necrosis and sloughing.
   C. Drowsiness, ataxia, nystagmus, and nausea may occur.

V. **Drug interactions.** The various drug interactions associated with chronic phenytoin dosing (ie, accelerated metabolism of other drugs) are not applicable to its acute emergency use.

VI. **Dosage and method of administration**
   A. **Parenteral.** Administer a loading dose of 15–20 mg/kg IV slowly at a rate not to exceed 50 mg/min (or 1 mg/kg/min in children). Do *not* administer by the intramuscular route.
   B. **Maintenance dose.** Give 5 mg/kg/d as a single oral dose of capsules or twice daily for other dosage forms and in children. Monitor serum phenytoin levels.

VII. **Formulations**
   A. **Parenteral.** Phenytoin sodium (Dilantin, others), 50 mg/mL, 10-mL ampules.
   B. **Oral.** Phenytoin sodium (Dilantin, others), 30- and 100-mg capsules.

PHYSOSTIGMINE

James F. Buchanan, PharmD

I. **Pharmacology.** Physostigmine is a reversible inhibitor of acetylcholinesterase, the enzyme that degrades acetylcholine. Physostigmine increases concentrations of acetylcholine, causing stimulation of both muscarinic and nicotinic receptors. The tertiary amine structure of physostigmine allows it to penetrate the blood-brain barrier and exert central cholinergic effects as well. After parenteral administration, the onset of action is within 3–8 minutes and the duration of effect is usually 30–60 minutes. The elimination half-life is 15–40 minutes.

II. **Indications**
   A. Physostigmine is used for the management of severe anticholinergic syndrome (agitated delirium, sinus tachycardia, hyperthermia with absent sweating). Its overall utility is limited, because most patients with anticholinergic poisoning can be managed supportively.
   B. Physostigmine is sometimes used diagnostically to differentiate functional psychosis from anticholinergic delirium.

III. **Contraindications**
   A. Physostigmine should *not* be used as an antidote for cyclic antidepressant overdose because it may worsen cardiac conduction disturbances, cause bradyarrhythmias or asystole, and aggravate or precipitate seizures.
   B. Do not use physostigmine with concurrent use of depolarizing neuromuscular blockers (eg, succinylcholine, decamethonium).

IV. **Adverse effects**

A. Bradycardia, heart block, asystole.
B. Seizures (particularly with rapid administration).
C. Nausea, vomiting, diarrhea.
D. Bronchorrhea, bronchospasm.
E. Fasciculations, muscle weakness.

V. **Drug interactions**
  A. Physostigmine may potentiate depolarizing neuromuscular blocking agents (eg, succinylcholine, decamethonium).
  B. It may have additive depressant effects on cardiac conduction in patients with cyclic antidepressant overdose.

VI. **Dosage and method of administration.** Parenteral: 0.5–2 mg slow IV push (children, 0.02 mg/kg); may repeat as needed every 20–30 minutes. Atropine (see p 293) should be kept nearby to reverse excessive muscarinic stimulation.

VII. **Formulation.** Parenteral: Physostigmine salicylate (Antilirium), 1 mg/mL.

PRALIDOXIME (2-PAM)

Olga F. Woo, PharmD

I. **Pharmacology.** Pralidoxime (2-PAM) reverses organophosphate poisoning by reactivating phosphorylated cholinesterase enzyme and protecting the enzyme from further inhibition. To be most effective, it should be given before the enzyme has been irreversibly bound ("aged") by the organophosphate (about 24 hours). The clinical effect of pralidoxime is most apparent at nicotinic receptors, with reversal of skeletal muscle weakness and muscle fasciculations. Its impact on muscarinic symptoms (salivation, sweating, bradycardia, bronchorrhea) is less pronounced than that of the antimuscarinic agent atropine (see p 293). Peak plasma concentrations are reached within 5–15 minutes after intravenous administration. Pralidoxime is eliminated by renal excretion and hepatic metabolism, with a half-life of 0.8–2.7 hours.

II. **Indications**
  A. Pralidoxime is used to treat poisoning caused by organophosphate insecticides. It is most effective if treatment is initiated within the first 24 hours following exposure.
  B. The use of pralidoxime in cases of carbamate poisoning remains controversial; it is probably not harmful, but because of the short duration of reversible effects due to carbamates, it is rarely used.

III. **Contraindications**
  A. Use in patients with myasthenia gravis may precipitate a myasthenic crisis.
  B. Use with caution and in reduced doses in patients with renal impairment.

IV. **Adverse effects**
  A. Nausea, headache, dizziness, diplopia, and hyperventilation may occur.
  B. Rapid intravenous administration may result in tachycardia, laryngospasm, muscle rigidity, and transient neuromuscular blockade.

V. **Drug interactions.** Symptoms of atropinization may occur more quickly when atropine and pralidoxime are administered concurrently.

VI. **Dosage and method of administration**
  A. Give 1–2 g IV (children, 25–50 mg/kg, maximum 1 g) over 5–10 minutes (rate not to exceed 200 mg/min in adults or 4 mg/kg/min in children), or give intravenous infusion in 100 mL of saline (1–2 mL/kg) over 15–30 minutes. Repeat dose in 1 hour if muscle weakness is not relieved.
  B. Repeat the initial dose every 4–12 hours as needed to control nicotinic symptoms. This is particularly important for treatment of lipid-soluble organophosphates such as fenthion, which may have prolonged effects.
  C. The intravenous route is preferred over oral therapy, particularly in the presence of gastrointestinal symptoms.

VII. **Formulation.** Parenteral: Pralidoxime chloride (Protopam), 1 g with 20 mL sterile water.

PROPRANOLOL

James F. Buchanan, PharmD

I. **Pharmacology.** Propranolol is a nonselective β-adrenergic blocker that acts on β_1-receptors in the myocardium and β_2-receptors in the lung, vascular smooth muscle, and kidney. Within the myocardium, propranolol depresses heart rate, conduction velocity, myocardial contractility, and automaticity. Although propranolol is effective orally, for toxicologic emergencies it is usually administered by the intravenous route. After intravenous injection, the onset of action is nearly immediate and the duration of effect is 10 minutes to 2 hours, depending on the cumulative dose. The drug is eliminated by hepatic metabolism, with a half-life of about 2–3 hours.

II. **Indications**
   A. To control excessive sinus tachycardia or ventricular arrhythmias caused by catecholamine excess (eg, theophylline, caffeine) or sympathomimetic drug intoxication (eg, amphetamines, ephedrine, cocaine).
   B. To control hypertension in patients with excessive β_1-mediated increase in heart rate and contractility; use in conjunction with a vasodilator (eg, phentolamine; see p 335) in patients with mixed α- and β-adrenergic hyperstimulation.
   C. To raise the diastolic blood pressure in patients with hypotension due to excessive β_2-mediated vasodilation (eg, theophylline or caffeine intoxication).

III. **Contraindications**
   A. Use with extreme caution in patients with asthma, congestive heart failure, sinus node dysfunction, or other cardiac conduction disease and in those receiving cardiac-depressant drugs.
   B. Do not use as single therapy for hypertension due to sympathomimetic overdose. Propranolol produces peripheral vascular beta-blockade, abolishing β_2-mediated vasodilation and leaving unopposed α-mediated vasoconstriction, resulting in paradoxic worsening of hypertension.

IV. **Adverse effects**
   A. Bradycardia, sinus and atrioventricular block.
   B. Hypotension, congestive heart failure.
   C. Bronchospasm in patients with asthma or bronchospastic chronic obstructive pulmonary disease.

V. **Drug interactions**
   A. Propranolol has an additive hypotensive effect with other antihypertensive agents.
   B. It may potentiate competitive neuromuscular blockers (see p 326).
   C. The drug has additive depressant effects on cardiac conduction and contractility when given with some calcium antagonists (eg, verapamil, diltiazem).
   D. Cimetidine reduces hepatic clearance of propranolol.

VI. **Dosage and method of administration**
   A. **Parenteral.** Give 0.5–3 mg IV (children, 0.01–0.02 mg/kg IV; maximum 1 mg/dose); dose may be repeated as needed after 5–10 minutes. The dose required for complete β-receptor blockade is 0.2 mg/kg.
   B. **Oral.** Oral dosing may be initiated after the patient is stabilized; the dosage range is about 1–5 mg/kg/d in 3–4 divided doses for both children and adults.

VII. **Formulations**
   A. **Parenteral.** Propranolol hydrochloride (Inderal), 1 mg/mL.
   B. **Oral.** Propranolol hydrochloride (Inderal, others), 60-, 80-, 120-, 160-mg capsules; 10-, 20-, 40-, 60-, 80-, 90-mg tablets.

PROTAMINE

James F. Buchanan, PharmD

I. **Pharmacology.** Protamine is a cationic protein that rapidly binds to and inactivates heparin. The onset of action after intravenous administration is nearly immediate (30–60 s).

II. **Indications**
   A. Protamine is used for the reversal of the anticoagulant effect of heparin when an excessively large dose has been inadvertently administered. Protamine is generally not needed for treatment of bleeding during standard heparin therapy because discontinuance of the heparin infusion is generally sufficient.
   B. It is used for reversal of regional anticoagulation in the hemodialysis circuit in cases in which anticoagulation of the patient would be contraindicated (ie, active gastrointestinal or central nervous system bleeding).

III. **Contraindications**
   A. Do not give protamine to patients with known sensitivity to the drug.
   B. Protamine reconstituted with benzyl alcohol should not be used in neonates because of suspected toxicity from the alcohol.

IV. **Adverse effects**
   A. Rapid intravenous administration is associated with hypotension, bradycardia, and anaphylactoid reactions.
   B. Rebound effect due to heparin may occur within 8 hours of protamine administration.

V. **Drug interactions.** The anticoagulant effect of heparin is inhibited by protamine.

VI. **Dosage and method of administration**
   A. Administer protamine by slow intravenous injection.
   B. The dose of protamine depends on the total dose and time since administration of heparin.
      1. Immediately after heparin administration, give 1–1.5 mg of protamine for each 100 units of heparin.
      2. At 30–60 minutes after heparin administration, give only 0.5–0.75 mg of protamine for each 100 units of heparin.
      3. Two hours after heparin administration, give only 0.25–0.375 mg of protamine for each 100 units of heparin.
      4. If heparin was administered by constant infusion, give 25–50 mg of protamine.

VII. **Formulation.** Parenteral: Protamine sulfate, 50 and 250 mg and 10 mg/mL.

PYRIDOXINE (VITAMIN B_6)

Kathryn H. Keller, PharmD

I. **Pharmacology.** Pyridoxine (vitamin B_6) is a water-soluble B-complex vitamin that acts as a cofactor in many enzymatic reactions. Overdose involving isoniazid or other monomethylhydrazines (eg, gyromitrin mushrooms, some rocket fuel) may cause seizures by interfering with pyridoxine utilization in the brain, and pyridoxine given in high doses can rapidly control these seizures. In ethylene glycol intoxication, pyridoxine theoretically may enhance metabolic conversion of the toxic metabolite, glyoxylic acid, to the nontoxic product, glycine. Pyridoxine is well absorbed orally but is usually given intravenously for urgent uses. The biologic half-life is about 15–20 days.

II. **Indications**
   A. Acute management of seizures caused by intoxication with isoniazid, *Gyromitra* mushrooms (monomethylhydrazine); or hydrazine (rocket fuel).

    B. Adjunct to therapy for ethylene glycol intoxication.

III. Contraindications. There are no known contraindications.

IV. Adverse effects

    A. Usually no adverse effects are noted from acute dosing of pyridoxine.

    B. Chronic excessive doses may result in peripheral neuropathy.

    C. Excessive pyridoxine use in pregnancy has resulted in pyridoxine-dependency seizures in neonates.

V. Drug interactions. No interactions are associated with acute dosing.

VI. Dosage and method of administration

    A. Isoniazid poisoning. Give 1 g of pyridoxine intravenously for each gram of isoniazid known to have been ingested. If ingested amount is unknown, administer 4–5 g IV empirically and repeat as needed.

    B. Monomethylhydrazine poisoning. Give 25 mg/kg IV; may repeat as necessary.

    C. Ethylene glycol poisoning. Give 50 mg IV or IM every 6 hours until intoxication is resolved.

VII. Formulation. Parenteral: Pyridoxine hydrochloride (Beesix, Hexa-Betalin), 100 mg/mL (10% solution).

THIAMINE (VITAMIN B₁)

James F. Buchanan, PharmD

    I. Pharmacology. Thiamine (vitamin B_1) is a water-soluble vitamin that acts as an essential cofactor for various pathways of carbohydrate metabolism. Thiamine also acts as a cofactor in the metabolism of glyoxylic acid (produced in ethylene glycol intoxication). Thiamine deficiency may result in beriberi and Wernicke-Korsakoff syndrome. Thiamine is rapidly absorbed after oral, intramuscular, or intravenous administration.

II. Indications

    A. Empirical therapy to prevent Wernicke-Korsakoff syndrome in alcoholic or malnourished patients.

    B. Adjunctive treatment in patients poisoned with ethylene glycol to possibly enhance the detoxification of glyoxylic acid.

III. Contraindications. Do not give to patients with known sensitivity to thiamine.

IV. Adverse effects

    A. Anaphylactoid reactions, vasodilation, hypotension, weakness, and angioedema following rapid intravenous injection.

    B. Acute pulmonary edema in patients with beriberi owing to sudden increase in vascular resistance.

V. Drug interactions. Theoretically, thiamine may enhance the effect of neuromuscular blockers, although the clinical significance is unclear.

VI. Dosage and method of administration. Parenteral: 100 mg (children, 50 mg) slowly IV (over 5 minutes) or IM; repeat every 6 hours.

VII. Formulation. Parenteral: Thiamine hydrochloride (Betalin, others), 100 and 200 mg/mL.

THIOSULFATE, SODIUM

Susan Kim, PharmD

    I. Pharmacology. Sodium thiosulfate is a sulfur donor that promotes the conversion of cyanide to less toxic thiocyanate by the sulfur transferase enzyme rhodanese. Thiosulfate is essentially nontoxic and may be given empirically in suspected cyanide poisoning.

II. Indications

    A. Acute cyanide poisoning.

    B. Suspected cyanide poisoning (ie, smoke inhalation victims).

III. Contraindications. There are no known contraindications.

  IV. Adverse effects. May produce burning sensation during infusion.
   V. Drug interactions. There are no known drug interactions.
  VI. Dosage and method of administration. Parenteral: Administer 12.5 g (50 mL
     of 25% solution) IV. The pediatric dose is 400 mg/kg (1.6 mL/kg of 25%
     solution) up to 50 mL. May be repeated in 30–60 minutes.
 VII. Formulation. Parenteral: Eli Lilly Cyanide Kit; thiosulfate sodium, 25%
     solution, 50 mL.

VITAMIN K₁ (PHYTONADIONE)

James F. Buchanan, PharmD

   I. Pharmacology. Vitamin K_1 is an essential cofactor in the hepatic synthesis
     of coagulation factors II, VII, IX, X, and prothrombin. In adequate doses,
     vitamin K_1 reverses the inhibitory effects of coumarin and indanedione
     derivatives on the synthesis of these factors. **Vitamin K_3 (menadione) is *not*
     effective** in reversing excessive anticoagulation caused by these agents.
     After parenteral vitamin K_1 administration, there is a 6- to 8-hour delay
     before vitamin K-dependent coagulation factors begin to achieve signifi-
     cant levels and peak effects are not seen until 1–2 days after initiation of
     therapy. The duration of effect is 1–2 weeks. The response to vitamin K_1 is
     variable; it is influenced by the potency of the ingested anticoagulant and
     the patient's hepatic biosynthetic capability. Fresh-frozen plasma or whole
     blood is indicated for immediate control of serious hemorrhage.
  II. Indications
    A. Excessive anticoagulation due to coumarin and indanedione deriva-
       tives.
    B. Vitamin K deficiency (eg, malnutrition, malabsorption) with coagulo-
       pathy.
    C. Hypoprothrombinemia due to salicylate intoxication.
 III. Contraindications. Do not use in patients with known hypersensitivity.
 IV. Adverse effects
    A. Anaphylactoid reactions have been reported after intravenous adminis-
       tration. Intravenous use should be restricted to true emergencies; the
       patient must be closely monitored in an intensive care setting.
    B. Intramuscular administration in anticoagulated patients may cause
       large, painful hematomas. This can be avoided by using oral or subcuta-
       neous routes.
    C. Patients receiving anticoagulants for medical reasons (eg, deep vein
       thrombosis, prosthetic heart valves) may experience untoward effects
       from complete reversal of their anticoagulation status. These patients
       should receive vitamin K_1 only if anticoagulation is dangerously exces-
       sive and then only with extremely small titrated doses (1–2 mg) until the
       prothrombin time is in the desired therapeutic range (eg, 1.5–2 times
       normal). Anticoagulation with heparin may be indicated until the de-
       sired prothrombin time is achieved.
   V. Drug interactions. Vitamin K_1 causes antagonism of coumadin and in-
     danedione derivatives.
  VI. Dosage and method of administration
    A. Oral. Oral therapy may be indicated with small ingestions of anticoagu-
       lants. The usual oral dose of vitamin K_1 is 10–25 mg in adults and 5–10
       mg in children. This dose may be repeated in 12–24 hours if needed. In
       intoxication with "superwarfarin" indanedione derivatives (see p 132),
       therapy should be continued for several weeks.
    B. Intramuscular and subcutaneous. Subcutaneous administration is the
       preferred route. The adult dose is 5–10 mg, and that for children is 1–5
       mg. May be repeated in 6–8 hours.
    C. Intravenous. Intravenous administration is used only when hemorrhage
       is present or imminent. The usual dose is 10–50 mg (5–20 mg in chil-

dren), depending on the severity of anticoagulation, in preservative-free dextrose or sodium chloride solution. Give slowly at a rate not to exceed 1 mg/min. Dose may be repeated every 4 hours as needed.

VII. Formulations
  A. Oral. Phytonadione (Mephyton), 5-mg tablets.
  B. Parenteral. Phytonadione (AquaMEPHYTON, Konakion) 2 and 10 mg/mL.

References

Gilman AG et al (editors): *Goodman & Gilman's The Pharmacological Basis of Therapeutics,* 7th ed. Macmillan, 1985.

Kastrup EK et al (editors): *Drug Facts & Comparisons 1988.* Lippincott, 1988.

Martindale W (editor): *The Extra Pharmacopoeia,* 28th ed. Rittenhouse, 1982.

McEnvoy GK (editor): *American Hospital Formulary Service Drug Information 1988.* American Society of Hospital Pharmacists, 1988.

US Pharmacopoeial Convention: *Drug Information for the Health Care Provider.* USPC, 1988.

Section IV. Environmental and Occupational Toxicology

EMERGENCY MEDICAL RESPONSE TO HAZARDOUS MATERIALS INCIDENTS

Frank J. Mycroft, PhD, Jeffrey R. Jones, MPH, CIH, and Kent R. Olson, MD

With the increasing numbers of accidental incidents involving hazardous materials, local emergency response providers must be prepared to handle victims who may be contaminated with chemical substances. Many local jurisdictions are developing Hazardous Materials (HazMat) teams, usually comprised of fire and paramedical personnel who are trained to identify hazardous situations quickly and to take the lead in organizing a response. Health care providers such as ambulance personnel, nurses, physicians, and local hospital officials should participate in emergency response planning with their local HazMat team before a chemical disaster occurs.

I. **General Considerations.** The most important elements of successful medical management of a hazardous materials incident are as follows:
- A. Use extreme caution when dealing with unknown or unstable conditions.
- B. Rapidly assess the potential acute hazard of the substances involved.
- C. Determine the potential for secondary contamination of downstream personnel and facilities.
- D. Perform any needed decontamination on scene ***before*** victim transport, if possible.

II. **Organization of the incident.** Most incidents are operated under the control of the Incident Commander, usually the senior fire chief or police or coast guard officer. The first priorities will be to secure the area, establish a command post, create hazard zones, and appoint a health and safety officer.
- A. **Hazard zones** (Fig IV–1) are determined by the nature of the spilled substance and wind and geographic conditions. In general, the command post and support area will be upwind and upgrade from the spill, with sufficient distance to allow rapid escape if conditions change.
  1. The **"hot" area** is the most dangerous and may require carefully selected personal protective gear as well as vigorous decontamination when leaving the area.
  2. Basic decontamination, if indicated, should be carried out in the **"contamination reduction"** area.
  3. Patients in the hot and contamination reduction areas will generally receive only rudimentary first aid such as cervical spine stabilization and placement on a backboard. Additional first aid or more sophisticated medical treatment will be provided in the **support area** after the victim has undergone basic decontamination.
- B. **Health and safety officer.** A predesignated person, usually a member of the HazMat team, will be in charge of health and safety. This person will determine the nature and degree of any hazard, the need for specialized personal protective gear, and the decontamination requirements; the officer will also monitor entry into and exit from the spill site.

III. **Assessment of hazard potential.** Be prepared to recognize dangerous situations and to respond appropriately. The potential for toxic or other injury depends on the identities of the chemicals involved, their toxicities, their chemical and physical properties, the conditions of exposure, and the

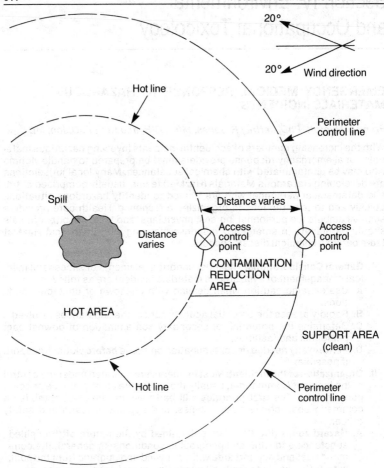

Figure IV-1. Control zones at a hazardous materials incident site.

circumstances surrounding their release. Be aware that a substance's reactivity, flammability, explosivity, or corrosivity may be a source of greater hazard than its systemic toxicity.

A. Identify the substances involved. Make inquiries and look for labels, warning placards, or shipping papers.

1. The **National Fire Protection Association (NFPA)** has developed a labeling system for describing chemical hazards that is widely used (Fig IV–2, p 345 and p 346).

2. The **US Department of Transportation (DOT)** has developed a system of warning placards for vehicles carrying hazardous materials. The DOT placards usually bear a 4-digit substance identification code and also a single-digit hazard classification code (Fig IV–3). Identification of the substance from the 4-digit code can be provided by the regional poison control center, Chemtrec, or the DOT manual (see **B,** below).

3. **Shipping papers,** which may include **Material Safety Data Sheets** (MSDSs), are usually carried by the driver or pilot or may be found in the cab of the truck.

	Color Code: BLUE		Color Code: RED		(Stability) Color Code: YELLOW
	Type of Possible Injury		Susceptibility of Materials to Burning		Susceptibility to Release of Energy
Signal		Signal		Signal	
4	Materials which on very short exposure could cause death or major residual injury even though prompt medical treatment were given.	4	Materials which will rapidly or completely vaporize at atmospheric pressure and normal ambient temperature, or which are readily dispersed in air and which will burn readily.	4	Materials which in themselves are readily capable of detonation or of explosive decomposition or reaction at normal temperatures and pressures.
3	Materials which on short exposure could cause serious temporary or residual injury even though prompt medical treatment were given.	3	Liquids and solids that can be ignited under almost all ambient temperature conditions.	3	Materials which in themselves are capable of detonation or explosive reaction but require a strong initiating source or which must be heated under confinement before initiation or which react explosively with water.
2	Materials which on intense or continued exposure could cause temporary incapacitation or possible residual injury unless prompt medical treatment is given.	2	Materials that must be moderately heated or exposed to relatively high ambient temperatures before ignition can occur.	2	Materials which in themselves are normally unstable and readily undergo violent chemical change but do not detonate. Also materials which may react violently with water or which may form potentially explosive mixtures with water.
1	Materials which on exposure would cause irritation but only minor residual injury even if no treatment is given.	1	Materials that must be preheated before ignition can occur.	1	Materials which in themselves are normally stable, but which can become unstable at elevated temperatures and pressures or which may react with water with some release of energy but not violently.
0	Materials which on exposure under fire conditions would offer no hazard beyond that of ordinary combustible material.	0	Materials that will not burn.	0	Materials which in themselves are normally stable, even under fire exposure conditions, and which are not reactive with water.

Figure IV-2. National Fire Protection Association (NFPA) identification of the hazards of materials. Continued on p 346. (Reproduced, with permission, from *Fire Protection Guide on Hazardous Materials*, 9th ed. National Fire Protection Association, 1986.)

NATIONAL FIRE PROTECTION ASSOCIATION
IDENTIFICATION OF THE FIRE HAZARDS OF MATERIALS

NFPA 704
HAZARD SIGNAL SYSTEM

Flammability (Red)

4 – Highly flammable and volatile
3 – Highly flammable
2 – Flammable
1 – Low flammability
0 – Does not burn

Health Hazard (Blue)

4 – Extremely hazardous
3 – Moderately hazardous
2 – Hazardous
1 – Slightly hazardous
0 – No health hazard

Reactivity (Yellow)

4 – Highly explosive, detonates readily
3 – Explosive, less readily detonated
2 – Violently reactive but does not detonate
1 – Not violently reactive
0 – Normally stable

Other Hazards

☢ – Radioactive

OX – Oxidizer

〰 – Water-reactive

Figure IV-2. National Fire Protection Association (NFPA) identification of the hazards of materials. (Continued)

B. **Obtain acute toxicity information.** Determine the acute health effects and obtain advice on general hazards, decontamination procedures, and medical management of victims. Resources include:
   1. **Regional poison control centers** (see Table I–41, p 51). The poison control center can provide information on immediate health effects, the need for decontamination or specialized protective gear, and specific treatment including the use of antidotes. The regional poison center can also provide consultation with a medical toxicologist.
   2. **Chemtrec** ([800] 424-9300). Operated by chemical manufacturing industries, this hotline can provide information on the identity and hazardous properties of chemicals and, when appropriate, can put the caller in touch with industry representatives.
   3. **Table IV–12** (p 365) and specific chemicals covered in Section II of this manual.
   4. A variety of texts, journals, and computerized information systems are available but are of uneven scope or depth. See the reference list at the end of this chapter.
C. **Recognize dangerous environments.** In general, environments likely to expose the rescuer to the same conditions that caused grave injury to the victim are not safe for unprotected entry. **These situations require trained and properly equipped rescue personnel.** Examples include the following:
   1. Any indoor environment where the victim was rendered unconscious or otherwise disabled.
   2. Environments causing acute onset of symptoms in rescuers such as chest tightness, shortness of breath, eye or throat irritation, coughing, dizziness, headache, nausea, or incoordination.
   3. Confined spaces such as large tanks or crawl spaces: their poor

EXAMPLE OF PLACARD AND PANEL WITH ID NUMBER

The Identification Number (ID No.) may be displayed on placards or on orange panels on tanks. Check the sides of the transport vehicle if the ID number is not displayed on the ends of the vehicle.

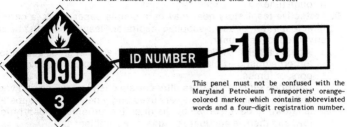

ID NUMBER → **1090**

This panel must not be confused with the Maryland Petroleum Transporters' orange-colored marker which contains abbreviated words and a four-digit registration number.

Figure IV-3. Example of US Department of Transportation (DOT) vehicle warning placard and panel with DOT identification number.

ventilation and small size can result in extremely high levels of airborne contaminants. In addition, such spaces permit only a slow or strenuous exit, which may become physically impossible for an intoxicated individual.

4. Spills involving substances with poor warning properties or high vapor pressures (see p 362), especially when they occur in an indoor or enclosed environment. Substances with poor warning properties can cause serious injury without any warning signs of exposure such as smell or eye irritation. High vapor pressures increase the likelihood that dangerous air concentrations may be present.

D. **Determine the potential for secondary contamination.** Although the threat of secondary contamination of emergency response personnel, equipment, and downstream facilities *may* be significant, it varies widely depending on the chemical, its concentration, and whether basic decontamination has already been performed. Not all toxic substances carry a risk of downstream contamination even though they may be extremely hazardous to rescuers in the hot zone.

1. Examples of substances with no significant risk for secondary contamination of personnel outside the hot zone are carbon monoxide gas, arsine gas, and chlorine gas.

2. Examples of substances with significant potential for secondary contamination and requiring extensive decontamination and protection of downstream personnel include chlorinated hydrocarbon insecticides, oily nitro compounds, and radioactive materials such as plutonium.

3. In most cases involving substances with a high potential for secondary contamination, this risk can be minimized by removal of soaked clothing and thorough decontamination in the contamination reduction corridor, including soap or shampoo wash. Following these measures, only *rarely* will the medical team face significant personal threat to their health from an exposed victim.

IV. **Personal protective equipment.** Personal protective equipment includes chemical-resistant clothing and gloves and respiratory protective gear. The use of such equipment should be supervised by experts in industrial hygiene or others with appropriate training and experience. Equipment that is incorrectly selected, improperly fitted, poorly maintained, or inappropriately used may provide a false sense of security and may fail, resulting in serious injury.

A. **Protective clothing** may be as simple as a disposable apron or as sophisticated as a fully encapsulated chemically resistant suit. However, no chemically resistant clothing is completely impervious to all chemicals over the full range of exposure conditions. Each suit is rated for its resistance to specific chemicals, and many are also rated for breakthrough time.

B. Protective respiratory gear may be a simple paper mask, a cartridge filter respirator, or an air-supplied respirator. Respirators must be properly fitted for each user.

    1. A paper mask provides partial protection against gross quantities of airborne dust particles but does not prevent exposure to gases, vapors, or fumes.

    2. Cartridge filter respirators filter certain chemical gases and vapors out of the ambient air. They are used only when the toxic substance is known to be adsorbed by the filter, the airborne concentration is low, and there is adequate oxygen in the ambient air.

    3. Air-supplied respirators provide an independent source of clean air. They may be fully self-contained units or masks supplied by a long hose. Self-contained breathing apparatus (SCBA) has a limited duration of air supply, from 5 to 30 minutes.

V. Victim management. Victim management includes rapid hot zone stabilization, initial decontamination, delivery to emergency medical services personnel at the clean zone perimeter, and medical assessment and treatment in the support area. Usually the HazMat team or other fire department personnel with appropriate training and protective gear will be responsible for rescue from the hot zone, where skin and respiratory protection is critical. Emergency medical personnel without such training must not enter the hot zone unless so advised by the incident commander or safety officer.

A. Stabilization in the hot zone. If there is suspicion of trauma, the patient should be placed on a backboard and a cervical collar applied if appropriate. Beyond this therapy, no significant medical intervention can be expected from rescuers who are wearing bulky suits, masks, and heavy gloves. Therefore, every effort should be made to get the seriously ill patient out of this area as quickly as possible.

B. Initial decontamination. Gross decontamination may take place in the hot zone (eg, brushing off chemical powder, removing soaked clothing), but most decontamination occurs in the contamination reduction corridor before delivery of the victim to waiting emergency medical personnel in the support area. Do not delay critical treatment while decontaminating the victim. Consult a regional poison control center (see Table I–41, p 51) for specific advice on decontamination. See also Section I, p 39.

    1. Pull or cut off contaminated clothing and flush exposed skin, hair, or eyes with copious plain water from a high-volume low-pressure fire hose. For oily substances, additional washing with soap or shampoo may be required.

    2. Double-bag and save all removed clothing and jewelry.

    3. Collect run-off water if possible, but rapid flushing of exposed skin or eyes should not be delayed because of environmental concerns.

    4. In the majority of incidents, basic victim decontamination as outlined above will substantially reduce or eliminate the potential for secondary contamination of downstream personnel or equipment. Procedures for cleaning equipment and people are contaminant-specific and depend on the risk of chemical persistence as well as toxicity.

C. Treatment in the support area. Once the patient is decontaminated and released into the support area, basic medical assessment and treatment by emergency medical providers may begin. In the majority of incidents, once the victim has been removed from the hot zone and is stripped and flushed, there is little or no risk of secondary contamination of these providers and sophisticated protective gear is not necessary. Simple surgical latex gloves and a plain apron or disposable outer clothing are generally sufficient.

1. Maintain a patent airway and assist breathing if necessary (see p 2). Administer supplemental oxygen.
2. Provide supportive care for shock, arrhyhthmias, coma, or seizures (see Fig 1–1, p 2).
3. Treat with specific antidotes if appropriate and available.
4. Further skin, hair, or eye washing may be necessary.
5. Take notes on the probable or suspected level of exposure for each victim, the initial symptoms and signs, and treatment provided. For chemicals with delayed toxic effects, this could be lifesaving.

VI. **Ambulance transport and hospital treatment.** No special precautions should be necessary if adequate decontamination has been carried out in the field prior to transport.

1. Patients who have ingested toxic substances may vomit en route; carry a large plastic-lined basin and extra towels to soak up spillage.
2. For those unpredictable situations in which a contaminated victim arrives at the hospital before decontamination, it is important to have a strategy ready that will minimize exposure to hospital personnel.
   a. Ask the local HazMat team to set up a contamination reduction area outside the hospital emergency department entrance.
   b. Prepare in advance a hose with 85 °F water, soap, and an old gurney for rapid decontamination *outside* the emergency department entrance. Have a child's inflatable pool or other container ready to collect water runoff, if possible.
   c. Do not bring patients soaked with volatile liquids into the emergency department until they have been stripped and flushed outside.
   d. For incidents involving radioactive materials or other highly contaminating substances that are not volatile, utilize the hospital's radiation accident protocol, which will generally include:
      (1) Restricted access zones.
      (2) Isolation of ventilation ducts leading out of the treatment room to prevent spreading the contamination throughout the hospital.
      (3) Paper covering for floors, using absorbent materials if liquids are involved.
      (4) Protective clothing for hospital staff (gloves, paper masks, shoe covers, caps, and gowns).
      (5) Double-bagging and saving all contaminated clothing and equipment.
      (6) Instituting monitoring to detect the extent and persistence of contamination (ie, a Geiger counter for radiation incidents).
      (7) Contacting appropriate local, state, and federal offices to notify them of the incident and to obtain advice on laboratory testing and decontamination of equipment.

VII. **Summary.** The emergency medical response to a hazardous materials incident requires prior training and planning to protect the health of response personnel and victims.
A. Response plans and training should be flexible. The hazard and the required actions vary greatly with the circumstances at the scene and the chemicals involved.
B. First responders should be able to:
   1. Recognize potentially hazardous situations.
   2. Take steps to protect themselves from injury.

3. Obtain accurate information about the identity and toxicity of each chemical substance involved.
4. Use appropriate protective gear.
5. Perform victim decontamination before transport to a hospital.
6. Provide appropriate first-aid and advanced supportive measures as needed.
7. Coordinate their actions with other responding agencies such as the HazMat team, police and fire departments, and regional poison control centers.

References

Bronstein AC, Currance PL: *Emergency Care for Hazardous Materials Exposure.* Mosby, 1988.
California Emergency Medical Services Authority and Toxics Epidemiology Program, Los Angeles County Department of Health Services: *Hazardous Materials Medical Management Protocols.* EMS Authority, 1989. (Contact EMS Authority, 1030 Fifteenth Street, Suite 202, Sacramento, CA 95814.)
Fire Protection Guide on Hazardous Materials, 9th ed. National Fire Protection Association, 1986.
A Guide to the Hospital Management of Injuries Arising From Exposure to or Involving Ionizing Radiation. American Medical Association, 1984.
OSHA: Hazardous waste operations and emergency response: Interim final rule. 29 CFR Part 1910.45653-.45775. *Fed Reg* 1986;**51**:45654.
Pol DR, Cheremisinoff PN: *Emergency Response to Hazardous Materials Incidents.* Technomic, 1984.
Research and Special Programs Administration, US Department of Transportation: *Hazardous Materials: Emergency Response Guide Book.* DOT P5800.**2**. US Government Printing Office, 1984.
Stutz DR, Janusz SJ: *Hazardous Materials Injuries: A Handbook for Prehospital Care,* 2nd ed. Bradford Communications, 1988.

INITIAL EVALUATION OF OCCUPATIONAL CHEMICAL EXPOSURES

Charles E. Becker, MD, and Kent R. Olson, MD

I. **General considerations**
   A. The patient with an occupational chemical exposure may come to the physician with a chronic work-related medical condition or with an acute illness requiring urgent medical attention. Chronic illness may not be correctly associated with work if there is no easily recognized temporal relationship between the work schedule and the disease. In addition, acute illnesses may not be recognized as work-related if there is a delay of more than a few hours before onset of symptoms or if there is no history of a dramatic incident at the workplace such as an explosion, fire, or major spill. Thus, it is important to maintain a high index of suspicion about occupational illness in any patient who is working.
   B. This chapter outlines the initial evaluation of the patient with an occupational chemical exposure. This material is designed for the emergency department or urgent care center physician rather than the practitioner who is providing continuing health care or workplace medical surveillance programs. For a more detailed discussion of occupational illness, refer to one of the several textbooks of occupational medicine listed in the references.
II. **Urgent evaluation of the patient**
   A. **Stabilize the patient**
      1. If the patient is acutely ill, refer immediately to Section I (p 2) of this handbook for step-by-step guidance on management of common

complications of poisoning. In general, establish a patent airway, assist ventilation if needed, give supplemental oxygen, and monitor the vital signs and electrocardiogram.

2. If the patient has not been decontaminated at the scene, determine whether the patient poses a risk of secondary contamination to the emergency department, office personnel, or facility. Simple removal of clothing and showering or flushing with copious amounts of water is satisfactory for most chemical exposures (see Section I, p 39).

B. **Obtain history of the incident**
1. **From the victim or a coworker.** The patient may be unable to provide accurate details about the incident. Determine whether the patient was accompanied by a coworker who can provide information about the specific incident and the work environment. Find out what activity the patient was involved in when the illness occurred. Determine whether there was a loss of consciousness, seizures, or other signs or symptoms, some of which may have resolved by the time medical attention was available. Ask about treatment already provided at the scene (eg, skin or eye irrigation, oxygen administration).
2. **Chemical identification.** Ask the patient or coworker to identify the chemicals involved in the incident. Often they may have only a vague idea of the chemicals used or may refer to them by common or slang terms (ie, "solvent" or "dopant"), so it is also important to contact the work site for the names of specific chemicals the worker may have been exposed to (see **3**, below). In addition, check Table IV–1 for a list of possible exposures associated with several common occupations.
3. **Work environment.** Obtain a description of the work environment. Was the room excessively hot or poorly ventilated? Was the patient working in an enclosed space or tank? These situations can cause

TABLE IV-1. SELECTED OCCUPATIONS AND SPECIFIC EXPOSURES

Occupation or Industry	Exposures (Syndrome)
Bakers	Flour, fungi, grain dust (asthma)
Battery manufacturing or repair	Lead
Butchers	Vinyl plastic fumes (asthma)
Carpenters	Wood dust, wood preservatives (skin problems, nasal cancer)
Cement workers	Potassium chromate, dichromate (asthma)
Coal miners	Dust, silica (lung disease)
Dentists	Mercury, waste anesthetic gases
Dry cleaners	Solvents (liver, skin, and neurologic disease [neuropathy])
Electronics workers	Toluene diisocyanate (asthma); solvent exposure, hydrofluoric acid (skin burns).
Electroplating	Cyanide, chromium, nickel
Explosives manufacturing	Nitrates (headache and rebound vasoconstriction)
Farm workers	Pesticides; infectious agents; NO_2, pentachlorophenol, H_2S

continued

TABLE IV-1. SELECTED OCCUPATIONS AND SPECIFIC EXPOSURES (Continued)

Occupation or Industry	Exposures (Syndrome)
Felt makers	Mercury (neuropathy)
Fire fighters	Carcinogens, smoke products (eg, CO, CN, asbestos)
Foundry workers	Silica (lung disease)
Fumigators	Methylbromide (encephalopathy, neuropathy), sulfuryl fluoride (pulmonary edema), organophosphates and carbamates
Hospital workers	Infectious agents, radiation, cleansers, ethylene oxide
Insulation industry	Formaldehyde, asbestos, fiberglass
Insulators	Asbestos, fiberglass
Jackhammer operators	Vibration (vascular disease)
Meat packing or weighing	Polyvinylchloride or papain (asthma, Q fever)
Miners	Dust (lung disease)
Office workers	Poorly designed workplace (joint and eye problems)
Painters	Solvents, lead, isocyanates
Pathology technicians	Fluorocarbons (palpitations)
Petroleum industry	Benzene (leukemia), NH_3 and H_2S, polycyclic aromatic hydrocarbons
Pottery industry	Silica, lead
Poultry workers	Asthma, psittacosis
Radiator repairmen	Lead
Rubber manufacturing	Ethylenediamine (asthma, bladder cancer)
Sausage makers	Garlic powder (asthma)
Seamen	Asbestos
Sewer workers	H_2S (hydrogen sulfide)
Shoe repairmen	Benzene (leukemia), benzidine (bladder cancer)
Spelunkers	Histoplasmosis, rabies
Sterilizer operators	Ethylene oxide (polyneuropathy)
Vintners	Arsenic (cancer and dermatitis)
Welders	Metal and polymer fume fever, ultraviolet radiation (skin and corneal burns), lead
Woodworkers	N-Hexane (neuropathy), dust (asthma)

heat exhaustion or hypoxia, which may masquerade as chemical intoxication.
4. **Protective gear.** Was the patient using protective gear? If the patient smelled an odor or experienced eye or throat irritation, this may suggest protective suit failure, improper fitting, or use of the wrong equipment. Also, be aware that fully encapsulated suits may not allow for proper ventilation or sweating, resulting in hypoxia or heat exhaustion.
5. **Work practices.** Ask whether there have been recent changes in work practices or manufacturing processes. Has the patient recently changed specific job duties? Has a new chemical been introduced?
6. **Other medical problems.** Consider preexisting medical conditions that may mimic or aggravate chemical intoxication, such as alcoholism, coronary artery disease, or chronic obstructive pulmonary disease.

C. **Obtain useful information from the work site**
1. **Work site contacts.** The following persons at the work site may have access to useful information: the work supervisor, the health and safety officer, the industrial hygienist, an on-site nurse or physician, a union health and safety representative, a company personnel representative.
2. **Chemical identification.** Have the work site contact obtain the **Material Safety Data Sheet** for information on chemical products used at the patient's workstation. If there is a Department of Transportation (DOT) identification placard (see p 347) on the container, check the index of this handbook to identify the chemical and then locate it in Table IV–12 or in Section II.
3. **Air measurements.** If an accidental overexposure has occurred, ask whether an industrial hygienist has measured air concentrations of the involved chemicals during or shortly after the incident. These measurements can be compared with recommended workplace exposure limits (Table IV–12). Generally, air levels at or below the permissible exposure limit (PEL) or threshold limit value (TLV) are not likely to be responsible for serious acute illness.
4. **Baseline health data.** Obtain information from the patient's company medical file on any previous baseline physical examination and laboratory testing (eg, cholinesterase levels, blood lead levels, pul-

TABLE IV-2. SELECTED OCCUPATIONAL SKIN DISORDERS

Skin Disorders	Selected Causes
Contact dermatitis Irritant	Fibrous glass, corrosives, soaps
Allergic	Nickel, chromates
Chemical burns	Corrosive acids and alkali, phenols, hydrofluoric acid, phosphorus
Acne	Oils, fats, tars
Chloracne	Polychlorinated biphenyls, dioxin
Pigmentary changes	Aniline, arsenic, phenols
Cancer	Ultraviolet radiation, arsenic
Hair loss	Thallium, arsenic, radiation

TABLE IV-3. OCCUPATIONAL EXPOSURE OF THE EYES, EARS, NOSE, AND THROAT

Warning Properties	Selected Examples
None	Carbon monoxide, diethylamine
Weak	Ethylene oxide, nitrogen oxides
Strong	Acetone, ammonia, chlorine

monary function tests, chest radiographs) that could be compared with current data.
- **D. Perform physical examination and laboratory testing**
  1. **Organ system evaluation.** In addition to the routine examination, emphasis should be placed on organ systems most likely to be affected by specific chemicals and those that yield the most clues to occupational exposures or illness. For acute illness, the most common sites affected are the central nervous system and the cardio-respiratory system. Tables IV–1 through IV–11 describe considerations for several organ systems affected by occupational exposures.
    a. **Skin.** The skin is the organ most commonly exposed to occupational toxins. Many chemicals are irritating to the skin, and some are sensitizers, capable of producing chronic allergic skin disorders. Solvents generally cause skin defatting, resulting in loss of the protective stratum corneum barrier and allowing enhanced penetration by toxic chemicals. Alkali, acids, and other corrosive materials cause chemical burns. Other chemicals may cause acne, chloracne, depigmentation, cancer, or hair loss (Table IV–2).
    b. **Eyes, ears, nose, and throat.** Many chemicals that are highly water-soluble rapidly dissolve in the moist mucous membranes of the eyes, nose, and throat, providing excellent warning properties of local irritation. Others may have distinctive odors, although this may be unreliable because of concurrent upper respiratory infection or olfactory fatigue (Table IV–3).
    c. **Lungs.** Along with the skin, the lungs are a very common route of chemical exposure. With highly water-soluble or irritating gases, early warning properties usually prevent prolonged exposure and

TABLE IV-4. SELECTED OCCUPATIONAL PULMONARY EXPOSURES

Lung Diseases	Selected Causes
Acute	
Wheezing, bronchitis, pulmonary edema	Sulfur dioxide, methyl isocyanate, chlorine, nitrogen oxides, ammonia, phosgene, formaldehyde, many others
Induction of asthma	Isocyanates, wood pulp dust, nickel
Extrinsic alveolitis	Woodworking, farming
Metal fume fever	Zinc oxides (welding galvanized steel)
Chronic	
Interstitial	Asbestosis, silicosis, coal dust
Granulomatous	Beryllium
Cancer	Asbestos, arsenic, bischloromethyl ether, cigarette smoke, chromates

TABLE IV-5. SELECTED OCCUPATIONAL MUSCULOSKELETAL DISORDERS

Disorders	Selected Causes
Local injuries	
Low back pain	Heavy labor, lifting
Reynaud's syndrome	Vibration, cold
Carpal tunnel syndrome	Vibration, assemblers, packers
Degenerative arthritis	Housekeeping, heavy labor
Systemic illnesses	
Scleroderma	Some organic solvents
Gout	Lead
Osteosclerosis	Fluoride
Aseptic necrosis	Scuba divers
Osteonecrosis	Phosphorus
Osteosarcoma	Radium

symptoms are most severe early after exposure. On the other hand, with less soluble gases symptoms may be delayed 6–24 hours. Several lung exposures have long latency periods before overt disease appears, such as asbestosis and other pneumoconioses (Table IV–4).

   d. **Musculoskeleton.** Injuries to the musculoskeletal system are the most common type of reported on-the-job injuries. Many types of work involving repetitive motion may cause acute tendinitis and, with cumulative trauma, may result in chronic pain syndromes. Consider that a chemical exposure (eg, solvent or pesticide) may enhance the risk of a mechanical accident (Table IV–5).

   e. **Nervous system.** The central and peripheral nervous systems are frequently involved in acute and chronic occupational chemical exposures. Ask about paresthesias, dysesthesias, local weakness, fatigue, disturbed sleep patterns, or headache (Table IV–6).

   f. **Gastrointestinal system.** Symptoms are often nonspecific. Gastroenteritis may be confused with viral or food-borne illness. Colic and constipation should suggest lead exposure. Many toxins can cause subtle or severe hepatic damage. Be sure to elicit a history of alcohol use or dependency, which may aggravate workplace chemical hepatitis (Table IV–7).

   g. **Cardiovascular system.** Workplace chemical exposures may

TABLE IV-6. SELECTED OCCUPATIONAL NEUROLOGIC DISORDERS

Disorders	Selected Causes
CNS tumors	Vinyl chloride
Parkinsonism	Manganese, carbon monoxide, carbon disulfide
Headache	Carbon monoxide, nitrites, solvents, methemoglobinemia
Acute encephalopathy	Carbon monoxide, solvents, lead, carbon disulfide, methyl bromide
Peripheral neuropathy	Lead, arsenic, mercury, thallium, n-hexane, methyl butyl ketone, methyl bromide, acrylamide, triorthocresyl phosphate

TABLE IV-7. SELECTED OCCUPATIONAL GASTROINTESTINAL DISORDERS

Disorders	Selected Causes
Nausea and vomiting	Organophosphates and carbamates, epoxy resins, copper fumes, zinc fumes, solvents
Diarrhea	Organophosphates and carbamates, arsenic, thallium, phosphorus
Jaundice	Hemolysis (eg, arsine), hepatitis (carbon tetrachloride, nitrobenzene, hydrazine, phosphorus, dioxin)

cause acute myocardial abnormalities (eg, cardiac ischemia or arrhythmias) or may affect peripheral vascular tone. Chronic exposures may be associated with a higher risk of coronary disease (Table IV-8).

   h. **Hematopoietic system.** The hematopoietic system can be affected by acute and chronic workplace chemical exposures. Exposures in the distant past may have a long latency period before causing cancer (eg, benzene; Table IV-9).

   i. **Renal system.** Many occupational chemical exposures produce acute or chronic kidney dysfunction and bladder abnormalities. Up to 60–70% of kidney function may be lost before the decrease is clinically apparent (Table IV-10).

   j. **Endocrine system.** Table IV-11 shows selected disorders of the endocrine and reproductive systems caused by occupational chemical exposures.

2. **General laboratory panel.** In general, the following empirical tests are recommended for most patients with an occupational chemical exposure.

   a. CBC (complete blood count).
   b. BUN (blood urea nitrogen) and creatinine.
   c. Glucose and electrolytes.
   d. Liver enzymes.
   e. Urinalysis.

3. **Specific laboratory tests.** If the exposure agent is known, order specific tests as recommended in Section II. In general, focus attention on the organ systems affected. For example, a chest radiograph and arterial blood gases (and possibly pulmonary function tests) would be appropriate after exposure to a pulmonary irritant gas, and an

TABLE IV-8. SELECTED OCCUPATIONAL CARDIOVASCULAR DISORDERS

Disorders	Selected Causes
Coronary artery disease	Cabon disulfide, carbon monoxide
Arrhythmias	Halogenated hydrocarbons, barium
Hypertension	Lead
Cor pulmonale	Fibrogenic restrictive lung disease
Angina pectoris	Carbon monoxide, methylene chloride
Hypotension	Nitrites, nitroglycerin

TABLE IV-9. SELECTED OCCUPATIONAL HEMATOPOIETIC DISORDERS

Disorders	Selected Causes
Hemolysis	Arsine, naphthalene, stibine
Methemoglobinemia	Nitrites, aniline, oxidizers
Bone marrow suppression	Arsenic, radiation, benzene
Porphyria	Hexachlorobenzene, lead
Neutropenia	Chlorinated hydrocarbons
Anemia	Lead

electrocardiogram or cardiac monitoring would be performed after exposure to a chlorinated solvent.
4. **Baseline tests.** Remember to check whether baseline tests are available in the patient's company file to compare with current data.
5. **Consultation.** A regional poison center (see p 51), medical toxicologist, or occupational medicine specialist may be able to assist in the selection and interpretation of laboratory tests.

III. **Treatment and disposition**
   A. **Treatment**
      1. Treatment recommendations are provided in Sections I and II for common complications of poisoning and for many specific chemicals and other toxic agents.
      2. Other sources of information on treatment of acute occupational poisoning are listed in the references.
   B. **Disposition**
      1. Remember that many chemicals may cause delayed-onset effects (for example, pulmonary edema may occur several hours after exposure to nitrogen dioxide). In such cases, prolonged observation in the emergency department or in the hospital may be necessary.
      2. Be sure that a method is established to notify the patient of laboratory test results, to explain abnormal findings, and to provide treatment when appropriate.
      3. Patients should be referred to a qualified occupational medicine specialist for follow-up. An occupational medicine physician may already be available at the work site or may be found through a local medical school or government agency.
   C. **Mandated reporting**
      1. There are a variety of specific legal requirements for reporting of occupational exposures to state and federal agencies. In some cases, specific laboratory testing and workplace exclusion are mandated by law (for example, for lead exposure).
      2. If you are not already familiar with local, state, or federal reporting

TABLE IV-10. SELECTED OCCUPATIONAL RENAL DISORDERS

Renal Disorders	Selected Causes
Acute tubular necrosis	Glycols, inorganic mercury, arsine
Chronic renal failure	Lead, cadmium, radiation
Bladder cancers	Benzidine, β-naphthylamine

TABLE IV-11. SELECTED OCCUPATIONAL ENDOCRINE AND REPRODUCTIVE DISORDERS

Disorders	Selected Causes
Thyroiditis	Polychlorinated biphenyls
Aspermia	Dibromochloropropane
Miscarriage	Lead, anesthetic gases

requirements, contact the local health officer or environmental health officer or a regional Occupational Safety and Health Administration (OSHA) office. Table IV-15 (see p 504) lists regional federal OSHA offices and their telephone numbers. Note: Some states have their own programs (eg, Cal-OSHA in California). Obtain referral from regional OSHA office.

3. Be certain to ensure strict confidentiality of all patient information other than that required by law to be reported.

4. Check to determine whether other workers have been affected. Some may have stayed at work or may have gone to other treatment facilities. If a potentially life-threatening hazard still exists at the work site, then workers may need to be evacuated and immediate reporting to local officials is mandatory.

5. Determine whether there has been potential contamination of the environment in the neighborhood of the workplace, which might necessitate evacuation of local residents. Once again, reporting of the incident to local officials is essential.

IV. **Summary: Characteristics of occupational exposures**
   A. There may be a delay in onset of symptoms.
   B. The exposure may be difficult to identify and quantify.
   C. Other workers may be exposed.
   D. Potential for contamination of health care providers and the environment should be determined.
   E. Expert consultation may be available through local agencies and federal OSHA offices.
   F. There may be special reporting requirements mandated by law.

References

LaDou J (editor): *Occupational Medicine.* Appleton & Lange, 1990.
National Institute of Occupational Safety and Health: *A Guide to the Work-Relatedness of Disease.* US Department of Health and Human Services/Centers for Disease Control, 1979.
National Institute of Occupational Safety and Health: *Recommendations for Occupational Safety and Health Standards 1988.* US Department of Health and Human Services/Centers for Disease Control, 1988.
Proctor NH, Hughes JP, Fischman ML: *Chemical Hazards of the Workplace,* 2nd ed. Lippincott, 1988.
Rom WN (editor): *Environmental and Occupational Medicine.* Little, Brown, 1983.

THE TOXIC HAZARDS OF INDUSTRIAL AND OCCUPATIONAL CHEMICALS

Frank J. Mycroft, PhD, and Patricia Hess Hiatt, BS

Table IV-12 provides basic information on the toxicity of many of the most commonly encountered and toxicologically significant industrial chemicals.

Table IV–12 is intended to expedite the recognition of potentially hazardous exposure situations and therefore provides information such as vapor pressures, warning properties, physical appearance, occupational exposure standards and guidelines, and hazard classification codes, which may also be useful in the assessment of an exposure situation. Table IV–12 is divided into 3 sections: **health hazards, exposure guidelines,** and **comments.** To use the table correctly, it is important to understand the scope and limitations of the information it provides.

The chemicals included in Table IV–12 were selected according to the following criteria: (1) toxicological significance; (2) common use; (3) public health interest; and (4) availability of toxicologic, regulatory, and physical/chemical properties information.

I. Health hazards information

A. The health hazards section focuses primarily on the basic hazards associated with inhalation of or skin exposures to chemicals that might occur in a workplace. It is based almost entirely on the occupational health literature. Most of our understanding of the potential effects of chemicals on human health derive from occupational exposures, which are typically many times greater than environmental exposures.

B. The information in the table unavoidably emphasizes *acute* health effects. Much more is known about the acute effects of chemicals on human health than about their chronic effects. The rapid onset of symptoms following exposure makes the causal association more readily apparent for acute health effects. To broaden the scope of the table, the findings of animal studies relating to the carcinogenic or developmental toxicity of a chemical are also included when available.

C. The table is *not* a comprehensive source of the toxicology and medical information needed to manage a severely symptomatic or poisoned patient. Medical management information and advice for poisonings are found in Section I (see pulmonary problems, pp 1–8, and pulmonary and skin decontamination, pp 39–40) and Section II (see caustics, p 114; gases, p 163; and hydrocarbons, p 165).

II. Problems in assessing health hazards

A. The nature and magnitude of the health hazards associated with occupational or environmental exposures to any chemical depend on its intrinsic toxicity and the conditions of exposure.

B. Characterization of these hazards is often difficult. Important considerations include the potency of the agent, the route of exposure, the level and temporal pattern of exposure, genetic susceptibility, overall health status, and life-style factors that may alter individual sensitivities (eg, alcohol consumption may cause "degreaser's flush" in workers exposed to trichloroethylene). Despite their value in estimating the likelihood and potential severity of an effect, quantitative measurements of the level of exposure are not often available.

C. Hazard characterizations cannot address undiscovered or unappreciated health effects. The limited information available on the health effects of most chemicals makes this a major concern. For example, of the more than 5 million compounds known to science, only about 90,000 have any listing in the *Registry of the Toxic Effects of Chemical Substances* published by the National Institute for Occupational Safety and Health (NIOSH). Of these 90,000 substances, only comparatively small numbers have any toxicity studies relating to their potential tumorigenic (3674 substances) or reproductive (4991 substances) effects in animals or humans. Because of these gaps, the absence of information does not imply the absence of hazard.

D. The predictive value of animal findings for humans is sometimes uncertain. For many effects, however, there is considerable concordance between test animals and humans. A discussion of the specific problems in the interpretation and use of carcinogenicity information is found on p 477.

E. The developmental toxicity information presented here is not a sufficient basis on which to make clinical judgments as to whether a given exposure might adversely affect a pregnancy. For most chemicals that are known to have adverse effects on fetal development in test animals, there are insufficient epidemiologic data in humans. The predictive value of these animal findings for humans, who are typically exposed to levels much lower than those used in animal tests, is thought to be poor. In general, so little is known about the effects of substances on fetal development that it is prudent to conservatively manage all chemical exposures. The information here is presented solely to identify those compounds for which available data further indicate the need to control exposures.

III. Exposure guidelines and National Fire Protection Association rankings
A. Threshold limit values (TLVs)
1. The TLVs are workplace exposure guidelines established by the American Conference of Governmental Industrial Hygienists (ACGIH), a professional society. Although the ACGIH has no regulatory authority, its recommendations are highly regarded by the members of the occupational health community and government agencies.
2. The toxicologic basis for each TLV varies. A TLV may be set on the basis of such diverse effects as respiratory sensitization, sensory irritation, narcosis, or asphyxia. Therefore, the TLV is not a relative index of toxicity. Because the degree of health hazard is a continuous function of exposure, TLVs are not fine lines separating safe from dangerous levels of exposure. The *Documentation of the Threshold Limit Values,* which is published by the ACGIH and describes in detail the rationale for each value, should be consulted for specific information on the toxicologic significance of a particular TLV.
3. The **Threshold Limit Value–Time-Weighted Average (TLV–TWA)** refers to airborne contaminants and is the time-weighted average concentration for a normal 8-hour workday and 40-hour workweek to which nearly all workers may be repeatedly exposed, day after day, without adverse effect. Unless otherwise indicated, the values listed under the ACGIH TLV heading are the TLV–TWA values. Common units for a TLV–TWA are **ppm** (parts of chemical per million parts of air) and **mg/m³** (milligrams of chemical per cubic meter of air). At standard temperature and pressure, **TLV values in ppm can be converted to their equivalent concentrations in mg/m³** by multiplying the TLV in ppm by the molecular weight of the chemical and dividing the result by 22.4 (1 mol of gas displaces 22.4 L of air at standard temperature and pressure):

$$mg/m^3 = \frac{ppm \times MW}{22.4}$$

4. The **threshold limit value ceiling (TLV-C)** is the airborne concentration that should not be exceeded during any part of a working exposure. Ceiling guidelines are often set for rapidly acting agents. TLV-Cs are listed under the ACGIH TLV heading and are noted by a **"(C)."** For compounds with both a TLV–TWA and a TLV-C, only the TLV–TWA is listed in the table.

5. Compounds for which **skin contact** is a significant route of exposure are designated with an **"S."**

6. The ACGIH classifies some substances as being *confirmed* **(A1)** or *suspected* **(A2) human carcinogens.** These designations are also provided in the table.

7. The TLVs are heavily based on workplace exposures and conditions occurring within the USA. Their application, which requires training in industrial hygiene, is therefore limited to similar exposures and conditions.

B. **Permissible exposure limits (PEL)**

1. The **PEL** is an airborne exposure standard set and enforced by the Occupational Safety and Health Administration (OSHA), an agency of the federal government. The PEL is analogous to the TLV–TWA, and many of the same considerations apply. It is the maximum 8-hour TWA air concentration to which workers may be exposed during a 40-hour workweek. Those PELs designated with a **"(C)"** are **ceiling values** that should not be exceeded during any part of a working exposure. In addition, substances for which **skin contact** is an important route of exposure are designated with an **"S."**

2. Substances that are specifically **regulated as carcinogens** by OSHA are indicated by **"OSHA CA"** under the PEL heading. For these carcinogens, additional regulations apply.

3. Some states operate their own occupational health and safety programs in cooperation with OSHA. In these states, other, stricter standards may apply.

4. Because exposure standards are often set to protect against discomfort, nonspecific minor health complaints including irritation, cough, nausea, and headache can be indicative of overexposure.

C. **Immediately dangerous to life or health. (IDLH)** The immediately dangerous to life or health (IDLH) level represents "a maximum concentration from which one could escape within 30 minutes without any escape-impairing symptoms or any irreversible health effects." These values were jointly set by OSHA and NIOSH for the purpose of respirator selection. The notation **"NIOSH CA"** under this heading identifies those chemicals that **NIOSH recommends be treated as potential human carcinogens.**

D. **National Fire Protection Association codes**

1. The National Fire Protection Association (NFPA) has created a system for identifying and ranking the potential fire hazards of materials. The system has 3 principal categories of hazard: **health (H), flammability (F),** and **reactivity (R).** Within each category, hazards are ranked from four (4), indicating a severe hazard, to zero (0), indicating no special hazard. The NFPA rankings for each substance are listed under their appropriate headings. The criteria for rankings within each category are found in Fig IV–2, p 345.

2. The NFPA health hazard category is based on both the intrinsic toxicity of a chemical and the toxicities of its combustion or breakdown products. The overall ranking is determined by the greater source of health hazard under fire or other emergency conditions. The common hazards from the ordinary combustion of materials are not considered in these rankings.

3. This system is intended to provide basic information to fire-fighting and emergency response personnel. Its application to specific situations requires skill. Conditions at the scene, such as the amount of material involved and its rate of release, wind conditions, and the proximity to various populations and their health status, are as important as the intrinsic properties of a chemical in determining the magnitude of hazard.

IV. Comments section

A. The comments section provides supplementary information on the physical and chemical properties of substances that would be helpful in assessing their health hazards. Information such as physical state and appearance, vapor pressures, warning properties, and potential breakdown products is included.

B. Information on physical state and appearance of a compound may help in its identification and indicate whether dusts, mists, vapors, or gases are likely means of airborne exposure. *Note:* For many products, especially pesticides, appearance and some hazardous properties vary with the formulation.

C. Chemicals possessing high vapor pressures, significant systemic toxicities, and poor warning properties are of special concern because harmful exposures to these substances may go unrecognized.

1. Vapor pressure. The vapor pressure of a substance determines its maximum air concentration and influences the degree of inhalation exposure. Vapor pressures fluctuate greatly with temperature.

a. Substances with high vapor pressures tend to volatilize more quickly and can reach higher maximum air concentrations than substances with low vapor pressures. Some substances have such low vapor pressures that only their dusts or mists pose an inhalation hazard.

b. Substances with a **saturated air concentration** below their TLVs do not pose a significant vapor inhalation hazard. Vapor pressures can be roughly converted to a saturated air concentration expressed in ppm by dividing by 760 mm Hg and then multiplying the result by 1 million to adjust for the original units of parts per million (a pressure of 1 equals 760 mm Hg):

$$\text{ppm} = \frac{\text{Vapor pressure (mm Hg)}}{760} \times 10^6$$

2. Warning properties. Warning properties, such as odor and sensory irritation, can be valuable indicators of exposure. However, because of olfactory fatigue and individual differences in odor thresholds, the sense of smell is often unreliable for many compounds. There is no correlation between the quality of an odor and its toxicity. Pleasant-smelling compounds are not necessarily less toxic than foul-smelling ones.

a. The warning property assessments found in the table are based on OSHA evaluations. For the purpose of this manual, chemicals described as having *good* warning properties can be detected at levels below the PEL by smell or irritation by most individuals. Chemicals described as having *adequate* warning properties can be detected at air levels near the PEL. Chemicals described as having *poor* warning properties can be detected only at levels significantly above the PEL or not at all.

b. Reported values for odor threshold in the literature vary greatly for many chemicals and are uncertain. These differences make assessments of warning qualities difficult.

3. Thermal breakdown products. Under fire conditions, many organic substances will break down to other toxic substances. The amounts, kinds, and distribution of breakdown products vary with the fire conditions and are not easily modeled. Information on the likely thermal decomposition products is included because of their importance in the assessment of health hazards under fire conditions.

a. In general, incomplete combustion of *any* organic material will produce some carbon monoxide.

b. The partial combustion of compounds containing sulfur, nitrogen, or phosphorus atoms will also release their oxides.

c. Compounds with chlorine atoms will release some hydrogen chloride or chlorine when exposed to high heat or fire; some chlorinated compounds may also generate phosgene.

d. Compounds containing the fluorine atom are similarly likely to break down to yield some hydrogen fluoride and fluorine.

e. Some compounds, such as polyurethane, which contain an unsaturated carbon-nitrogen bond, will release cyanide during their decomposition.

f. Polychlorinated aromatic compounds may yield polychlorinated dibenzodioxins and polychlorinated dibenzofurans when heated.

g. In addition, smoke from a chemical fire is likely to contain large amounts of the volatilized original chemical and still other poorly characterized partial breakdown products.

h. The thermal breakdown product information found in Table IV–12 is derived primarily from data found in the literature and the general considerations described immediately above. Aside from the NFPA codes, Table IV–12 does not otherwise cover the chemical reactivities and compatibilities of substances.

V. Summary. Table IV–12 provides basic information that describes the potential health hazards associated with exposure to several hundred chemicals. The table is not a comprehensive listing of all the possible health hazards for each chemical. The information compiled here comes from a wide variety of respected sources (see references) and focuses on the more likely or commonly reported health effects. Publications from the National Institute for Occupational Safety and Health, the Occupational Safety and Health Administration, the American Conference of Governmental Industrial Hygienists, the Hazard Evaluation System and Information Service of the State of California, and the National Fire Protection Association; major textbooks in the fields of toxicology and occupational health; and major review articles were the primary sources of the information found here. Refer to the original sources for more complete information.

Table IV–12 is intended primarily to guide users in the quick qualitative assessment of common toxic hazards. Its application to specific situations requires skill. Because of the many data gaps in the toxicologic literature, exposures should generally be managed conservatively. Contact a regional poison control center (see Table I–41) for expert assistance in managing specific emergency exposures.

References

Air contaminants: Permissible exposure limits. *Fed Reg* 1989;**54**:2923.

Barlow SM, Sullivan FM (editors): *Reproductive Hazards of Industrial Chemicals.* Academic Press, 1982.

Chemical Emergency Preparedness Program: Interim Guidance. US Environmental Protection Agency, 1985.

Code of Federal Regulations. 29 CFR Chapter XVIII 1910.1000 (1985).

Fire Protection Guide on Hazardous Materials, 9th ed. National Fire Protection Association, 1986.

Hayes WJ Jr: *Pesticides Studied in Man.* Williams & Wilkins, 1982.

IARC Monographs on the Evaluation of the Carcinogenic Risk of Chemicals to Humans. 42 vols. World Health Organization, 1972–1988.

Morgan DP: *Recognition and Management of Pesticide Poisonings,* 3rd ed. US Environmental Protection Agency, 1982.

National Toxicology Program: *Fourth Annual Report on Carcinogens.* US Department of Health and Human Services, 1985.

NIOSH: *Occupational Diseases: A Guide to Their Recognition.* US Department of Health and Human Services, 1977.

NIOSH: Recommendations for occupational safety and health standards. *MMWR* 1986;**35(Suppl 1S).**

NIOSH/OSHA: *Occupational Health Guidelines for Chemical Hazards.* DHHS (NIOSH) Publication No. 81-123. US Department of Health and Human Services, 1981.

NIOSH/OSHA: *Pocket Guide to Chemical Hazards.* NIOSH Publication No. 78-210. US Department of Health and Human Services, 1985.

Proctor NH, Hughes JP, Fischman ML: *Chemical Hazards of the Workplace,* 2nd ed. Lippincott, 1988.

Rumack BH (editor): *Poisindex.* Vol 56. Micromedex, 1988.

Schardein JL: *Chemically Induced Birth Defects.* Marcel Dekker, 1985.

Schardein JL, Schwetz BA, Kenel MF: Species sensitivities and prediction of teratogenic potential. *Environ Health Perspect* 1985;**61:**55.

Sittig M: *Handbook of Toxic and Hazardous Chemicals.* Noyes, 1985.

Threshold Limit Values and Biological Exposure Indices, 5th ed. American Council of Governmental Industrial Hygienists, 1986.

Threshold Limit Values and Biological Exposure Indices, 6th ed. American Council of Governmental Industrial Hygienists, 1987.

IV: THE TOXIC HAZARDS OF INDUSTRIAL AND OCCUPATIONAL CHEMICALS   **365**

TABLE IV-12. HEALTH HAZARD SUMMARIES FOR INDUSTRIAL AND OCCUPATIONAL CHEMICALS

Abbreviations and designations used in this table are defined as follows:

TLV = Threshold Limit Value–Time-Weighted Average (TLV-TWA air concentration (see p 360).	A1 = An ACGIH-confirmed human carcinogen (see p 478).
PEL = Permissible Exposure Limit (time-weighted average) air concentration (see p 361).	A2 = An ACGIH-suspected human carcinogen (see p 478).
	NIOSH CA = Judged by NIOSH to be a known or suspected human carcinogen (see p 479).
IDLH = Immediately Dangerous to Life or Health air concentration (see p 361).	OSHA CA = Regulated by OSHA as an occupational carcinogen (see p 479).
	NFPA Codes = National Fire Protection Association hazard classification codes (see p 361 and Fig IV-2, p 345). 0 (no hazard) <—> 4 (severe hazard)
ppm = Parts of chemical per million parts of air.	H = Health hazard
mg/m³ = Milligrams of chemical per cubic meter of air.	F = Fire hazard
mppcf = Million particles of dust per cubic foot of air.	R = Reactivity hazard
(C) = Ceiling air concentration (TLV-C) that should not be exceeded at any time.	OX = Oxidizing agent
S = Skin absorption can be significant route of exposure.	W = Water-reactive substance

Health Hazard Summaries	ACGIH TLV	PEL	IDLH	NFPA Codes H F R	Comments
Acetaldehyde (CAS: 75-07-0): Corrosive; severe burns to eyes and skin may occur. Vapors strongly irritating to eyes and upper respiratory tract; pulmonary edema may result. A carcinogen in test animals.	100 ppm	100 ppm	10,000 ppm	2 4 2	Colorless liquid. Fruity odor and irritation are both adequate warning properties. Vapor pressure is 750 mm Hg at 20 °C (68 °F). Highly flammable.
Acetic acid (vinegar acid [CAS: 64-19-7]: Concentrated solutions are corrosive; severe burns to eyes and skin may occur. Vapors irritating to eyes and respiratory tract; delayed pulmonary edema may result from very high exposures.	10 ppm	10 ppm	1000 ppm	2 2 1	Colorless liquid. Pungent, vinegarlike odor and irritation both occur near the PEL and are adequate warning properties. Vapor pressure is 11 mm Hg at 20 °C (68 °F). Flammable.

continued

TABLE IV-12. HEALTH HAZARD SUMMARIES FOR INDUSTRIAL AND OCCUPATIONAL CHEMICALS (Continued)

Health Hazard Summaries	ACGIH TLV	PEL	IDLH	NFPA Codes H F R	Comments
Acetic anhydride (CAS: 108-24-7): Corrosive; severe burns to eyes and skin may result. Vapors highly irritating to eyes and respiratory tract; pulmonary edema may result.	5 ppm (C)	5 ppm (C)	1000 ppm	2 2 1 W	Colorless liquid. Odor and irritation both occur below the PEL and are good warning properties. Vapor pressure is 4 mm Hg at 20 °C (68 °F). Flammable. Evolves heat upon contact with water.
Acetone (dimethyl ketone, 2-propanone [CAS: 67-64-1]: Vapors mildly irritating to eyes and respiratory tract. Defats the skin, producing a dermatitis. A CNS depressant at high levels. Eye irritation and headache are common symptoms of moderate overexposure.	750 ppm	750 ppm	20,000 ppm	1 3 0	Coloress liquid with a sharp, aromatic odor. Eye irritation is an adequate warning property. Vapor pressure is 266 mm Hg at 25 °C (77 °F). Highly flammable.
Acetonitrile (methyl cyanide, cyanomethane, ethanenitrile [CAS: 75-05-8]): Vapors mildly irritating to eyes and respiratory tract. Inhibits several metabolic enzyme systems. Dermal absorption occurs. Slowly metabolized to cyanide; fatalities have resulted. Symptoms include headache, nausea, vomiting, weakness, and stupor. See p 134.	40 ppm S	40 ppm	4000 ppm	2 3 0	Colorless liquid. Etherlike odor, detectable at the PEL, is an adequate warning property. Vapor pressure is 73 mm Hg at 20 °C (68 °F). Flammable. Thermal breakdown products include oxides of nitrogen and cyanide.
Acetylene tetrabromide (tetrabromoethane [CAS: 79-27-6]): Direct contact is irritating to eyes and skin. Vapors irritating to eyes and respiratory tract. Dermal absorption occurs. Highly hepatotoxic; liver injury can result from low-level exposures.	1 ppm	1 ppm	10 ppm	3 0 1	Viscous, pale yellow liquid. Pungent, chloroform-like odor. Vapor pressure is less than 0.1 mm Hg at 20 °C (68 °F). Not combustible. Thermal breakdown products include hydrogen bromide and carbonyl bromide.
Acrolein (acrylaldehyde, 2-propenal [CAS: 107-02-8]): Highly corrosive; severe burns to eyes or skin may result. Vapors extremely irritating to eyes, skin, and respiratory tract; pulmonary edema has been reported. Permanent pulmonary function changes may result.	0.1 ppm	0.1 ppm	5 ppm	3 3 2	Colorless to yellow liquid. An unpleasant odor. Eye irritation occurs at low levels and provides a good warning property. Vapor pressure is 214 mm Hg at 20 °C (68 °F). Highly flammable.

Chemical and comments		NFPA (H F R)	Physical properties
Acrylamide (propenamide, acrylic amide) [CAS: 79-06-1]: Slightly irritating upon direct contact with concentrated solutions. Well absorbed by all routes. A potent neurotoxin causing peripheral neuropathy. Contact dermatitis also reported. Testicular toxicity and carcinogenicity in animals. See p 481.	0.03 mg/m³ S, A2 0.03 mg/m³ S	...	Colorless solid. Vapor pressure is 0.007 mm Hg at 20 °C (68 °F). Not flammable. Decomposes around 80 °C (176 °F). Breakdown products include oxides of nitrogen.
Acrylic acid (propenoic acid) [CAS: 79-10-7]: Corrosive; severe burns may result. Vapors highly irritating to eyes, skin, and respiratory tract. Limited evidence of adverse effects on fetal development at high doses in animals. Based on structural analogies, compounds containing the acrylate moiety may be carcinogens.	10 ppm S 10 ppm S	3 2 2	Colorless liquid with characteristic acrid odor. Vapor pressure is 31 mm Hg at 25 °C (77 °F). Flammable. Inhibitor added to prevent explosive self-polymerization. TLV under review.
Acrylonitrile (cyanoethylene, vinyl cyanide, propenenitrile [CAS: 107-13-1]: Direct contact can be strongly irritating to eyes and skin. Well absorbed by all routes. A CNS depressant at high levels. Slowly metabolized to cyanide. Moderate acute overexposure will produce headache, weakness, nausea, and vomiting. Evidence of adverse effects on fetal development at high doses in animals. A carcinogen in animals. Limited epidemiologic evidence for carcinogenicity in humans. See pp 134 and 481.	2 ppm S, A2 OSHA CA 4000 ppm NIOSH CA	4 3 2	Colorless liquid with a mild odor. Vapor pressure is 83 mm Hg at 20 °C (68 °F). Flammable. Polymerizes rapidly. Thermal decomposition products include hydrogen cyanide and oxides of nitrogen.
Aldrin [CAS: 309-00-2]: Minor skin irritant. Convulsant. Hepatotoxin. Well absorbed dermally. Limited evidence of carcinogenicity in animals. See pp 117 and 481.	0.25 mg/m³ S 100 mg/m³ NIOSH CA	3 1 0 (solutions) 2 0 0 (dry)	Tan to dark brown solid. A mild chemical odor. Vapor pressure is 0.000006 mm Hg at 20 °C (68 °F). Not flammable but breaks down, yielding hydrogen chloride gas.

continued

(C) = ceiling air concentration (TLV-C); S = skin absorption can be significant; A1 = ACGIH-confirmed human carcinogen; A2 = ACGIH-suspected human carcinogen; NFPA Hazard Codes: H = health, F = fire, R = reactivity, OX = oxidizer, 0 (none) <—> 4 (severe). See expanded definitions on p 365.

TABLE IV-12. HEALTH HAZARD SUMMARIES FOR INDUSTRIAL AND OCCUPATIONAL CHEMICALS (Continued)

Health Hazard Summaries	ACGIH TLV	PEL	IDLH	NFPA Codes H F R	Comments
Allyl alcohol (2-propen-1-ol)[CAS: 107-18-6]: Strongly irritating to eyes and skin; severe burns may result. Vapors highly irritating to eyes and respiratory tract; corneal necrosis and pulmonary edema could result. Systemic poisoning can result from dermal exposures. May cause liver and kidney injury.	2 ppm S	2 ppm S	150 ppm	3 3 0	Colorless liquid. Mustardlike odor and irritation occur near the PEL and serve as good warning properties. Vapor pressure is 17 mm Hg at 20 °C (68 °F). Flammable.
Allyl chloride (3-chloro-1-propene [CAS: 107-05-1]): Highly irritating to eyes and skin. Vapors highly irritating to eyes and respiratory tract; pulmonary edema may occur. Well absorbed by the skin, producing both superficial and penetrating irritation and pain. Causes liver and kidney injury in animals.	1 ppm	1 ppm	300 ppm	3 3 1	Colorless, yellow, or purple liquid. Pungent, disagreeable odor and irritation occur only at levels far above the PEL, so exposure is accompanied by poor warning. Vapor pressure is 295 mm Hg at 20 °C (68 °F). Highly flammable. Breakdown products include hydrogen chloride and phosgene.
Allyl glycidyl ether (AGE [CAS: 106-92-3]): Highly irritating to eyes and skin; severe burns may result. Vapors irritating to eyes and respiratory tract; delayed pulmonary edema may occur. Sensitization dermatitis has been reported. Hematopoietic and testicular toxicity occurs in animals at modest doses. Well absorbed through the skin.	5 ppm S	5 ppm	270 ppm	...	Colorless liquid. Unpleasant odor. Vapor pressure is 2 mm Hg at 20 °C (68 °F). Flammable.
Allyl propyl disulfide (onion oil [CAS: 2179-59-1]): Mucous membrane irritant and lacrimator.	2 ppm	2 ppm	...	...	Liquid with a pungent, irritating odor. Thermal breakdown products include sulfur oxide fumes.

Chemical and toxic effects				NFPA	Physical description
α-Alumina (aluminum oxide [CAS: 1344-28-1]): Nuisance dust and physical irritant.	10 mg/m³	10 mg/m³ (total dust) 5 mg/m³ (respirable fraction)	...	...	
Aluminum metal [CAS: 7429-90-5]: Dusts can cause mild eye and respiratory tract irritation. Long-term inhalation of large amounts of fine aluminum powders has been reported to cause pulmonary fibrosis.	10 mg/m³ (metal and oxide) 5 mg/m³ (pyrophoric dusts) 2 mg/m³ (soluble salts)	15 mg/m³ (metal and oxide) 5 mg/m³ (respirable fraction, pyropowders, welding fumes) 2 mg/m³ (soluble salts)	...	0 1 1	Oxidizes readily. Fine powders and flakes are flammable and explosive when mixed with air. Reacts with acids and caustic solutions to produce flammable hydrogen gas.
4-Aminodiphenyl (p-aminobiphenyl, p-phenylaniline [CAS: 92-67-1]): Potent bladder carcinogen in humans. See p 482.	S, A1	OSHA CA	NIOSH CA	...	Colorless crystals.
2-Aminopyridine [CAS: 504-29-0]: Mild irritant. Potent CNS convulsant. Very well absorbed by inhalation and skin contact. Symptoms include headache, dizziness, nausea, elevated blood pressure, and convulsions.	0.5 ppm	0.5 ppm	5 ppm	...	Colorless solid with a distinctive odor with a very low vapor pressure at 20 °C (68 °F). Combustible.
Amitrole (3-amino-1,2,4-triazole [CAS: 61-82-5]): Mildly irritating upon direct contact. Well absorbed by inhalation and skin contact. Shows antithyroid activity in animals. Evidence of adverse effects on fetal development in animals. A carcinogen in animals. See p 482.	0.2 mg/m³	0.2 mg/m³	...	...	Crystalline solid. Appearance and some hazardous properties vary with the formulation.

(C) = ceiling air concentration (TLV-C); S = skin absorption can be significant; A1 = ACGIH-confirmed human carcinogen; A2 = ACGIH-suspected human carcinogen; NFPA Hazard Codes: H = health, F = fire, R = reactivity, OX = oxidizer, W = water-reactive, 0 (none) <—> 4 (severe). See expanded definitions on p 365.

continued

TABLE IV-12. HEALTH HAZARD SUMMARIES FOR INDUSTRIAL AND OCCUPATIONAL CHEMICALS (Continued)

Health Hazard Summaries	ACGIH TLV	PEL	IDLH	NFPA Codes H F R	Comments
Ammonia (CAS: 7664-41-7): Corrosive; severe burns to eyes and skin result. Vapors highly irritating to eyes and respiratory tract; pulmonary edema has been reported. See p 60.	25 ppm	50 ppm	500 ppm	3 1 0 (liquid) 2 1 0 (gas)	Colorless gas or aqueous solution. Pungent odor and irritation are good warning properties. Flammable. Breakdown products include oxides of nitrogen.
n-Amyl acetate (CAS: 628-63-7): Defats the skin, producing a dermatitis. Vapors mildly irritating to eyes and upper respiratory tract. A CNS depressant at very high levels. Reversible liver and kidney injury may occur at very high exposures.	100 ppm	100 ppm	4000 ppm	1 3 0	Colorless liquid. Its bananalike odor detectable below the PEL is a good warning property. Vapor pressure is 4 mm Hg at 20 °C (68 °F). Flammable.
sec-Amyl acetate [CAS: 628-38-0]: Defats the skin, producing a dermatitis. Vapors irritating to eyes and upper respiratory tract. A CNS depressant at very high levels. Reversible liver and kidney injury may occur at high-level exposures.	125 ppm	125 ppm	9000 ppm	1 3 0	Colorless liquid. A fruity odor occurs below the PEL and is a good warning property. Vapor pressure is 7 mm Hg at 20 °C (68 °F). Flammable.
Aniline (aminobenzene, phenylamine [CAS: 62-53-3]): Mildly irritating to eyes upon direct contact, with corneal injury possible. Potent inducer of methemoglobinemia (see p 204). Well absorbed via inhalation and dermal routes. A carcinogen in animals.	2 ppm S	2 ppm S	100 ppm	3 2 0	Colorless to brown viscous liquid. Distinctive amine odor and mild eye irritation occur well below the PEL and are good warning properties. Vapor pressure is 0.6 mm Hg at 20 °C (68 °F). Combustible. Breakdown products include oxides of nitrogen.
o-Anisidine (o-methoxyaniline [CAS: 29191-52-4]): Mild skin sensitizer causing dermatitis. Causes methemoglobinemia (see p 204). Well absorbed through skin. Headaches and vertigo are signs of exposure. Possible liver and kidney injury in animals. See p 482.	0.1 ppm S	0.5 mg/m³	50 mg/m³	2 1 0	Colorless, red, or yellow liquid with the fishy odor of amines. Vapor pressure is less than 0.1 mm Hg at 20 °C (68 °F). Combustible.

Chemical					Appearance/Comments
Antimony and salts (antimony trichloride, antimony trioxide, antimony pentachloride [CAS: 7440-36-0]): Dusts and fumes irritating to eyes and skin, producing blisters on moist areas of skin. Inhaled dusts or fumes are irritating to the respiratory tract; pneumoconiosis has been reported. Chronic overexposure may be cardiotoxic and cause liver injury. See p 74.	0.5 mg/m³ (as Sb)	0.5 mg/m³ (as Sb)	80 mg/m³ (as Sb)	…	The metal is silver-white and has a very low vapor pressure. Some chloride salts release HCl upon contact with water.
ANTU (α-naphthylthiourea [CAS: 86-88-4]): Well absorbed by skin contact and inhalation. Pulmonary edema and liver injury may result. Repeated exposures can injure the thyroid and adrenals, producing hypothyroidism. Possible slight contamination with a 2-naphthylamine, a human bladder carcinogen.	0.3 mg/m³	0.3 mg/m³	100 mg/m³	…	Colorless to gray solid powder. Odorless. Breakdown products include oxides of nitrogen and sulfur dioxide.
Arsenic (CAS: 7440-38-2): Irritating to eyes and skin; hyperpigmentation, hyperkeratoses, and skin cancers have been described. A general protoplasmic poison. May cause bone marrow suppression, peripheral neuropathy, and gastrointestinal, liver, and cardiac injury. Some arsenic compounds have adverse effects on fetal development in animals. Dust inhalation linked to respiratory tract cancers in workers. See pp 82 and 482.	0.2 mg/m³ (as As) OSHA CA	0.5 mg/m³ (as As)	NIOSH CA	…	Elemental forms vary in appearance. Crystals are gray. Amorphous forms may be yellow or black. Vapor pressure is very low—about 1 mm Hg at 372 °C (701 °F).
Arsenic trioxide (CAS: 1327-53-3): Highly irritating to eyes, skin, and mucous membranes. Perforation of the nasal septum, hyperpigmentation, and hyperkeratosis have been reported. Associated with lung cancer in workers. See pp 82 and 482.	A2	…	…		White powder; not combustible.

(C) = ceiling air concentration (TLV-C); S = skin absorption can be significant; A1 = ACGIH-confirmed human carcinogen; A2 = ACGIH-suspected human carcinogen; NFPA Hazard Codes: H = health, F = fire, R = reactivity, OX = oxidizer, W = water-reactive, 0 (none) < —> 4 (severe). See expanded definitions on p 365.

continued

TABLE IV–12. HEALTH HAZARD SUMMARIES FOR INDUSTRIAL AND OCCUPATIONAL CHEMICALS (Continued)

Health Hazard Summaries	ACGIH TLV	PEL	IDLH	NFPA Codes H F R	Comments
Arsine (CAS: 7784-42-1): Extremely toxic hemolytic agent. Symptoms include abdominal pain, jaundice, hemoglobinuria, and renal failure. Low-level chronic exposures reported to cause anemia. See p 83.	0.05 ppm	0.05 ppm	6 ppm NIOSH CA	...	Colorless gas with an unpleasant garliclike odor. Flammable. Breakdown products include arsenic trioxide and arsenic fumes.
Asbestos (chrysotile, amosite, crocidolite, tremolite, anthophyllite): Effects of exposure include asbestosis (fibrosis of the lung), lung cancer, mesothelioma, and possible digestive tract cancer. Signs of toxicity are usually delayed at least 15-20 years. See pp 84 and 483.	See comments A1	0.2 fibers/cm³ OSHA CA	NIOSH CA	...	Fibrous materials. Not combustible. The TLV-TWA values vary with the mineral: amosite, 0.5 fibers/cm³; crocidolite, 0.2 fibers/cm³; chrysotile and other forms, 2 fibers/cm³.
Asphalt fumes (CAS: 8052-42-4): Vapors and fumes irritating to eyes, skin, and respiratory tract. Skin contact can produce hyperpigmentation, dermatitis, or photosensitization. Some constituents are carcinogenic in animals. See p 483.	5 mg/m³	...	...	0 1 0	Smoke with an acrid odor.
Azinphos-methyl (Guthion [CAS: 86-50-0]): Organophosphate anticholinesterase insecticide. Requires metabolic activation. Dermal toxicity is low. See p 225.	0.2 mg/m³ S	0.2 mg/m³ S	...	...	Brown waxy solid with a negligible vapor pressure. Not combustible. Breakdown products include sulfur dioxide, oxides of nitrogen, and phosphoric acid.
Barium and soluble compounds (CAS: 7440-39-3): Powders irritating to eyes, skin, and upper respiratory tract. Upon ingestion, soluble forms of barium stimulate and then paralyze smooth, skeletal, and cardiac muscle. Cardiac arrhythmias may occur. See p 87.	0.5 mg/m³ (as Ba)	0.5 mg/m³	250 mg/m³	...	Most soluble barium compounds are odorless white solids. Elemental barium spontaneously ignites on contact with air and reacts with water to form flammable hydrogen gas.

Chemical	TLV	PEL/OSHA	NIOSH/IDLH	NFPA (H F R)	Physical description
Benomyl (methyl 1-(butylcarbamoyl)-2-benzimidazolecarbamate, Benlate [CAS: 17804-35-2]): A carbamate cholinesterase inhibitor. Mildly irritating to eyes and skin. Of low systemic toxicity in animals by all routes. Limited evidence of adverse effects on fetal development in animals at high doses. See p 106.	0.8 ppm	10 mg/m³ (total dust) 5 mg/m³ (respirable fraction)	...	...	White crystalline solid with a negligible vapor pressure at 20 °C (68 °F). Appearance and some hazardous properties vary with the formulation.
Benzene [CAS: 71-43-2]: Vapors mildly irritating to eyes and respiratory tract. Well absorbed by all routes. A CNS depressant at high levels. Symptoms include headache, nausea, tremors, and coma. High levels may sensitize the myocardium to the arrhythmogenic effects of epinephrine. Chronic exposure may result in hematopoietic system depression, aplastic anemia, and leukemia. See pp 89 and 483.	10 ppm A2	10 ppm OSHA CA	2000 ppm NIOSH CA	2 3 0	Colorless liquid. Aromatic hydrocarbon odor. Vapor pressure is 75 mm Hg at 20 °C (68 °F). Flammable.
Benzidine (p-diaminodiphenyl [CAS: 92-87-5]): Extremely well absorbed by inhalation and through skin. Caused bladder cancer in exposed workers. See p 483.	S, A1	OSHA CA	NIOSH CA	...	White or reddish solid crystals. Breakdown products include oxides of nitrogen.
Benzoyl peroxide [CAS: 94-36-0]: Dusts cause skin, eye, and respiratory tract irritation. A skin sensitizer.	5 mg/m³	5 mg/m³	1000 mg/m³	1 4 4 OX	White granules or crystalline solids with a very faint odor. Vapor pressure is negligible at 20 °C (68 °F). Strong oxidizer, reacting with combustible materials. Decomposes at 75 °C (167 °F). Unstable and explosive at high temperatures.
Benzyl chloride (α-chlorotoluene, (chloro-methyl)benzene [CAS: 100-44-7]): Highly irritating to skin and eyes. A potent lacrimator. Vapors highly irritating to respiratory tract; pulmonary edema could result. CNS complaints include weakness, headache, and irritability. May injure liver.	1 ppm	1 ppm	10 ppm	2 2 1	Colorless liquid with a pungent odor. Vapor pressure is 0.9 mm Hg at 20 °C (68 °F). Combustible. Breakdown products include phosgene and hydrogene chloride.

(C) = ceiling air concentration (TLV-C); S = skin absorption can be significant; A1 = ACGIH-confirmed human carcinogen; A2 = ACGIH-suspected human carcinogen; NFPA Hazard Codes: H = health, F = fire, R = reactivity, OX = oxidizer, 0 (none) <—> 4 (severe). See expanded definitions on p 365.

continued

TABLE IV-12. HEALTH HAZARD SUMMARIES FOR INDUSTRIAL AND OCCUPATIONAL CHEMICALS (Continued)

Health Hazard Summaries	ACGIH TLV	PEL	IDLH	NFPA Codes H F R	Comments
Beryllium (CAS: 7440–41–7): Dusts and fumes cause eye, skin, and respiratory tract irritation; may cause pulmonary edema. Chronic low-level exposures to beryllium oxide dusts have produced interstitial lung disease (berylliosis). Soluble salts are sensitizers and cause severe mucous membrane irritation. A carcinogen in animals. There is limited evidence of carcinogenicity in humans. See p 483.	0.002 mg/m³ A2	0.002 mg/m³	NIOSH CA	4 1 0	Silver-white metal or dusts. Reacts with some acids to produce flammable hydrogen gas.
Biphenyl (diphenyl) (CAS: 92–52–4): Fumes mildly irritating to eyes. Chronic overexposures can cause bronchitis and liver injury. Peripheral neuropathy and CNS injury have also been reported.	0.2 ppm	0.2 ppm	300 mg/m³	2 1 0	White crystals. Unusual but pleasant odor. Combustible. Vapor pressure is 0.005 mm Hg at 20°C (68°F).
Bismuth telluride (bismuth tritelluride (CAS: 1304–82–1)): Based on limited studies, an inert or nuisance dust. Inhalation produces mild and reversible pulmonary effects in animals.	10 mg/m³ 5 mg/m³ (selenium doped)	15 mg/m³ (total dust) 5 mg/m³ (respirable fraction)	...	...	Gray platelets or crystals. Vapor pressure is negligible at 20 °C (68 °F).
Borates (anhydrous sodium tetraborate, borax (CAS: 1303–96–4)): Contact with dusts is highly irritating to eyes, skin, and respiratory tract. Contact with tissue moisture may cause thermal burns because hydration of borates generates heat. See p 94.	1 mg/m³ (anhydrous and pentahydrate) 5 mg/m³ (decahydrate)	10 mg/m³	...	...	White or light gray solid crystals. Odorless.

Chemical			NFPA	
Boron oxide (boric anhydride, boric oxide [CAS: 1303-86-2]): Contact with moisture generates boric acid. Direct eye or skin contact with dusts is irritating. Occupational inhalation exposure has caused sore throat and cough. Evidence for adverse effects on the testes in animals. See p 94.	10 mg/m³	10 mg/m³ (total dust) 5 mg/m³ (respirable fraction)	...	Colorless glassy granules, flakes, or powder. Odorless. Not combustible.
Boron tribromide (CAS: 10294-33-4): Corrosive; decomposed by tissue moisture to hydrogen bromide and boric acid. Severe skin and eye burns may result from direct contact. Vapors highly irritating to eyes and respiratory tract; delayed pulmonary edema may result. See p. 94.	1 ppm (C)	1 ppm (C)	...	Colorless fuming liquid. Reacts with water, forming hydrogen bromide and boric acid. Vapor pressure is 40 mm Hg at 14 °C (57 °F).
Boron trifluoride (CAS: 7637-07-2): Corrosive; decomposed by tissue moisture to hydrogen fluoride and boric acid. Severe skin and eye burns may result. Vapors highly irritating to eyes, skin, and respiratory tract; may cause delayed pulmonary edema. See p 94.	1 ppm (C)	100 ppm	3 0 1	Colorless gas. Dense white irritating fumes produced on contact with moist air. These fumes contain boric acid and hydrogen fluoride.
Bromine (CAS: 7726-95-6): Corrosive; severe skin and eye burns may result. Vapors highly irritating to eyes and respiratory tract; delayed-onset pulmonary edema may result. Measleslike eruptions may appear on the skin several hours after a severe exposure.	0.1 ppm	10 ppm	4 0 0 OX	Heavy red-brown fuming liquid. Odor and irritation thresholds are below the PEL and are adequate warning properties. Vapor pressure is 175 mm Hg at 20 °C (68 °F). Not combustible.
Bromine pentafluoride (CAS: 7789-30-2): Corrosive; severe skin and eye burns may result. Vapors extremely irritating to eyes and upper respiratory tract; pulmonary edema may result. Chronic overexposures caused severe liver and kidney injury in animals. See p 114.	0.1 ppm	...	4 0 3 W, OX	Pale yellow liquid. Pungent odor. Not combustible. Highly reactive, igniting most organic materials and corroding many metals. Highly reactive with acids. Breakdown products include bromine and fluorine.

(C) = ceiling air concentration (TLV-C); S = skin absorption can be significant; A1 = ACGIH-confirmed human carcinogen; A2 = ACGIH-suspected human carcinogen; NFPA Hazard Codes: H = health, F = fire, R = reactivity, OX = oxidizer, W = water-reactive, 0 (none) <—> 4 (severe). See expanded definitions on p 365.

continued

TABLE IV-12. HEALTH HAZARD SUMMARIES FOR INDUSTRIAL AND OCCUPATIONAL CHEMICALS (Continued)

Health Hazard Summaries	ACGIH TLV	PEL	IDLH	NFPA Codes H F R	Comments
Bromoform (tribromomethane [CAS: 75-25-2]): Vapors highly irritating to eyes and respiratory tract. Well absorbed by inhalation and skin contact. CNS depressant. Liver and kidney injury may occur. Two preliminary tests indicate that it may be an animal carcinogen.	0.5 ppm S	0.5 ppm S	...	...	Colorless to yellow liquid. Chloroformlike odor and irritation are adequate warning properties. Vapor pressure is 5 mm Hg at 20 °C (68 °F). Not combustible. Thermal breakdown products include hydrogen bromide and bromine.
1,3-Butadiene (CAS: 106-99-0): Contact with liquid can cause dermatitis and frostbite. Vapors mildly irritating. A CNS depressant at very high levels. Evidence of adverse effects on fetal development in animals at high doses. Animal carcinogen. See p 484.	10 ppm A2	1000 ppm	20,000 ppm NIOSH CA	2 4 2	Colorless gas. Mild aromatic odor is a good warning property. Readily polymerizes. Inhibitor added to prevent peroxide formation. PEL under review.
2-Butoxyethanol (ethylene glycol monobutyl ether, butyl cellosolve [CAS: 111-76-2]): Liquid very irritating to eyes and slightly irritating to skin. Vapors irritating to eyes and upper respiratory tract. Mild CNS depressant. A hemolytic agent in animals. Well absorbed dermally. Liver and kidney toxicity in animals. See p 151.	25 ppm S	25 ppm S	700 ppm	...	Colorless liquid with a mild etherlike odor. Irritation occurs below the PEL and is a good warning property. Vapor pressure is 0.6 mm Hg at 20 °C (68 °F). Flammable.
n-Butyl acetate (CAS: 123-86-4): Defatting agent causing dermatitis. Vapors irritating to eyes and upper respiratory tract. A CNS depressant at high levels.	150 ppm	150 ppm	10,000 ppm	1 3 0	Colorless liquid. Fruity odor is a good warning property. Vapor pressure is 10 mm Hg at 20 °C (68 °F). Flammable.
sec-Butyl acetate (2-butanol acetate [CAS: 105-46-4]): Defatting agent causing dermatitis. Vapors irritating to eyes and upper respiratory tract. A CNS depressant at high levels.	200 ppm	200 ppm	10,000 ppm	1 3 0	Colorless liquid with a fruity odor. Vapor pressure is 10 mm Hg at 20 °C (63 °F). Flammable.

Chemical				NFPA	Comments
tert-Butyl acetate (tert-butyl ester of acetic acid [CAS: 540-88-5]): Defatting agent causing dermatitis. Vapors irritating to eyes and upper respiratory tract. A CNS depressant at high levels.	200 ppm	200 ppm	8000 ppm	...	Colorless liquid with a fruity odor. Flammable.
Butyl acrylate (CAS: 141-32-2): Highly irritating to skin and eyes; corneal necrosis may result. Vapors highly irritating to eyes and respiratory tract. Based on structural analogies, compounds containing the acrylate moiety may be carcinogens.	10 ppm	10 ppm	...	2 2 2	Colorless liquid. Vapor pressure is 3.2 mm Hg at 20 °C (68 °F). Flammable. Usually contains inhibitor to prevent polymerization.
n-Butyl alcohol (CAS: 71-36-3): Irritating upon direct contact. A defatting agent causing dermatitis. Vapors mildly irritating to eyes and upper respiratory tract. A CNS depressant at very high levels. Chronic occupational overexposures associated with hearing loss and vestibular impairment.	50 ppm (C) S	50 ppm (C) S	8000 ppm	1 3 0	Colorless liquid. Strong odor and irritation occur below the PEL and are both good warning properties. Flammable. Vapor pressure is 4.4 mm Hg at 20 °C (68 °F).
sec-Butyl alcohol (CAS: 78-92-2): Defatting agent causing dermatitis. Vapors mildly irritating to eyes and upper respiratory tract. A CNS depressant at high levels.	100 ppm	100 ppm	10,000 ppm	1 3 0	Colorless liquid. Pleasant odor occurs well below the PEL and is an adequate warning property. Vapor pressure is 13 mm Hg at 20 °C (68 °F). Flammable.
tert-Butyl alcohol (CAS: 75-65-0): Defatting agent causing dermatitis. Vapors mildly irritating to eyes and upper respiratory tract. A CNS depressant at high levels.	100 ppm	100 ppm	8000 ppm	1 3 0	Colorless liquid. Camphorlike odor and irritation occur slightly below the PEL and are good warning properties. Vapor pressure is 31 mm Hg at 20 °C (68 °F). Flammable.

(C) = ceiling air concentration (TLV-C); S = skin absorption can be significant; A1 = ACGIH-confirmed human carcinogen; A2 = ACGIH-suspected human carcinogen; NFPA Hazard Codes: H = health, F = fire, R = reactivity, OX = oxidizer, W = water-reactive, 0 (none) < — > 4 (severe). See expanded definitions on p 365.

continued

TABLE IV-12. HEALTH HAZARD SUMMARIES FOR INDUSTRIAL AND OCCUPATIONAL CHEMICALS (Continued)

Health Hazard Summaries	ACGIH TLV	PEL	IDLH	NFPA Codes H F R	Comments
Butylamine (CAS: 109-73-9): Caustic alkali. Liquid highly irritating to eyes and skin upon direct contact; severe burns may result. Vapors highly irritating to eyes and upper respiratory tract; pulmonary edema may result. May cause histamine release. Symptoms of poisoning in animals included restlessness and convulsions.	5 ppm (C) S	5 ppm (C) S	2000 ppm	2 3 0	Colorless liquid. Ammonia or fishlike odor occurs below the PEL and is an adequate warning property. Vapor pressure is about 82 mm Hg at 20 °C (68 °F). Flammable.
***tert*-Butyl chromate (CAS: 1189-85-1):** Liquid highly irritating to eyes and skin; severe burns may result. Vapors or mists irritating to eyes and respiratory tract. A liver and kidney toxin. By analogy to other Cr(VI) compounds, a possible carcinogen. See pp 124 and 485.	0.1 mg/m³ (C) S (as CrO₃)	0.1 mg/m³ (C) S	...	...	Liquid. Reacts with moisture.
***n*-Butyl glycidyl ether (BGE, glycidylbutylether, 1,2-epoxy-3-butoxy propane [CAS: 2426-08-6]):** Liquid irritating to eyes and skin. Vapors irritating to the respiratory tract. A CNS depressant. Causes sensitization dermatitis upon repeated exposures. Testicular atrophy and hematopoietic injury at modest doses in animals.	25 ppm	25 ppm	3500 ppm	...	Colorless liquid. Vapor pressure is 3 mm Hg at 20 °C (68 °F).
***n*-Butyl lactate (CAS: 138-22-7):** Vapors irritating to eyes and respiratory tract. Workers have complained of sleepiness, headache, coughing, nausea, and vomiting.	5 ppm	5 ppm	...	1 2 0	Colorless liquid. Vapor pressure is 0.4 mm Hg at 20 °C (68 °F). Combustible.
***n*-Butyl mercaptan (butanethiol [CAS: 109-79-5]):** Vapors mildly irritating to eyes and respiratory tract. Pulmonary edema occurred at high exposure levels in animals. A CNS depressant at very high levels. See p 169.	0.5 ppm	0.5 ppm	2500 ppm	2 3 0	Colorless liquid. Strong, offensive garliclike odor. Vapor pressure is 35 mm Hg at 20 °C (68 °F). Flammable.

Chemical				Description
o-sec-Butylphenol (CAS: 89-72-5): Irritating to skin upon direct, prolonged contact; burns have resulted. Vapors mildly irritating to eyes and respiratory tract.	5 ppm S	5 ppm S	...	A liquid.
p-tert-Butyltoluene (CAS: 98-51-1): Mild skin irritant upon direct contact. Defatting agent causing dermatitis. Vapors irritating to eyes and respiratory tract. A CNS depressant. May sensitize the myocardium to the arrhythmogenic effects of epinephrine. Decreased blood pressure, increased pulse rate, tremor, and anxiety may occur. Limited evidence of adverse effects on fetal development in animals at high doses.	10 ppm	10 ppm	...	Colorless liquid. Gasolinelike odor and irritation occur below the PEL and are both good warning properties. Vapor pressure is less than 1 mm Hg at 20 °C (68 °F). Combustible.
Cadmium and compounds: Fumes and dusts highly irritating to respiratory tract; pulmonary edema has been reported. Chronic exposures associated with kidney and lung injury. Adverse effects on the testes and on fetal development in animals. Cadmium and some of its compounds are carcinogenic in animals. Limited direct evidence for carcinogenicity in humans. See pp 99 and 484.	0.05 mg/m³ (as Cd)	0.1 mg/m³ (fume) 0.2 mg/m³ (dust)	...	40 mg/m³ NIOSH CA	Compounds vary in color. Give off fumes when heated or burned. Generally poor warning properties. Metal has a vapor pressure of about 1 mm Hg at 394 °C (741 °F) and reacts with acids to produce flammable hydrogen gas. TLV and PEL under review.
Calcium cyanamide (calcium carbimide, lime nitrogen [CAS: 156-62-7]): Dusts highly irritating to eyes, skin, and respiratory tract. Causes sensitization dermatitis. Systemic symptoms include nausea, fatigue, headache, chest pain, and shivering. A disulfiramlike interaction with alcohol, "cyanamide flush," may occur in exposed workers. See p 143.	0.5 mg/m³	0.5 mg/m³	...	...	Gray crystalline material. Reacts with water, generating ammonia and flammable acetylene.
Calcium hydroxide (hydrated lime, caustic lime [CAS: 1305-62-0]): Corrosive; severe eye and skin burns may result. Dusts moderately irritating to eyes and respiratory tract.	5 mg/m³	5 mg/m³	...	...	White, deliquescent crystalline powder. Odorless.

(C) = ceiling air concentration (TLV-C); S = skin absorption can be significant; A1 = ACGIH-confirmed human carcinogen; A2 = ACGIH-suspected human carcinogen; NFPA Hazard Codes: H = health, F = fire, R = reactivity, OX = oxidizer, W = water-reactive, 0 (none) < — > 4 (severe). See expanded definitions on p 365.

continued

TABLE IV-12. HEALTH HAZARD SUMMARIES FOR INDUSTRIAL AND OCCUPATIONAL CHEMICALS (Continued)

Health Hazard Summaries	ACGIH TLV	PEL	IDLH	NFPA Codes H F R	Comments
Calcium oxide (lime, quicklime, burnt lime [CAS: 1305-78-8]): Corrosive. Exothermic reactions with moisture. Highly irritating to eyes and skin upon direct contact. Dusts highly irritating to skin, eyes, and upper respiratory tract; pulmonary edema has been reported.	2 mg/m³	5 mg/m³	250 mg/m³	1 0 1	White or gray solid powder. Odorless. Hydration generates heat.
Camphor, synthetic (CAS: 76-22-2): Irritating to eyes and skin upon direct contact. Vapors irritating to eyes and nose; may cause loss of sense of smell. A convulsant at high levels. See p 104.	2 ppm	2 mg/m³	200 mg/m³	0 2 0	Colorless glassy solid. Sharp, obnoxious, aromatic odor near the PEL is an adequate warning property. Vapor pressure is 0.18 mm Hg at 20 °C (68 °F). Combustible.
Caprolactam (CAS: 105-60-2): Highly irritating to eyes and skin upon direct contact. Vapors, dusts, and fumes highly irritating to eyes and upper respiratory tract. Convulsant activity in animals.	1 mg/m³ (dust) 4.3 ppm (vapor)	1 mg/m³ (dust) 5 ppm (vapor)	...	...	White solid crystals. Unpleasant odor. Vapor pressure is 6 mm Hg at 120 °C (248 °F). Thermal breakdown products include oxides of nitrogen. TLV under review.
Captafol (Difolatan [CAS: 2425-06-1]): Dusts irritating to eyes, skin, and respiratory tract. A skin and respiratory tract sensitizer. May cause photoallergic dermatitis. Evidence of carcinogenicity in animals.	0.1 mg/m³ S	0.1 mg/m³	...	...	White solid crystals. Distinctive, pungent odor. Thermal breakdown products include hydrogen chloride and oxides of nitrogen or sulfur.
Carbaryl (1-naphthyl N-methylcarbamate, Sevin [CAS: 63-25-2]): A carbamate-type cholinesterase inhibitor. Evidence of adverse effects on fetal development in animals at high doses. See p 106.	5 mg/m³	5 mg/m³	625 mg/m³	...	Colorless, white, or gray solid. Odorless. Vapor pressure is 0.005 mm Hg at 20 °C (68 °F). Breakdown products include oxides of nitrogen and methylamine.

Substance	PEL	TLV	IDLH	NFPA Codes (H F R)	Comments
Carbofuran (2,3-dihydro-2,2'-dimethyl-7-benzofuranyl-methylcarbamate, Furadan [CAS: 1563-66-2]): A carbamate-type cholinesterase inhibitor. Not well absorbed by skin contact. See p 106.	0.1 mg/m³	0.1 mg/m³	…		White solid crystals. Odorless. Vapor pressure is 0.00005 mm Hg at 33 °C (91 °F). Thermal breakdown products include oxides of nitrogen.
Carbon disulfide (CAS: 75-15-0): Irritating upon prolonged contact. Vapors mildly irritating to eyes and upper respiratory tract. A CNS depressant causing coma at high concentrations. Well absorbed by all routes. Acute symptoms include headaches, dizziness, nervousness, and fatigue. Peripheral and cranial neuropathies, parkinsonianlike syndromes, and psychosis may occur. A liver and kidney toxin. A possible atherogenic agent. Adversely affects male and female reproductive systems in animals and humans. Evidence for adverse effects on fetal development in animals.	10 ppm S	4 ppm S	500 ppm	2 3 0	Colorless to pale yellow liquid. Disagreeable odor occurs below the PEL and is a good warning property. Vapor pressure is 300 mm Hg at 20 °C (68 °F). Highly flammable.
Carbon monoxide (CAS: 630-08-0): Binds to hemoglobin, forming carboxyhemoglobin and causing cellular hypoxia. Persons with heart disease are more susceptible. Symptoms include headache, dizziness, coma, and convulsions. Permanent CNS impairment and adverse effects on fetal development may occur after severe posioning. See p 109.	50 ppm	35 ppm	1500 ppm	2 4 0	Colorless, odorless gas. No warning properties.
Carbon tetrabromide (tetrabromomethane) [CAS: 558-13-4]): Highly irritating to eyes upon direct contact. Vapors highly irritating to eyes and respiratory tract; delayed pulmonary edema may occur. The liver and kidneys are also likely target organs.	0.1 ppm	0.1 ppm	…		White to yellow-brown solid. Vapor pressure is 40 mm Hg at 96 °C (204 °F). Nonflammable; thermal breakdown products may include hydrogen bromide and bromine.

(C) = ceiling air concentration (TLV-C); S = skin absorption can be significant; A1 = ACGIH-confirmed human carcinogen; A2 = ACGIH-suspected human carcinogen; NFPA Hazard Codes: H = health, F = fire, R = reactivity, OX = oxidizer, W = water-reactive, 0 (none) <—> 4 (severe). See expanded definitions on p 365.

continued

TABLE IV-12. HEALTH HAZARD SUMMARIES FOR INDUSTRIAL AND OCCUPATIONAL CHEMICALS (Continued)

Health Hazard Summaries	ACGIH TLV	PEL	IDLH	NFPA Codes H F R	Comments
Carbon tetrachloride (tetrachloromethane [CAS: 56-23-5]): Mildly irritating upon direct contact. A CNS depressant. Highly toxic to kidney and liver. Alcohol abuse increases risk of liver toxicity. May cause cardiac arrhythmias. A carcinogen in animals. See pp 111 and 484.	5 ppm S, A2	2 ppm	300 ppm NIOSH CA	3 0 0	Colorless. Etherlike odor is a poor warning property. Vapor pressure is 91 mm Hg at 20 °C (68 °F). Not combustible. Breakdown products include hydrogen chloride, chlorine gas, and phosgene.
Carbonyl fluoride (COF_2 [CAS: 353-50-4]): Extremely irritating to eyes and respiratory tract; delayed pulmonary edema may result. Toxicity results from its hydrolysis to hydrofluoric acid. See p 167.	2 ppm	2 ppm	...	...	Colorless, odorless gas. Decomposes upon contact with water to produce hydrofluoric acid.
Catechol (1,2-benzenediol [CAS: 120-80-9]): Highly irritating upon direct contact; severe eye and deep skin burns result. Well absorbed by skin. Systemic toxicity similar to that of phenol (see p 234); however, catechol may be more likely to cause convulsions and hypertension. At high doses, renal and liver injury may occur.	5 ppm	5 ppm S	...	...	Colorless solid crystals.
Cesium hydroxide (cesium hydrate [CAS: 21351-79-1]): Corrosive. Highly irritating upon direct contact; severe burns may result. Dusts are irritating to eyes and upper respiratory tract.	2 mg/m³	2 mg/m³	...	...	Colorless or yellow crystals that absorb moisture. Negligible vapor pressure.
Chlordane (CAS: 57-74-9): Irritating to skin. A CNS convulsant. Skin absorption is rapid and has caused convulsions and death. Hepatotoxic. There is equivocal evidence of carcinogenicity in animals. See p 117.	0.5 mg/m³ S	0.5 mg/m³ S	500 mg/m³	...	Viscous amber liquid. Formulations vary in appearance. A chlorinelike odor. Vapor pressure is 0.00001 mm Hg at 20 °C (68 °F). Not combustible. Thermal breakdown products include hydrogen chloride, phosgene, and chlorine gas.

Chemical				NFPA	Description
Chlorinated camphene (toxaphene) [CAS: 8001-35-2]: Moderately irritating upon direct contact. A CNS convulsant. Acute symptoms include nausea, confusion, tremors, and convulsions. Well absorbed by skin. Potential liver and kidney injury. See p 117.	0.5 mg/m³ S	0.5 mg/m³ S	200 mg/m³	...	Waxy amber-colored solid. Formulations vary in appearance. Turpentinelike odor. Vapor pressure is about 0.3 mm Hg at 20 °C (68 °F).
Chlorinated diphenyl oxide [CAS: 55720-99-5]: Chloracne may result from even small exposures. A hepatotoxin in chronically exposed animals. Symptoms include gastrointestinal upset, jaundice, and fatigue.	0.5 mg/m³	0.5 mg/m³	5 mg/m³	...	Waxy solid or liquid. Vapor pressure is 0.00006 mm Hg at 20 °C (68 °F).
Chlorine [CAS: 7782-50-5]: Extremely irritating to eyes, skin, and respiratory tract; severe burns and pulmonary edema may occur. Symptoms include lacrimation, sore throat, headache, coughing, and wheezing. High concentrations may cause rapid tissue swelling and airway obstruction. See p 119.	1 ppm	0.5 ppm	25 ppm	3 0 0 OX	Amber liquid or greenish-yellow gas. Irritating odor and irritation occur near the PEL and are both good warning properties.
Chlorine dioxide (chlorine peroxide) [CAS: 10049-04-4]: Extremely irritating to eyes and respiratory tract; delayed pulmonary edema and severe bronchitis (acute and chronic) have been reported. See p 119.	0.1 ppm	0.1 ppm	10 ppm	...	Yellow-green gas or liquid. Sharp odor at the PEL is a good warning property. Reacts with water to produce perchloric acid. Decomposes explosively in sunlight, with heat, or with shock to produce chlorine gas.
Chlorine trifluoride (chlorine fluoride) [CAS: 7790-91-2]: Upon contact with moist tissues, hydrolyzes to chlorine, hydrogen fluoride, and chlorine dioxide. Extremely irritating to eyes, skin, and respiratory tract; severe burns or delayed pulmonary edema could result. See pp 119 and 167.	0.1 ppm (C)	0.1 ppm (C)	20 ppm	4 0 3 W	Greenish-yellow or colorless liquid or gas. Possesses a suffocating, sweet odor. Not combustible. Water-reactive, yielding hydrogen fluoride and chlorine gas.

continued

(C) = ceiling air concentration (TLV-C); S = skin absorption can be significant; A1 = ACGIH-confirmed human carcinogen; A2 = ACGIH-suspected human carcinogen; NFPA Hazard Codes: H = health, F = fire, R = reactivity, OX = oxidizer, W = water-reactive, 0 (none) < — > 4 (severe). See expanded definitions on p 365.

TABLE IV-12. HEALTH HAZARD SUMMARIES FOR INDUSTRIAL AND OCCUPATIONAL CHEMICALS (Continued)

Health Hazard Summaries	ACGIH TLV	PEL	IDLH	NFPA Codes H F R	Comments
Chloroacetaldehyde [CAS: 107-20-0]: Extremely corrosive upon direct contact; severe burns will result. Vapors extremely irritating to eyes, skin, and upper respiratory tract; delayed pulmonary edema may occur at high levels.	1 ppm (C)	1 ppm (C)	250 ppm	...	Colorless liquid with a pungent, irritating odor. Vapor pressure is 100 mm Hg at 20 °C (68 °F). Combustible. Readily polymerizes. Thermal breakdown products include phosgene and hydrogen chloride.
α-Chloroacetophenone (tear gas, chemical Mace [CAS: 532-27-4]): Extremely irritating to eyes and respiratory tract; delayed pulmonary edema has been reported. A potent skin sensitizer.	0.05 ppm	0.05 ppm	100 mg/m³	2 1 0	Sharp, irritating odor and irritation occur near the PEL and are adequate warning properties. Vapor pressure is 0.012 mm Hg at 20 °C (68 °F).
Chlorobenzene (monochlorobenzene [CAS: 108-90-7]): Irritating; skin burns may result from prolonged contact. Vapors irritating to eyes and upper respiratory tract. A CNS depressant. May sensitize myocardium to arrhythmogenic effects of epinephrine. Prolonged exposure to high levels has caused lung, liver, and kidney injury in animals. Lacks the hematopoietic toxicity of benzene.	75 ppm	75 ppm	2400 ppm	2 3 0	Colorless liquid. Aromatic odor occurs below the PEL and is a good warning property. Vapor pressure is 8.8 mm Hg at 20 °C (68 °F). Flammable. Thermal breakdown products include hydrogen chloride and phosgene. TLV under review.
o-Chlorobenzylidenemalononitrile (tear gas, OCBM, CS [CAS: 2698-41-1]): Highly irritating on contact; severe burns may result. Aerosols and vapors very irritating to eyes and upper respiratory tract. Potent skin sensitizer. Symptoms include headache, nausea and vomiting, severe eye and nose irritation, excess salivation, coughing, and wheezing.	0.05 ppm (C) S	0.05 ppm (C) S	2 mg/m³	...	White solid crystals. Pepperlike odor. Vapor pressure is much less than 1 mm Hg at 20 °C (68 °F).

Chemical				Comments
Chlorobromomethane (bromochloromethane, Halon 1011 [CAS: 74-97-5]): Irritating upon direct contact; dermatitis may result from defatting action. Vapors mildly irritating to eyes and respiratory tract. A CNS depressant. Disorientation, nausea, headache, seizures, and coma have been reported at high exposure. May sensitize the myocardium to arrhythmogenic effects of epinephrine. Chronic high doses caused liver and kidney injury in animals.	200 ppm	200 ppm	5000 ppm	...	Colorless to pale yellow liquid. Sweet, pleasant odor detectable far below the PEL. Vapor pressure is 117 mm Hg at 20 °C (68 °F). Thermal breakdown products include hydrogen chloride, hydrogen bromide, and phosgene.
Chlorodifluoromethane (Freon 22 [CAS: 75-45-6]): Irritating upon direct contact; prolonged contact causes defatting dermatitis. Vapors mildly irritating to eyes and respiratory tract. A CNS depressant and cardiac sensitizer only at very high levels in animals. At high doses, there is evidence for adverse effects on fetal development in animals. See p 161.	1000 ppm	1000 ppm	...	Colorless, almost odorless gas. Nonflammable. Thermal breakdown products may include hydrogen fluoride. Vapor pressure is 10 mm Hg at 20 °C (68 °F).
Chloroform (trichloromethane [CAS: 67-66-3]): Mildly irritating upon direct contact; dermatitis may result from prolonged exposure. Vapors slightly irritating to eyes and respiratory tract. A CNS depressant. Can cause cardiac arrhythmias by sensitizing the heart to epinephrine. Can produce liver and kidney damage. Evidence of adverse effects on fetal development in animals. A carcinogen in animals. See pp 120 and 485.	10 ppm A2	2 ppm	1000 ppm NIOSH CA	2 0 0	Colorless liquid. Pleasant, sweet odor. Not combustible. Vapor pressure is 160 mm Hg at 20 °C (68 °F). Breakdown products include hydrogen chloride, phosgene, and chlorine gas.
bis(Chloromethyl) ether (BCME [CAS: 542-88-1]): A human and animal carcinogen. See p 485.	0.001 ppm A1	OSHA CA	NIOSH CA	...	Colorless liquid with a suffocating odor. Vapor pressure is 100 mm Hg at 20 °C (68 °F).

(C) = ceiling air concentration (TLV-C); S = skin absorption can be significant; A1 = ACGIH-confirmed human carcinogen; A2 = ACGIH-suspected human carcinogen; NFPA Hazard Codes: H = health, F = fire, R = reactivity, OX = oxidizer, W = water-reactive, 0 (none) < —> 4 (severe). See expanded definitions on p 365.

continued

TABLE IV-12. HEALTH HAZARD SUMMARIES FOR INDUSTRIAL AND OCCUPATIONAL CHEMICALS (Continued)

Health Hazard Summaries	ACGIH TLV	PEL	IDLH	NFPA Codes H F R	Comments
Chloromethyl methyl ether (CMME, methyl chloromethyl ether [CAS: 107-30-2]): Vapors irritating to eyes and upper respiratory tract. Workers show increased risk of lung cancer, possibly owing to contamination of CMME with 1–7% BCME. See p 485.	A2	OSHA CA	NIOSH CA	...	Combustible. Breakdown products include oxides of nitrogen and hydrogen chloride.
1-Chloro-1-nitropropane (CAS: 600-25-9): Based on animal studies, vapors highly irritating to eyes and respiratory tract and may cause pulmonary edema. Based on high-dose animal studies, may injure cardiac muscle, liver, and kidney.	2 ppm	2 ppm	2000 ppm	2 3	Colorless liquid. Unpleasant odor and tearing occur near the PEL and are good warning properties. Vapor pressure is 5.8 mm Hg at 20 °C (68 °F).
Chloropentafluoroethane (fluorocarbon 115 [CAS: 76-15-3]): Irritating upon direct contact; prolonged contact causes defatting dermatitis. Vapors mildly irritating to eyes and respiratory tract. A CNS depressant and cardiac sensitizer only at very high levels in animals. See p 161.	1000 ppm	1000 ppm	...	...	Colorless, odorless gas. Thermal breakdown products include hydrogen fluoride and hydrogen chloride.
Chloropicrin (trichloronitromethane [CAS: 76-06-2]): Extremely irritating upon direct contact; severe burns may result. Vapors extremely irritating to eyes, skin, and respiratory tract; delayed pulmonary edema has been reported. Kidney and liver injuries have been observed in animals.	0.1 ppm	0.1 ppm	4 ppm	4 0 3	Colorless, oily liquid. Sharp, penetrating odor and tearing occur near the PEL and are good warning properties. Vapor pressure is 20 mm Hg at 20 °C (68 °F). Breakdown products include oxides of nitrogen, phosgene, nitrosyl chloride, and chlorine gas.

Chemical	TLV	NIOSH/CA	NFPA (H F R)	Physical properties
β-Chloroprene (2-chloro-1,3-butadiene [CAS: 126-99-8]): Irritating upon direct contact. Vapors irritating to eyes and respiratory tract. A CNS depressant at high levels. Liver and kidneys are major target organs. Limited evidence for adverse effects on fetal development in animals. Equivocal evidence of carcinogenicity in animals. See p 485.	10 ppm S	400 ppm NIOSH CA	2 3 0	Colorless liquid with an etherlike odor. Vapor pressure is 179 mm Hg at 20 °C (68 °F). Highly flammable. Breakdown products include hydrogen chloride.
o-Chlorotoluene (2-chloro-1-methylbenzene [CAS: 95-49-8]): Workplace exposures not known to cause adverse effects from inhalation or direct contact. May sensitize the myocardium to the arrhythmogenic effects of epinephrine. In animals, direct contact produced skin and eye irritation; high vapor exposures resulted in tremors, convulsions, and coma.	50 ppm	50 ppm	2 2 0	Colorless liquid. Vapor pressure is 10 mm Hg at 43 °C (109 °F). Flammable.
Chlorpyrifos (Dursban, O,O-diethyl-O-(3,5,6-trichloro-2-pyridinyl [CAS: 2921-88-2]): An organophosphate-type cholinesterase inhibitor. See p 225.	0.2 mg/m³ S	0.2 mg/m³ S	⋯	White solid crystals. Vapor pressure is 0.00002 mm Hg at 25 °C (77 °F).
Chromic acid and chromates (chromium trioxide, sodium dichromate, potassium chromate): Highly irritating upon direct contact; severe eye and skin ulceration (chrome ulcers) may result. Dusts and mists highly irritating to eyes and respiratory tract. Skin and respiratory sensitization may occur. The kidney is a major target organ. Chromium trioxide is a teratogen in animals. Certain hexavalent chromium compounds are carcinogenic in animals and humans. See pp 124 and 485.	0.5 mg/m³ (CrII and III compounds) 0.05 mg/m³ (CrVI compounds) A1	0.1 ppm (C)	⋯	Soluble chromate compounds are water-reactive.

(C) = ceiling air concentration (TLV-C); S = skin absorption can be significant; A1 = ACGIH-confirmed human carcinogen; A2 = ACGIH-suspected human carcinogen; NFPA Hazard Codes: H = health, F = fire, R = reactivity, OX = oxidizer, W = water-reactive, 0 (none) <—> 4 (severe). See expanded definitions on p 365.

continued

TABLE IV-12. HEALTH HAZARD SUMMARIES FOR INDUSTRIAL AND OCCUPATIONAL CHEMICALS (Continued)

Health Hazard Summaries	ACGIH TLV	PEL	IDLH	NFPA Codes H F R	Comments
Chromium metal and insoluble chromium salts: Irritating upon direct contact with skin and eyes; dermatitis may result. Ferrochrome alloys associated with pneumoconiotic changes. See p 124.	0.5 mg/m³ (metal, as Cr) 0.05 mg/m³ (CrVI compounds, as Cr) A1	1 mg/m³ (metal)	...	...	Chromium metal, silver luster; copper chromite, greenish-blue solid. Odorless.
Chromyl chloride (CAS: 14977-61-8): Hydrolyzes upon contact with moisture to produce chromic trioxide, HCl, chromic trichloride, and chlorine. Highly irritating upon direct contact; severe burns may result. Mists and vapors highly irritating to eyes and respiratory tract; pulmonary edema may result. Certain hexavalent chromium VI compounds are carcinogenic in animals and humans. See pp 124 and 485.	0.025 ppm	...	NIOSH CA	3 0 1	Dark red fuming liquid. Water-reactive, yielding hydrogen chloride, chlorine gas, chromic acid, and chromic chloride.
Coal tar pitch volatiles (particulate polycyclic aromatic hydrocarbons [CAS: 65996-93-2]): Irritating upon direct contact. Contact dermatitis, acne, hypermelanosis, and photosensitization may occur. Fumes irritating to eyes and respiratory tract. A carcinogen in animals and humans. See p 485.	0.2 mg/m³ A1	0.2 mg/m³	400 mg/m³ NIOSH CA	0 1 0	A complex mixture composed of a high percentage of polycyclic aromatic hydrocarbons. A smoky odor. Combustible.
Cobalt and compounds: Irritating upon direct contact; dermatitis and skin sensitization may occur. Fumes and dusts irritate the upper respiratory tract; chronic interstitial pneumonitis and respiratory tract sensitization reported. Cardiotoxicity associated with ingestion.	0.05 mg/m³ (metal dust and fume, as Co)	0.05 mg/m³	20 mg/m³	...	Elemental cobalt is a black or gray, odorless solid with a negligible vapor pressure.

Cobalt hydrocarbonyl (CAS: 16842-03-8): In animal testing, overexposure produces symptoms similar to those of nickel carbonyl and iron pentacarbonyl. Effects include headache, nausea, vomiting, dizziness, fever, and pulmonary edema.	0.1 mg/m³ (as Co)	...	0.1 mg/m³	...	Flammable gas.
Copper fumes, dusts, and salts: Irritation upon direct contact varies with the compound. The salts are more irritating and can cause corneal ulceration. Allergic contact dermatitis is rare. Dusts and mists irritating to the respiratory tract; nasal ulceration has been described. Metal fume fever (see p 201) can result from overexposure to fumes or fine dusts. Particles embedded in the eye can cause discoloration. See p 131.	1 mg/m³ (dusts and mists) 0.2 mg/m³ (copper fume)	...	1 mg/m³ (dusts and mists) 0.1 mg/m³ (copper fume)	...	Salts vary in color. Generally odorless.
Cotton dust: Chronic exposure causes a respiratory syndrome called byssinosis. Symptoms include cough and wheezing, typically appearing on the first day of the workweek and continuing for a few days or all week, although they may subside within an hour after leaving work. Can lead to irreversible obstructive airway disease.	0.2 mg/m³	500 mg/m³	1 ppm (cotton waste processing)	...	The TLV-TWA is 0.2 mg/m³ of the lint-free dust.

(C) = ceiling air concentration (TLV-C); S = skin absorption can be significant; A1 = ACGIH-confirmed human carcinogen; A2 = ACGIH-suspected human carcinogen; NFPA Hazard Codes: H = health, F = fire, R = reactivity, OX = oxidizer, W = water-reactive, 0 (none) < → 4 (severe). See expanded definitions on p 365.

continued

TABLE IV-12. HEALTH HAZARD SUMMARIES FOR INDUSTRIAL AND OCCUPATIONAL CHEMICALS (Continued)

Health Hazard Summaries	ACGIH TLV	PEL	IDLH	NFPA Codes H F R	Comments
Creosote (coal tar creosote [CAS: 8001-58-9]): A primary irritant, photosensitizer, and corrosive. Direct eye contact can cause severe keratitis and corneal scarring. Prolonged skin contact can cause chemical acne, pigmentation changes, and severe penetrating burns. Exposure to the fumes or vapors causes irritation of respiratory tract; pulmonary edema may result. Systemic toxicity is due to phenolic and cresolic constituents; ingestion causes severe gastrointestinal irritation, headache, transitory CNS stimulation, and seizures. Liver and kidney injury may occur. A carcinogen in animals. Some evidence for carcinogenicity in humans. See p 486.	...	...	NIOSH CA	2 2 0	Oily, dark liquid. Appearance and some hazardous properties vary with the formulation. Sharp, penetrating smoky odor. Combustible.
Cresol (methylphenol, cresylic acid, hydroxymethylbenzene [CAS: 1319-77-3]): Corrosive. Skin and eye contact can cause severe burns. Exposure may be prolonged by a local anesthetic action on skin. Dermal absorption is a major route of systemic poisoning. Symptoms include headache, nausea and vomiting, tinnitus, dizziness, weakness, and confusion. Severe liver and kidney injury may occur. See p 234.	5 ppm S	5 ppm S	250 ppm	3 2 0 *(ortho)* 3 1 0 *(meta, para)*	Colorless, yellow, or pink liquid with a phenolic odor. Vapor pressure is 0.2 mm Hg at 20 °C (68 °F). Combustible.
Crotonaldehyde (2-butenal [CAS: 4170-30-3]): Highly irritating upon direct contact; severe burns may result. Vapors highly irritating to eyes and respiratory tract; delayed pulmonary edema may occur.	2 ppm	2 ppm	400 mg/m³	3 3 2	Colorless to straw-colored liquid. Pungent, irritating odor occurs below the PEL and is an adequate warning property. Vapor pressure is 30 mm Hg at 20 °C (68 °F). Flammable. Polymerizes when heated.

Substance	TLV	PEL	IDLH	NFPA Codes (H-F-R)	Comments
Crufomate (4-tert-butyl-2-chlorophenyl N-methyl O-methylphosphoramidate [CAS: 299-86-5]): An organophosphate cholinesterase inhibitor. See p 225.	5 mg/m³	5 mg/m³	...	...	Crystals or yellow oil. Pungent odor. Flammable.
Cumene (isopropylbenzene [CAS: 98-82-8]): Mildly irritating upon direct contact. A CNS depressant at moderate levels. Well absorbed through skin.	50 ppm S	50 ppm S	8000 ppm	2 3 0	Colorless liquid. Sharp, aromatic odor below the PEL is a good warning property. Vapor pressure is 8 mm Hg at 20 °C (68 °F). Flammable.
Cyanamide (carbodiimide [CAS: 420-04-2]): Causes transient vasomotor flushing. Highly irritating and caustic to eyes and skin. Has a disulfiramlike interaction with alcohol, producing flushing, headache, and dyspnea. See p 143.	2 mg/m³	2 mg/m³	...	4 1 3	Combustible. Thermal breakdown products include oxides of nitrogen.
Cyanide salts (sodium cyanide, potassium cyanide): Potent and rapidly fatal metabolic asphyxiants that inhibit cytochrome oxidase and stop cellular respiration. Caustic action on skin can promote dermal absorption. See p 134.	5 mg/m³ (as cyanide) S	5 mg/m³ (as cyanide)	50 mg/m³ (as cyanide)	...	Solids. Mild, almondlike odor. In presence of moisture or acids, hydrogen cyanide may be released. Odor is a poor indicator of exposure to hydrogen cyanide.
Cyanogen (dicyan, oxalonitrile [CAS: 460-19-5]): Hydrolyzes to release hydrogen cyanide and cyanic acid. Toxicity similar to that of hydrogen cyanide. Vapors irritating to eyes and upper respiratory tract. Animal testing suggests cyanogen is 10-fold less toxic than hydrogen cyanide. See p 134.	10 ppm	10 ppm	...	4 4 2	Colorless gas. Pungent, almondlike odor. Breaks down on contact with water to yield hydrogen cyanide and cyanate. Flammable.
Cyanogen chloride (CAS: 506-77-4): Vapors highly irritating to eyes and respiratory tract; conjunctivitis and delayed pulmonary edema may result. Cyanide interferes with cellular respiration. See p 134.	0.3 ppm (C)	0.3 ppm (C)	...	...	Colorless liquid or gas with a pungent odor. Thermal breakdown products include hydrogen cyanide and hydrogen chloride.

(C) = ceiling air concentration (TLV-C); S = skin absorption can be significant; A1 = ACGIH-confirmed human carcinogen; A2 = ACGIH-suspected human carcinogen; NFPA Hazard Codes: H = health, F = fire, R = reactivity, 0 (none) <—> 4 (severe). See expanded definitions on p 365.

continued

TABLE IV-12. HEALTH HAZARD SUMMARIES FOR INDUSTRIAL AND OCCUPATIONAL CHEMICALS (Continued)

Health Hazard Summaries	ACGIH TLV	PEL	IDLH	NFPA Codes H F R	Comments
Cyclohexane (CAS: 110-82-7): Mildly irritating upon direct contact; defatting agent causing dermatitis. Vapors irritating to eyes and upper respiratory tract. A CNS depressant at high levels. Chronically exposed animals developed liver and kidney injury.	300 ppm	300 ppm	10,000 ppm	1 3 0	Colorless liquid with a sweet, chloroformlike odor. Vapor pressure is 95 mm Hg at 20 °C (68 °F). Highly flammable.
Cyclohexanol (CAS: 108-93-0): Irritating upon direct contact; defatting agent causing dermatitis. Vapors irritating to eyes and respiratory tract. Well absorbed by skin. A CNS depressant at high levels. Based on animal tests, it may injure the liver and kidney at high doses.	50 ppm S	50 ppm S	3500 ppm	1 2 0	Colorless viscous liquid. Mild camphorlike odor. Irritation occurs near the PEL and is a good warning property. Vapor pressure is 1 mm Hg at 20 °C (68 °F). Combustible.
Cyclohexanone (CAS: 108-94-1): Irritating upon direct contact; defatting agent causing dermatitis. Vapors irritate the eyes and upper respiratory tract. A CNS depressant at very high levels. Chronic, moderate doses caused slight liver injury in animals.	25 ppm S	25 ppm S	5000 ppm	1 2 0	Clear to pale yellow liquid with peppermintlike odor. Vapor pressure is 2 mm Hg at 20 °C (68 °F). Flammable.
Cyclohexene (1,2,3,4-tetrahydrobenzene (CAS: 110-83-8)): By structural analogy to cyclohexane, may cause respiratory tract irritation. A CNS depressant.	300 ppm	300 ppm	10,000 ppm	1 3 0	Colorless liquid with a sweet odor. Vapor pressure is 67 mm Hg at 20 °C (68 °F). Flammable. Readily forms peroxides and polymerizes.
Cyclohexylamine (aminocyclohexane [CAS: 108-91-8]): Corrosive and highly irritating upon direct contact. Vapors highly irritating to eyes and respiratory tract. Pharmacologically active, possessing sympathomimetic activity. Weak methemoglobin-forming activity (see p 204). Animal studies suggest brain, liver, and kidneys are target organs.	10 ppm	10 ppm	…	2 3 0	Liquid with an obnoxious, fishy odor. Flammable. Vapor pressure is 15 mm Hg at 30 °C (86 °F).

Chemical			NFPA	Comments
Cyclonite (RDX, trinitrotrimethylenetriamine [CAS: 121-82-4]): Dermal and inhalation exposures affect the CNS with symptoms of confusion, headache, nausea, vomiting, convulsions, and coma.	1.5 mg/m³ S	1.5 mg/m³ S	...	...	Crystalline solid. Vapor pressure is negligible at 20 °C (68 °F). Thermal breakdown products include oxides of nitrogen. Explosive.
Cyclopentadiene [CAS: 542-92-7]: Mildly irritating upon direct contact; defatting agent causing dermatitis. Vapors irritating to eyes and upper respiratory tract. A CNS depressant at high levels. Animal studies suggest some potential for kidney and liver injury.	75 ppm	75 ppm	2000 ppm	...	Colorless liquid. Sweet, turpentinelike odor. Irritation occurs near the PEL and is a good warning property. Vapor pressure is high at 20 °C (68 °F). Flammable.
Cyclopentane [CAS: 287-92-3]: Mildly irritating upon direct contact; defatting agent causing dermatitis. Vapors irritating to eyes and upper respiratory tract. A CNS depressant at very high levels. Solvent mixtures containing cyclopentane and possibly *n*-hexane have caused peripheral neuropathy.	600 ppm	600 ppm	...	1 3 0	Colorless liquid with a faint hydrocarbon odor. Vapor pressure is about 400 mm Hg at 31 °C (88 °F). Flammable.
DDT (dichlorodiphenyltrichloroethane [CAS: 50-29-3]): Dusts irritating to eyes. Ingestion may cause tremor and convulsions. May sensitize the myocardium to the arrhythmogenic effects of epinephrine. Chronic low-level exposure results in bioaccumulation with no discernible adverse effects. A carcinogen in animals. See pp 117 and 487.	1 mg/m³ S	1 mg/m³ S	NIOSH CA	...	Colorless, white, or yellow solid crystals with a faint aromatic odor. Vapor pressure is 0.0000002 mm Hg at 20 °C (68 °F). Combustible.
Decaborane (CAS: 17702-41-9): A potent CNS toxin. Symptoms include headache, dizziness, nausea, loss of coordination, and fatigue. Symptoms may be delayed in onset for 1-2 days; convulsions occur in more severe poisonings. Systemic poisonings often result from dermal absorption. Animal studies suggest a potential for liver and kidney injury.	0.05 ppm S	0.05 ppm S	20 ppm	3 2 1	Colorless solid crystals with a pungent odor. Vapor pressure is 0.05 mm Hg at 25 °C (77 °F). Combustible. Reacts with water to produce flammable hydrogen gas.

(Cl) = ceiling air concentration (TLV-C); S = skin absorption can be significant; A1 = ACGIH-confirmed human carcinogen; A2 = ACGIH-suspected human carcinogen; NFPA Hazard Codes: H = health, F = fire, R = reactivity, OX = oxidizer, W = water-reactive, 0 (none) < — > 4 (severe). See expanded definitions on p 365.

continued

TABLE IV-12. HEALTH HAZARD SUMMARIES FOR INDUSTRIAL AND OCCUPATIONAL CHEMICALS (Continued)

Health Hazard Summaries	ACGIH TLV	PEL	IDLH	NFPA Codes H F R	Comments
Demeton (Systox, mercaptophos [CAS: 8065-48-3]): An organophosphate-type cholinesterase inhibitor. See p 225.	0.01 ppm S	0.1 mg/m³ S	20 mg/m³	...	A sulfurlike odor. A very low vapor pressure at 20 °C (68 °F). Thermal breakdown products include oxides of sulfur.
Diacetone alcohol (4-hydroxy-4-methyl-2-pentanone [CAS: 123-42-2]): Irritating upon direct contact; defatting agent causing dermatitis. Vapors very irritating to eyes and respiratory tract. A CNS depressant at high levels. Some hemolytic activity.	50 ppm	50 ppm	2100 ppm	1 2 0	Colorless liquid with an agreeable odor. Vapor pressure is 0.8 mm Hg at 20 °C (68 °F). Flammable.
Diazinon (O,O-diethyl O-2-isopropyl-4-methyl-6-pyrimidinyl thiophosphate [CAS: 333-41-5]): An organophosphate-type cholinesterase inhibitor. Well absorbed dermally. See p 225.	0.1 mg/m³ S	0.1 mg/m³ S	...	...	Commercial grades are yellow to brown liquids with a faint odor. Vapor pressure is 0.00014 mm Hg at 20 °C (68 °F). Thermal breakdown products include oxides of nitrogen and sulfur.
Diazomethane (azimethylene, diazirine [CAS: 334-88-3]): Extremely irritating to eyes and respiratory tract; pulmonary edema has been reported. Immediate symptoms include cough, chest pain, and respiratory distress. A potent methylating agent and respiratory sensitizer.	0.2 ppm	0.2 ppm	10 ppm	...	Yellow gas with a musty odor. Air mixtures and compressed liquids can be explosive when heated or shocked.
Diborane (boron hydride [CAS: 19287-45-7]): Extremely irritating to the respiratory tract; delayed pulmonary edema may result. Repeated exposures have been associated with headache, fatigue, and dizziness; muscle weakness or tremors; and chills or fever. Animal studies suggest the liver and kidney are also target organs.	0.1 ppm	0.1 ppm	40 ppm	3 4 3 W	Colorless gas. Obnoxious, nauseatingly sweet odor. Highly flammable. Water-reactive; ignites spontaneously with moist air at room temperatures. A strong reducing agent. Breakdown products include boron oxide fumes.

Substance [CAS]: toxicity	TLV	PEL	IDLH	H	F	R	Comments
1,2-Dibromo-3-chloropropane (DBCP) [CAS: 96-12-8]: Irritant of eyes and respiratory tract. Has caused sterility (aspermia, oligospermia) in overexposed men. Well absorbed by skin contact and inhalation. A carcinogen in animals. See p 487.	...	OSHA CA	...		...		Brown liquid with a pungent odor. Combustible. Thermal breakdown products include hydrogen bromide amd hydrogen chloride.
Dibutyl phosphate (di-n-butyl phosphate) [CAS: 107-66-4]: A moderately strong acid likely to be irritating upon direct contact. Vapors and mists are irritating to the respiratory tract and have been associated with headache at low levels.	1 ppm	1 ppm	125 ppm		...		Colorless to brown liquid. Odorless. Vapor pressure is much less than 1 mm Hg at 20 °C (68 °F). Decomposes at 100 °C (212 °F) to produce phosphoric acid fumes.
Dibutyl phthalate [CAS: 84-74-2]: Mildly irritating upon direct contact. Ingestion has produced nausea, dizziness, photophobia, and lacrimation but no permanent effects. Adverse effects on fetal development in animals at very high doses.	5 mg/m³	5 mg/m³	9300 mg/m³	0	1	0	Colorless, oily liquid with a faint aromatic odor. Vapor pressure is less than 0.01 mm Hg at 20 °C (68 °F). Combustible.
1,2-Dichloroacetylene [CAS: 7572-29-4]: Vapors extremely irritating to eyes and respiratory tract; pulmonary edema may result. CNS toxicity includes nausea and vomiting, headache, involvement of trigeminal nerve and facial muscles.	0.1 ppm (C)	0.1 ppm (C)	...		...		Colorless liquid.
o-Dichlorobenzene (1,2-dichlorobenzene) [CAS: 95-50-1]: Irritating upon direct contact; skin blisters and hyperpigmentation may result from prolonged contact. Vapor also irritating to eyes and upper respiratory tract. May sensitize the myocardium to the arrhythmogenic effects of epinephrine. Highly hepatotoxic in animals. Animal studies also suggest the blood (methemoglobinemia) and kidneys are target organs.	50 ppm (C)	50 ppm (C)	1700 ppm	2	2	0	Colorless to pale yellow liquid. Aromatic odor and eye irritation occur well below the PEL and are adequate warning properties. Thermal breakdown products include hydrogen chloride and chlorine gas.

(C) = ceiling air concentration (TLV-C); S = skin absorption can be significant; A1 = ACGIH-confirmed human carcinogen; A2 = ACGIH-suspected human carcinogen; NFPA Hazard Codes: H = health, F = fire, R = reactivity, OX = oxidizer, W = water-reactive, 0 (none) < — > 4 (severe). See expanded definitions on p 365.

continued

TABLE IV-12. HEALTH HAZARD SUMMARIES FOR INDUSTRIAL AND OCCUPATIONAL CHEMICALS (Continued)

Health Hazard Summaries	ACGIH TLV	PEL	IDLH	NFPA Codes H F R	Comments
p-Dichlorobenzene (1,4-dichlorobenzene [CAS: 106-46-7]: Irritating upon direct contact with the solid. Vapors irritating to eyes and upper respiratory tract. Systemic effects include headache, nausea, vomiting, and liver injury. May sensitize the myocardium to the arrhythmogenic effects of epinephrine. The ortho isomer is more toxic to the liver. Evidence of carcinogenicity in animals. See p 213.	75 ppm	75 ppm	1000 ppm	2 2 0	Colorless or white solid. Mothball odor and irritation occur near the PEL and are adequate warning properties. Vapor pressure is 0.4 mm Hg at 20 °C (68 °F). Combustible. Thermal breakdown products include hydrogen chloride.
3,3'-Dichlorobenzidine (CAS: 91-94-1): Well absorbed by the dermal route. Animal studies suggest that severe eye injury and respiratory tract irritation may occur. A potent carcinogen in animals. See p 487.	S, A2	OSHA CA	NIOSH CA	...	Crystalline needles with a faint odor.
Dichlorodifluoromethane (Freon 12, fluorocarbon 12 [CAS: 75-71-8]): Defatting action may cause dermatitis. Vapor inhalation produces CNS depression at very high levels. Other effects of extremely high exposures include respiratory tract irritation and sensitization of the myocardium to the arrhythmogenic effects of epinephrine. See p 161.	1000 ppm	1000 ppm	50,000 ppm	...	Colorless gas. Etherlike odor is a poor warning property. Vapor pressure is 5.7 mm Hg at 20 °C (68 °F). Not combustible. Decomposes slowly on contact with water or heat to produce hydrogen chloride, hydrogen fluoride, and phosgene.
1,3-Dichloro-5,5-dimethylhydantoin (Halane, Dactin [CAS: 118-52-5]): Releases hypochlorous acid and chlorine gas on contact with moisture. Direct contact with the dust or concentrated solutions irritating to eyes, skin, and respiratory tract. See p 119.	0.2 mg/m³	0.2 mg/m³	5 mg/m³	...	White solid with a chlorinelike odor. Odor and eye irritation occur below the PEL and are adequate warning properties. Not combustible. Thermal breakdown products include hydrogen chloride, phosgene, oxides of nitrogen, and chlorine gas.

Chemical				NFPA	Comments
1,1-Dichloroethane (ethylidene chloride) [CAS: 75-34-3]: Mild eye and skin irritant; defatting action can cause dermatitis. Vapors irritating to the respiratory tract. A CNS depressant at high levels. Animal studies suggest slight potential for kidney and liver injury. May sensitize the myocardium to the arrhythmogenic effects of epinephrine.	200 ppm	100 ppm	4000 ppm	2 3 0	Colorless, oily liquid. Chloroformlike odor occurs at the PEL. Vapor pressure is 182 mm Hg at 20 °C (68 °F). Flammable. Thermal breakdown products include vinyl chloride, hydrogen chloride and phosgene.
1,2-Dichloroethane (ethylene dichloride [CAS: 107-06-2]: Irritating upon prolonged contact; burns may occur. Vapors irritating to eyes and respiratory tract; pulmonary edema may occur at very high levels of exposure. Highly hepatotoxic. Severe liver and kidney injury has been reported. A CNS depressant at high levels. May sensitize the myocardium to the arrhythmogenic effects of epinephrine. Well absorbed dermally. A carcinogen in animals. See p 489.	10 ppm	1 ppm	1000 ppm, NIOSH CA	2 3 0	Flammable. Thermal breakdown products include hydrogen chloride and phosgene.
1,1-Dichloroethylene (vinylidine chloride [CAS: 75-35-4]: Irritating upon direct contact. Vapors irritating to eyes and respiratory tract. In animals, damages the liver and kidneys. May sensitize the myocardium to the arrhythmogenic effects of epinephrine. Limited evidence of carcinogenicity in animals. See p 500.	5 ppm	1 ppm	NIOSH CA	2 4 2	Colorless liquid. Sweet, etherlike or chloroformlike odor occurs below the PEL and is a good warning property. Polymerizes readily.
1,2-Dichloroethene (1,2-dichloroethene, acetylene dichloride [CAS: 540-59-0]: Defatting action can cause dermatitis. Vapors mildly irritating to respiratory tract. A CNS depressant at high levels; once used as an anesthetic agent. Low hepatotoxicity. May sensitize the myocardium to the arrhythmogenic effects of epinephrine.	200 ppm	200 ppm	4000 ppm	2 3 2	Colorless liquid with a slightly acrid, etherlike or chloroformlike odor. Vapor pressure is about 220 mm Hg at 20 °C (68 °F). Thermal breakdown products include hydrogen chloride and phosgene.

(C) = ceiling air concentration (TLV-C); S = skin absorption can be significant; A1 = ACGIH-confirmed human carcinogen; A2 = ACGIH-suspected human carcinogen; NFPA Hazard Codes: H = health, F = fire, R = reactivity, OX = oxidizer, W = water-reactive, 0 (none) < — > 4 (severe). See expanded definitions on p 365.

continued

TABLE IV-12. HEALTH HAZARD SUMMARIES FOR INDUSTRIAL AND OCCUPATIONAL CHEMICALS (Continued)

Health Hazard Summaries	ACGIH TLV	PEL	IDLH	NFPA Codes H F R	Comments
Dichloroethyl ether (bis[2-chloroethyl] ether, dichloroethyl oxide [CAS: 111-44-4]): Irritating upon direct contact; corneal injury may result. Vapors highly irritating to respiratory tract; pulmonary edema may result. Defatting action may cause dermatitis. Dermal absorption occurs. Animal studies suggest the liver and kidneys are target organs at high exposures. Limited evidence for carcinogenicity in animals.	5 ppm S	5 ppm S	250 ppm	2 2 0	Colorless liquid. Obnoxious, chlorinated solvent odor occurs at the PEL and is a good warning property. Flammable. Breaks down on contact with water. Thermal breakdown products include hydrogen chloride.
Dichlorofluoromethane (fluorocarbon 21, Freon 21 [CAS: 75-43-4]): Contact with liquid may cause frostbite. Animal studies suggest much greater hepatotoxicity than most common fluorocarbons. Causes CNS depression, respiratory irritation, and sensitization of the myocardium to the arrhythmogenic effects of epinephrine at extremely high air levels. See p 161.	10 ppm	10 ppm	50,000 ppm	...	Colorless liquid or gas with a faint etherlike odor. Thermal breakdown products include hydrogen chloride, hydrogen fluoride, and phosgene.
1,1-Dichloro-1-nitroethane [CAS: 594-72-9]: Based on animal studies, highly irritating upon direct contact. Vapors highly irritating to eyes, skin, and respiratory tract; delayed pulmonary edema may result. In animals, lethal doses also injured the liver, heart, and kidneys.	2 ppm	2 ppm	150 ppm	2 2 3	Colorless liquid. Obnoxious odor and tearing occur only at dangerous levels and are poor warning properties. Vapor pressure is 15 mm Hg at 20 °C (68 °F).
2,4-Dichlorophenoxyacetic acid (2,4-D [CAS: 94-75-9]): Direct skin contact can produce a rash. Overexposed workers have rarely experienced peripheral neuropathy. Rabdomyolysis and minor liver and kidney injury may occur. Adverse effects on fetal development at high doses in animals. See p 121.	10 mg/m³	10 mg/m³	500 mg/m³	...	White to yellow crystals. Appearance and some hazardous properties vary with the formulation. Odorless. Vapor pressure is negligible at 20 °C (68 °F). Thermal breakdown products include hydrogen chloride and phosgene.

Chemical			NFPA (H F R)	Physical Description
1,3-Dichloropropene (1,3-dichloropropylene, Telone [CAS: 542-75-6]): Based on animal studies, irritating upon direct contact. Well absorbed dermally. Vapors irritating to eyes and upper respiratory tract; delayed pulmonary edema may result. In animals, moderate doses caused severe injuries to the liver, pancreas, and kidneys. A carcinogen in animals. See p 487.	1 ppm S	1 ppm S	2 3 0	Colorless or straw-colored liquid. Sharp, chloroformlike odor. Polymerizes readily. Vapor pressure is 28 mm Hg at 25 °C (77 °F). Thermal breakdown products include hydrogen chloride and phosgene.
2,2-Dichloropropionic acid (CAS: 75-99-0): Corrosive upon direct contact with concentrate; severe burns may result. Vapors mildly irritating to eyes and respiratory tract.	1 ppm	1 ppm	…	Colorless liquid. The sodium salt is a solid.
Dichlorotetrafluoroethane (fluorocarbon 114 [CAS: 76-14-2]): Contact with liquid may cause frostbite. Vapors may cause respiratory irritation, CNS depression, and cardiac sensitization to the arrhythmogenic effects of epinephrine at very high levels of exposure. See p 161.	1000 ppm	1000 ppm	50,000 ppm	Colorless gas with a mild etherlike odor. Thermal breakdown products include hydrogen chloride, hydrogen fluoride, and phosgene.
Dichlorvos (DDVP, 2,2-dichlorovinyl dimethyl phosphate [CAS: 62-73-7]): An organophosphate-type cholinesterase inhibitor. Extremely well absorbed through skin. Evidence of carcinogenicity in animals. See p 225.	0.1 ppm S	…	200 mg/m³	Colorless to amber liquid with a slight chemical odor. Vapor pressure is 0.032 mm Hg at 32 °C (90 °F).
Dicrotophos (dimethyl *cis*-2-dimethylcarbamoyl-1-methylvinyl phosphate, Bidrin [CAS: 141-66-2]): An organophosphate cholinesterase inhibitor. Dermal absorption occurs. See p 225.	0.25 mg/m³ S	0.25 mg/m³ S	…	Brown liquid with a mild ester odor.

(C) = ceiling air concentration (TLV-C); S = skin absorption can be significant; A1 = ACGIH-confirmed human carcinogen; A2 = ACGIH-suspected human carcinogen; NFPA Hazard Codes: H = health, F = fire, R = reactivity, OX = oxidizer, W = water-reactive, 0 (none) < — > 4 (severe). See expanded definitions on p 365.

continued

TABLE IV-12. HEALTH HAZARD SUMMARIES FOR INDUSTRIAL AND OCCUPATIONAL CHEMICALS (Continued)

Health Hazard Summaries	ACGIH TLV	PEL	IDLH	NFPA Codes H F R	Comments
Dieldrin (CAS: 60-57-1): Minor skin irritant. Potent convulsant and hepatotoxin. Dermal absorption is a major route of systemic poisoning. Overexposures produce headache, dizziness, twitching, and convulsions. Limited evidence for adverse effects on fetal development and carcinogenicity in animals. See pp 117 and 468.	0.25 mg/m³ S	0.25 mg/m³ S	450 mg/m³ NIOSH CA	. . .	Light brown solid flakes with a mild chemical odor. Appearance and some hazardous properties vary with the formulation. Vapor pressure is 0.0000002 mm Hg at 32 °C (90 °F). Not combustible.
Diethylamine (CAS: 109-89-7): Caustic. Highly irritating upon direct contact; severe burns may result. Vapors highly irritating to eyes and respiratory tract; pulmonary edema may occur. Subacute animal studies suggest liver and heart may be target organs.	10 ppm	10 ppm	2000 ppm	2 3 0	Colorless liquid. Fishy, ammonialike odor occurs below the PEL and is a good warning property. Vapor pressure is 195 mm Hg at 20 °C (68 °F). Highly flammable. Thermal breakdown products include oxides of nitrogen.
2-Diethylaminoethanol (N,N-diethylethanolamine, DEAE): Based on animal studies, highly irritating upon direct contact and a skin sensitizer. Vapors likely irritating to eyes, skin, and respiratory tract. Reports of nausea and vomiting after a momentary exposure to 100 ppm.	10 ppm S	10 ppm S	500 ppm	3 2 0	Colorless liquid. Weak to nauseating ammonia odor. Flammable. Thermal breakdown products include oxides of nitrogen.
Diethylenetriamine (DETA [CAS: 111-40-0]): Caustic; highly irritating upon direct contact; severe burns may result. Vapors highly irritating to eyes and respiratory tract; delayed pulmonary edema may occur. Dermal and respiratory sensitization frequently occurs.	1 ppm S	1 ppm	. . .	3 1 0	Viscous yellow liquid with an ammonialike odor. Vapor pressure is 0.37 mm Hg at 20 °C (68 °F). Combustible. Thermal breakdown products include oxides of nitrogen.
Diethyl ketone (3-pentanone [CAS: 96-22-0]): Mildly irritating upon direct contact; defatting action may cause dermatitis. Vapors mildly irritating to eyes and respiratory tract.	200 ppm	200 ppm	. . .	1 3 0	Colorless liquid with an acetonelike odor. Flammable. Vapor pressure is 27 mm Hg at 20 °C (68 °F).

Difluorodibromomethane (dibromodifluoromethane, Freon 12B2 [CAS: 75-61-6]): Based on animal tests, vapors irritate the respiratory tract. A CNS depressant. May sensitize the myocardium to the arrhythmogenic effects of epinephrine. In animals, high-level chronic exposures caused lung, liver, and CNS injury. See p 161.

100 ppm   100 ppm   ...   Heavy, volatile, colorless liquid with an obnoxious, distinctive odor. Vapor pressure is 620 mm Hg at 20 °C (68 °F). Not combustible. Thermal breakdown products include hydrogen bromide and hydrogen fluoride.

Diglycidyl ether (di[2,3-epoxypropyl-ether, DGE [CAS: 2238-07-5]): Extremely irritating upon direct contact; severe burns result. Vapors highly irritating to eyes and respiratory tract; delayed pulmonary edema may result. Testicular atrophy and adverse effects on the hematopoietic system at low doses in animals. CNS depression also noted. An alkylating agent and a carcinogen in animals.

0.1 ppm   0.1 ppm   ...   Colorless liquid with a very irritating odor. Vapor pressure is 0.09 mm Hg at 25 °C (77 °F).

Diisobutyl ketone (2,6-dimethyl-4-heptanone [CAS: 108-83-8]): Mildly irritating upon direct contact. Vapors mildly irritate eyes and respiratory tract. A CNS depressant at high levels.

25 ppm   25 ppm   1 2 0   Colorless liquid with a weak, etherlike odor. Vapor pressure is 1.7 mm Hg at 20 °C (68 °F).

Diisopropylamine (CAS: 108-18-9): Caustic. Highly irritating upon direct contact; severe burns may result. Vapors very irritating to eyes and respiratory tract; pulmonary edema may result. Workers exposed to levels 5- to 10-fold above the TLV complained of hazy vision, nausea, and headache.

5 ppm   5 ppm   3 3 0   Colorless liquid with an ammonialike odor. Vapor
S   S   pressure is 60 mm Hg at 20 °C (68 °F). Flammable. Thermal breakdown products include oxides of nitrogen.

Dimethylacetamide (DMAC [CAS: 127-19-5]): Potent hepatotoxin. Inhalation and skin contact are major routes of absorption. In a therapeutic trial, 400 mg/kg caused confusion, lethargy, and hallucinations. Limited evidence for adverse effects on fetal development in animals at high doses.

10 ppm   10 ppm   2 2 0   Colorless liquid with a weak ammonialike odor.
S   S   Vapor pressure is 1.5 mm Hg at 20 °C (68 °F). Combustible. Thermal breakdown products include oxides of nitrogen.

(C) = ceiling air concentration (TLV-C); S = skin absorption can be significant; A1 = ACGIH-confirmed human carcinogen; A2 = ACGIH-suspected human carcinogen; NFPA Hazard Codes: H = health, F = fire, R = reactivity, OX = oxidizer, W = water-reactive, 0 (none) <—> 4 (severe). See expanded definitions on p 365.

continued

TABLE IV-12. HEALTH HAZARD SUMMARIES FOR INDUSTRIAL AND OCCUPATIONAL CHEMICALS (Continued)

Health Hazard Summaries	ACGIH TLV	PEL	IDLH	NFPA Codes H F R	Comments
Dimethylamine (DMA [CAS: 124-40-3]): Corrosive upon direct contact; severe burns may result. Vapors extremely irritating to eyes and respiratory tract; pulmonary edema may result. Animal studies suggest liver is a target organ.	10 ppm	10 ppm	2000 ppm	3 4 0	Colorless liquid or gas. Fishy or ammonialike odor far below PEL is a good warning property. Flammable. Thermal breakdown products include oxides of nitrogen. Vapor pressure is 1.72 mm Hg at 20 °C (68 °F).
***N,N*-Dimethylaniline (CAS: 121-69-7]):** Causes methemoglobinemia and secondary tissue anoxia. A CNS depressant. Well absorbed dermally. See p 204.	5 ppm S	5 ppm S	100 ppm	3 2 0	Straw- to brown-colored liquid with an aminelike odor. Vapor pressure is less than 1 mm Hg at 20 °C (68 °F). Combustible. Thermal breakdown products include oxides of nitrogen.
Dimethylcarbamoyl chloride (CAS: 79-44-7]): Rapidly hydrolyzed by moisture to dimethylamine, carbon dioxide, and hydrochloric acid. Expected to be extremely irritating upon direct contact or by inhalation. A carcinogen in animals. See p 489.	A2	...	...	...	Liquid. Rapidly reacts with moisture to yield dimethylamine and hydrogen chloride.
***N,N*-Dimethylformamide (DMF [CAS: 68-12-2]):** Defatting agent producing dermatitis. Dermally well absorbed. Symptoms of overexposure include abdominal pain, nausea, and vomiting. Hepatotoxicity has been observed. Interferes with ethanol to cause disulfiramlike reactions. Limited epidemiologic association with an increased risk of testicular cancer.	10 ppm S	10 ppm S	3500 ppm	1 2 0	Colorless to pale yellow liquid. Faint ammonialike odor is a poor warning property. Vapor pressure is 2.7 mm Hg at 20 °C (68 °F). Flammable. Thermal breakdown products include oxides of nitrogen.

Substance				NFPA (H F R)	Comments
1,1-Dimethylhydrazine: Corrosive upon direct contact; severe burns may result. Vapors extremely irritating to eyes and respiratory tract; delayed pulmonary edema may occur. Well absorbed through the skin. A convulsant, hemolytic agent, hepatotoxin, and carcinogen in animals. See p 489.	0.5 ppm S, A2	0.5 ppm S	50 ppm NIOSH CA	3 3 1	Colorless liquid with yellow fumes. Amine odor. Vapor pressure is 103 mm Hg at 20 °C (68 °F). Thermal breakdown products include oxides of nitrogen. TLV under review.
Dimethyl sulfate (CAS: 77-78-1): Powerful vesicant action; hydrolyzes to sulfuric acid and methanol. Extremely irritating upon direct contact; severe burns have resulted. Vapors irritating to eyes and respiratory tract; delayed pulmonary edema may result. Skin absorption is rapid. A carcinogen in animals. See p 489.	0.1 ppm S, A2	0.1 ppm S	10 ppm	4 2 0	Colorless, oily liquid. Very mild onion odor is barely perceptible and is a poor warning property. Vapor pressure is 0.5 mm Hg at 20 °C (68 °F). Combustible. Thermal breakdown products include sulfur oxides.
Dinitrobenzene: May stain tissues yellow upon direct contact. Vapors are irritating to respiratory tract. Potent inducer of methemoglobinemia (see p 204). Chronic exposures may result in anemia and liver damage. Very well absorbed through the skin.	0.15 ppm S	1 mg/m³ S	200 mg/m³	3 1 4	Pale yellow crystals. Explosive; detonated by heat or shock. Vapor pressure is much less than 1 mm Hg at 20 °C (68 °F). Thermal breakdown products include oxides of nitrogen.
Dinitro-o-cresol (2-methyl-4,6-dinitrophenol [CAS: 534-52-1]): Highly toxic; uncouples oxidative phosphorylation in mitochondria, increasing metabolic rate and leading to fatigue, sweating, rapid breathing, tachycardia, and fever. Liver and kidney injury may occur. Symptoms may last for days as dinitro-o-cresol is very slowly excreted. Poisonings may result from dermal exposure. See p 231.	0.2 mg/m³ S	0.2 mg/m³ S	5 mg/m³	…	Yellow solid crystals. Dust is explosive. Odorless. Vapor pressure is 0.00005 mm Hg at 20 °C (68 °F). Thermal breakdown products include oxides of nitrogen.

(C) = ceiling air concentration (TLV-C); S = skin absorption can be significant; A1 = ACGIH-confirmed human carcinogen; A2 = ACGIH-suspected human carcinogen; NFPA Hazard Codes: H = health, F = fire, R = reactivity, OX = oxidizer, W = water-reactive, 0 (none) < — > 4 (severe). See expanded definitions on p 365.

continued

TABLE IV-12. HEALTH HAZARD SUMMARIES FOR INDUSTRIAL AND OCCUPATIONAL CHEMICALS (Continued)

Health Hazard Summaries	ACGIH TLV	PEL	IDLH	NFPA Codes H F R	Comments
2,4-Dinitrotoluene (DNT [CAS: 121-14-2]): Causes methemoglobinemia upon overexposure. Uncouples oxidative phosphorylation, leading to increased metabolic rate and hyperthermia, tachycardia, and fatigue. A hepatotoxin. Dermal absorption occurs. A carcinogen in animals. See pp 204 and 489.	1.5 mg/m³ S	1.5 mg/m³ S	200 mg/m³ NIOSH CA	3 1 3	Orange-yellow solid (pure) or oily liquid with a characteristic odor. Explosive. Thermal breakdown products include oxides of nitrogen. Vapor pressure is 1 mm Hg at 20 °C (68 °F).
1,4-Dioxane (1,4-diethylene dioxide [CAS: 123-91-1]): Defatting action may cause dermatitis. Vapors irritating to eyes and respiratory tract. Inhalation or dermal exposures may cause gastrointestinal upset and liver and kidney injury. A carcinogen in animals. See p 489.	25 ppm S	25 ppm S	200 ppm NIOSH CA	2 3 1	Colorless liquid. Mild etherlike odor occurs only at dangerous levels and is a poor warning property. Vapor pressure is 29 mm Hg at 20 °C (68 °F). Flammable.
Dioxathion (2,3-p-dioxanedithiol S,S-bis(O,O-diethyl phosphorodithioate) [CAS: 78-34-2]): An organophosphate-type cholinesterase inhibitor. Well absorbed dermally. See p 225.	0.2 mg/m³ S	0.2 mg/m³ S	…	…	Amber liquid. Vapor pressure is negligible at 20 °C (68 °F). Thermal breakdown products include oxides of sulfur.
Dipropylene glycol methyl ether (DPGME [CAS: 34590-94-8]): Mildly irritating to eyes upon direct contact. A CNS depressant at very high levels.	100 ppm S	100 ppm S	…	0 2 0	Colorless liquid with a mild etherlike odor. Nasal irritation is a good warning property. Vapor pressure is 0.3 mm Hg at 20 °C (68 °F). Combustible.

Chemical	TWA	PEL	IDLH	H	F	R	Comments
Diquat (1,1'-ethylene-2,2'-dipyridinium dibromide, Reglone, Dextrone [CAS: 85-00-7]): Corrosive in high concentrations. Poisoning produces brain stem and cerebral hemorrhagic infarction and abdominal distention. Acute renal failure and reversible liver injury may occur. Chronic feeding studies caused cataracts in animals. See p 230.	0.5 mg/m³	0.5 mg/m³	…				Yellow solid crystals. Appearance and some hazardous properties vary with the formulation.
Disulfiram (tetraethylthiuram disulfide, Antabuse [CAS: 97-77-8]): Inhibits aldehyde dehydrogenase, an enzyme involved in ethanol metabolism. Exposure to disulfiram and alcohol will produce flushing, headache, and hypotension. See p 143.	2 mg/m³	2 mg/m³	…				Crystalline solid. Thermal breakdown products include oxides of sulfur.
Disulfoton (O,O-diethyl-S-ethylmercapto-ethyl dithiophosphate [CAS: 298-04-4]): An organophosphate-type cholinesterase inhibitor. Dermally well absorbed. See p 225.	0.1 mg/m³ S	0.1 mg/m³ S	…				Vapor pressure is 0.00018 mm Hg at 20 °C (68 °F). Thermal breakdown products include oxides of sulfur.
Divinylbenzene (DVB, vinylstyrene [CAS: 1321-74-0]): Mildly irritating upon direct contact. Vapors mildly irritating to eyes and respiratory tract.	10 ppm	10 ppm	…	2	2	2	Pale yellow liquid. Combustible. Must contain inhibitor to prevent explosive polymerization.
Emery (corundum, impure aluminum oxide [CAS: 112-62-9]): An abrasive, nuisance dust causing physical irritation to eyes, skin, and respiratory tract.	10 mg/m³ (total dust) 5 mg/m³ (respirable fraction)	10 mg/m³	…				Solid crystals of aluminum oxide.
Endosulfan [CAS: 115-29-7]: Inhalation and skin absorption are major routes of exposure. Symptoms include nausea, confusion, excitement, twitching, and convulsions. Animal studies suggest liver and kidney injury from very high exposures. See p 117.	0.1 mg/m³ S	0.1 mg/m³ S	200 mg/m³				Tan, waxy solid with a mild sulfur dioxide odor. Thermal breakdown products include oxides of sulfur and hydrogen chloride.

(C) = ceiling air concentration (TLV-C); S = skin absorption can be significant; A1 = ACGIH-confirmed human carcinogen; A2 = ACGIH-suspected human carcinogen; NFPA Hazard Codes: H = health, F = fire, R = reactivity, OX = oxidizer, W = water-reactive, 0 (none) < — > 4 (severe). See expanded definitions on p 365.

continued

TABLE IV–12. HEALTH HAZARD SUMMARIES FOR INDUSTRIAL AND OCCUPATIONAL CHEMICALS (Continued)

Health Hazard Summaries	ACGIH TLV	PEL	IDLH	NFPA Codes H F R	Comments
Endrin (CAS: 72-20-8): Endrin is the stereoisomer of dieldrin, and its toxicity is very similar. Well absorbed through skin. Overexposure may produce headache, dizziness, nausea, confusion, twitching, and convulsions. Adverse effects on fetal development in animals. See p 117.	0.1 mg/m³ S	0.1 mg/m³ S	200 mg/m³ ...		Colorless, white, or tan solid. A mild chemical odor and negligible vapor pressure of 0.0000002 mm Hg at 20 °C (68 °F). Not combustible. Thermal breakdown products include hydrogen chloride.
Epichlorohydrin (chloropropylene oxide) [CAS: 106-89-8]: Extremely irritating upon direct contact; severe burns may result. Vapors highly irritating to eyes and respiratory tract; pulmonary edema has been reported. Other effects include nausea, vomiting, and abdominal pain. Sensitization has been occasionally reported. Animal studies suggest a potential for liver and kidney injury. High doses reduce fertility in animals. A carcinogen in animals. See p 489.	2 ppm S	2 ppm S	100 ppm NIOSH CA	3 2 2	Colorless liquid. The irritating, chloroformlike odor is detectable only at extremely high exposures and is a poor warning property. Vapor pressure is 13 mm Hg at 20 °C (68 °F). Flammable. Thermal breakdown products include hydrogen chloride and phosgene.
EPN (O-ethyl O-p-nitrophenyl phenylphosphonothioate [CAS: 2104-64-5]): An organophosphate-type cholinesterase inhibitor. See p 225.	0.5 mg/m³ S	0.5 mg/m³ S	50 mg/m³ ...		Yellow solid or brown liquid. Vapor pressure is 0.0003 mm Hg at 100 °C (212 °F).
Ethanolamine (2-aminoethanol [CAS: 141-43-5]): Highly irritating upon direct contact; severe burns may result. Prolonged contact with skin is irritating. Animal studies suggest that, at high levels, vapors are irritating to eyes and respiratory tract and liver and kidney injury may occur.	3 ppm	3 ppm	1000 ppm	2 2 0	Colorless liquid. A mild ammonialike odor occurs at the PEL and is an adequate warning property. Vapor pressure is less than 1 mm Hg at 20 °C (68 °F). Combustible. Thermal breakdown products include oxides of nitrogen.

Chemical	TLV	PEL	IDLH	NFPA (H F R)	Comments
Ethion (phosphorodithioic acid [CAS: 563-12-2]): An organophosphate-type cholinesterase inhibitor. Well absorbed dermally. See p 225.	0.4 mg/m³ S	0.4 mg/m³ S	...	...	Colorless, odorless liquid when pure. Technical products have an objectionable odor. Vapor pressure is 0.000002 mm Hg at 20 °C (68 °F). Thermal breakdown products include oxides of sulfur.
2-Ethoxyethanol (ethylene glycol monoethyl ether, EGEE, Cellosolve [CAS: 110-80-5]): Mildly irritating on direct contact. Lung, liver, testes, kidney, and spleen injury in animals. Skin contact is a major route of absorption. Overexposures may reduce sperm counts in men. A potent teratogen in both rats and rabbits. See p 151.	5 ppm S	200 ppm	6000 ppm	2 2 0	Colorless liquid. Very mild, sweet odor occurs only at very high levels and is a poor warning property. Vapor pressure is 4 mm Hg at 20 °C (68 °F). PEL under review.
2-Ethoxyethyl acetate (ethylene glycol monoethyl ether acetate, Cellosolve acetate): Mildly irritating upon direct contact. May produce CNS depression and kidney injury. Skin contact is a major route of absorption. Metabolized to 2-ethoxyethanol. Adverse effects on fertility and fetal development in animals. See p 151.	5 ppm S	100 ppm	2500 ppm	1 2	Colorless liquid. Mild etherlike odor occurs at the PEL and is a good warning property. Flammable. PEL under review. Vapor pressure is 1.2 mm Hg at 20 °C (68 °F).
Ethyl acetate (CAS: 141-78-6): Slightly irritating to eyes and skin. Vapors irritating to eyes and respiratory tract. A CNS depressant at very high levels.	400 ppm	400 ppm	10,000 ppm	1 3 0	Colorless liquid. Fruity odor occurs at the PEL and is a good warning property. Vapor pressure is 76 mm Hg at 20 °C (68 °F). Flammable.
Ethyl acrylate (CAS: 140-88-5): Extremely irritating upon direct contact; severe burns may result. A skin sensitizer. Vapors highly irritating to eyes and respiratory tract; delayed pulmonary edema may result. In animal tests, heart, liver, and kidney damage was observed at high doses. Limited evidence for adverse effects on fetal development in animals at high doses. A carcinogen in animals. See p 489.	5 ppm S	2000 ppm	5 ppm S	2 3 2	Colorless liquid. Acrid odor occurs below the PEL and is a good warning property. Vapor pressure is 29.5 mm Hg at 20 °C (68 °F). Flammable. Contains an inhibitor to prevent dangerous selfpolymerization. TLV under review.

(C) = ceiling air concentration (TLV-C); S = skin absorption can be significant; A1 = ACGIH-confirmed human carcinogen; A2 = ACGIH-suspected human carcinogen; NFPA Hazard Codes: H = health, F = fire, R = reactivity, OX = oxidizer, W = water-reactive, 0 (none) < —> 4 (severe). See expanded definitions on p 365.

continued

TABLE IV-12. HEALTH HAZARD SUMMARIES FOR INDUSTRIAL AND OCCUPATIONAL CHEMICALS (Continued)

Health Hazard Summaries	ACGIH TLV	PEL	IDLH	NFPA Codes H F R	Comments
Ethyl alcohol (alcohol, grain alcohol, ethanol, EtOH [CAS: 64-17-5]): Irritating to eyes upon direct contact with high concentrations. At high levels, vapors irritating to eyes and respiratory tract. A CNS depressant at high levels of exposure. Strong evidence for adverse effects on fetal development in animals and humans (fetal alcohol syndrome). See p 148.	1000 ppm	1000 ppm	...	0 3 0	Colorless liquid with a mild, sweet odor. Vapor pressure is 43 mm Hg at 20 °C (68 °F). Flammable.
Ethylamine (CAS: 75-04-7): Corrosive upon direct contact; severe burns may result. Vapors highly irritating to eyes skin, and respiratory tract; delayed pulmonary edema may result. Animal studies suggest potential for liver and kidney injury at moderate doses.	10 ppm	10 ppm	4000 ppm	3 4 0	Colorless liquid or gas with an ammonialike odor. Highly flammable. Thermal breakdown products include oxides of nitrogen. Vapor pressure is 400 mm Hg at 20 °C (68 °F).
Ethyl amyl ketone (5-methyl-3-heptanone [CAS: 541-85-5]): Irritating to eyes upon direct contact. Defatting action may cause dermatitis. Vapors irritating to eyes and respiratory tract. A CNS depressant at high levels.	25 ppm	25 ppm	...	...	Colorless liquid with a strong, distinctive odor. Flammable. Vapor pressure is 2.7 mm Hg at 20 °C (68 °F).
Ethylbenzene (CAS: 100-41-4): Mildly irritating to eyes upon direct contact. May cause skin burns upon prolonged contact. Dermally well absorbed. Vapors irritating to eyes and respiratory tract. A CNS depressant at high levels of exposure. May sensitize the myocardium to the arrhythmogenic effects of epinephrine.	100 ppm	100 ppm	2000 ppm	2 3 0	Colorless liquid. Aromatic odor and irritation occur at levels close to the PEL and are adequate warning properties. Vapor pressure is 7.1 mm Hg at 20 °C (68 °F). Flammable.

Chemical and health effects			NFPA	Properties
Ethyl bromide (CAS: 74-96-4): Irritating to skin upon direct contact. Irritating to respiratory tract. A CNS depressant at high levels. Former use as an anesthetic agent was discontinued because of fatal liver, kidney, and myocardial injury. May sensitize the myocardium to the arrhythmogenic effects of epinephrine.	200 ppm	200 ppm 3500 ppm	2 1 0	Colorless to yellow liquid. Etherlike odor detectable only at high, dangerous levels. Vapor pressure is 375 mm Hg at 20 °C (68 °F). Highly flammable. Thermal breakdown products include hydrogen bromide and bromine gas.
Ethyl butyl ketone (3-heptanone) (CAS: 106-35-4): Mildly irritating to eyes upon direct contact. Defatting action may cause dermatitis. Vapors irritating to eyes and respiratory tract. A CNS depressant at high levels.	50 ppm	50 ppm 3000 ppm	1 2 0	Colorless liquid. Fruity odor is a good warning property. Vapor pressure is 4 mm Hg at 20 °C (68 °F). Flammable.
Ethyl chloride (CAS: 75-00-3): Mildly irritating to eyes and respiratory tract. A CNS depressant at high levels. May cause cardiac arrhythmias by sensitizing the myocardium to epinephrine at high levels. Animal studies suggest the kidneys and liver are target organs at high doses. Structurally similar to the carcinogenic chloroethanes.	1000 ppm	1000 ppm 20,000 ppm	2 4 0	Colorless liquid or gas (at room temperature) with a pungent, etherlike odor. Highly flammable. Thermal breakdown products include hydrogen chloride and phosgene.
Ethylene chlorohydrin (2-chloroethanol) (CAS: 107-07-3): Irritating to eyes upon direct contact. Skin contact is extremely hazardous because it is not irritating and absorption is rapid. Vapors irritating to eyes and respiratory tract; pulmonary edema has been reported. Systemic effects include CNS depression, myocardiopathy, shock, and liver and kidney damage.	1 ppm (C) S	1 ppm (C) 10 ppm S	3 2 0	Colorless liquid with a weak etherlike odor. Vapor pressure is 5 mm Hg at 20 °C (68 °F). Combustible. Thermal breakdown products include hydrogen chloride and phosgene.
Ethylenediamine (CAS: 107-15-3): Highly irritating upon direct contact; burns may result. Respiratory and dermal sensitization may occur. Vapors irritating to eyes and respiratory tract; pulmonary edema may occur. Animal studies suggest potential for kidney injury at high doses.	10 ppm	10 ppm 2000 ppm	3 2 0	Colorless viscous liquid or solid. Ammonialike odor occurs at the PEL and is an adequate warning property. Vapor pressure is 10 mm Hg at 20 °C (68 °F). Flammable. Thermal breakdown products include oxides of nitrogen.

(C) = ceiling air concentration (TLV-C); S = skin absorption can be significant; A1 = ACGIH-confirmed human carcinogen; A2 = ACGIH-suspected human carcinogen; NFPA Hazard Codes: H = health, F = fire, R = reactivity, OX = oxidizer, W = water-reactive, 0 (none) < — > 4 (severe). See expanded definitions on p 365.

continued

TABLE IV-12. HEALTH HAZARD SUMMARIES FOR INDUSTRIAL AND OCCUPATIONAL CHEMICALS (Continued)

Health Hazard Summaries	ACGIH TLV	PEL	IDLH	NFPA Codes H	F	R	Comments
Ethylene dibromide (1,2-dibromoethane, EDB [CAS: 106-93-4]): Highly irritating upon direct contact; severe burns result. Highly toxic by all routes. Vapors highly irritating to eyes and respiratory tract; delayed pulmonary edema may occur. Severe liver and kidney injury may occur. A CNS depressant. Adverse effects on the testes in animals. A carcinogen in animals. See pp 150 and 489.	S, A2	20 ppm	400 ppm NIOSH CA	3	0	0	Colorless liquid. Mild, sweet odor is a poor warning property. Vapor pressure is 11 mm Hg at 20 °C (68 °F). Not combustible. Thermal breakdown products include hydrogen bromide and bromine gas. PEL under review.
Ethylene glycol (antifreeze [CAS: 107-21-1]): A CNS depressant. Metabolized to oxalic acid; acidosis may result. Precipitation of calcium oxalate crystals in tissues can cause extensive injury. Adversely affects fetal development in animals at very high doses. Not well absorbed dermally. See p 151.	50 ppm (C)	50 ppm (C)	...	1	1	0	Colorless viscous liquid. Odorless with a very low vapor pressure.
Ethylene glycol dinitrate (EGDN [CAS: 628-96-6]): Causes vasodilation similar to other nitrite compounds. Headache, hypotension, flushing, palpitation, delirium, and CNS depression may develop by all routes. Well absorbed by all routes. Tolerance and dependence may develop to vasodilatory effects; cessation after repeated exposures may cause angina pectoris and sudden death. See p 216.	0.05 ppm S	S	80 ppm	...			Yellow oily liquid. Vapor pressure is 0.05 mm Hg at 20 °C (68 °F). Explosive.
Ethyleneimine (CAS: 151-56-4): Strong caustic. Highly irritating upon direct contact; severe burns may result. Vapors irritating to eyes and respiratory tract; delayed-onset pulmonary edema may occur. Overexposures have resulted in nausea, vomiting, headache, and dizziness. Well absorbed dermally. A carcinogen in animals. See p 490.	0.5 ppm S	OSHA CA	NIOSH CA	3	3	2	Colorless liquid with an aminelike odor. Vapor pressure is 160 mm Hg at 20 °C (68 °F). Flammable. Contains inhibitor to prevent explosive self-polymerization.

Chemical	TLV	PEL	IDLH	H	F	R	Comments
Ethylene oxide (CAS: 75-21-8): Highly irritating upon direct contact; rapid evaporation may also cause frostbite. Vapors irritating to eyes and respiratory tract; delayed pulmonary edema has been reported. A CNS depressant at very high levels. Chronic overexposures can cause peripheral neuropathy and possible permanent CNS impairment. Adverse effects on fetal development and fertility in animals and limited evidence in humans. A carcinogen in animals. Limited evidence of carcinogenicity in humans. See pp 153 and 490.	1 ppm A2	OSHA CA	800 ppm NIOSH CA	2	4	3	Colorless. Highly flammable. Etherlike odor is a poor warning property.
Ethyl ether (diethyl ether [CAS: 60-29-7]): Defatting action may cause dermatitis. Vapors irritating to eyes and respiratory tract. A CNS depressant and anesthetic agent; tolerance may develop to this effect. Overexposure produces nausea, headache, dizziness, anesthesia, and respiratory arrest.	400 ppm	400 ppm	19,000 ppm	2	4	1	Colorless liquid. Etherlike odor occurs at low levels and is a good warning property. Vapor pressure is 439 mm Hg at 20 °C (68 °F). Highly flammable.
Ethyl formate (CAS: 109-94-4): Slightly irritating to the skin upon direct contact. Vapors mildly irritating to eyes and upper respiratory tract. In animals, very high levels cause rapid narcosis and pulmonary edema.	100 ppm	100 ppm	8000 ppm	2	3	0	Colorless liquid. Fruity odor and irritation occur near the PEL and are good warning properties. Vapor pressure is 194 mm Hg at 20 °C (68 °F). Highly flammable.
Ethyl mercaptan (ethanethiol [CAS: 75-08-1]): Vapors mildly irritating to eyes and respiratory tract. Respiratory paralysis and CNS depression at very high levels. Headache, nausea, and vomiting are likely owing to its strong odor. See p 169.	0.5 ppm	0.5 ppm	2500 ppm	2	4	0	Colorless liquid. Penetrating, offensive, mercaptanlike odor. Vapor pressure is 442 mm Hg at 20 °C (68 °F).

(C) = ceiling air concentration (TLV-C); S = skin absorption can be significant; A1 = ACGIH-confirmed human carcinogen; A2 = ACGIH-suspected human carcinogen; NFPA Hazard Codes: H = health, F = fire, R = reactivity, OX = oxidizer, W = water-reactive, 0 (none) < — > 4 (severe). See expanded definitions on p 365.

continued

TABLE IV-12. HEALTH HAZARD SUMMARIES FOR INDUSTRIAL AND OCCUPATIONAL CHEMICALS (Continued)

Health Hazard Summaries	ACGIH TLV	PEL	IDLH	NFPA Codes H F R	Comments
N-Ethylmorpholine [CAS: 100-74-3]: Irritating to eyes upon direct contact. Vapors irritating to eyes and respiratory tract. Workers exposed to levels near the TLV reported drowsiness and temporary visual disturbances, including corneal edema. Animal testing suggests potential for skin absorption.	5 ppm S	5 ppm S	2000 ppm	2 3 0	Colorless liquid with ammonialike odor. Vapor pressure is 5 mm Hg at 20 °C (68 °F). Flammable. Thermal breakdown products include oxides of nitrogen.
Ethyl silicate (tetraethyl orthosilicate) [CAS: 78-10-4]: Irritating upon direct contact. Vapors irritating to eyes and respiratory tract. All human effects noted at vapor exposures above the odor threshold. In subchronic animal testing, the vapor produced liver, lung, and kidney damage, and delayed onset pulmonary edema.	10 ppm	10 ppm	1000 ppm	2 2 0	Colorless liquid. Faint alcohollike odor and irritation are good warning properties. Vapor pressure is 2 mm Hg at 20 °C (68 °F). Flammable.
Fenamiphos (ethyl 3-methyl-4-(methylthio)phenyl(1-methylethyl)phosphoramide [CAS: 22224-92-6]: An organophosphate-type cholinesterase inhibitor. Well absorbed dermally. See p 225.	0.1 mg/m³ S	0.1 mg/m³ S	...	...	Tan, waxy solid. Vapor pressure is 0.000001 mm Hg at 30 °C (86 °F).
Fensulfothion (O,O-diethyl O-[4-(methyl-sulfinyl)phenyl] phosphorothioate [CAS: 115-90-2]: An organophosphate-type cholinesterase inhibitor. See p 225.	0.1 mg/m³	0.1 mg/m³	...	...	Brown liquid.
Fenthion (O,O-dimethyl O-[3-methyl-4-(methylthio)phenyl] phosphorothioate [CAS: 55-38-9]: An organophosphate-type cholinesterase inhibitor. Dermal absorption is rapid. Highly lipid soluble; toxicity may be prolonged. See p 225.	0.2 mg/m³ S	0.2 mg/m³ S	...	...	Yellow to tan viscous liquid with a mild garliclike odor. Vapor pressure is 0.00003 mm Hg at 20 °C (68 °F).

Chemical	TLV	NFPA (H F R)	Appearance/Notes
Ferbam (ferric dimethyldithiocarbamate [CAS: 14484-64-1]): Dusts irritating upon direct contact; causes dermatitis in persons sensitized to sulfur. Dusts are mild upper respiratory tract irritants. Limited evidence for adverse effects on fetal development in animals.	10 mg/m³	...	Odorless, black solid. Vapor pressure is negligible at 20 °C (68 °F). Thermal breakdown products include oxides of nitrogen and sulfur.
Ferrovanadium dust (CAS: 12604-58-9): Mild irritant of eyes and respiratory tract.	10 mg/m³ (total dust) 5 mg/m³ (respirable fraction)	...	Odorless, dark-colored powders.
Fibrous glass dust: Human exposures have not produced any effects other than those associated with "nuisance" dusts, notably respiratory irritation at high concentrations. Limited experimental and epidemiologic evidence for carcinogenicity.	1 mg/m³	...	Continuous fibers or woollike batts.
Fluoride dust (as fluoride): Irritating to eyes and upper respiratory tract. Workers exposed to levels 4 times the TLV suffered nasal irritation and bleeding. Lower exposures have produced nausea and eye and respiratory tract irritation. Chronic overexposures may result in skin rashes and minor-to-major changes in bones and teeth. See p 154.	10 mg/m³	...	Appearance varies with the compound. Sodium fluoride is a colorless to blue solid.
Fluorine (CAS: 7782-41-4): Rapidly reacts with moisture to form ozone and hydrofluoric acid. The gas is a severe eye, skin, and respiratory tract irritant; severe penetrating burns and pulmonary edema have resulted. See p 167.	2.5 mg/m³ (as F)	...	Pale yellow gas. Sharp odor is a poor warning property. Highly reactive; will ignite many oxidizable materials.
Fonofos (O-ethyl S-phenyl ethylphosphono-thiolothionate, Dyfonate [CAS: 944-22-9]): An organophosphate-type cholinesterase inhibitor. Highly toxic; oral toxicity in animals ranged from 3 to 13 mg/kg for rats, and rabbits died after eye instillation. See p 225.	2.5 mg/m³ (as F) 1 ppm 0.1 ppm 0.1 mg/m³ S	4 0 3 W	Vapor pressure is 0.00021 mm Hg at 20 °C (68 °F). Thermal breakdown products include oxides of sulfur.

(C) = ceiling air concentration (TLV-C); S = skin absorption can be significant; A1 = ACGIH-confirmed human carcinogen; A2 = ACGIH-suspected human carcinogen; NFPA Hazard Codes: H = health, F = fire, R = reactivity, OX = oxidizer, W = water-reactive, 0 (none) <—> 4 (severe). See expanded definitions on p 365.

continued

TABLE IV-12. HEALTH HAZARD SUMMARIES FOR INDUSTRIAL AND OCCUPATIONAL CHEMICALS (Continued)

Health Hazard Summaries	ACGIH TLV	PEL	IDLH	NFPA Codes H F R	Comments
Formaldehyde (formic aldehyde, methanal, HCHO, formalin [CAS: 50-00-0]): Highly irritating to eyes upon direct contact; severe burns result. Irritating to skin; may cause a sensitization dermatitis. Vapors highly irritating to eyes and respiratory tract; fatal pulmonary edema has been reported. Respiratory sensitization may occur. A carcinogen in animals. See pp 160 and 490.	1 ppm A2	1 ppm OSHA CA	100 ppm NIOSH CA	2 4 0 (gas) 2 2 0 (formalin)	Colorless gas with a suffocating odor. Combustible. Formalin (37% methanol) solutions are flammable. TLV under review.
Formamide (methanamide [CAS: 75-12-7]): In animal tests, mildly irritating upon direct contact. Adverse effects on fetal development in animals at very high doses.	10 ppm S	20 ppm	...	2 1	Clear, viscous liquid. Odorless. Vapor pressure is 2 mm Hg at 70 °C (158 °F). Combustible. Thermal breakdown products include oxides of nitrogen.
Formic acid (CAS: 64-18-6): Acid is corrosive; severe burns may result from contact of eyes and skin with concentrated acid. Vapors highly irritating to eyes and respiratory tract; pulmonary edema may result. See also p 202.	5 ppm	5 ppm	100 ppm	3 2 0	Colorless liquid. Pungent odor and irritation occur near the PEL and are adequate warning properties. Vapor pressure is 30 mm Hg at 20 °C (68 °F). Combustible.
Furfural (bran oil [CAS: 98-01-1]): Highly irritating upon direct contact; burns may result. Vapors highly irritating to eyes and respiratory tract; pulmonary edema may result. Animal studies indicate the liver is a target organ. Hyperreflexia and convulsions occur at large doses in animals.	2 ppm S	2 ppm S	250 ppm	2 2 0	Colorless to light brown liquid. Almondlike odor occurs below the PEL and is a good warning property. Vapor pressure is 2 mm Hg at 20 °C (68 °F). Combustible. Thermal breakdown products include oxides of nitrogen.

Chemical					Physical Properties
Furfuryl alcohol (CAS: 98-00-0): Defatting action may cause dermatitis. Dermal absorption occurs. Vapors irritating to eyes and respiratory tract. A CNS depressant at high air levels.	10 ppm S	10 ppm S	250 ppm	1 2 1	Clear, colorless liquid. Upon exposure to light and air, changes color to red or brown. Vapor pressure is 0.53 mm Hg at 20 °C (68 °F). Combustible.
Gasoline (CAS: 8006-61-9): Although exact composition varies, the acute toxicity of all gasolines is similar. Defatting action may cause dermatitis. Vapors irritating to eyes and respiratory tract at high levels. A CNS depressant; symptoms include incoordination, dizziness, headaches, and nausea. Benzene (< 1%) is the most significant chronic health hazard. Other additives such as ethylene dibromide and tetraethyl and tetramethyl lead are present in low amounts or are only slightly volatile. Limited evidence for carcinogenicity in animals. See p 165.	300 ppm	300 ppm	...	...	Clear to amber liquid with a characteristic odor. Highly flammable.
Germanium tetrahydride (CAS: 7782-65-2): A hemolytic agent with effects similar to but less potent than arsine in animals. Symptoms include abdominal pain, hematuria, anemia, and jaundice.	0.2 ppm	0.2 ppm	...	...	Colorless gas. Highly flammable.
Glutaraldehyde (1,5-pentandial (CAS: 111-30-8]): The purity and therefore the toxicity of glutaraldehyde varies widely. Allergic dermatitis may occur. Highly irritating on contact; severe burns may result. Vapors highly irritating to eyes and respiratory tract; pulmonary edema and respiratory sensitization may occur. In animals, the liver is a target organ at high doses.	0.2 ppm (C)	0.2 ppm (C)	...	...	Colorless solid crystals. Vapor pressure is 0.0152 mm Hg at 20 °C (68 °F). Can undergo hazardous self-polymerization.
Glycidol (2,3-epoxy-1-propanol [CAS: 556-52-5]): Highly irritating to eyes on contact; burns may result. Moderately irritating to skin and respiratory tract; pulmonary edema may result.	25 ppm	25 ppm	500 ppm	...	Colorless liquid. Vapor pressure is 0.9 mm Hg at 25 °C (77 °F). Combustible.

(C) = ceiling air concentration (TLV-C); S = skin absorption can be significant; A1 = ACGIH-confirmed human carcinogen; A2 = ACGIH-suspected human carcinogen; NFPA Hazard Codes: H = health, F = fire, R = reactivity, OX = oxidizer, W = water-reactive, 0 (none) < —> 4 (severe). See expanded definitions on p 365.

continued

TABLE IV-12. HEALTH HAZARD SUMMARIES FOR INDUSTRIAL AND OCCUPATIONAL CHEMICALS (Continued)

Health Hazard Summaries	ACGIH TLV	PEL	IDLH	NFPA Codes H F R	Comments
Hafnium (CAS: 7440-58-6): Based on animal studies, dusts are mildly irritating to eyes and skin. Liver injury may occur at very high doses.	0.5 mg/m³	0.5 mg/m³	250 mg/m³	...	The metal is a gray solid. Other compounds vary in appearance.
Heptachlor (CAS: 76-44-8): CNS convulsant. Skin absorption is rapid and has caused convulsions and death. Hepatotoxic. Stored in fatty tissues. Limited evidence for adverse effects on fetal development in animals at high doses. Evidence of carcinogenicity in animals. See p 117.	0.5 mg/m³ S	0.5 mg/m³ S	100 mg/m³	...	White or light tan, waxy solid with a camphorlike odor. Vapor pressure is 0.0003 mm Hg at 20 °C (68 °F). Thermal breakdown products include hydrogen chloride. Not combustible.
n-Heptane (CAS: 142-82-5): Defatting action may cause dermatitis. Vapors only slightly irritating to eyes and respiratory tract. A CNS depressant at high levels. May sensitize myocardium to arrhythmogenic effects of epinephrine.	400 ppm	400 ppm	4250 ppm	1 3 0	Colorless clear liquid. Mild gasolinelike odor occurs below the PEL and is a good warning property. Vapor pressure is 40 mm Hg at 20 °C (68 °F). Flammable.
Hexachlorobutadiene (CAS: 87-68-3): Based on animal studies, rapid dermal absorption is expected. Kidney is the major target organ. Animal carcinogen. See p 490.	0.02 ppm S, A2	0.02 ppm	...	2 1 1	Heavy, colorless liquid. Thermal breakdown products include hydrogen chloride and phosgene.
Hexachlorocyclopentadiene (CAS: 77-47-4): Vapors extremely irritating to eyes and respiratory tract; lacrimation, salivation, and pulmonary edema may occur. In animals, a potent kidney and liver toxin. At higher levels the brain, heart, and adrenal glands were affected. Tremors occurred at high doses. Evidence of carcinogenicity in animals.	0.01 ppm	0.01 ppm	...	...	Yellow to amber liquid with a pungent odor. Vapor pressure is 0.08 mm Hg at 20 °C (68 °F). Not combustible.

Chemical			NFPA (H F R)	Comments
Hexachloroethane (perchloroethane) [CAS: 67-72-1]: Hot fumes irritating to eyes, skin, and mucous membranes. Based on animal studies, a CNS depressant causing weakness, muscle twitching, and kidney and liver injury at high doses. Limited evidence of carcinogenicity in animals. See p 491.	10 ppm	1 ppm S; 300 ppm NIOSH CA	...	White solid with a camphorlike odor. Vapor pressure is 0.22 mm Hg at 20 °C (68 °F). Not combustible. Thermal breakdown products include phosgene, chlorine gas, and hydrogen chloride.
Hexachloronaphthalene (Halowax 1014 [CAS: 1335-87-1]): Based on workplace experience, a potent toxin causing severe chloracne and severe, occasionally fatal, liver injury. Skin absorption can occur.	0.2 mg/m³ S	0.2 mg/m³ S	...	Light yellow solid with an aromatic odor. Vapor pressure is less than 1 mm Hg at 20 °C (68 °F). Not combustible.
Hexamethylphosphoramide (CAS: 680-31-9): Low-level exposures produce nasal cavity cancer in rats. See p 491.	S, A2	...	...	Colorless liquid with an aromatic odor. Vapor pressure is 0.07 mm Hg at 20 °C (68 °F). Thermal breakdown products include oxides of nitrogen.
_n_-Hexane (normal hexane [CAS: 110-54-3]): Defatting action may cause dermatitis. Vapors mildly irritating to eyes and respiratory tract. A CNS depressant at high levels, producing headache, dizziness, and gastrointestinal upset. Occupational overexposures have resulted in peripheral neuropathies. Methyl ethyl ketone potentiates this toxicity.	50 ppm	50 ppm	5000 ppm	1 3 0	Colorless, clear liquid with a mild gasoline odor. Vapor pressure is 124 mm Hg at 20 °C (68 °F). Highly flammable.
Hexane isomers (other than _n_-hexane): Defatting action may cause dermatitis. Vapors mildly irritating to eyes and respiratory tract. A CNS depressant at high levels, producing headache, dizziness, and gastrointestinal upset.	500 ppm	500 ppm	...	Colorless liquids with a mild petroleum odor. Vapor pressures are high at 20 °C (68 °F). Highly flammable.
sec-Hexyl acetate (1,3-dimethylbutyl acetate [CAS: 108-84-9]): At low levels, vapors irritating to eyes and respiratory tract. Based on animal studies, a CNS depressant at high levels.	50 ppm	50 ppm	4000 ppm	1 2 0	Colorless liquid. Unpleasant fruity odor and irritation are both good warning properties. Vapor pressure is 4 mm Hg at 20 °C (68 °F). Flammable.

(C) = ceiling air concentration (TLV-C); S = skin absorption can be significant; A1 = ACGIH-confirmed human carcinogen; A2 = ACGIH-suspected human carcinogen; NFPA Hazard Codes: H = health, F = fire, R = reactivity, OX = oxidizer, W = water-reactive, 0 (none) <—> 4 (severe). See expanded definitions on p 365.

continued

TABLE IV-12. HEALTH HAZARD SUMMARIES FOR INDUSTRIAL AND OCCUPATIONAL CHEMICALS (Continued)

Health Hazard Summaries	ACGIH TLV	PEL	IDLH	NFPA Codes H F R	Comments
Hexylene glycol (2-methyl-2,4-pentanediol [CAS: 107-41-5]): Irritating upon direct contact; vapors irritating to eyes and respiratory tract. A CNS depressant at very high doses in animal studies.	25 ppm (C)	25 ppm (C)	...	1 1 0	Liquid with a faint sweet odor. Vapor pressure is 0.05 mm Hg at 20 °C (68 °F). Combustible.
Hydrazine (diamine [CAS: 302-01-2]): Corrosive upon direct contact; severe burns result. Vapors extremely irritating to eyes and respiratory tract; pulmonary edema may occur. Highly hepatotoxic. A convulsant and hemolytic agent in animal studies. Kidneys are also target organs. Well absorbed by all routes. A carcinogen in animals. See p 491.	0.1 ppm S, A2	0.1 ppm S	80 ppm NIOSH CA	3 3 2 (vapors explosive)	Colorless, fuming, viscous liquid with an amine odor. Vapor pressure is 10 mm Hg at 20 °C (68 °F). Flammable. Thermal breakdown products include oxides of nitrogen. TLV under review.
Hydrogen bromide (HBr [CAS: 10035-10-6]): Direct contact with concentrated solutions may cause acid burns. Vapors highly irritating to eyes and respiratory tract; pulmonary edema may result.	3 ppm (C)	3 ppm (C)	50 ppm	3 0 0	Colorless gas or pressurized liquid. Acrid odor and irritation occur near the PEL and are adequate warning properties. Not combustible.
Hydrogen chloride (muriatic acid, HCl [CAS: 7647-01-0]): Direct contact with concentrated solutions may cause acid burns. Vapors highly irritating to eyes and respiratory tract; pulmonary edema has resulted. Repeated or prolonged exposures may cause erosion of the teeth. See p 163.	5 ppm (C)	5 ppm (C)	100 ppm	3 0 0	Colorless gas with a pungent, choking odor. Irritation occurs near the PEL and is a good warning property. Not combustible.

continued

Chemical	PEL	TLV	IDLH	H	F	R		Comments
Hydrogen cyanide (hydrocyanic acid, prussic acid, HCN [CAS: 74-90-8]): A rapidly acting, potent metabolic asphyxiant that inhibits cytochrome oxidase and stops cellular respiration. See p 134.	10 ppm (C); S		60 mg/m³; S	4	4	2		Colorless to pale blue liquid or colorless gas with a sweet, bitter almond smell that is an inadequate warning property even for those sensitive to it. Vapor pressure is 620 mm Hg at 20 °C (68 °F).
Hydrogen fluoride (hydrofluoric acid, HF [CAS: 7664-39-3]): Produces severe, penetrating burns to eyes, skin, and deeper tissues upon direct contact with solutions. Pain and erythema may be delayed as much as 24 hours. As a gas, highly irritating to the eyes and respiratory tract; pulmonary edema has resulted. Chronic overexposures may cause fluorosis. See p 167.	3 ppm (C) (as F)	3 ppm	20 ppm	4	0	0		Colorless fuming liquid or gas. Irritation occurs at levels below the PEL and is an adequate warning property. Vapor pressure is 760 mm Hg at 20 °C (68 °F). Not combustible.
Hydrogen peroxide: A strong oxidizing agent. Direct contact with concentrated solutions can produce severe eye damage and skin irritation, including erythema and vesicle formation. Vapors irritating to eyes, skin, and mucous membranes.	1 ppm	1 ppm	75 ppm	2	0	3	OX	Colorless liquid with a slightly sharp, distinctive odor. Vapor pressure is 5 mm Hg at 30 °C (86 °F). Because of instability, usually found in aqueous solutions. Not combustible but a very powerful oxidizing agent.
Hydrogen selenide (CAS: 7783-07-5): Vapors extremely irritating to eyes and respiratory tract; delayed-onset pulmonary edema may result. Systemic symptoms from low-level exposure include nausea and vomiting, fatigue, metallic taste in mouth, and a garlicky breath odor. Animal studies indicate hepatotoxicity.	0.05 ppm	0.05 ppm	2 ppm				...	Colorless gas. The strongly offensive odor and irritation occur only at levels far above the PEL and are poor warning properties. Water-reactive.
Hydrogen sulfide (CAS: 7783-06-4): Vapors irritating to eyes and respiratory tract; pulmonary edema may result. Keratitis and corneal vesiculation have been reported. Potent systemic toxin causing rapid respiratory paralysis and death. Systemic effects of low-level exposure include headache, cough, nausea, and vomiting. See p 169.	10 ppm	10 ppm	300 ppm	3	4	0		Colorless gas. Although the strong rotten egg odor can be detected at very low levels, olfactory fatigue occurs. Odor is therefore a poor warning property. Flammable.

(C) = ceiling air concentration (TLV-C); S = skin absorption can be significant; A1 = ACGIH-confirmed human carcinogen; A2 = ACGIH-suspected human carcinogen; NFPA Hazard Codes: H = health, F = fire, R = reactivity, OX = oxidizer, W = water-reactive, 0 (none) < — > 4 (severe). See expanded definitions on p 365.

TABLE IV-12. HEALTH HAZARD SUMMARIES FOR INDUSTRIAL AND OCCUPATIONAL CHEMICALS (Continued)

Health Hazard Summaries	ACGIH TLV	PEL	IDLH	NFPA Codes H F R	Comments
Hydroquinone (1,4-dihydroxybenzene [CAS: 123-31-9]): Highly irritating to eyes upon direct contact. Chronic occupational exposures may cause partial discoloration of the cornea and conjunctiva, local corneal opacity, and structural changes in the cornea that affect visual acuity. The only systemic effects reported result from ingestion and include tinnitus, headache, dizziness, gastrointestinal upset, and CNS excitation.	2 mg/m³	2 mg/m³	200 mg/m³	2 1 0	White solid crystals. Vapor pressure is less than 0.001 mm Hg at 20 °C (68 °F). Combustible.
2-Hydroxypropyl acrylate (HPA [CAS: 999-61-1]): Highly irritating upon direct contact; severe burns may result. Vapors highly irritating to eyes and respiratory tract. Based on structural analogies, compounds containing the acrylate moiety may be carcinogens.	0.5 ppm S	0.5 ppm S	...	3 1 1	Combustible liquid.
Indene (CAS: 95-13-6): Repeated direct contact with the skin produced a dry dermatitis but no systemic effects. Vapors likely irritating to eyes and respiratory tract. Based on animal studies, high air levels may cause liver and kidney damage.	10 ppm	10 ppm	...	...	Colorless liquid.
Indium (CAS: 7440-74-6): Based on animal studies, the soluble salts are extremely irritating to eyes upon direct contact. Dusts irritating to eyes and respiratory tract; alveolar edema and acute pneumonitis may result. In animals, indium compounds are highly toxic parenterally but much less toxic orally.	0.1 mg/m³	0.1 mg/m³	...	...	Appearance varies with the compound. The elemental metal is a silverwhite lustrous solid.

continued

Substance				NFPA H	NFPA F	NFPA R	Comments
Iodine (CAS: 7553-56-2): Extremely irritating upon direct contact; severe burns result. Vapors extremely irritating and corrosive to eyes and respiratory tract; pulmonary edema may result. Rarely, a skin sensitizer. See p 174.	0.1 ppm (C)	0.1 ppm (C)	10 ppm				Violet-colored solid crystals. Sharp, characteristic odor is a poor warning property. Vapor pressure is 0.3 mm Hg at 20 °C (68 °F). Not combustible.
Iron oxide fume (CAS: 1309-37-1): Fumes and dusts can produce a benign pneumoconiosis (siderosis) with shadows on chest radiographs.	5 mg/m³ (as Fe)	10 mg/m³	. . .				Red-brown fume with a metallic taste. Vapor pressure is negligible at 20 °C (68 °F).
Iron pentacarbonyl (iron carbonyl) (CAS: 13463-40-6): Acute toxicity resembles that of nickel carbonyl. Inhalation of vapors can cause lung and systemic injury without warning signs. Symptoms of overexposure include headache, nausea and vomiting, and dizziness. Symptoms of severe poisoning are fever, extreme weakness, and pulmonary edema; effects may be delayed for up to 36 hours.	0.1 ppm	0.1 ppm	. . .				Colorless to yellow viscous liquid. Vapor pressure is 40 mm Hg at 30.3 °C (86.5 °F). Highly flammable.
Iron salts: Dusts or mists irritating to the respiratory tract.	1 mg/m³ (as Fe)	1 mg/m³ (as Fe)	. . .				. . .
Isoamyl acetate (banana oil, 3-methyl butyl acetate) (CAS: 123-92-2]: May be irritating to skin upon prolonged contact. Vapors mildly irritating to eyes and respiratory tract; at very high levels, pulmonary edema may result. Symptoms in men exposed to 950 ppm for 0.5 hour included headache, weakness, dyspnea, and irritation of the nose and throat. A CNS depressant at high doses in animals.	100 ppm	100 ppm	3000 ppm	1	3	0	Colorless liquid. Bananalike odor and irritation occur at low levels and are good warning properties. Vapor pressure is 4 mm Hg at 20 °C (68 °F). Flammable.
Isoamyl alcohol (3-methyl-1-butanol) [CAS: 123-51-3]: A defatting agent causing dermatitis. Vapors irritating to eyes and upper respiratory tract. A CNS depressant at high levels.	100 ppm	100 ppm	8000 ppm	1	2	0	Colorless liquid. Irritating alcohollike odor and irritation are good warning properties. Vapor pressure is 2 mm Hg at 20 °C (68 °F). Flammable.

(C) = ceiling air concentration (TLV-C); S = skin absorption can be significant; A1 = ACGIH-confirmed human carcinogen; A2 = ACGIH-suspected human carcinogen; NFPA Hazard Codes: H = health, F = fire, R = reactivity, OX = oxidizer; W = water-reactive, 0 (none) <—> 4 (severe). See expanded definitions on p 365.

TABLE IV-12. HEALTH HAZARD SUMMARIES FOR INDUSTRIAL AND OCCUPATIONAL CHEMICALS (Continued)

Health Hazard Summaries	ACGIH TLV	PEL	IDLH	NFPA Codes H F R	Comments
Isobutyl acetate (2-methylpropyl acetate) [CAS: 110-19-0]: A defatting agent causing dermatitis. Vapors mildly irritating to eyes and respiratory tract. A CNS depressant at high levels.	150 ppm	150 ppm	7500 ppm	1 3 0	Colorless liquid. Pleasant fruity odor is a good warning property. Vapor pressure is 13 mm Hg at 20 °C (68 °F). Flammable.
Isobutyl alcohol (2-methyl-1-propanol) [CAS: 78-83-1]: Defatting action may cause dermatitis. A CNS depressant at high levels.	50 ppm	50 ppm	8000 ppm	1 3 0	Colorless liquid. Mild characteristic odor is a good warning property. Vapor pressure is 9 mm Hg at 20 °C (68 °F). Flammable.
Isophorone (trimethylcyclohexenone) [CAS: 78-59-1]: Defatting action may cause dermatitis. Vapors irritating to eyes and respiratory tract. Workers exposed to 5-8 ppm complained of fatigue and malaise after 1 month. Higher exposures result in nausea, headache, dizziness, and a feeling of suffocation at 200-400 ppm.	5 ppm (C)	4 ppm	800 ppm	2 2 0	Colorless liquid with a camphorlike odor. Vapor pressure is 0.2 mm Hg at 20 °C (68 °F). Flammable.
Isophorone diisocyanate (CAS: 4098-71-9): Based on animal studies, extremely irritating upon direct contact; severe burns may result. By analogy with other isocyanates, vapors or mists likely to be potent respiratory sensitizers. See p 179.	0.005 ppm S	0.005 ppm S	...	...	Colorless to pale yellow liquid. Vapor pressure is 0.0003 mm Hg at 20 °C (68 °F). Possible thermal breakdown products include oxides of nitrogen and hydrogen cyanide.
2-Isopropoxyethanol (isopropyl Cellosolve, ethylene glycol monoisopropyl ether) [CAS: 109-59-1]: A defatting agent causing dermatitis. In animal tests, vapor exposures increase the osmotic fragility of erythrocytes and cause anemia. See p 151.	25 ppm	25 ppm	...	...	Clear colorless liquid with a characteristic odor.

Chemical	TLV	IDLH	H	F	R	Properties
Isopropyl acetate (CAS: 108-21-4): A defatting agent causing dermatitis. Vapors irritating to the eyes and respiratory tract. A weak CNS depressant.	250 ppm	16,000 ppm	1	3	0	Colorless liquid. Fruity odor and irritation are good warning properties. Vapor pressure is 43 mm Hg at 20 °C (68 °F). Flammable.
Isopropyl alcohol (isopropanol, 2-propanol [CAS: 67-63-0]): A defatting agent causing dermatitis. Vapors produce mild eye and upper respiratory tract irritation. High exposures can produce CNS depression. See p 181.	400 ppm	20,000 ppm	1	3	0	Rubbing alcohol. Sharp odor and irritation are adequate warning properties. Vapor pressure is 33 mm Hg at 20 °C (68 °F). Flammable.
Isopropylamine (2-aminopropane [CAS: 75-31-0]): Corrosive upon direct contact; severe burns may result. Vapors highly irritating to the eyes and respiratory tract; pulmonary edema may occur. Exposure to vapors can cause transient corneal edema.	5 ppm	4000 ppm	3	4	0	Colorless liquid. Strong ammonia odor and irritation are good warning properties. Vapor pressure is 478 mm Hg at 20 °C (68 °F). Highly flammable. Thermal breakdown products include oxides of nitrogen.
Isopropyl ether (diisopropyl ether [CAS: 108-20-3]): A skin irritant upon prolonged contact with liquid. Vapors mildly irritating to the eyes and respiratory tract. A CNS depressant.	250 ppm	10,000 ppm	2	3	1	Colorless liquid. Offensive and sharp etherlike odor and irritation are good warning properties. Vapor pressure is 119 mm Hg at 20 °C (68 °F). Highly flammable. Contact with air causes formation of explosive peroxides.
Isopropyl glycidyl ether (CAS: 4016-14-2): Irritating upon direct contact. Allergic dermatitis may occur. Vapors irritating to eyes and respiratory tract. In animals, a CNS depressant at high oral doses; chronic exposures produced liver injury. Some glycidyl ethers possess hematopoietic and testicular toxicity.	50 ppm	1500 ppm	…			Flammable. Vapor pressure is 9.4 mm Hg at 25 °C (77 °F).

(C) = ceiling air concentration (TLV-C); S = skin absorption can be significant; A1 = ACGIH-confirmed human carcinogen; A2 = ACGIH-suspected human carcinogen; NFPA Hazard Codes: H = health, F = fire, R = reactivity, OX = oxidizer, W = water-reactive, 0 (none) < — > 4 (severe). See expanded definitions on p 365.

continued

TABLE IV-12. HEALTH HAZARD SUMMARIES FOR INDUSTRIAL AND OCCUPATIONAL CHEMICALS (Continued)

Health Hazard Summaries	ACGIH TLV	PEL	IDLH	NFPA Codes H F R	Comments
Kepone (chlordecone [CAS: 143-50-0]): Neurotoxin; slurred speech, memory impairment, incoordination, weakness, tremor, and convulsions. Causes infertility in males. Hepatotoxic. Well absorbed by all routes. Adverse fetal effects in animals. A carcinogen in animals. See pp 117 and 491.	...	...	NIOSH CA	...	A solid.
Ketene [CAS: 463-51-4]: Vapors extremely irritating to the eyes and respiratory tract; pulmonary edema may result and can be delayed for up to 72 hours. Toxicity similar to that of phosgene in both magnitude and time course.	0.5 ppm	0.5 ppm	25 ppm	...	Colorless gas with a sharp odor. Polymerizes readily. Acetylating agent. Water-reactive.
Lead (inorganic compounds, dusts, and fumes): Toxic to CNS and peripheral nerves, kidneys, and heme synthesis. Toxicity may result from acute or chronic exposures. Inhalation and ingestion are the major routes of absorption. Symptoms include abdominal pain, constipation, anemia, and peripheral neuropathy. Encephalopathy may develop with high blood levels. Adversely affects reproductive functions in men and women. Adverse effects on fetal development in animals. Some lead compounds are carcinogenic in animals. See pp 184 and 491.	0.15 ppm	...	...	...	The elemental metal is dark gray. Vapor pressure is low, about 2 mm Hg at 1000 °C (1832 °F).
Lead arsenate (CAS: 10102-48-4): Most common acute poisoning symptoms are due to arsenic, with lead being responsible for chronic toxicity. Symptoms include abdominal pain, headache, vomiting, diarrhea, nausea, itching, and lethargy. Liver and kidney damage may also occur. See pp 82 and 184.	0.15 mg/m³	...	300 mg/m³	2 0 0	White powder often dyed pink. Not combustible.

Chemical				
Lead chromate (chrome yellow) [CAS: 7758–97–6]: Toxicity may result from both the chromium and the lead components. Lead chromate is a suspect human carcinogen owing to the carcinogenicity of Cr(VI) compounds. See pp 124, 184 and 491.	0.05 mg/m³ (as Cr) A2	...	...	Yellow pigment in powder or crystal form.
Lindane (gamma-hexachlorocyclohexane [CAS: 58–89–9]): A CNS stimulant and convulsant. Vapors irritating to the eyes and mucous membranes and produce severe headaches and nausea. Well absorbed by all routes. Animal feeding studies have resulted in lung, liver, and kidney damage. Equivocal evidence of carcinogenicity in animals. See p 117.	0.5 mg/m³ S	1000 mg/m³	2 1 0 (solution) 2 0 0 (solid)	White crystalline substance with a musty odor if impure. Not combustible. Vapor is 0.0000094 mm Hg at 20 °C (68 °F).
Lithium hydride (CAS: 7580–67–8): Strong vesicant and alkaline corrosive. Extremely irritating upon direct contact; severe burns result. Dusts extremely irritating to eyes and respiratory tract; pulmonary edema may develop. Symptoms of systemic toxicity include nausea, tremors, confusion, blurring of vision, and coma. See p 114.	0.025 mg/m³	50 mg/m³	3 4 2 W	Off-white, translucent solid powder that darkens on exposure. Odorless. Highly water-reactive, yielding highly flammable hydrogen gas and caustic lithium hydroxide. Finely dispersed powder may ignite spontaneously.
LPG (liquified petroleum gas [CAS: 68476–85–7]): Direct contact with the liquid may produce irritation and frostbite. A simple asphyxiant and possible CNS depressant. Flammability dangers greatly outweigh toxicity concerns.	1000 ppm	19,000 ppm	...	Colorless gas. An odorant is usually added as the pure product is odorless. Highly flammable.
Magnesium oxide fume (CAS: 1309–48–4): Slightly irritating to eyes and upper respiratory tract. Based on animal studies, may cause metal fume fever similar to that caused by zinc oxide. See p 201.	10 mg/m³ (total dust) 5mg/m³ (respirable fraction)	10 mg/m³	...	White fume.

(C) = ceiling air concentration (TLV-C); S = skin absorption can be significant; A1 = ACGIH-confirmed human carcinogen; A2 = ACGIH-suspected human carcinogen; NFPA Hazard Codes: H = health, F = fire, R = reactivity, OX = oxidizer, W = water-reactive, 0 (none) <—> 4 (severe). See expanded definitions on p 365.

continued

TABLE IV-12. HEALTH HAZARD SUMMARIES FOR INDUSTRIAL AND OCCUPATIONAL CHEMICALS (Continued)

Health Hazard Summaries	ACGIH TLV	PEL	IDLH	NFPA Codes H F R	Comments
Malathion (*O,O*-dimethyl dithiophosphate of diethyl mercaptosuccinate [CAS: 121-75-5]): An organophosphate-type cholinesterase inhibitor. May cause skin sensitization. Absorbed dermally. See p 225.	10 mg/m³ S	10 mg/m³ (total dust) 5 mg/m³ (respirable fraction)	5000 mg/m³	...	Colorless to brown liquid with mild skunklike odor. Vapor pressure is 0.00004 mm Hg at 20 °C (68 °F). Thermal breakdown products include oxides of sulfur and phosphorus.
Maleic anhydride (2,5-furandione): Extremely irritating upon direct contact; severe burns may result. Vapors and mists extremely irritating to eyes, skin, and upper respiratory tract; pulmonary edema may develop. A skin and respiratory tract sensitizer.	0.25 ppm	0.25 ppm	...	3 1 1	Colorless to white solid. Strong, penetrating odor. Eye irritation occurs at the PEL and is an adequate warning property. Vapor pressure is 0.16 mm Hg at 20 °C (68 °F). Combustible.
Manganese (CAS: 7439-96-5): Chronic overexposure results in an insidious, progressive toxicity similar to parkinsonism. Acute exposure can produce symptoms similar to those of metal fume fever. See pp 195 and 201.	5 mg/m³ (C) (dusts and compounds, as Mn) 1 mg/m³ (fume, as Mn)	5 mg/m³ (C) (as Mn) 1 mg/m³ (fume)	10,000 mg/m³	...	Elemental metal is a gray, hard, brittle solid. Other compounds vary in appearance.
Mercury (quicksilver) [CAS: 7439-97-6]): Acute exposures to high vapor levels cause respiratory tract irritation; pulmonary edema has been reported. Well absorbed by inhalation. Skin contact can produce irritation and sensitization dermatitis. Mercury salts but not metallic mercury are toxic by acute ingestion. High acute or chronic overexposures can result in severe kidney injury, organic brain injury, and peripheral neuropathies. Some inorganic mercury compounds have adverse effects on fetal development in animals. See p 197.	0.05 mg/m³ (metal) S 0.1 mg/m³ (aryl and inorganic compounds, as Hg) S	0.1 mg/m³ (C) (metal and inorganic compounds, as Hg) 0.05 mg/m³ (vapor) S	28 mg/m³	...	Elemental metal is a dense, silvery liquid. Odorless. Vapor pressure is 0.0012 mm Hg at 20 °C (68 °F).

Substance			NFPA	Description
Mercury, alkyl compounds (dimethylmercury, diethyl mercury, ethylmercuric chloride): Irritating upon direct contact; some compounds may cause burns. Well absorbed by all routes. Slow excretion may allow accumulation to occur. Readily crosses blood-brain barrier and placenta. High acute or chronic overexposures can cause kidney damage, organic brain disease, and peripheral neuropathy. Methylmercury is teratogenic in humans. See p 197.	0.01 mg/m³ (alkyl compounds, as Hg) S	0.01 mg/m³ (alkyl compounds, as Hg) S	10 mg/m³	...	Colorless liquids or solids. Many alkyl compounds have a disagreeable odor.
Mesityl oxide (4-methyl-3-penten-2-one [CAS: 141-79-7]): Causes dermatitis upon prolonged contact. Vapors very irritating to eyes and respiratory tract; pulmonary edema may develop. Based on animal tests, a CNS depressant and renal toxin at high levels.	15 ppm	15 ppm	5000 ppm	3 3 0	Colorless viscous liquid with a peppermintlike odor. Irritation is an adequate warning property. Vapor pressure is 8 mm Hg at 20 °C (68 °F). Flammable. Readily forms peroxides.
Methacrylic acid (2-methylpropenoic acid [CAS: 79-41-4]): Corrosive upon direct contact; severe burns result. Vapors highly irritating to eyes and, possibly, respiratory tract. Based on structural analogies, compounds containing the acrylate moiety may be carcinogens.	20 ppm	20 ppm S	...	3 2 2	Liquid with an acrid, disagreeable odor. Vapor pressure is less than 0.1 mm Hg at 20 °C (68 °F). Combustible. Polymerizes above 15 °C (59 °F).
Methomyl (S-methyl N(methylcarbamoyl)oxy] thioacetimidate, Lannate, Nudrin [CAS: 16752-77-5]): A carbamate-type cholinesterase inhibitor. See p 106.	2.5 mg/m³	2.5 mg/m³	...	...	A slight sulfur odor. Vapor pressure is 0.00005 mm Hg at 20 °C (68 °F). Thermal breakdown products include oxides of nitrogen and sulfur.
Methoxychlor (dimethoxy-DDT, 2,2-bis(p-methoxyphenol)-1,1,1-trichloroethane [CAS: 72-43-5]): A convulsant at very high doses in animals. Limited evidence for adverse effects on fetal development in animals. See p 117.	10 mg/m³	10 mg/m³ (total dust) 5 mg/m³ (respirable fraction)	7500 mg/m³	...	Colorless to tan solid with a mild fruity odor. Appearance and some hazardous properties vary with the formulation. Vapor pressure is very low at 20 °C (68 °F).

continued

(C) = ceiling air concentration (TLV-C); S = skin absorption can be significant; A1 = ACGIH-confirmed human carcinogen; A2 = ACGIH-suspected human carcinogen; NFPA Hazard Codes: H = health, F = fire, R = reactivity, OX = oxidizer, W = water-reactive, 0 (none) <—> 4 (severe). See expanded definitions on p 365.

TABLE IV-12. HEALTH HAZARD SUMMARIES FOR INDUSTRIAL AND OCCUPATIONAL CHEMICALS (Continued)

Health Hazard Summaries	ACGIH TLV	PEL	IDLH	NFPA Codes H F R	Comments
2-Methoxyethanol (ethylene glycol mono-methyl ether, methyl cellosolve [CAS: 109-86-4]): Workplace overexposures have resulted in depression of the hematopoietic system and encephalopathy. Symptoms include disorientation, lethargy, and anorexia. Well absorbed dermally. Animal testing revealed testicular atrophy and teratogenicity at low doses. Overexposure associated with reduced sperm counts in workers. See p 151.	5 ppm S	25 ppm	2000 ppm	2 2 0	Clear, colorless liquid with a faint odor. Vapor pressure is 6 mm Hg at 20 °C (68 °F). Flammable. PEL under review.
2-Methoxyethyl acetate (ethylene glycol monomethyl ether acetate, methyl cellosolve acetate [CAS: 110-49-6]): Mildly irritating to eyes upon direct contact. Dermally well absorbed. Vapors slightly irritating to the respiratory tract. A CNS depressant at high levels. Based on animal studies, may cause kidney damage, leukopenia, testicular atrophy, and birth defects. See p 151.	5 ppm S	25 ppm	4500 ppm	1 2	Colorless liquid with a mild, pleasant odor. Flammable. PEL under review. Vapor pressure is 3.3 mm Hg at 20°C (68° F).
Methyl acetate (CAS: 79-20-9): Defatting action may cause dermatitis. Vapors moderately irritating to the eyes and respiratory tract. A CNS depressant at high levels. Hydrolyzed to methanol in the body with possible consequent neurotoxicity similar to that of methanol. See p 202.	200 ppm	200 ppm	10,000 ppm	1 3 0	Colorless liquid with a pleasant, fruity odor that is a good warning property. Vapor pressure is 173 mm Hg at 20 °C (68 °F). Flammable.
Methyl acetylene (propyne [CAS: 74-99-7]): A CNS depressant and respiratory irritant at very high air concentrations in animals.	1000 ppm	1000 ppm	11,000 ppm	2 4 2	Colorless gas with sweet odor. Flammable.

			H	F	R	
Methyl acrylate (2-propenoic acid methyl ester [CAS: 96-33-3]): Highly irritating upon direct contact; severe burns may result. A possible skin sensitizer. Vapors highly irritating to the eyes and respiratory tract; delayed-onset pulmonary edema may result. Based on structural analogies, compounds containing the acrylate moiety may be carcinogens.	10 ppm S	1000 ppm	2	3	2	Colorless liquid with a sharp, fruity odor. Vapor pressure is 68.2 mm Hg at 20 °C (68 °F). Inhibitor included to prevent violent polymerization.
Methylacrylonitrile (2-methyl-2-pro-penenitrile, methacrylonitrile [CAS: 126-98-7]): Mildly irritating upon direct contact. Defatting action may cause dermatitis. Well absorbed dermally. In animal tests, acute inhalation at high levels caused death without signs of irritation, probably by a mechanism similar to that of acrylonitrile. Lower levels produced convulsions and loss of motor control in hind limbs.	1 ppm S	1 ppm	…			Liquid. Vapor pressure is 40 mm Hg at 13 °C (55 °F).
Methylal (dimethoxymethane [CAS: 109-87-5]): Defatting action may cause dermatitis. Mildly irritating to eyes and respiratory tract. A CNS depressant at very high levels. Animal studies suggest a potential to injure heart, liver, kidney, and lung at very high air levels.	1000 ppm	10,000 ppm	2	3	2	Colorless liquid with pungent, chloroformlike odor. Highly flammable. Vapor pressure is 330 mm Hg at 20 °C (68 °F).
Methyl alcohol (methanol, wood alcohol [CAS: 67-56-1]): Mildly irritating to eyes and skin; defatting action may cause dermatitis. Systemic toxicity may result from absorption by all routes. A CNS depressant. Symptoms include headache, nausea, abdominal pain, dizziness, shortness of breath, metabolic acidosis, and coma. Visual disturbances range from blurred vision to blindness. See p 202.	200 ppm S	25,000 ppm	1	3	0	Colorless liquid. Distinctive odor is a poor warning property. Vapor pressure is 100 mm Hg at 21 °C (70 °F). Highly flammable.

(C) = ceiling air concentration (TLV-C); S = skin absorption can be significant; A1 = ACGIH-confirmed human carcinogen; A2 = ACGIH-suspected human carcinogen; NFPA Hazard Codes: H = health, F = fire, R = reactivity, OX = oxidizer, W = water-reactive, 0 (none) < — > 4 (severe). See expanded definitions on p 365.

continued

TABLE IV-12. HEALTH HAZARD SUMMARIES FOR INDUSTRIAL AND OCCUPATIONAL CHEMICALS (Continued)

Health Hazard Summaries	ACGIH TLV	PEL	IDLH	NFPA Codes H F R	Comments
Methylamine [CAS: 74-89-5]: Caustic. Highly irritating to eyes, skin, and respiratory tract; severe burns and delayed pulmonary edema may result.	10 ppm	10 ppm	100 ppm	3 4 0	Colorless gas with a fishy or ammonialike odor. Odor is a poor warning property owing to olfactory fatigue. Flammable.
Methyl n-amyl ketone (2-heptanone) [CAS: 110-43-0]: Defatting action may cause dermatitis. Vapors are irritating to eyes and respiratory tract; pulmonary edema may result from very high exposure. A CNS depressant.	50 ppm	100 ppm	4000 ppm	1 2 0	Colorless or white liquid with a fruity odor. Vapor pressure is 2.6 mm Hg at 20 °C (68 °F). Flammable.
N-methyl aniline [CAS: 100-61-8]: A potent inducer of methemoglobinemia. Well absorbed by all routes. Animal studies suggest potential for pulmonary edema and liver and kidney injury. See p 204.	0.5 ppm S	...	100 ppm	3 2 0	Yellow to light brown liquid with a weak ammonialike odor. Vapor pressure is less than 1 mm Hg at 20 °C (68 °F). Thermal breakdown products include oxides of nitrogen.
Methyl bromide (bromomethane) [CAS: 74-83-9]: Causes severe irritation and burns upon direct contact. Vapors irritating to the lung; pulmonary edema may result. The CNS, liver, and kidneys are major target organs; acute poisoning causes nausea, vomiting, delirium, and convulsions. Both inhalation and skin exposure may cause systemic toxicity. Chronic exposures associated with peripheral neuropathy. Limited evidence of carcinogenicity in animals. See pp 206 and 492, and Chloropicrin in this table.	5 ppm S	5 ppm S	2000 ppm NIOSH CA	3 1 0	Colorless liquid with a low boiling point (3.6 °C [38.5 °F]); a gas at room temperature. Mild chloroformlike odor that is a poor warning property. Chloropicrin, a lacrimator, is often added as a warning agent.
Methyl n-butyl ketone (2-hexanone) [CAS: 591-78-6]: Vapors irritating to eyes and upper respiratory tract at high levels. A CNS depressant at high doses. Causes peripheral neuropathy by a mechanism thought to be the same as that of n-hexane. Well absorbed by all routes.	5 ppm	5 ppm	5000 ppm	2 3 0	Colorless liquid with an acetonelike odor. Vapor pressure is 3.8 mm Hg at 20 °C (68 °F). Flammable.

Chemical (CAS Number) and Comments	TLV		IDLH	NFPA (H F R)	Physical Properties
Methyl chloride (CAS: 74-87-3): Once used as a local anesthetic. Symptoms include headache, confusion, ataxia, convulsions, and coma. Liver, kidney, and bone marrow are other target organs. May sensitize the myocardium to the arrhythmogenic effects of epinephrine. Limited evidence for adverse effects on fetal development in animals at high doses. A suspected carcinogen. See p 492.	50 ppm	50 ppm	10,000 ppm NIOSH CA	2 4 0	Colorless gas with a mild, sweet odor that is a poor warning property. Highly flammable.
Methyl-2-cyanoacrylate (CAS: 137-05-3): Vapors irritating to the eyes and upper respiratory tract. A strong and fast-acting glue. Direct contact with the eye may result in mechanical injury if the immediate bonding of the eyelids is followed by forced separation.	2 ppm	2 ppm	…	…	Colorless viscous liquid.
Methylcyclohexane (CAS: 108-87-2): Irritating upon direct contact. Vapors irritating to eyes and respiratory tract. A CNS depressant at high levels. Based on animal studies, some liver and kidney injury may occur at chronic high doses.	400 ppm	400 ppm	10,000 ppm	2 3 0	Colorless liquid with a faint benzenelike odor. Vapor pressure is 37 mm Hg at 20 °C (68 °F). Highly flammable.
Methylcyclohexanol (CAS: 25639-42-3): Based on animal studies, irritating upon prolonged direct contact. Vapors irritating to eyes and upper respiratory tract at high levels. A CNS depressant. Liver and kidneys also may be target organs at very high doses.	50 ppm	50 ppm	10,000 ppm	0 2 0	Colorless to straw-colored liquid with a mild coconutlike odor that is a poor warning property. Vapor pressure is less than 1 mm Hg at 20 °C (68 °F). Combustible.
o-Methylcyclohexanone (CAS: 583-60-8): Based on animal studies, irritating upon direct contact. Dermal absorption occurs. Vapors irritating to eyes and upper respiratory tract. A CNS depressant at high levels.	50 ppm S	50 ppm S	2500 ppm	2 0	Colorless liquid with mild peppermint odor. Irritation is a good warning property. Vapor pressure is about 1 mm Hg at 20 °C (68 °F). Flammable.

(C) = ceiling air concentration (TLV-C); S = skin absorption can be significant; A1 = ACGIH-confirmed human carcinogen; A2 = ACGIH-suspected human carcinogen; NFPA Hazard Codes: H = health, F = fire, R = reactivity, OX = oxidizer, W = water-reactive, 0 (none) <—> 4 (severe). See expanded definitions on p 365.

continued

TABLE IV-12. HEALTH HAZARD SUMMARIES FOR INDUSTRIAL AND OCCUPATIONAL CHEMICALS (Continued)

Health Hazard Summaries	ACGIH TLV	PEL	IDLH	NFPA Codes H F R	Comments
Methyl demeton (*O,O*-dimethyl 2-ethylmercaptoethyl thiophosphate [CAS: 8022-00-2]): An organophosphate-type cholinesterase inhibitor. See p 225.	0.5 mg/m³ S	0.5 mg/m³ S	...	...	Colorless to pale yellow liquid with an unpleasant odor. Vapor pressure is 0.00036 mm Hg at 20 °C (68 °F). Thermal breakdown products include oxides of sulfur and phosphorus.
4,4'-Methylene-bis(2-chloroaniline) (MOCA [CAS: 101-14-4]): A carcinogen in test animals. Dermal absorption occurs. See p 492.	0.02 ppm S, A2	0.02 ppm	NIOSH CA	...	Tan solid. Thermal breakdown products include oxides of nitrogen and hydrogen chloride.
Methylene bis(4-cyclohexylisocyanate [CAS: 5124-30-1]): A strong irritant and skin sensitizer. Based on analogy to other isocyanates, vapors are likely to be potent respiratory tract irritants and sensitizers. See p 179.	0.005 ppm	0.01 ppm (C)	...	...	White to pale yellow solid flakes. Odorless. Possible thermal breakdown products include oxides of nitrogen and hydrogen cyanide.
Methylene bisphenyl isocyanate (4,4-di-phenylmethane diisocyanate, MDI [CAS: 101-68-8]): Irritating upon direct contact. Vapors and dusts highly irritating to eyes and upper respiratory tract; pulmonary edema may occur. Potent respiratory tract sensitizer. See p 179.	0.005 ppm	0.02 ppm (C)	10 ppm	...	White to pale yellow flakes. Odorless. Vapor pressure is 0.05 mm Hg at 20 °C (68 °F). Possible thermal breakdown products include oxides of nitrogen and hydrogen cyanide.
Methylene c̲̲ride (methylene dichloride, dichloromethane [CAS: 75-0̲-2]): Irritating upon prolonged direct contact. Dermal absorption occurs. Vapors irritating to eyes and upper respiratory tract; pulmonary edema may develop. A CNS depressant. Sensitizes the myocardium to arrhythmogenic effects of epinephrine. Liver and kidney injury at high concentrations. Metabolized to carbon monoxide with resultant carboxyhemoglobin formation. A carcinogen in animals. See pp 207 and 492.	50 ppm A2	OSHA CA	5000 ppm NIOSH CA	2 1 0	Heavy colorless liquid with a chloroformlike odor that is a poor warning property. Vapor pressure is 350 mm Hg at 20 °C (68 °F). Possible thermal breakdown products include phosgene and hydrogen chloride.

Chemical / Toxicity			NFPA (H F R)	Physical properties
4,4'-Methylene dianiline (4,4'-diaminodiphenylmethane) [CAS: 101-77-9]: Vapors highly irritating to eyes and respiratory tract. Systemic toxicity may result from inhalation, ingestion, or skin contact. Methemoglobinemia (see p 204), kidney injury, and evidence of carcinogenicity in animals. See p 492.	0.1 ppm S, A2	... NIOSH CA	3 1 0	Light brown crystals with a faint amine odor. Combustible. Thermal breakdown products include oxides of nitrogen.
Methyl ethyl ketone, MEK [CAS: 78-93-3]: Defatting action may cause skin irritation. Vapors irritating to eyes and respiratory tract. A CNS depressant at high levels. Potentiates neurotoxicity of methyl butyl ketone and *n*-hexane.	200 ppm	200 ppm 3000 ppm	1 3 0	Colorless liquid with a mild acetone odor. Vapor pressure is 77 mm Hg at 20 °C (68 °F). Flammable.
Methyl ethyl ketone peroxide [CAS: 1338-23-4]: Based on chemical reactivity, highly irritating upon direct contact; severe burns may result. Vapors or mists likely to be highly irritating to the eyes and respiratory tract; pulmonary edema may result. In animals, overexposure resulted in liver, kidney, and lung damage.	0.2 ppm (C)	0.7 ppm (C) ...	...	Colorless liquid with a characteristic odor. Shock sensitive. Breaks down above 50 °C (122 °F). Explodes upon rapid heating. May contain additives such as dimethyl phthalate, cyclohexanone peroxide, or diallylphthalate to add stability.
Methyl formate [CAS: 107-31-3]: Vapors highly irritating to eyes and respiratory tract; pulmonary edema may develop. Based on animal data, a CNS depressant at high levels. Exposure has been associated with visual disturbances, including temporary blindness.	100 ppm	100 ppm 5000 ppm	2 4 0	Colorless liquid with a pleasant odor at high levels. Odor is a poor warning property. Vapor pressure is 476 mm Hg at 20 °C (68 °F). Highly flammable.
Methylhydrazine (monomethylhydrazine) [CAS: 60-34-4]: Based on animal studies, similar to hydrazine in toxic actions. Vapors likely to be highly irritating to the eyes and respiratory tract. Causes methemoglobinemia (see p 204) and hemolytic anemia. Highly hepatotoxic. Causes kidney injury. A convulsant. A carcinogen in animals. See p 492.	0.2 ppm (C) S, A2	0.2 ppm (C) S 5 ppm NIOSH CA	3 3 2	Colorless clear liquid. Vapor pressure is 36 mm Hg at 20 °C (68 °F). Flammable. TLV under review.

(C) = ceiling air concentration (TLV-C); S = skin absorption can be significant; A1 = ACGIH-confirmed human carcinogen; A2 = ACGIH-suspected human carcinogen; NFPA Hazard Codes: H = health, F = fire, R = reactivity, OX = oxidizer, W = water-reactive, 0 (none) < — > 4 (severe). See expanded definitions on p 365.

continued

TABLE IV-12. HEALTH HAZARD SUMMARIES FOR INDUSTRIAL AND OCCUPATIONAL CHEMICALS (Continued)

Health Hazard Summaries	ACGIH TLV	PEL	IDLH	NFPA Codes H F R	Comments
Methyl iodide: (Iodomethane [CAS: 74-88-4]): An alkylating agent. Based on chemical properties, likely to be highly irritating upon direct contact; severe burns may result. Dermal absorption is likely. Vapors highly irritating to respiratory tract; pulmonary edema has resulted. Neurotoxic; symptoms include nausea, vomiting, dizziness, slurred speech, visual disturbances, ataxia, tremor, irritability, convulsions, and coma. Delusions and hallucinations may last for weeks during recovery. Severe hepatic injury may also occur. Limited evidence of carcinogenicity in animals. See p 492.	2 ppm S, A2	2 ppm S	800 ppm NIOSH CA	...	Colorless, yellow, red, or brown liquid. Not combustible. Vapor pressure is 375 mm Hg at 20 °C (68 °F). Thermal breakdown products include iodine and hydrogen iodide.
Methyl isoamyl ketone (5-methyl-2-hexanone [CAS: 110-12-3]): Defatting action may cause dermatitis. By analogy to other aliphatic ketones, vapors are likely to be irritating to eyes and upper respiratory tract. Likely to be a CNS depressant.	50 ppm	50 ppm	...	1 2 0	Colorless liquid with a pleasant odor. Vapor pressure is 4.5 mm Hg at 20 °C (68 °F). Flammable.
Methyl isobutyl ketone (4-methyl-2-pentanone, hexone [CAS: 108-10-1]): Irritating to eyes upon direct contact. Defatting action may cause dermatitis. Vapors irritating to eyes and upper respiratory tract. Reported systemic symptoms in humans are weakness, dizziness, ataxia, nausea, vomiting, and headache. High-dose studies in animals suggest a potential for liver and kidney injury.	50 ppm	50 ppm	3000 ppm	2 3 0	Colorless liquid with a mild odor. Vapor pressure is 7.5 mm Hg at 25 °C (77 °F). Flammable.

Chemical			NFPA	Comments
Methyl isocyanate (CAS: 624-83-9): Highly reactive; highly corrosive upon direct contact. Vapors extremely irritating to eyes, skin, and respiratory tract; severe burns and pulmonary edema have resulted. A sensitizing agent. See p 179.	0.02 ppm S	20 ppm	2 3 W	Colorless liquid with a sharp, disagreeable odor that is a poor warning property. Vapor pressure is 348 mm Hg at 20 °C (68 °F). Flammable. Reacts with water to release methylamine. Polymerizes upon heating. Thermal breakdown products include hydrogen cyanide and oxides of nitrogen.
Methyl mercaptan (CAS: 74-93-1): Causes delayed-onset pulmonary edema. CNS effects include narcosis and convulsions. See p 169.	0.5 ppm	400 ppm	2 4 0	Colorless liquid with an offensive rotten egg odor. Odor and irritation are good warning properties.
Methyl methacrylate (CAS: 80-62-6): Irritating upon direct contact. Vapors irritating to the eyes, skin, and upper respiratory tract. A sensitizer. At very high levels may produce headache, nausea, vomiting, dizziness. Limited evidence for adverse effects on fetal development in animals at very high doses.	100 ppm	4000 ppm	2 3 2	Colorless liquid with a pungent, acrid, fruity odor. Vapor pressure is 35 mm Hg at 20 °C (68 °F). Flammable. Contains inhibitors to prevent self-polymerization.
Methyl parathion (O,O-dimethyl O-p-nitro-phenylphosphorothioate) [CAS: 298-00-0]: An organophosphate cholinesterase inhibitor. See p 225.	0.2 mg/m³ S	0.2 mg/m³ S	4 1 2 (solid) / 4 3 2 (in xylene)	Tan liquid with a strong garliclike odor. Vapor pressure is 0.5 mm Hg at 20 °C (68 °F).
Methyl propyl ketone (2-pentanone) [CAS: 107-87-9]: Defatting action may cause dermatitis. Vapors irritating to eyes and respiratory tract. A CNS depressant at high levels.	200 ppm	5000 ppm	2 3 0	Colorless liquid with a characteristic odor. Vapor pressure is 27 mm Hg at 20 °C (68 °F). Flammable.
Methyl silicate (tetramethoxy silane) [CAS: 681-84-5]: Highly reactive; corrosive upon direct contact; severe burns and loss of vision may result. Vapors extremely irritating to eyes and respiratory tract; severe eye burns and pulmonary edema may result.	1 ppm	...	...	Colorless crystals. Reacts with water, forming silicic acid and methanol.

(C) = ceiling air concentration (TLV-C); S = skin absorption can be significant; A1 = ACGIH-confirmed human carcinogen; A2 = ACGIH-suspected human carcinogen; NFPA Hazard Codes: H = health, F = fire, R = reactivity, OX = oxidizer, W = water-reactive, 0 (none) <—> 4 (severe). See expanded definitions on p 365.

continued

TABLE IV-12. HEALTH HAZARD SUMMARIES FOR INDUSTRIAL AND OCCUPATIONAL CHEMICALS (Continued)

Health Hazard Summaries	ACGIH TLV	PEL	IDLH	NFPA Codes H F R	Comments
α-Methylstyrene (CAS: 98-83-9): Slightly irritating upon direct contact. Vapors irritating to eyes and upper respiratory tract. A CNS depressant at high levels.	50 ppm	50 ppm	5000 ppm	2 2 1	Colorless liquid with a characteristic odor. Irritation is an adequate warning property. Vapor pressure is 1.9 mm Hg at 20 °C (68 °F). Flammable.
Metribuzin (4-amino-6-[1,1-dimethylethyl]-3[methylthio]-1,2,4-triazin-5[4H]-one [CAS: 21087-64-9]): Human data available reveal no irritation or sensitization after dermal exposure. In animal testing, was poorly absorbed through the skin and produced no direct skin or eye irritation. Repeated high doses caused CNS depression and liver and thyroid effects.	5 mg/m³	5 mg/m³	...	...	Vapor pressure is 0.00001 mm Hg at 20 °C (68 °F). Thermal breakdown products include oxides of sulfur and nitrogen.
Mevinphos (2-carbomethoxy-1-methylvinyl dimethyl phosphate, phosdrin, phosdrin [CAS: 7786-34-7]): An organophosphate cholinesterase inhibitor. Well absorbed by all routes. Repeated exposures to low levels can accumulate to produce symptoms. See p 225.	0.01 ppm S	...	40 mg/m³	...	Colorless or yellow liquid with a faint odor. Vapor pressure is 0.0022 mm Hg at 20 °C (68 °F). Combustible. Thermal breakdown products include phosphoric acid mist.
Mica (CAS: 12001-25-2): Dusts can cause pneumoconiosis upon chronic inhalation. Symptoms include cough, dyspnea, weakness, and weight loss.	3 mg/m³ (respirable dust)	3 mg/m³ (respirable dust)	...	...	Colorless solid flakes or sheets. Odorless. Vapor pressure is negligible at 20 °C (68 °F). Noncombustible.

Chemical			NFPA	Description
Monocrotophos (dimethyl 2-methylcarbamoyl-1-methyl-vinyl phosphate [CAS: 6923-22-4]: An organophosphate-type cholinesterase inhibitor. Limited human data indicate it is well absorbed through the skin but is rapidly metabolized and excreted. See p 225. 0.25 mg/m³ | 0.25 mg/m³ | ... | ...				Reddish-brown solid with a mild odor.
Morpholine (tetrahydro-1,4-oxazine [CAS: 110-91-8]): Caustic; extremely irritating upon direct contact; severe burns may result. Well absorbed dermally. Vapors irritating to eyes and upper respiratory tract. Exposure to vapors has caused transient corneal edema. May cause pulmonary edema and severe liver and kidney injury. 20 ppm S | 20 ppm S | 8000 ppm | 2 3 0				Colorless liquid with mild ammonialike odor. Vapor pressure is 7 mm Hg at 20 °C (68 °F). Flammable. Thermal breakdown products include oxides of nitrogen.
Naled (dibrom, 1,2-dibromo-2,2-dichloroethyl dimethyl phosphate [CAS: 300-76-... ...n organophosphate anticholinesterase agent. Hi... irritating upon contact; eye injury is likely. Dermal s... ization can occur. Well absorbed dermally; localized muscular twitching results within minutes of contact. See p 225. 3 mg/m³ S | ... | ... | ...				Has a pungent odor. Vapor pressure is 0.002 mm Hg at 20 °C (68 °F). Not combustible. Thermal breakdown products include hydrogen bromide, hydrogen chloride, and phosphoric acid.
Naphthalene [CAS: 91-20-3]: Highly irritating to eyes upon direct contact. Vapors are irritating to eyes and may cause cataracts upon chronic exposure. Dermally well absorbed; both skin exposure and ingestion have produced headache, nausea, methemoglobinemia, and hemolytic anemia. See p 213. 10 ppm | 10 ppm | 500 ppm | 2 2 0				White to brown solid. The mothball odor and respiratory tract irritation are good warning properties. Vapor pressure is 0.05 mm Hg at 20 °C (68 °F). Combustible.
β-Naphthylamine (2-aminonaphthalene [CAS: 91-59-8]): Acute overexposures can cause methemoglobinemia (see p 357r) or acute hemorrhagic cystitis. Well absorbed through skin. Known human bladder carcinogen. See p 493. A1 | OSHA CA | NIOSH CA | 2 1 0				White to reddish crystals. Vapor pressure is 1 mm Hg at 108 °C (226 °F). Combustible.

(C) = ceiling air concentration (TLV-C); S = skin absorption can be significant; A1 = ACGIH-confirmed human carcinogen; A2 = ACGIH-suspected human carcinogen; NFPA Hazard Codes: H = health, F = fire, R = reactivity, OX = oxidizer, W = water-reactive, 0 (none) <—> 4 (severe). See expanded definitions on p 365.

continued

TABLE IV-12. HEALTH HAZARD SUMMARIES FOR INDUSTRIAL AND OCCUPATIONAL CHEMICALS (Continued)

Health Hazard Summaries	ACGIH TLV	PEL	IDLH	NFPA Codes H F R	Comments
Nickel metal and soluble inorganic salts (nickel chloride, nickel sulfate, nickel nitrate, nickel oxide): May cause a severe sensitization dermatitis, "nickel itch," upon repeated contact. Fumes highly irritating to the respiratory tract; pulmonary edema may occur. The TLV may not protect all individuals from dermatitis or sensitization. Some compounds have adverse effects on fetal development in animals. Some compounds are suspected human nasal and lung carcinogens. See p 493.	1 mg/m³ (metal) 0.1 mg/m³ (soluble inorganic compounds, as Ni)	1 mg/m³ (metal) 0.1 mg/m³ (soluble inorganic compounds, as Ni)	NIOSH CA (metal)	. . .	Gray metallic powder or green solids. All forms are odorless.
Nickel carbonyl (nickel tetracarbonyl) [CAS: 13463-39-3]: Inhalation of vapors can cause severe lung and systemic injury without warning signs. Symptoms include headache, nausea, vomiting, fever, and extreme weakness. Pulmonary edema may be delayed up to 36 hours. Based on animal studies, liver and brain damage may occur. Adverse effects on fetal development in animals. A carcinogen in animals.	0.05 ppm	0.001 ppm	0.001 ppm	4 3 3	Colorless liquid or gas. The musty odor is a poor warning property. Vapor pressure is 321 mm Hg at 20 °C (68 °F). Highly flammable. TLV under review.
Nicotine [CAS: 54-11-5]: A potent nicotinic cholinergic receptor agonist. Well absorbed by all routes of exposure. Symptoms include dizziness, confusion, weakness, nausea and vomiting, tachycardia and hypertension, tremors, convulsions, and muscle paralysis. Death from respiratory paralysis can be very rapid. Adverse effects on fetal development in animals. See p 214.	0.5 mg/m³ S	0.5 mg/m³ S	35 mg/m³	4 1 0	Pale yellow to dark brown viscous liquid with a fishy or aminelike odor. Vapor pressure is 0.0425 mm Hg at 20 °C (68 °F). Combustible. Thermal breakdown products include oxides of nitrogen.

Chemical	TLV	PEL	IDLH	NFPA (H F R)	Comments
Nitric acid (aqua fortis, engraver's acid) [CAS: 7697-37-2]: Concentrated solutions corrosive to eyes and skin; very severe penetrating burns result. Vapors highly irritating to eyes and respiratory tract; delayed pulmonary edema has resulted. Chronic inhalation exposure can produce bronchitis and erosion of the teeth. See p 217.	2 ppm	2 ppm	100 ppm	3 0 0 OX	Colorless, yellow, or red fuming liquid with an acrid, suffocating odor. Vapor pressure is approximately 62 mm Hg at 25 °C (77 °F). Not combustible.
Nitric oxide (NO, nitrogen monoxide) [CAS: 10102-43-9]: Nitric oxide slowly converts to nitrogen dioxide in air; eye and mucous membrane irritation and delayed pulmonary edema are likely due to nitrogen dioxide. Based on animal studies, may cause methemoglobinemia. See p 217.	25 ppm	25 ppm	100 ppm	....	Colorless or brown gas. The sharp, sweet odor occurs below the PEL and is a good warning property.
p-Nitroaniline [CAS: 100-01-6]: Irritating to eyes upon direct contact; may injure cornea. Well absorbed by all routes. Overexposure results in headache, weakness, respiratory distress, and methemoglobinemia. Symptoms may be delayed up to 4 hours. Liver damage may also result. See p 204.	3 mg/m³ S	3 mg/m³ S	300 mg/m³	3 1 3	Yellow solid with an ammonialike odor that is a poor warning property. Vapor pressure is much less than 1 mm Hg at 20 °C (68 °F). Combustible. Thermal breakdown products include oxides of nitrogen.
Nitrobenzene [CAS: 98-95-3]: Irritating upon direct contact; sensitization dermatitis may occur. Well absorbed by all routes. Causes methemoglobinemia. Symptoms include headache, cyanosis, weakness, and gastrointestinal upset. May injure liver. Limited evidence for adverse effects on fetal development in animals. See p 204.	1 ppm S	1 ppm S	200 ppm	3 2 0	Pale yellow to dark brown viscous liquid. Shoe polishlike odor is a good warning property. Vapor pressure is much less than 1 mm Hg at 20 °C (68 °F). Combustible. Thermal breakdown products include oxides of nitrogen.
p-Nitrochlorobenzene [CAS: 100-00-5]: Irritating upon direct contact; sensitization dermatitis may occur upon repeated exposures. Well absorbed by all routes. Causes methemoglobinemia. Symptoms include headache, cyanosis, weakness, and gastrointestinal upset. May cause liver and kidney injury. See p 204.	0.1 ppm S	1 mg/m³ S	1000 ppm	2 1 3	Yellow solid with a sweet odor. Vapor pressure is 0.009 mm Hg at 25 °C (77 °F). Combustible. Thermal breakdown products include oxides of nitrogen and hydrogen chloride.

(C) = ceiling air concentration (TLV-C); S = skin absorption can be significant; A1 = ACGIH-confirmed human carcinogen; A2 = ACGIH-suspected human carcinogen; NFPA Hazard Codes: H = health, F = fire, R = reactivity, OX = oxidizer, W = water-reactive, 0 (none) < – > 4 (severe). See expanded definitions on p 365.

continued

TABLE IV-12. HEALTH HAZARD SUMMARIES FOR INDUSTRIAL AND OCCUPATIONAL CHEMICALS (Continued)

Health Hazard Summaries	ACGIH TLV	PEL	IDLH	NFPA Codes H F R	Comments
4-Nitrodiphenyl (4-nitrobiphenyl [CAS: 92-93-3]): Extremely well absorbed through skin. Produces bladder cancer in dogs and rabbits. Metabolized to 4-aminodiphenyl, a potent carcinogen in humans. See p 494.	A1	OSHA CA	NIOSH CA	...	White solid with a sweet odor. Thermal break-down products include oxides of nitrogen.
Nitroethane [CAS: 79-24-3]: Defatting action may cause dermatitis. Based on high-exposure studies in animals. Vapors are irritating to the respiratory tract; pulmonary edema may result. A CNS depressant. Causes liver injury at high levels of exposure in animals. A structurally similar compound, 2-nitropropane, is a carcinogen.	100 ppm	100 ppm	1000 ppm	1 3 3 (explodes on heating)	Colorless viscous liquid with a fruity odor that is a poor warning property. Vapor pressure is 15.6 mm Hg at 20 °C (68 °F). Flammable. Thermal breakdown products include oxides of nitrogen.
Nitrogen dioxide (CAS: 10102-44-0): Gases and vapors irritating to eyes and respiratory tract; fatal pulmonary edema has resulted. Initial symptoms include cough and dyspnea. Pulmonary edema may appear after a delay of several hours. The acute phase may be followed by a fatal secondary stage, with fever and chills, dyspnea, cyanosis, and recurring pulmonary edema. See p 217.	3 ppm	See Comments	50 ppm	...	Dark brown fuming liquid or gas. Pungent odor and irritation occur at 10–20 ppm. Vapor pressure is 720 mm Hg at 20 °C (68 °F). No PEL; 15-minute Short-Term Exposure Limit (STEL) is 1 ppm.
Nitrogen trifluoride (nitrogen fluoride [CAS: 7783-54-2]): Vapors may cause eye irritation. Based on animal studies, may cause methemoglobinemia (see p 204). Liver and kidney damage. Chronic exposures may cause fluorosis. See p 167.	10 ppm	10 ppm	2000 ppm	...	Colorless gas with a moldy odor that is a poor warning property. Not combustible. Highly reactive and explosive under a number of conditions.

Chemical	TLV	OSHA	NIOSH	NFPA	Properties
Nitroglycerin (glycerol trinitrate [CAS: 55-63-0]): Causes vasodilation, including coronary arteries. Headache and drop in blood pressure are common. Well absorbed by all routes. Tolerance to vasodilation can occur; cessation of exposure may precipitate angina pectoris in pharmacologically dependent workers. See p 216.	0.05 ppm S	...	...	2 2 4	Pale yellow viscous liquid. Vapor pressure is 0.00026 mm Hg at 20 °C (68 °F). Highly explosive.
Nitromethane [CAS: 75-52-5]: Defatting action may cause dermatitis. Based on high-dose animal studies, may cause ataxia, weakness, convulsions, respiratory tract irritation, and liver and kidney injury.	100 ppm	100 ppm	1000 ppm	1 3 3	Colorless liquid with a faint fruity odor that is a poor warning property. Vapor pressure is 27.8 mm Hg at 20 °C (68 °F). Thermal breakdown products include oxides of nitrogen.
1-Nitropropane [CAS: 108-03-2]: Vapors irritating to eyes and respiratory tract; based on animal studies, pulmonary edema may result from very high exposures. At high doses, liver and kidney injury may occur.	25 ppm	25 ppm	2300 ppm	1 3 1 (may explode on heating)	Colorless liquid with a faint fruity odor that is a poor warning property. Vapor pressure is 7.5 mm Hg at 20 °C (68 °F). Flammable. Thermal breakdown products include oxides of nitrogen.
2-Nitropropane [CAS: 79-46-9]: Vapors irritating to respiratory tract; pulmonary edema may develop. Workers exposed to high vapor concentrations complained of respiratory irritation, headaches, and gastrointestinal upset. Highly hepatotoxic; fatalities have resulted. Well absorbed by all routes. High-dose animal tests indicate that methemoglobinemia (see p 204) and kidney and heart injury may occur. Limited evidence for adverse effects on fetal development in animals. A carcinogen in animals. See p 494.	10 ppm A2	10 ppm	2300 ppm NIOSH CA	2 3 1 (may explode on heating)	Colorless liquid. Vapor pressure is 12.9 mm Hg at 20 °C (68 °F). Flammable. Thermal breakdown products include oxides of nitrogen.
N-Nitrosodimethylamine (dimethylnitrosamine [CAS: 62-75-9]): Overexposed workers suffered severe liver damage. Based on animal studies, well absorbed by all routes. A potent animal carcinogen producing liver, kidney, and lung cancers. See p 495.	A2, S	OSHA CA	NIOSH CA	...	Yellow viscous liquid. Combustible.

(C) = ceiling air concentration (TLV-C); S = skin absorption can be significant; A1 = ACGIH-confirmed human carcinogen; A2 = ACGIH-suspected human carcinogen; NFPA Hazard Codes: H = health, F = fire, R = reactivity, OX = oxidizer, W = water-reactive, 0 (none) < — > 4 (severe). See expanded definitions on p 365.

continued

TABLE IV-12. HEALTH HAZARD SUMMARIES FOR INDUSTRIAL AND OCCUPATIONAL CHEMICALS (Continued)

Health Hazard Summaries	ACGIH TLV	PEL	IDLH	NFPA Codes H F R	Comments
Nitrotoluene o-, m-, p-nitrotoluene [CAS: 99-08-1]: May cause methemoglobinemia, but this is rare. By analogy to structurally similar compounds, dermal absorption is likely to occur.	2 ppm S	2 ppm S	200 ppm	3 1 0	Ortho and meta, yellow liquid or solid. Para, yellow solid. All isomers have a weak, aromatic odor. Vapor pressure is approximately 0.15 mm Hg at 20 °C (68 °F). Thermal breakdown products include oxides of nitrogen.
Nitrous oxide [CAS: 10024-97-2]: A CNS depressant. There is evidence that it may have an adverse effect on human fertility and fetal development.. See p 220.	...	...	...	...	Colorless gas. Sweet odor. Not combustible.
Nonane [CAS: 111-84-2]: Defatting action may cause dermatitis. Based on animal data, likely to be a CNS depressant at high levels.	200 ppm	200 ppm	...	0 3 0	Colorless flammable liquid. Vapor pressure is 10 mm Hg at 38 °C (100 °F).
Octachloronaphthalene (Halowax 1051 [CAS: 2234-13-1]): By analogy to other chlorinated naphthalenes, workers overexposed by inhalation or skin contact may experience chloracne and liver damage.	0.1 mg/m³ S	0.1 mg/m³ S	200 mg/m³	...	Pale yellow solid with an aromatic odor. Vapor pressure is less than 1 mm Hg at 20 °C (68 °F). Not combustible. Thermal breakdown products include hydrogen chloride.
Octane [CAS: 111-65-9]: Defatting action may cause dermatitis. Vapors mildly irritating to eyes and respiratory tract. A CNS depressant at very high concentrations.	300 ppm	300 ppm	3750 ppm	0 3 0	Colorless liquid. Gasolinelike odor and irritation are good warning properties. Vapor pressure is 11 mm Hg at 20 °C (68 °F). Flammable.

Chemical			NFPA codes	Physical description
Osmium tetroxide (osmic acid) [CAS: 20816-12-0]: Corrosive upon direct contact; severe burns may result. Fumes are highly irritating to eyes and respiratory tract. Based on high-dose animal studies, pulmonary edema, bone marrow injury, and kidney damage may occur.	0.0002 ppm / 0.0002 ppm	1 mg/m³	...	Colorless to pale yellow solid with a sharp and irritating odor like chlorine. Vapor pressure is 7 mm Hg at 20 °C (68 °F). Not combustible.
Oxalic acid (ethanedioic acid) [CAS: 144-62-7]: A strong acid; corrosive to eyes and to skin upon direct contact. Fumes irritating to upper respiratory tract. Highly toxic upon ingestion; precipitation of calcium oxalate crystals can cause hypocalcemia and renal damage. See p 227.	1 mg/m³ / 1 mg/m³	500 mg/m³	1 1 0 (nonfire) 2 1 0 (fire)	Colorless or white solid. Odorless. Vapor pressure is less than 0.001 mm Hg at 20 °C (68 °F).
Oxygen difluoride, fluorine monoxide [CAS: 7783-41-7]: Extremely irritating to the eyes, skin, and respiratory tract; pulmonary edema may occur. Based on animal studies, may injure kidney, internal genitalia, and other organs. Workers have complained of intractable headaches after low-level exposures. See p 167.	0.05 ppm (C) / 0.05 ppm (C)	0.5 ppm	...	Colorless gas with a strong and foul odor. Olfactory fatigue is common, so odor is a poor warning property. A strong oxidizing agent.
Ozone (triatomic oxygen [CAS: 10028-15-6]): Irritating to eyes and upper and lower respiratory tract; delayed pulmonary edema has been reported.	0.1 ppm / 0.1 ppm	10 ppm	...	Colorless or bluish gas. Sharp, distinctive odor is an adequate warning property. A strong oxidizing agent.
Paraquat (1,1'-dimethyl-4,4'-bipyridinium dichloride [CAS: 4687-14-7]): Commercial high-concentration preparations extremely irritating upon direct contact; severe corrosive burns may result. A potent toxin causing delayed, progressive fatal pulmonary fibrosis after ingestion. Can also cause serious kidney and liver injury. See p 230.	0.1 mg/m³ / 0.1 mg/m³ S	1.5 mg/m³	...	Odorless white to yellow solid. Vapor pressure is negligible at 20 °C (68 °F). Not combustible. Thermal breakdown products include oxides of nitrogen and sulfur and hydrogen chloride.

(C) = ceiling air concentration (TLV-C); S = skin absorption can be significant; A1 = ACGIH-confirmed human carcinogen; A2 = ACGIH-suspected human carcinogen; NFPA Hazard Codes: H = health, F = fire, R = reactivity, OX = oxidizer, W = water-reactive, 0 (none) <—> 4 (severe). See expanded definitions on p 365.

continued

TABLE IV-12. HEALTH HAZARD SUMMARIES FOR INDUSTRIAL AND OCCUPATIONAL CHEMICALS (Continued)

Health Hazard Summaries	ACGIH TLV	PEL	IDLH	NFPA Codes H F R	Comments
Parathion (*O,O*-diethyl *O-p*-nitrophenyl phosphorothioate [CAS: 56-38-2]): Highly potent organophosphate cholinesterase inhibitor. Systemic toxicity has resulted from inhalation, ingestion, and dermal exposures. See p 225.	0.1 mg/m^3 S	0.1 mg/m^3	20 mg/m^3	4 1 2	Yellow to dark brown liquid with garliclike odor. Odor threshold of 0.04 ppm suggests it has good warning properties. Vapor pressure is 0.0004 mm Hg at 20 °C (68 °F). Thermal breakdown products include oxides of sulfur, nitrogen, and phosphorus.
Pentaborane [CAS: 19624-22-7]: Highly irritating upon direct contact; severe burns may result. Vapors irritating to the respiratory tract. A potent CNS toxin; symptoms include headache, nausea, weakness, confusion, hyperexcitability, tremors, seizures, and coma. Mental (loss of memory, poor judgment) and psychic effects may persist. Liver and kidney injury may also occur.	0.005 ppm	0.005 ppm	3 ppm	3 3 2	Colorless liquid. Vapor pressure is 171 mm Hg at 20 °C (68 °F). The pungent sour-milk odor occurring only at air levels well above the PEL is a poor warning property. May ignite spontaneously. Reacts violently with halogenated extinguishing media. Thermal breakdown products include boron acids.
Pentachloronaphthalene (Halowax 1013 [CAS: 1321-64-8]): Chloracne results from prolonged skin contact or inhalation. May cause severe, potentially fatal liver injury or necrosis by all routes of exposure.	0.5 mg/m^3 S	0.5 mg/m^3 S	···	···	Pale yellow waxy solid with a pleasant aromatic odor. Odor threshold not known. Vapor pressure is less than 1 mm Hg at 20 °C (68 °F). Not combustible. Thermal breakdown products include hydrogen chloride fumes.
Pentachlorophenol (Penta, PCP [CAS: 87-86-5]): Irritating upon direct contact; burns may result. Vapors irritating to eyes and respiratory tract. A potent metabolic poison; uncouples oxidative phosphorylation. Well absorbed by all routes. Adverse effects on fetal development in animals. See p 231.	0.5 mg/m^3 S	0.5 mg/m^3 S	150 mg/m^3	3 2 0 (solutions) 3 0 0 (dry)	Eye and nose irritation occur slightly above the PEL and are good warning properties. Vapor pressure is 0.0002 mm Hg at 20 °C (68 °F). Not combustible. Thermal breakdown products include hydrogen chloride, chlorinated phenols, and octachlorodibenzodioxin.

Chemical				NFPA	Description
Pentane (n-pentane) [CAS: 109-66-0]: Defatting agent causing dermatitis. Vapors mildly irritating to eyes and respiratory tract. A CNS depressant at high levels.	600 ppm	600 ppm	5000 ppm	1 4 0	Colorless liquid with a gasolinelike odor that is an adequate warning property. Vapor pressure is 426 mm Hg at 20 °C (68 °F). Flammable.
Perchloromethyl mercaptan (trichloromethyl sulfur chloride [CAS: 594-42-3]): Extremely irritating upon direct contact; severe burns may result. Vapors highly irritating to eyes and respiratory tract. Fatal exposures have involved pulmonary edema and liver and kidney injury.	0.1 ppm	0.1 ppm	10 ppm	...	Pale yellow to orange-red oily liquid with a foul and acrid odor at low levels. Vapor pressure is 65 mm Hg at 20 °C (68 °F). Not combustible. Reacts with hot water. Thermal breakdown products include carbon tetrachloride, sulfur monochloride, and sulfur dioxide.
Perchloryl fluoride (chlorine oxyfluoride [CAS: 7616-94-6]): Highly irritating upon direct contact; severe burns may result. Vapors extremely irritating to eyes and respiratory tract; pulmonary edema may result. Based on high-dose animal studies, fluorosis and methemoglobinemia may occur. See pp 167 and 204.	3 ppm	3 ppm	385 ppm	...	Colorless gas. Usually stored in cylinders as a pressurized liquid. The distinctive sweet odor is a poor warning property. A strong oxidizing agent. Thermal breakdown products include hydrogen fluoride and chlorine gas.
Petroleum distillates (petroleum naphtha, petroleum ether): Defatting action may cause dermatitis. Vapors irritating to eyes and respiratory tract. A CNS depressant. If n-hexane or benzene is present, those hazards should be addressed. See p 165.	400 ppm (rubber solvent)	400 ppm	10,000 ppm	1 4 0 (petroleum naphtha)	Colorless liquid. Kerosenelike odor at levels below the PEL serves as a warning property. Highly flammable. Vapor pressure is about 40 mm Hg at 20 °C (68 °F).
Phenol (carbolic acid, hydroxybenzene [CAS: 108-95-2]): Corrosive acid and protein denaturant. Direct eye or skin contact causes severe tissue damage or blindness. Deep skin burns can occur without warning pain. Systemic toxicity by all routes; percutaneous absorption of vapor occurs. Vapors highly irritating to eyes and respiratory tract. Symptoms include nausea, vomiting, circulatory collapse, convulsions, and coma. Toxic to liver and kidney. A tumor promoter. See p 234.	5 ppm S	5 ppm S	100 ppm	3 2 0	Colorless to pink crystalline solid, or viscous liquid. Its odor has been described as being distinct, acrid, and aromatic or as being sweet and tarry. As the odor is detected at or below the PEL, it is a good warning property. Vapor pressure is 0.36 mm Hg at 20 °C (68 °F). Combustible.

(C) = ceiling air concentration (TLV); S = skin absorption can be significant; A1 = ACGIH-confirmed human carcinogen; A2 = ACGIH-suspected human carcinogen; NFPA Hazard Codes: H = health, F = fire, R = reactivity, OX = oxidizer, W = water-reactive, 0 (none) <—> 4 (severe). See expanded definitions on p 365.

continued

TABLE IV-12. HEALTH HAZARD SUMMARIES FOR INDUSTRIAL AND OCCUPATIONAL CHEMICALS (Continued)

Health Hazard Summaries	ACGIH TLV	PEL	IDLH	NFPA Codes H F R	Comments
Phenylenediamine (p-aminoaniline, p-aminoaniline [CAS: 106-50-3]): Irritating upon direct contact. May cause skin and respiratory tract sensitization. Occupational asthma has been described. Inflammatory reactions of larynx and pharynx have often been noted in exposed workers.	0.1 mg/m³ S	0.1 mg/m³ S	25 mg/m³	...	White to light purple or brown solid, depending on degree of oxidation. Combustible. Thermal breakdown products include oxides of nitrogen.
Phenyl ether (diphenyl ether [CAS: 101-84-8]): Mildly irritating upon prolonged direct contact. Vapors irritating to eyes and respiratory tract. Based on high-dose experiments in animals, liver and kidney damage may occur after ingestion.	1 ppm	1 ppm	...	...	Colorless liquid or solid. Mildly disagreeable odor detected below the PEL serves as a good warning property. Vapor pressure is 0.02 mm Hg at 25 °C (77 °F). Combustible.
Phenyl glycidyl ether (PGE, 1,2-epoxy-3-phenoxypropane [CAS: 122-60-1]): Irritating upon direct contact. A skin sensitizer. Based on animal studies, vapors are very irritating to eyes and respiratory tract. In high-dose animal studies, a CNS depressant producing liver, kidney, spleen, testes, thymus, and hematopoietic system injury.	1 ppm	1 ppm	...	...	Colorless liquid with an unpleasant, sweet odor. Vapor pressure is 0.01 mm Hg at 20 °C (68 °F). Combustible. Readily forms peroxides.
Phenylhydrazine [CAS: 100-63-0]): A strong base and corrosive upon direct contact. A potent skin sensitizer. Dermal absorption occurs. Vapors irritating to eyes and respiratory tract; pulmonary edema may result. Can cause hemolytic anemia with secondary kidney damage. Limited evidence of carcinogenicity in animals. See p 496.	5 ppm S, A2	5 ppm S	250 ppm NIOSH CA	3 2 0	Pale yellow crystals or oily liquid with a weakly aromatic odor. Darkens upon exposure to air and light. Vapor pressure is less than 0.1 mm Hg at 20 °C (68 °F). Combustible. Thermal breakdown products include oxides of nitrogen. TLV under review.

Chemical				NFPA (H F R)	Description
Phenylphosphine (CAS: 638-21-1): In animals, subchronic inhalation at 2 ppm caused loss of appetite, diarrhea, tremor, hemolytic anemia, dermatitis, and irreversible testicular degeneration.	0.05 ppm (C)	0.05 ppm (C)	...	...	Crystalline solid. Spontaneously combustible at high air concentrations.
Phorate (O,O-diethyl S-(ethylthio)methyl phosphorodithioate, Thimet [CAS: 298-02-2]): An organophosphate-type cholinesterase inhibitor. Well absorbed by all routes. See p 225.	0.05 mg/m³ S	0.05 mg/m³ S	...	...	Clear liquid. Vapor pressure is 0.002 mm Hg at 20 °C (68 °F).
Phosgene (carbonyl chloride, COCl₂ [CAS: 75-44-5]): Irritating to the respiratory tract; delayed pulmonary edema may occur. Exposure can be insidious because irritation and smell are inadequate as warning properties for pulmonary injury. Higher levels cause irritation of the eyes, skin, and mucous membranes. See p 241.	0.1 ppm	0.1 ppm	2 ppm	4 0 0	Colorless gas. Sweet haylike odor at low concentrations; sharp and pungent odor at high concentrations. Dangerous concentrations may not be detected by odor.
Phosphine (hydrogen phosphide [CAS: 7803-51-2]): Extremely irritating to the respiratory tract; fatal pulmonary edema has resulted. Symptoms in moderately overexposed workers included diarrhea, nausea, vomiting, cough, headache, and dizziness. See p 242.	0.3 ppm	0.3 ppm	200 ppm	3 4 1	Colorless gas. A fishy or garliclike odor detected well below the PEL is considered to be a good warning property. May ignite spontaneously on contact with air.
Phosphoric acid (CAS: 7664-38-2): A strong corrosive acid; severe burns may result from direct contact. Mist or vapors irritating to eyes and upper respiratory tract.	1 mg/m³	1 mg/m³	...	2 0 0	Colorless, syrupy, odorless liquid. Solidifies at temperatures below 20 °C (68 °F). Vapor pressure is 0.03 mm Hg at 20 °C (68 °F). Not combustible.

(C) = ceiling air concentration (TLV-C); S = skin absorption can be significant; A1 = ACGIH-confirmed human carcinogen; A2 = ACGIH-suspected human carcinogen; NFPA Hazard Codes: H = health, F = fire, R = reactivity, OX = oxidizer, 0 (none) < -- > 4 (severe). See expanded definitions on p 365.

continued

TABLE IV-12. HEALTH HAZARD SUMMARIES FOR INDUSTRIAL AND OCCUPATIONAL CHEMICALS (Continued)

Health Hazard Summaries	ACGIH TLV	PEL	IDLH	NFPA Codes H F R	Comments
Phosphorus (yellow phosphorus, white phosphorus, P [CAS: 7723-14-0]): Severe, penetrating burns may result upon direct contact. Material may ignite upon contact with skin. Fumes irritating to eyes and respiratory tract; pulmonary edema may occur. Systemic symptoms include abdominal pain, jaundice, and garlic odor on the breath; chronic poisoning can involve jaw bone necrosis (phossy jaw). See p 243.	0.1 mg/m^3	0.1 mg/m^3	...	3 3 1	White to yellow, waxy or crystalline solid with acrid fumes. Flammable. Vapor pressure is 0.026 mm Hg at 20 °C (68 °F). Ignites spontaneously on contact with air. Thermal breakdown products include phosphoric acid fume.
Phosphorus oxychloride (CAS: 10025-87-3): Reacts with moisture to release phosphoric and hydrochloric acids; highly corrosive upon direct contact. Fumes extremely irritating to eyes and respiratory tract; pulmonary edema may occur. Systemic symptoms include headache, dizziness, dyspnea, and nephritis. See p 163.	0.1 ppm	0.1 ppm	...	3 0 2 W	Clear colorless to pale yellow, fuming liquid possessing a pungent odor. Vapor pressure is 40 mm Hg at 27.3 °C (81 °F). Not combustible.
Phosphorus pentachloride (CAS: 10026-13-8): Reacts with moisture to release phosphoric and hydrochloric acids; highly corrosive upon direct contact. Fumes extremely irritating to eyes and respiratory tract; pulmonary edema may result.	0.1 ppm	1 mg/m^3	200 mg/m^3	...	Pale yellow solid with a hydrochloric acidlike odor. Not combustible.
Phosphorus pentasulfide (CAS: 1314-80-3): Rapidly reacts with moisture and moist tissues to form hydrogen sulfide and phosphoric acid. Severe burns may result from prolonged contact with tissues. Dusts or fumes extremely irritating to eyes and respiratory tract. Systemic toxicology is predominantly caused by hydrogen sulfide. See p 169.	1 mg/m^3	1 mg/m^3	750 mg/m^3	...	Greenish-yellow solid with odor of rotten eggs. Olfactory fatigue reduces value of smell as a warning property. Thermal breakdown products include sulfur dioxide, hydrogen sulfide, phosphorus pentoxide, and phosphoric acid fumes.

Substance				NFPA	Comments
Phosphorus trichloride (CAS: 7719-12-2): Reacts with moisture to release phosphoric and hydrochloric acids; highly corrosive upon direct contact. Fumes extremely irritating to eyes and respiratory tract; pulmonary edema may occur.	0.2 ppm	0.2 ppm	50 ppm	3 0 2 W	Fuming colorless to yellow liquid. Irritation provides a good warning property. Vapor pressure is 100 mm Hg at 20 °C (68 °F). Not combustible.
Phthalic anhydride (phthalic acid anhydride [CAS: 85-44-9]): Extremely irritating upon direct contact; chemical burns occur after prolonged contact. Dusts and vapors extremely irritating to respiratory tract. A potent skin and respiratory tract sensitizer.	1 ppm	1 ppm	10,000 ppm	2 1 0	White crystalline solid with choking odor at very high air concentrations. Vapor pressure is 0.05 mm Hg at 20 °C (68 °F). Combustible. Thermal breakdown products include phthalic acid fumes.
Picloram (4-amino-3,5,6-trichloropicolinic acid [CAS: 1918-02-1]): Dusts mildly irritating to skin, eyes, and respiratory tract. Has low oral toxicity in animals.	10 mg/m^3	10 mg/m^3 (total dust) 5 mg/m^3 (respirable fraction)	...	...	White powder possessing a bleachlike odor. Vapor pressure is 0.0000006 mm Hg at 35 °C (95 °F). Thermal breakdown products include oxides of nitrogen and hydrogen chloride.
Picric acid (2,4,6-trinitrophenol [CAS: 88-89-1]): Irritating upon direct contact. Dust stains skin yellow and can cause a sensitization dermatitis. Symptoms of low-level exposure are headache, dizziness, and gastrointestinal upset. Ingestion of large amounts causes hemolysis, nephritis, and hepatitis. Staining of the conjunctiva and aqueous humor can give vision a yellow hue. A weak uncoupler of oxidative phosphorylation.	0.1 mg/m^3 S	0.1 mg/m^3 S	100 mg/m^3	2 4 4	Pale yellow crystalline solid or paste. Odorless. Vapor pressure is much less than 1 mm Hg at 20 °C (68 °F). Decomposes explosively above 120 °C (248 °F). May detonate when shocked. Contact with metals, ammonia, or calcium compounds can form salts that are much more sensitive to shock detonation.
Pindone (Pival, 2-pivaloyl-1,3-indanedione [CAS: 83-26-1]): A vitamin K antagonist anticoagulant. See p 132.	0.1 mg/m^3	0.1 mg/m^3	200 mg/m^3	...	Bright yellow crystalline substance.

(C) = ceiling air concentration (TLV-C); S = skin absorption can be significant; A1 = ACGIH-confirmed human carcinogen; A2 = ACGIH-suspected human carcinogen; NFPA Hazard Codes: H = health, F = fire, R = reactivity, OX = oxidizer, W = water-reactive, 0 (none) < — > 4 (severe). See expanded definitions on p 365.

continued

TABLE IV-12. HEALTH HAZARD SUMMARIES FOR INDUSTRIAL AND OCCUPATIONAL CHEMICALS (Continued)

Health Hazard Summaries	ACGIH TLV	PEL	IDLH	NFPA Codes H F R	Comments
Piperazine dihydrochloride (CAS: 142-64-3): Irritating upon direct contact; burns may result. A moderate skin and respiratory sensitizer. Nausea, vomiting, and diarrhea are side effects of medicinal use. Overdosage has caused confusion, lethargy, coma, and seizures.	5 mg/m^3	5 mg/m^3	...	...	White crystalline solid with a mild fishy odor.
Piperidine (CAS: 110-89-4): Highly irritating upon direct contact; severe burns may result. Vapors irritating to eyes and upper respiratory tract. Small doses initially stimulate autonomic ganglia; larger doses depress them. A 30–60 mg/kg dose may produce symptoms in humans.	...	...	...	2 3 3	Flammable.
Platinum—soluble salts (sodium chloroplatinate; ammonium chloroplatinate, platinum tetrachloride): Sensitizers causing asthma and dermatitis. Metallic platinum does not share these effects. Soluble platinum compounds are also highly irritating to eyes, mucous membranes, and upper respiratory tract.	0.002 mg/m^3 (as Pt)	0.002 mg/m^3 (as Pt)	...	...	Appearance varies with the compound. Thermal breakdown products of some chloride salts include chlorine gas.
Polychlorinated biphenyls (chlorodiphenyls, PCBs): Exposure to high concentrations is irritating to eyes, nose, and throat. Chronically overexposed workers suffer from chloracne and liver injury. Reported symptoms are anorexia, gastrointestinal upset, and peripheral neuropathies. Some health effects may be due to contaminants or thermal decomposition products. Adverse effects on fetal development and fertility in animals. A carcinogen in animals. See pp 252 and 496.	1 mg/m^3 (42% chlorine) S 0.5 mg/m^3 (54% chlorine) S	1 mg/m^3 (42% chlorine) S 0.5 mg/m^3 (54% chlorine) S	10 mg/m^3 (42% chlorine) NIOSH CA 5 mg/m^3 (54% chlorine) NIOSH CA	...	42% chlorinated: a colorless to dark brown liquid with a slight hydrocarbon odor and a vapor pressure of 0.001 mm Hg at 20 °C (68 °F). 54% chlorinated: light yellow oily liquid with a slight hydrocarbon odor and a vapor pressure of 0.00006 mm Hg at 20 °C (68 °F). Thermal breakdown products include chlorinated dibenzofurans and chlorodibenzodioxins.

Polytetrafluoroethylene decomposition products: Overexposures result in polymer fume fever, a disease with flulike symptoms including chills, fever, and cough. See p 201.

... | ... | | | Produced by pyrolysis of Teflon and related materials. Perisofluorobutylene and carbonyl fluoride are among the pyrolysis products.

Polyvinyl chloride decomposition products: Fumes are irritating to the respiratory tract and may cause "meat wrapper's" asthma.

... | ... | | | Produced by the high-temperature partial breakdown of polyvinyl chloride plastics.

Portland cement (a mixture of mostly tricalcium silicate and dicalcium silicate with some alumina, calcium aluminate, and iron oxide): Irritant of the eyes, nose, and skin; corrosive burns may occur. Long-term heavy exposure has been associated with dermatitis and bronchitis.

10 mg/m³ (<1% quartz) | 10 mg/m³ (total dust) 5 mg/m³ (respirable fraction) | | | Gray powder. Odorless.

Potassium hydroxide (KOH [CAS: 1310-58-3]): A caustic alkali causing severe burns to tissues upon direct contact. Exposure to dust or mist causes eye, nose, and respiratory tract irritation. See p 114.

2 mg/m³ (C) | 2 mg/m³ (C) | 3 | 0 | 1 | White solid that absorbs moisture. Vapor pressure is negligible at 20 °C (68 °F). Gives off heat and a corrosive mist when in contact with water.

Propargyl alcohol (2-propyn-1-ol [CAS: 107-19-7]): Irritating to skin upon direct contact. Dermally well absorbed. A CNS depressant. Causes liver and kidney injury in animals.

1 ppm S | 1 ppm S | 3 | 3 | 3 | Light to straw-colored liquid with a geraniumlike odor. Vapor pressure is 11.6 mm Hg at 20 °C (68 °F). Flammable.

Propionic acid (CAS: 79-09-4): Irritating to eyes and skin upon direct contact with concentrated solutions; burns may result. Vapors irritating to eyes, skin, and respiratory tract. A food additive of low systemic toxicity.

10 ppm | 10 ppm | 2 | 2 | 0 | Colorless oily liquid with a pungent, somewhat rancid odor. Vapor pressure is 10 mm Hg at 39.7 °C (103.5 °F). Flammable.

(C) = ceiling air concentration (TLV-C); S = skin absorption can be significant; A1 = ACGIH-confirmed human carcinogen; A2 = ACGIH-suspected human carcinogen; NFPA Hazard Codes: H = health, F = fire, R = reactivity, OX = oxidizer, W = water-reactive, 0 (none) <—> 4 (severe). See expanded definitions on p 365.

continued

TABLE IV-12. HEALTH HAZARD SUMMARIES FOR INDUSTRIAL AND OCCUPATIONAL CHEMICALS (Continued)

Health Hazard Summaries	ACGIH TLV	PEL	IDLH	NFPA Codes H F R	Comments
Propoxur (o-isopropoxyphenyl N-methylcarbamate, DDVP, Baygon [CAS: 114-26-1]): A carbamate anticholinesterase insecticide. Limited evidence for adverse effects on fetal development in animals. See p 106.	0.5 mg/m³	0.5 mg/m³	...	...	White crystalline solid with a faint characteristic odor. Vapor pressure is 0.01 mm Hg at 120 °C (248 °F).
n-Propyl acetate (CAS: 109-60-4): Defatting action may cause dermatitis. Vapors irritating to eyes and respiratory tract. Excessive inhalation may cause weakness, nausea, and chest tightness. Based on high-exposure studies in animals, a CNS depressant.	200 ppm	200 ppm	8000 ppm	1 3 0	Colorless liquid. Mild fruity odor and irritant properties provide good warning properties. Vapor pressure is 25 mm Hg at 20 °C (68 °F). Flammable.
Propyl alcohol (1-propanol [CAS: 71-23-8]): Defatting action may cause dermatitis. Vapors mildly irritating to eyes and respiratory tract. A CNS depressant.	200 ppm	200 ppm	4000 ppm	1 3 0	Colorless volatile liquid. Vapor pressure is 15 mm Hg at 20 °C (68 °F). Mild alcohollike odor is an adequate warning property.
Propylene dichloride (1,2-dichloropropane [CAS: 78-87-5]): Defatting action may cause dermatitis. Vapors very irritating to eyes and respiratory tract; based on high-exposure studies in animals, pulmonary edema may occur. Causes CNS depression and severe liver and kidney damage at modest doses in animals.	75 ppm	75 ppm	2000 ppm	2 3 0	Colorless liquid. Chloroformlike odor is considered to be an adequate warning property. Vapor pressure is 40 mm Hg at 20 °C (68 °F). Flammable. Thermal breakdown products include hydrogen chloride.
Propylene glycol dinitrate (1,2-propylene glycol dinitrate, PGDN [CAS: 6423-43-4]): Mildly irritating upon direct contact. Dermal absorption occurs. Causes methemoglobinemia (see p 204). Potent vasodilator causing hypotension and headache. See p 216.	0.05 ppm S	0.05 ppm	...	...	Colorless liquid with an unpleasant odor. Thermal breakdown products include oxides of nitrogen.

Chemical				NFPA (H F R)	Comments
Propylene glycol monomethyl ether (1-methoxy-2-propanol) [CAS: 107-98-2]: Defatting action may cause dermatitis. Vapors very irritating to the eyes and possibly the respiratory tract. A mild CNS depressant.	100 ppm	100 ppm	…	0 3 0	Colorless, flammable liquid.
Propylene imine (2-methylaziridine) [CAS: 75-55-8]: Very irritating upon direct contact; severe burns may result. Vapors highly irritating to eyes and respiratory tract; pulmonary edema may occur. May also injure liver and kidneys. Well absorbed dermally. A carcinogen in animals. See p 497.	2 ppm S, A2	2 ppm S	500 ppm	…	A fuming colorless liquid with a strong ammonia-like odor. Flammable. Thermal breakdown products include oxides of nitrogen.
Propylene oxide (2-epoxypropane) [CAS: 75-56-9]: Highly irritating upon direct contact; severe burns result. Quick evaporative cooling can cause frostbite. Vapors highly irritating to eyes and respiratory tract; pulmonary edema may occur. Based on high-dose animal studies, a mild CNS depressant. A carcinogen in animals. See p 497.	20 ppm	20 ppm	2000 ppm	2 4 2	Colorless liquid. Its sweet, etherlike odor is considered to be an adequate warning property. Vapor pressure is 442 mm Hg at 20 °C (68 °F). Highly flammable. Polymerizes violently.
n-Propyl nitrate (nitric acid n-propyl ester [CAS: 627-13-4]): Vasodilator causing headaches and hypotension. Causes methemoglobinemia. See pp 204 and 216.	25 ppm	25 ppm	2000 ppm	2 4 3 OX	Pale yellow liquid with an unpleasant sweet odor. Vapor pressure is 18 mm Hg at 20 °C (68 °F). Flammable. Thermal breakdown products include oxides of nitrogen.
Pyrethrum (pyrethrin I or II; cinerin I or II; jasmolin I or II): Dusts cause primary contact dermatitis and skin and respiratory tract sensitization. Of very low systemic toxicity. See p 254.	5 mg/m³	5 mg/m³	5000 mg/m³	…	Vapor pressure is negligible at 20 °C (68 °F). Combustible.

(C) = ceiling air concentration (TLV-C); S = skin absorption can be significant; A1 = ACGIH-confirmed human carcinogen; A2 = ACGIH-suspected human carcinogen; NFPA Hazard Codes: H = health, F = fire, R = reactivity, OX = oxidizer, W = water-reactive, 0 (none) <—> 4 (severe). See expanded definitions on p 365.

continued

TABLE IV-12. HEALTH HAZARD SUMMARIES FOR INDUSTRIAL AND OCCUPATIONAL CHEMICALS (Continued)

Health Hazard Summaries	ACGIH TLV	PEL	IDLH	NFPA Codes H F R	Comments
Pyridine (CAS: 110-86-1): Irritating upon prolonged direct contact; occasional reports of skin sensitization. Vapors irritating to eyes and respiratory tract. A CNS depressant. Chronic ingestion of small amounts has caused fatal liver and kidney injury. Workers exposed to 6—12 ppm have complained of headache, dizziness, and gastrointestinal upset. Dermally well absorbed.	5 ppm	5 ppm	3600 ppm	2 3 0	Colorless or yellow liquid with a nauseating odor and a definite "taste" that serves as a good warning property. Vapor pressure is 18 mm Hg at 20 °C (68 °F). Flammable. Thermal breakdown products include oxides of nitrogen and cyanide.
Pyrogallol (1,2,3-trihydroxybenzene; pyrogallic acid (CAS: 87-66-1): Highly irritating upon direct contact; severe burns may result. Potent reducing agent. May cause methemoglobinemia (see p 204). Attacks heart, lung, liver, kidney, red blood cells, bone marrow, and muscle. May cause sensitization dermatitis. Deaths have resulted from the topical application of salves containing pyrogallol.	...	...	...	...	White to gray odorless solid.
Quinone (1,4-cyclohexadienedione, p-benzoquinone (CAS: 106-51-4]): A severe irritant of the eyes and respiratory tract. Acute overexposure to dust or vapors can cause conjunctival irritation and discoloration, corneal edema, ulceration, and scarring. Chronic exposures can permanently reduce visual acuity. Skin contact can cause irritation, ulceration, and staining.	0.1 ppm	0.1 ppm	75 ppm	1 2 1	Pale yellow crystalline solid. The acrid odor is not a reliable warning property. Vapor pressure is 0.1 mm Hg at 20 °C (68 °F). Sublimes when heated.
Resorcinol (1,3-dihydroxybenzene [CAS: 108-46-3]): Corrosive acid and protein denaturant; extremely irritating upon direct contact; severe burns result. May cause methemoglobinemia. A sensitizer. Dermally well absorbed. See pp 204 and 234.	10 ppm	10 ppm	...	1 0	White crystalline solid with a faint odor. May turn pink on contact with air. Vapor pressure is 1 mm Hg at 108 °C (226 °F). Combustible.

Ronnel (O,O-dimethyl-O-(2,4,5-trichlorophenyl)phosphorothioate [CAS: 299-84-3]): One of the least toxic organophosphate anticholinesterase insecticides. See p 225.

10 mg/m³ | 10 mg/m³ | 5000 mg/m³ | ...

Vapor pressure is 0.0008 mm Hg at 20 °C (68 °F). Not combustible. Unstable above 149 °C (300 °F); harmful gases such as sulfur dioxide, dimethyl sulfide, and trichlorophenol may be released.

Rotenone (tubatoxin, cube root, derris root, derrin [CAS: 83-79-4]): Irritating upon direct contact. Dusts irritate the respiratory tract. A metabolic poison; depresses cellular respiration and inhibits mitotic spindle formation. Ingestion of large doses numbs oral mucosa and causes nausea and vomiting, muscle tremors, and convulsions. Chronic exposure caused liver and kidney damage in animals.

5 mg/m³ | 5 mg/m³ | 5000 mg/m³ | ...

White to red crystalline solid. Vapor pressure is negligible at 20 °C (68 °F). A natural product extracted from such plants as cube, derris, and timbo. Odorless. Decomposes upon contact with air or light. Unstable to alkali.

Selenium and inorganic compounds (as selenium): Fumes, dusts, and vapors irritating to eyes, skin, and respiratory tract; pulmonary edema may occur. Many compounds are well absorbed dermally. A general protoplasmic poison. Chronic intoxication causes depression, nervousness, dermatitis, gastrointestinal upset, metallic taste in mouth and garlicky odor of breath, excess caries, and loss of fingernails or hair. The liver and kidney are also target organs. Some selenium compounds have been found to cause birth defects and cancers in animals. See p 267.

0.2 mg/m³ (as Se) | 0.2 mg/m³ | 100 mg/m³ | ...

Elemental selenium is a black, gray, or red crystalline or amorphous solid and is odorless.

Selenium dioxide (selenium oxide [CAS: 7446-08-4]): Strong vesicant; severe burns result from direct contact. Converted to selenious acid in the presence of moisture. If penetrates under fingernails, causes an excruciating inflammatory reaction. Well absorbed dermally. Fumes and dusts very irritating to eyes and respiratory tract; metal fume fever or delayed pulmonary edema may occur. See pp 201 and 267.

... | ... | ... | ...

White solid. Reacts with water to form selenious acid.

(C) = ceiling air concentration (TLV-C); S = skin absorption can be significant; A1 = ACGIH-confirmed human carcinogen; A2 = ACGIH-suspected human carcinogen; NFPA Hazard Codes: H = health, F = fire, R = reactivity, OX = oxidizer, W = water-reactive, 0 (none) <-> 4 (severe). See expanded definitions on p 365.

continued

TABLE IV-12. HEALTH HAZARD SUMMARIES FOR INDUSTRIAL AND OCCUPATIONAL CHEMICALS (Continued)

Health Hazard Summaries	ACGIH TLV	PEL	IDLH	NFPA Codes H F R	Comments
Selenium hexafluoride [CAS: 7783-79-1]: Vesicant. Reacts with moisture to form selenium acids and hydrofluoric acid; severe HF burns may result from direct contact. Fumes highly irritating to eyes and respiratory tract; pulmonary edema may result. See pp 167 and 267.	0.05 ppm	0.05 ppm (as Se)	5 ppm	...	Colorless gas. Not combustible.
Selenium oxychloride [CAS: 7791-23-3]: Strong vesicant. Direct contact can cause severe burns. Dermally well absorbed. Fumes extremely irritating to eyes and respiratory tract; delayed pulmonary edema may result. See p 267.	...	...	...	...	Colorless to yellow liquid. Hydrogen chloride fumes produced on contact with moisture.
Silane (silicon tetrahydride [CAS: 7803-62-5]: Little is known concerning its human health effects. Thought to be less toxic than other gaseous metallic hydrides (arsine, stibine) that cause hemolysis. The potential of silane to cause hemolysis is unknown.	5 ppm	...	...	1 4 2	Colorless gas with unpleasant odor. Flammable. Slowly reacts with moisture to form hydrogen gas and silicic acid.
Silica, amorphous (diatomaceous earth, precipitated and gel silica): Possesses little or no potential to cause silicosis. Most sources of amorphous silica contain quartz. If greater than 1% quartz is present, the quartz hazard must be addressed. When strongly heated (calcined) with limestone, diatomaceous earth becomes crystalline and can cause silicosis (see below).	10 mg/m^3	6 mg/m^3	...	...	White to gray powders. Odorless with a negligible vapor pressure. The TLV for dusts is 10 mg/m^3 if no asbestos and less than 1% quartz are present.

Substance			NFPA	Description
Silica, crystalline (quartz); fused amorphous silica; cristobolite; tridymite; tripoli [CAS: 14464-46-1]: Inhalation of dusts causes silicosis, a progressive, fibrotic scarring of the lung that can cause death by impairing lung function. Individuals with silicosis are much more susceptible to tuberculosis. Some forms of crystalline silica are carcinogenic. See p 497.	0.1 mg/m³ (quartz, fused silica, tripoli) 0.05 mg/m³ (cristobolite, tridymite)	0.1 mg/m³ (quartz, fused silica, tripoli) 0.05 mg/m³ (cristobolite, tridymite)	...	Colorless, odorless solid with a negligible vapor pressure. A component of many mineral dusts.
Silicon [CAS: 7440-21-3]: A biologically inert dust not causing silicosis or pulmonary fibrosis.	10 mg/m³	10 mg/m³ (total dust) 5 mg/m³ (respirable fraction)	1 4 2	Gray to black, lustrous needlelike crystals. Vapor pressure is negligible at 20 °C (68 °F).
Silicon tetrachloride [CAS: 10026-04-7]: Generates hydrochloric acid upon contact with moisture; severe burns may result. Extremely irritating to eyes and respiratory tract; pulmonary edema may result. See p 163.	...	...	...	Not combustible.
Silver [CAS: 7440-22-4]: Silver compounds cause argyria, a blue-gray discoloration of tissues, which may be generalized throughout the viscera or localized to the conjunctiva, nasal septum, and gums. Silver nitrate is corrosive upon direct contact with tissues.	0.01 mg/m³ (soluble compounds as Ag) 0.1 mg/m³ (metal)	0.01 mg/m³	...	Compounds vary in appearance. Silver nitrate is a strong oxidizer.
Sodium azide (hydrazoic acid, sodium salt; NaN₃ [CAS: 26628-22-8]: Potent cellular toxin; inhibits cytochrome oxidase in mitochondria. Eye irritation, bronchitis, headache, hypotension, and collapse have been reported in overexposed workers.	0.1 ppm (C)	0.3 ppm (C)	...	White, odorless, crystalline solid.

(C) = ceiling air concentration (TLV-C); S = skin absorption can be significant; A1 = ACGIH-confirmed human carcinogen; A2 = ACGIH-suspected human carcinogen; NFPA Hazard Codes: H = health, F = fire, R = reactivity, OX = oxidizer, W = water-reactive, 0 (none) < — > 4 (severe). See expanded definitions on p 365.

continued

TABLE IV-12. HEALTH HAZARD SUMMARIES FOR INDUSTRIAL AND OCCUPATIONAL CHEMICALS (Continued)

Health Hazard Summaries	ACGIH TLV	PEL	IDLH	NFPA Codes H F R	Comments
Sodium bisulfide (NaSH [CAS: 16721-80-5]): Decomposes in the presence of water to form hydrogen sulfide and sodium hydroxide. Highly corrosive and irritating to eyes, skin, and respiratory tract. See p 169.	...	...	...	...	White crystalline substance with a slight odor of sulfur dioxide.
Sodium bisulfite (sodium hydrogen sulfite, NaHSO₃ [CAS: 7631-90-5]): Irritating to eyes, skin, and respiratory tract. Hypersensitivity reactions (angioedema, bronchospasm, or anaphylaxis) are more frequent in asthmatics.	5 mg/m³	5 mg/m³	...	...	White crystalline solid with a slight sulfur dioxide odor and disagreeable taste.
Sodium fluoroacetate (compound 1080 [CAS: 62-74-8]): A highly toxic metabolic poison. Metabolized to fluorocitrate, which prevents the oxidation of acetate in the Krebs cycle. Human lethal oral dose ranges from 2 to 10 mg/kg. See p 155.	0.05 mg/m³ S	0.05 mg/m³ S	5 mg/m³	...	Fluffy white solid or a fine white powder. Sometimes dyed black. Hygroscopic. Odorless. Vapor pressure is negligible at 20 °C (68 °F). Not combustible. Thermal breakdown products include hydrogen fluoride.
Sodium hydroxide (NaOH [CAS: 1310-73-2]): A caustic alkali; may cause severe burns. Fumes or mists are highly irritating to eyes, skin, and upper respiratory tract; pulmonary edema may result from very high exposures. See p 114.	2 mg/m³ (C)	2 mg/m³ (C)	200 mg/m³	3 0 1	White solid that absorbs moisture. Odorless. Evolves great heat upon solution in water. Soda lye is an aqueous solution.
Sodium metabisulfite (sodium pyrosulfite [CAS: 7681-57-4]): Very irritating to eyes and skin upon direct contact. Dusts irritating to eyes and respiratory tract; pulmonary edema may result. Hypersensitivity reactions more frequent in asthmatics. See p 275.	5 mg/m³	5 mg/m³	...	...	White powder or crystalline material with a slight odor of sulfur dioxide. Reacts to form sulfur dioxide in the presence of moisture.

Substance				NFPA	Comments
Stibine (antimony hydride) [CAS: 7803-52-3]: A potent hemolytic agent similar to arsine. Gases irritating to the lung; pulmonary edema may occur. Liver and kidney are secondary target organs. See p 74.	0.1 ppm	0.1 ppm	40 ppm	...	Colorless gas. Odor similar to that of hydrogen sulfide but may not be a reliable warning property. Formed when acid solutions of antimony are treated with zinc or strong reducing agents.
Stoddard solvent (mineral spirits, a mixture of aliphatic and aromatic hydrocarbons [CAS: 8052-41-3]: Defatting action may cause dermatitis. Dermal absorption can occur. Vapors irritating to eyes and respiratory tract. A CNS depressant. Chronic overexposures associated with headache, fatigue, bone marrow hypoplasia, and jaundice. May contain a small amount of benzene. See p 165.	100 ppm	100 ppm	5000 ppm	...	Colorless liquid. Kerosenelike odor and irritation are good warning properties. Vapor pressure is approximately 2 mm Hg at 20 °C (68 °F). Flammable.
Strychnine [CAS: 57-24-9]: Causes muscular hyperrigidity, opisthotonus, and muscle breakdown. See p 274.	0.15 mg/m³	0.15 mg/m³	3 mg/m³	...	White solid. Odorless. Vapor pressure is negligible at 20 °C (68 °F). Thermal breakdown products include oxides of nitrogen.
Styrene monomer (vinylbenzene [CAS: 100-42-5]: Irritating upon direct contact; defatting action may cause dermatitis. Dermal absorption occurs. Vapors irritating to upper respiratory tract. A CNS depressant. Symptoms include headache, nausea, dizziness, and fatigue. Limited evidence for adverse effects on fetal development in animals.	50 ppm S	50 ppm	5000 ppm	2 3 2	Colorless viscous liquid. Sweet aromatic odor at low concentrations is an adequate warning property. Odor at high levels is acrid. Vapor pressure is 4.5 mm Hg at 20 °C (68 °F). Flammable. Inhibitor must be included to avoid explosive polymerization.
Subtilisins (proteolytic enzymes of *Bacillus subtilis* [CAS: 1395-21-7]: Primary skin and respiratory tract irritants. Potent sensitizers causing primary bronchoconstriction and respiratory allergies.	0.06 µg/m³ (C)	0.06 µg/m³ (C)	...	...	Light-colored powder.

(C) = ceiling air concentration (TLV-C); S = skin absorption can be significant; A1 = ACGIH-confirmed human carcinogen; A2 = ACGIH-suspected human carcinogen; NFPA Hazard Codes: H = health, F = fire, R = reactivity, OX = oxidizer; W = water-reactive, 0 (none) < — > 4 (severe). See expanded definitions on p 365.

continued

TABLE IV-12. HEALTH HAZARD SUMMARIES FOR INDUSTRIAL AND OCCUPATIONAL CHEMICALS (Continued)

Health Hazard Summaries	ACGIH TLV	PEL	IDLH	NFPA Codes H F R	Comments
Sulfur dioxide (CAS: 7446-09-5): Forms sulfurous acid upon contact with moisture. Strongly irritating to eyes and skin; burns may result. Extremely irritating to the respiratory tract; fatal pulmonary edema has resulted. See p 275.	2 ppm	2 ppm	100 ppm	...	Colorless gas. Pungent, suffocating odor with a "taste" and irritative effects that are good warning properties.
Sulfur hexafluoride (CAS: 2551-62-4): Considered to be essentially a nontoxic gas. Asphyxiation by the displacement of air is suggested as the greatest hazard.	1000 ppm	1000 ppm	...	...	Odorless, colorless dense gas.
Sulfuric acid (oil of vitriol, H$_2$SO$_4$ (CAS: 7664-93-9): Highly corrosive upon direct contact; severe burns may result. Breakdown may release sulfur dioxide. Exposure to the mist can irritate the eyes, skin, and respiratory tract. Chronic exposures can cause permanent injury to the lungs and teeth. See p 114.	1 mg/m^3	1 mg/m^3	80 mg/m^3	3 0 2 W	Colorless to dark brown heavy, oily liquid. Odorless. Eye irritation may be an adequate warning property. A strong oxidizer. Addition of water creates strong exothermic reaction. Vapor pressure is less than 0.001 mm Hg at 20 °C (68 °F).
Sulfur monochloride (CAS: 10025-67-9): Forms hydrochloric acid and sulfur dioxide upon contact with water; direct contact can cause burns. Vapors highly irritating to the eyes, skin, and primarily the upper respiratory tract; inhalation of high air concentrations can cause pulmonary edema. See p 275.	1 ppm (C)	1 ppm (C)	10 ppm	2 1 1	Fuming, amber to red, oily liquid with a pungent, irritating, sickening odor. Eye irritation is a good warning property. Vapor pressure is 6.8 mm Hg at 20 °C (68 °F). Combustible. Breakdown products include hydrogen sulfide, hydrogen chloride, and sulfur dioxide.

Substance				Description
Sulfur pentafluoride (disulfur decafluoride) [CAS: 5714-22-7]: Vapors are extremely irritating to the lungs; causes pulmonary edema at low levels (0.5 ppm) in animals. See pp 167 and 275.	0.01 ppm	0.01 ppm (C)	1 ppm (C)	Colorless liquid or vapor with a sulfur dioxidelike odor. Vapor pressure is 561 mm Hg at 20 °C (68 °F). Not combustible. Thermal breakdown products include sulfur dioxide and hydrogen fluoride.
Sulfur tetrafluoride (SF₄, [CAS: 7783-60-0]: Readily hydrolyzed by moisture to form sulfur dioxide and hydrogen fluoride. Extremely irritating to the respiratory tract; pulmonary edema may occur. Vapors also highly irritating to eyes and skin.	0.1 ppm	0.1 ppm (C)	...	Colorless gas. Reacts with moisture to form sulfur dioxide and hydrogen fluoride.
Sulfuryl fluoride (Vikane, SO_2F_2 [CAS: 2699-79-8]: Irritating to eyes and respiratory tract; delayed, fatal pulmonary edema has resulted. Acute high exposure causes tremors, convulsions, coma, and pulmonary edema in animals; chronic exposures cause kidney and liver injury.	5 ppm	5 ppm	1000 ppm	Colorless, odorless gas with no warning properties. Chloropicrin, a lacrimator, is often added to provide a warning property. Thermal breakdown products include sulfur dioxide and hydrogen fluoride.
Sulprofos [O-ethyl O-(4-(methylthio)phenyl] S-propylphosphorodithioate [CAS: 35400-43-2]: An organophosphate anticholinesterase insecticide. See p 225.	1 mg/m³	1 mg/m³	...	Tan-colored liquid with a characteristic sulfide odor.
Tantalum compounds (as tantalum): Of low acute toxicity. Dusts mildly irritating to the lungs.	5 mg/m³ (metal and oxide)	5 mg/m³ (as Ta)	...	Metal is a gray-black solid—platinum-white if polished. Odorless. Tantalum pentoxide is a colorless solid.

(C) = ceiling air concentration (TLV-C); S = skin absorption can be significant; A1 = ACGIH-confirmed human carcinogen; A2 = ACGIH-suspected human carcinogen; NFPA Hazard Codes: H = health, F = fire, R = reactivity, OX = oxidizer, W = water-reactive, 0 (none) < — > 4 (severe). See expanded definitions on p 365.

continued

TABLE IV-12. HEALTH HAZARD SUMMARIES FOR INDUSTRIAL AND OCCUPATIONAL CHEMICALS (Continued)

Health Hazard Summaries	ACGIH TLV	PEL	IDLH	NFPA Codes H F R	Comments
Tellurium and compounds (as tellurium): Complaints of sleepiness, nausea, metallic taste, and garlicky odor on breath and perspiration associated with workplace exposures. Neuropathies have been noted in high-dose studies. Hydrogen telluride causes pulmonary irritation and hemolysis; however, its ready decomposition reduces likelihood of a toxic exposure. Some tellurium compounds are fetotoxic or teratogenic in animals.	0.1 mg/m³ (as Te)	0.1 mg/m³ (as Te)	…	…	Metallic tellurium is a solid with a silvery-white or grayish luster.
Tellurium hexafluoride (CAS: 7783-80-4): Slowly hydrolyzes to release hydrofluoric acid and telluric acid. Extremely irritating to the eyes and respiratory tract; pulmonary edema may occur. Has caused headaches, dyspnea, and garlicky odor on the breath of overexposed workers. See p 167.	0.02 ppm	0.02 ppm	1 ppm	…	Colorless gas. Offensive odor. Not combustible. Thermal breakdown products include hydrogen fluoride.
Temephos (Abate, *O,O,O',O'*-tetramethyl *O,O*-thiodi-*p*-phenylene phosphorothioate [CAS: 3383-96-8]): Primary irritant of eyes, skin, and respiratory tract; a moderately toxic organophosphate-type cholinesterase inhibitor. Well absorbed by all routes. See p 225.	10 mg/m³	10 mg/m³ (total dust) 5 mg/m³ (respirable fraction)	…	…	…
Terphenyls (diphenyl benzenes, triphenyls [CAS: 26140-60-3]): Irritating upon direct contact. Vapors and mists irritating to respiratory tract; pulmonary edema has occurred at very high levels in animals. Animal studies also suggest a slight potential for liver and kidney injury.	0.5 ppm (C)	0.5 ppm (C)	3500 mg/m³	0 1 0	White to light yellow crystalline solids. Irritation is a possible warning property. Vapor pressure is very low at 20 °C (68 °F). Combustible. Commercial grades are mixtures of *o-*, *m-*, *p*-isomers.

1,1,1,2-Tetrachloro-2,2-difluoroethane (halocarbon 112a; refrigerant 112a [CAS: 76-11-9]): Of low acute toxicity. Defatting action may cause dermatitis. Very high air levels irritating to the eyes and respiratory tract. A CNS depressant at high levels. May cause cardiac sensitization to the arrhythmogenic effects of epinephrine. High-dose studies in animals suggest possible kidney and liver injury. See p 161.	500 ppm	15,000 ppm	...	Colorless liquid or solid with a slight etherlike odor. Vapor pressure is 40 mm Hg at 20 °C (68 °F). Not combustible. Thermal breakdown products include hydrogen chloride and hydrogen fluoride.
1,1,2,2-Tetrachloro-1,2-difluoroethane (halocarbon 112; refrigerant 112 [CAS: 76-12-0]): Of low acute toxicity. Once used as an anthelmintic. Very high air levels cause CNS depression. Vapors mildly irritating. May cause cardiac sensitization to the arrhythmogenic effects of epinephrine. Defatting agent. See p 161.	500 ppm	15,000 ppm	...	Colorless liquid or solid with a slight etherlike odor. Odor is of unknown value as a warning property. Vapor pressure is 40 mm Hg at 20 °C (68 °F). Not combustible. Thermal breakdown products include hydrogen chloride and hydrogen fluoride.
1,1,2,2-Tetrachloroethane (acetylene tetrachloride [CAS: 79-34-5]): Defatting action may cause dermatitis. Dermal absorption may cause systemic toxicity. Vapors very irritating to the eyes and upper respiratory tract. A CNS depressant. May cause hepatic or renal injury. May sensitize the myocardium to arrhythmogenic effects of epinephrine. Limited evidence of carcinogenicity in animals. See pp 282 and 498.	1 ppm S	150 ppm NIOSH CA	...	Colorless to light yellow liquid. Sweet, suffocating, chloroformlike odor is a good warning property. Vapor pressure is 8 mm Hg at 20 °C (68 °F). Not combustible. Thermal breakdown products include hydrogen chloride and phosgene.
Tetrachloroethylene (perchloroethylene [CAS: 127-18-4]): Irritating upon prolonged contact; mild burns may result. Vapors irritating to eyes and respiratory tract. A CNS depressant. May sensitize the myocardium to arrhythmogenic effects of epinephrine. Chronic overexposure may cause short-term memory loss and personality changes, liver and kidney injury. Limited evidence for carcinogenicity in animals. See pp 282 and 498.	25 ppm	50 ppm	500 ppm NIOSH CA	2 0 0	Colorless liquid. Chloroformlike or etherlike odor and eye irritation are adequate warning properties. Vapor pressure is 14 mm Hg at 20 °C (68 °F). Not combustible. Thermal breakdown products include phosgene and hydrochloric acid.

(C) = ceiling air concentration (TLV-C); S = skin absorption can be significant; A1 = ACGIH-confirmed human carcinogen; A2 = ACGIH-suspected human carcinogen; NFPA Hazard Codes: H = health, F = fire, R = reactivity, OX = oxidizer, W = water-reactive, 0 (none) < — > 4 (severe). See expanded definitions on p 365.

continued

TABLE IV-12. HEALTH HAZARD SUMMARIES FOR INDUSTRIAL AND OCCUPATIONAL CHEMICALS (Continued)

Health Hazard Summaries	ACGIH TLV	PEL	IDLH	NFPA Codes H F R	Comments
Tetrachloronaphthalene (Halowax [CAS: 1335-88-2]): Causes chloracne and jaundice. Stored in body fat. Dermal absorption occurs.	2 mg/m³	2 mg/m³ S	20 mg/m³	...	White to light yellow solid. Aromatic odor of unknown value as a warning property. Vapor pressure is less than 1 mm Hg at 20 °C (68 °F). Thermal breakdown products include hydrogen chloride and phosgene.
Tetraethyl-di-thionopyrophosphate (TEDP, sulfotepp [CAS: 3689-24-5]): An organophosphate anticholinesterase insecticide. Well absorbed dermally. See p 225.	...	...	35 mg/m³	...	Yellow liquid with garlic odor. Not combustible. Thermal breakdown products include sulfur dioxide and phosphoric acid mist.
Tetraethyl lead (CAS: 78-00-2): A potent CNS toxin. Dermally well absorbed. Can cause psychosis, mania, convulsions, and coma. Unlike the case with inorganic lead poisoning, red blood cells are not affected. Reports of reduced sperm counts and impotence in overexposed workers. See p 184.	0.1 mg/m³ (as Pb) S	0.075 mg/m³ (as Pb) S	40 mg/m³ (as Pb)	3 3 3	Colorless liquid. May be dyed blue, red, or orange. Slight musty odor of unknown value as a warning property. Vapor pressure is 0.2 mm Hg at 20 °C (68 °F). Combustible. Decomposes in light.
Tetraethyl pyrophosphate (TEPP [CAS: 107-49-3]): A potent organophosphate cholinesterase inhibitor. Rapidly absorbed through skin. See p 225.	0.004 ppm S	...	10 mg/m³	...	Colorless to amber liquid with a faint fruity odor. Slowly hydrolyzed in water. Vapor pressure is 1 mm Hg at 140 °C (284 °F). Not combustible. Thermal breakdown products include phosphoric acid mist.

Chemical				NFPA (H F R)	Comments
Tetrahydrofuran (THF, diethylene oxide) [CAS: 109-99-9]: Defatting action causes dermatitis. Mildly irritating upon direct contact. Vapors mildly irritating to eyes and upper respiratory tract. A CNS depressant at high levels. A liver and kidney toxin at high doses in animals.	200 ppm	200 ppm	20,000 ppm	2 3 1	Colorless liquid. The etherlike odor detectable well below the PEL provides a good warning property. Flammable. Vapor pressure is 145 mm Hg at 20 °C (68 °F).
Tetramethyl lead [CAS: 75-74-1]: A potent CNS toxin thought to be similar to tetraethyl lead. See p 184.	0.15 mg/m³ (as Pb) S	0.075 mg/m³ (as Pb) S	40 mg/m³ (as Pb)	3 3 3	Colorless liquid. May be dyed red, orange, or blue. Slight musty odor is of unknown value as a warning property. Vapor pressure is 22 mm Hg at 20 °C (68 °F).
Tetramethyl succinonitrile [CAS: 3333-52-6]: A potent convulsant. Headaches, nausea, dizziness, convulsions, and coma have occurred in overexposed workers.	0.5 ppm S	0.5 ppm S	5 ppm	…	Colorless, odorless solid. Thermal breakdown products include oxides of nitrogen.
Tetranitromethane [CAS: 509-14-8]: Highly irritating upon direct contact; mild burns may result. Vapors extremely irritating to eyes and respiratory tract; pulmonary edema has been reported. Causes methemoglobinemia (see p 204). Liver, kidney, and CNS injury in animals at high doses. Overexposure associated with headaches, fatigue, dyspnea. See p 216.	1 ppm	1 ppm	5 ppm	…	Colorless to light yellow liquid or solid with a pungent, acrid odor. Irritative effects are a good warning property. Vapor pressure is 8.4 mm Hg at 20 °C (68 °F). Not combustible. A weak explosive and oxidizer. Highly explosive in the presence of impurities.
Tetrasodium pyrophosphate [CAS: 7722-88-5]: Alkaline; dusts are mild irritants of eyes, skin, and upper respiratory tract.	5 mg/m³	5 mg/m³	…	…	White powder. Alkaline in aqueous solution.
Tetryl (2,4,6-trinitrophenylmethylnitramine [CAS: 479-45-8]): Causes severe sensitization dermatitis. Dusts extremely irritating to the eyes and upper respiratory tract. Stains tissues bright yellow. May injure the liver and kidneys. Overexposures also associated with malaise, headache, nausea, and vomiting.	1.5 mg/m³	0.1 mg/m³ S	…	…	White to yellow solid. Odorless. A strong oxidizer. Vapor pressure is much less than 1 mm Hg at 20 °C (68 °F). Explosive used in detonators and primers.

(C) = ceiling air concentration (TLV-C); S = skin absorption can be significant; A1 = ACGIH-confirmed human carcinogen; A2 = ACGIH-suspected human carcinogen; NFPA Hazard Codes: H = health, F = fire, R = reactivity, OX = oxidizer, W = water-reactive, 0 (none) < — > 4 (severe). See expanded definitions on p 365.

continued

TABLE IV-12. HEALTH HAZARD SUMMARIES FOR INDUSTRIAL AND OCCUPATIONAL CHEMICALS (Continued)

Health Hazard Summaries	ACGIH TLV	PEL	IDLH	NFPA Codes H F R	Comments
Thallium, soluble compounds (thallium sulfate, thallium acetate, thallium nitrate): A potent toxin causing diverse chronic effects, including psychosis, peripheral neuropathy, abdominal pain, irritability, and weight loss. Liver and kidney injury may occur. Ingestion causes severe hemorrhagic gastroenteritis. Absorption possible by all routes. See p 276.	0.1 mg/m³ (as Tl) S	0.1 mg/m³ (as Tl) S	20 mg/m³ (as Tl)	...	Appearance varies with the compound. The elemental form is a bluish-white, ductile heavy metal with a negligible vapor pressure.
Thioglycolic acid (mercaptoacetic acid [CAS: 68-11-1]): Skin or eye contact with concentrated acid causes severe burns. Vapors irritating to eyes and respiratory tract.	1 ppm S	1 ppm S	...	...	Colorless liquid. Unpleasant mercaptanlike odor. Vapor pressure is 10 mm Hg at 18 °C (64 °F).
Thiram (tetramethylthiuram disulfide [CAS: 137-26-8]): Dusts mildly irritating to eyes, skin, and upper respiratory tract. A moderate allergen and a potent skin sensitizer. Has disulfiramlike effects in exposed persons who consume alcohol (see p 143). A goitrogen. Adverse effects on fetal development in animals.	1 mg/m³	5 mg/m³	1500 mg/m³	...	White to yellow powder with a characteristic odor. May be dyed blue. Vapor pressure is negligible at 20 °C (68 °F). Thermal breakdown products include sulfur dioxide and carbon disulfide.
Tin, metal and inorganic compounds: Dusts irritating to the eyes, nose, throat, and skin. Prolonged inhalation may cause a benign pneumoconiosis. Some compounds react with water to form acids (tin tetrachloride, stannous chloride, and stannous sulfate) or bases (sodium and potassium stannate).	2 mg/m³ (as Sn)	2 mg/m³ (as Sn)	400 mg/m³ (as Sn)	...	Metallic tin is odorless with a dull, silvery color.

Chemical	TLV	PEL	IDLH	H	F	R	Comments
Tin, organic compounds: Highly irritating upon direct contact; burns may result. Dusts, fumes, or vapors highly irritating to the eyes and upper respiratory tract. Triethyltin is a potent neurotoxin; triphenyltin acetate is highly hepatotoxic. Trialkyltins are the most toxic, followed in order by the dialkyltins and monoalkyltins. Within each of these classes, the ethyltin compounds are the most toxic. All are well absorbed dermally.	0.1 mg/m³ (as Sn) S	0.1 mg/m³ (as Sn)	200 mg/m³ (as Sn)				There are many kinds of organotin compounds: mono-, di-, tri-, and tetra-alkyltin and -aryltin compounds exist. Combustible.
Titanium dioxide (CAS: 13463-67-7): A mild pulmonary irritant. Chronic heavy overexposures have been associated with mild pulmonary fibrosis.	10 mg/m³	10 mg/m³ (total dust) 5 mg/m³ (respirable fraction)	...				White odorless powder. Rutile is a common crystalline form. Vapor pressure is negligible.
Tolidine (o-tolidine, 3,3'-dimethylbenzidine [CAS: 119-93-7]): A carcinogen in animals. See p 499.	S, A2	...	NIOSH CA	3	2	0	White to reddish solid. Oxides of nitrogen are among thermal breakdown products.
Toluene (toluol, methylbenzene [CAS: 108-88-3]): Defatting action may cause dermatitis. Vapors mildly irritating to eyes and upper respiratory tract. A CNS depressant. May sensitize the myocardium to the arrhythmogenic effects of epinephrine. Abusive sniffing during pregnancy associated with birth defects. See p 281.	100 ppm	100 ppm	2000 ppm	2	3	0	Colorless liquid. Aromatic, benzenelike odor detectable at very low levels. Irritation serves as a good warning property. Vapor pressure is 22 mm Hg at 20 °C (68 °F). Flammable.
Toluene 2,4-diisocyanate (CAS: 584-84-9): A potent respiratory tract sensitizer and potent irritant of the eyes, skin, and respiratory tract. Pulmonary edema has resulted. A carcinogen in animals. See pp 179 and 499.	0.005 ppm	0.005 ppm	10 ppm	3	1	1	Colorless needles or a liquid with a sharp, pungent odor. Vapor pressure is approximately 0.04 mm Hg at 20 °C (68 °F). Combustible.

(C) = ceiling air concentration (TLV-C); S = skin absorption can be significant; A1 = ACGIH-confirmed human carcinogen; A2 = ACGIH-suspected human carcinogen; NFPA Hazard Codes: H = health, F = fire, R = reactivity, OX = oxidizer, W = water-reactive, 0 (none) < — > 4 (severe). See expanded definitions on p 365.

continued

TABLE IV-12. HEALTH HAZARD SUMMARIES FOR INDUSTRIAL AND OCCUPATIONAL CHEMICALS (Continued)

Health Hazard Summaries	ACGIH TLV	PEL	IDLH	NFPA Codes H F R	Comments
o-Toluidine (2-methylaniline [CAS: 95-53-4]): A corrosive alkali; can cause severe burns. Causes methemoglobinemia. Dermal absorption occurs. A carcinogen in animals. See pp 204 and 499.	2 ppm S, A2	5 ppm S	100 ppm	3 2 0	Colorless to pale yellow liquid. The weak aromatic odor is thought to be a good warning property. Vapor pressure is less than 1 mm Hg at 20 °C (68 °F).
m-Toluidine (3-methylaniline [CAS: 108-44-1]): A corrosive alkali; can cause severe burns. Causes methemoglobinemia. Dermal absorption occurs. See p 204.	2 ppm S	2 ppm S	...	...	Pale yellow liquid. Vapor pressure is less than 1 mm Hg at 20 °C (68 °F).
p-Toluidine (4-methylaniline [CAS: 106-49-0]): A corrosive alkali; can cause severe burns. Causes methemoglobinemia. Dermal exposure occurs. A carcinogen in animals. See pp 204 and 499.	2 ppm S, A2	2 ppm S	...	...	White solid. Vapor pressure is 1 mm Hg at 20 °C (68 °F).
Tributyl phosphate (CAS: 126-73-8): Highly irritating upon direct contact; causes severe eye injury and skin irritation. Vapors or mists irritating to the eyes and respiratory tract; high exposure in animals caused pulmonary edema. Weak anticholinesterase activity. Headache and nausea are reported.	0.2 ppm	0.2 ppm	1300 mg/m³	2 1 0	Colorless to pale yellow liquid. Odorless. Vapor pressure is very low at 20 °C (68 °F). Combustible. Thermal breakdown products include phosphoric acid fume.
Trichloroacetic acid (CAS: 76-03-9): A strong acid. A protein denaturant. Corrosive to eyes and skin upon direct contact.	1 ppm	1 ppm	...	...	Deliquescent crystalline solid. Vapor pressure is 1 mm Hg at 51 °C (128.3 °F). Thermal breakdown products include hydrochloric acid and phosgene.

Chemical			NFPA (H F R)	Description
1,2,4-Trichlorobenzene (CAS: 120–82–1): Prolonged or repeated contact can cause skin and eye irritation. Vapors irritating to the eyes, skin, and respiratory tract. High-dose animal exposures injure the liver, kidney, lung, and CNS. Does not cause chloracne.	5 ppm (C)	5 ppm (C)	2 1 0	A colorless liquid with an unpleasant, mothball-like odor. Vapor pressure is 1 mm Hg at 38.4 °C (101.1 °F). Combustible. Thermal breakdown products include hydrogen chloride and phosgene.
1,1,1-Trichloroethane (methyl chloroform, TCA [CAS: 71–55–6]): Defatting action may cause dermatitis. Vapors mildly irritating to eyes and respiratory tract. A CNS depressant. May sensitize the heart to the arrhythmogenic effects of epinephrine. Some dermal absorption occurs. Liver and kidney injury may occur. See p 282.	350 ppm	350 ppm	1000 ppm	3 1 1	Colorless liquid. Vapor pressure is 100 mm Hg at 20 °C (68 °F). Not combustible. Thermal breakdown products include hydrogen chloride and phosgene.
1,1,2-Trichloroethane (CAS: 79–00–5): Defatting action may cause dermatitis. Dermal absorption may occur. Vapors mildly irritating to eyes and respiratory tract. A CNS depressant. May sensitize the heart to the arrhythmogenic effects of epinephrine. Causes liver and kidney injury in animals. A carcinogen in animals. See p 282.	10 ppm S	10 ppm S	500 ppm NIOSH CA	...	Colorless liquid. Sweet, chloroformlike odor is of unknown value as a warning property. Vapor pressure is 19 mm Hg at 20 °C (68 °F). Not combustible. Thermal breakdown products include phosgene and hydrochloric acid.
Trichloroethylene (trichloroethene, TCE [CAS: 79–01–6]): Defatting action may cause dermatitis. Dermal absorption may occur. Vapors mildly irritating to eyes and respiratory tract. A CNS depressant. May rarely cause cranial and peripheral neuropathies. May damage the liver. Has a disulfiramlike effect (see p 143). Reported to cause liver and lung cancers in mice. See pp 282 and 499.	50 ppm	50 ppm	1000 ppm NIOSH CA	2 1 0	Colorless liquid. Sweet chloroformlike odor. Vapor pressure is 58 mm Hg at 20 °C (68 °F). Not combustible at room temperatures. Decomposition products include hydrogen chloride and phosgene.

(C) = ceiling air concentration (TLV-C); S = skin absorption can be significant; A1 = ACGIH-confirmed human carcinogen; A2 = ACGIH-suspected human carcinogen; NFPA Hazard Codes: H = health, F = fire, R = reactivity, OX = oxidizer, W = water-reactive, 0 (none) <–> 4 (severe). See expanded definitions on p 365.

continued

TABLE IV-12. HEALTH HAZARD SUMMARIES FOR INDUSTRIAL AND OCCUPATIONAL CHEMICALS (Continued)

Health Hazard Summaries	ACGIH TLV	PEL	IDLH	NFPA Codes H F R	Comments
Trichlorofluoromethane (Freon 11 [CAS: 75-69-4]): Vapors mildly irritating to eyes and respiratory tract. A CNS depressant. Very high air levels may sensitize the heart to the arrhythmogenic effects of epinephrine. See p 161.	1000 ppm (C)	...	10,000 ppm	...	Colorless liquid or gas at room temperature. Vapor pressure is 690 mm Hg at 20 °C (68 °F). Not combustible. Thermal breakdown products include hydrogen chloride and hydrogen fluoride.
Trichloronaphthalene (Halowax [CAS: 1321-65-9]): Causes chloracne. A hepatotoxin at low doses, causing jaundice. Stored in body fat. Systemic toxicity may occur following dermal exposure.	5 mg/m³ S	5 mg/m³ S	50 mg/m³	...	Colorless to pale yellow solid with an aromatic odor of uncertain value as a warning property. Vapor pressure is less than 1 mm Hg at 20 °C (68 °F). Flammable. Decomposition products include phosgene and hydrogen chloride.
2,4,5-Trichlorophenoxyacetic acid (2,4,5-T [CAS: 93-76-5]): Moderately irritating to eyes, skin, and respiratory tract. Ingestion can cause gastroenteritis and injury to the CNS, muscle, kidney, and liver. A weak uncoupler of oxidative phosphorylation. Polychlorinated dibenzodioxin compounds are contaminants (see p 142). There are reports of sarcomas occurring in applicators. See p 121.	10 mg/m³	10 mg/m³	5000 mg/m³	...	Colorless to tan solid. Appearance and some hazardous properties vary with the formulation. Odorless. Vapor pressure is negligible at 20 °C (68 °F). Not combustible. Thermal breakdown products include hydrogen chloride and dioxins.
1,1,2-Trichloro-1,2,2-trifluoroethane (Freon 113): Rapid evaporation from skin may cause frostbite. Vapors mildly irritating to eyes and mucous membranes. Very high air levels cause CNS depression and may injure the liver. Sensitizes the myocardium to the arrhythmogenic effects of epinephrine at air concentrations as low as 2000 ppm in animals. See p 161.	1000 ppm	1000 ppm	4500 ppm	...	Colorless liquid. Sweetish, chloroformlike odor occurs only at very high concentrations and is a poor warning property. Vapor pressure is 284 mm Hg at 20 °C (68 °F). Not combustible. Thermal breakdown products include hydrogen chloride, hydrogen fluoride, and phosgene.

Triethylamine (CAS: 121-44-8): An alkaline corrosive; highly irritating to eyes and skin; severe burns may occur. Vapors very irritating to eyes and respiratory tract; pulmonary edema may occur. High doses in animals cause heart, liver, and kidney injury. CNS stimulation possibly due to inhibition of monoamine oxidase.

| | 10 ppm | 10 ppm | 1000 ppm | 2 3 0 | Colorless liquid with a fishy, ammonialike odor of unknown value as a warning property. Vapor pressure is 54 mm Hg at 20 °C (68 °F). Flammable. |

Trifluorobromomethane (Halon 1301; Freon 13B1 [CAS: 75-63-8]): Extremely high air levels cause CNS depression and may sensitize the myocardium to the arrhythmogenic effects of epinephrine. See p 161.

| | 1000 ppm | 1000 ppm | 50,000 ppm | ... | Colorless gas with a weak etherlike odor at high levels and poor warning properties. Not combustible. |

Trifluoromethane (Freon 23 [CAS: 75-46-7]): Rapid evaporation from skin may cause frostbite. Vapors mildly irritating to the eyes and mucous membranes. Very high air levels cause CNS depression and may sensitize the heart to the arrhythmogenic effects of epinephrine. See p 161.

| | ... | ... | ... | ... | Not combustible. |

Trimellitic anhydride (TMAN [CAS: 552-30-7]): Dusts and vapors extremely irritating to eyes, nose, throat, and skin. Extremely severe pulmonary irritant and sensitizer.

| | 0.005 ppm | 0.005 ppm | ... | ... | Colorless solid. Hydrolyzes to trimellitic acid in aqueous solutions. Vapor pressure is 0.000004 mm Hg at 25 °C (77 °F). |

Trimethylamine (CAS: 75-50-3): An alkaline corrosive; highly irritating upon direct contact; severe burns may occur. Vapors very irritating to respiratory tract; pulmonary edema may occur.

| | 10 ppm | 10 ppm | ... | 2 4 0 | Highly flammable gas with a pungent, fishy, ammonialike odor. May be used as a warning agent in natural gas. |

Trimethyl phosphite (phosphorous acid trimethylester [CAS: 121-45-9]): Very irritating upon direct contact; severe burns may result. Vapors highly irritating to respiratory tract. Cataracts have developed in animals exposed to high air levels.

| | 2 ppm | 2 ppm | ... | 0 2 0 | Colorless liquid with a characteristic, strong, fishy, or ammonialike odor. Hydrolyzed in water. Vapor pressure is 24 mm Hg at 25 °C (77 °F). Combustible. |

(C) = ceiling air concentration (TLV-C); S = skin absorption can be significant; A1 = ACGIH-confirmed human carcinogen; A2 = ACGIH-suspected human carcinogen; NFPA Hazard Codes: H = health, F = fire, R = reactivity, OX = oxidizer, W = water-reactive, 0 (none) <—> 4 (severe). See expanded definitions on p 365.

continued

TABLE IV-12. HEALTH HAZARD SUMMARIES FOR INDUSTRIAL AND OCCUPATIONAL CHEMICALS (Continued)

Health Hazard Summaries	ACGIH TLV	PEL	IDLH	NFPA Codes H F R	Comments
Trinitrotoluene (2,4,6-trinitrotoluene, TNT [CAS: 118-96-7]): Irritating upon direct contact. Stains tissues yellow. Causes sensitization dermatitis. Vapors irritating to the upper respiratory tract. May cause liver injury, methemoglobinemia, and aplastic anemia. Occupational overexposure associated with cataracts.	0.5 mg/m³ S	0.5 mg/m³ S	...	2 4 4	White to light yellow crystalline solid. Odorless. Vapor pressure is 0.05 mm Hg at 85 °C (185 °F). Explosive upon heating or shock.
Triorthocresyl phosphate (TOCP [CAS: 78-30-8]): Potent neurotoxin causing delayed, partially reversible peripheral neuropathy by all routes. Inhibits acetylcholinesterase. See p 225.	0.1 mg/m³ S	0.1 mg/m³ S	40 mg/m³	...	Colorless viscous liquid. Odorless. Not combustible.
Triphenyl phosphate [CAS: 115-86-6]: Weak anticholinesterase activity in humans. Delayed neuropathy reported in animals.	3 mg/m³	3 mg/m³	...	2 1 0	Colorless solid. Faint phenolic odor. Not combustible. Thermal breakdown products include phosphoric acid fumes.
Tungsten and compounds: Few reports of human toxicity. Some salts may release acid upon contact with moisture. Chronic exposure to tungsten carbide in the hard-metals industry may be associated with fibrotic lung disease.	5 mg/m³ (insoluble compounds) 1 mg/m³ (soluble compounds)	5 mg/m³ 1 mg/m³	...	...	Elemental tungsten is a gray, hard, brittle metal. Finely divided powders are flammable.
Turpentine [CAS: 8006-64-2]: Irritating to eyes upon direct contact. Defatting action may cause dermatitis; dermal sensitizer. Dermal absorption occurs. Vapors irritating to upper respiratory tract. A CNS depressant at high air levels. See p 165.	100 ppm	100 ppm	1900 ppm	1 3 0	Colorless to pale yellow liquid with a characteristic paintlike odor that serves as a good warning property. Vapor pressure is 5 mm Hg at 20 °C (68 °F). Flammable.

Substance and health effects				H	F	R	Physical description
Uranium compounds: Many salts are irritating to the respiratory tract; soluble salts can cause injury to the kidneys. Uranium is a weakly radioactive element (alpha emitter); decays to the radionuclide, thorium 230. Uranium has the potential to cause radiation injury to the lungs, tracheobronchial lymph nodes, bone marrow, and skin.	0.2 mg/m³ (insoluble compounds, as U) 0.2 mg/m³ (soluble compounds, as U)	0.2 mg/m³ 0.05 mg/m³	30 mg/m³ 20 mg/m₃	…			Dense, silvery-white, lustrous metal. Finely divided powders are pyrophoric. Radioactive.
Valeraldehyde (pentanal) [CAS: 110-62-3]: Very irritating to eyes and skin; severe burns may result. Vapors highly irritating to the eyes and respiratory tract.	50 ppm	50 ppm	…	1	3	0	Colorless liquid with a fruity odor. Flammable.
Vanadium pentoxide (CAS: 1314-62-1): Dusts or fumes highly irritating to eyes, skin, and respiratory tract. Sensitization dermatitis reported. Tracheobronchitis, emphysema, and pulmonary edema may occur. Low-level exposure may cause a greenish discoloration of the tongue, metallic taste, and cough.	0.05 mg/m³	0.05 mg/m³ (C) (as V)	70 mg/m³ (as V)	…			Yellow-orange to rust-brown crystalline powder or dark gray flakes. Odorless. Not combustible.
Vinyl acetate (CAS: 108-05-4): Highly irritating upon direct contact; severe skin and eye burns may result. Vapors irritating to the eyes and respiratory tract. Mild CNS depressant at high levels.	10 ppm	10 ppm	…	2	3	2	Volatile liquid with a pleasant fruity odor at low levels. Vapor pressure is 115 mm Hg at 25 °C (77 °F). Flammable. Polymerizes readily. Must contain inhibitor to prevent polymerization.
Vinyl bromide (CAS: 593-60-2): At high air levels, an eye and respiratory tract irritant and CNS depressant; a kidney and liver toxin. Animal carcinogen. See p 500.	5 ppm A2	5 ppm	NIOSH CA	2	0	1	Colorless, highly flammable gas with a distinctive odor.

(C) = ceiling air concentration (TLV-C); S = skin absorption can be significant; A1 = ACGIH-confirmed human carcinogen; A2 = ACGIH-suspected human carcinogen; NFPA Hazard Codes: H = health, F = fire, R = reactivity, OX = oxidizer, W = water-reactive, 0 (none) < — > 4 (severe). See expanded definitions on p 365.

continued

TABLE IV-12. HEALTH HAZARD SUMMARIES FOR INDUSTRIAL AND OCCUPATIONAL CHEMICALS (Continued)

Health Hazard Summaries	ACGIH TLV	PEL	IDLH	NFPA Codes H F R	Comments
Vinyl chloride (CAS: 75-01-4): An eye and respiratory tract irritant at high air levels. Degeneration of distal phalanges with Raynaud's disease and scleroderma, thrombocytopenia, and liver injury have each been associated with workplace overexposures. A CNS depressant at high levels. May sensitize myocardium to the arrhythmogenic effects of epinephrine. Causes angiosarcoma of the liver in humans. See p 500.	5 ppm A1	...	NIOSH CA	2 4 1	Colorless, highly flammable gas with a sweet etherlike odor. Polymerizes readily.
Vinyl cyclohexene dioxide (vinylhexane dioxide [CAS: 106-87-6]): Moderately irritating upon direct contact; severe burns may result. Vapors highly irritating to eyes and respiratory tract. Testicular atrophy, leukemia, and necrosis of the thymus in animals. Topical application causes skin cancer in animals. See p 500.	10 ppm S, A2	10 ppm S	...	...	Colorless liquid. Vapor pressure is 0.1 mm Hg at 20 °C (68 °F).
Vinyl toluene (methylstyrene [CAS: 25013-15-4]): Defatting action may cause dermatitis. Vapors irritating to eyes and upper respiratory tract. A CNS depressant at high levels. Hepatic, renal, and hematologic toxicities observed at high doses in animals.	50 ppm	100 ppm	5000 ppm	2 2 1	Colorless liquid. Strong, unpleasant odor is considered to be an adequate warning property. Vapor pressure is 1.1 mm Hg at 20 °C (68 °F). Flammable. Inhibitor added to prevent explosive polymerization.
VM&P naphtha (varnish makers' and printers' naphtha; ligroin [CAS: 8030-30-6]): Defatting action may cause dermatitis. Vapors irritating to eyes and respiratory tract. A CNS depressant at high levels. May contain a small amount of benzene.	300 ppm	300 ppm	...	...	Colorless volatile liquid.

Warfarin (CAS: 81-81-2): An anticoagulant. Medicinal dosages associated with adverse effects on fetal development in animals and humans. See p 132.	0.1 mg/m³	0.1 mg/m³	…	Colorless crystalline substance. Odorless.
Xylene (mixture of *o*-, *m*-, *p*-dimethylbenzenes [CAS: 1330-20-7]): Defatting action may cause dermatitis. Vapors irritating to eyes and primarily the upper respiratory tract. A CNS depressant at high levels. May injure kidneys. See p 281.	100 ppm	10,000 ppm	2 3 0	Colorless liquid or solid. Weak, somewhat sweet, aromatic odor. Irritant effects are adequate warning properties. Vapor pressure is approximately 8 mm Hg at 20 °C (68 °F). Flammable.
Xylidine (dimethylaniline [CAS: 1300-73-8]): Causes methemoglobinemia of possible insidious onset. Dermal absorption may occur. Liver and kidney damage seen in animals. See p 204.	2 ppm S	150 ppm	3 1 0	Pale yellow to brown liquid. Weak, aromatic amine odor is an adequate warning property. Vapor pressure is less than 1 mm Hg at 20 °C (68 °F). Combustible. Thermal breakdown products include oxides of nitrogen. TLV under review.
Yttrium and compounds (yttrium metal; yttrium nitrate hexahydrate; yttrium chloride; yttrium oxide): Dusts irritating to the eyes and respiratory tract.	1 mg/m³ (as Y)	…	…	Appearance varies with compound.
Zinc chloride (CAS: 7646-85-7): Caustic and highly irritating upon direct contact; severe burns may result. Ulceration of exposed skin from exposure to fumes has been reported. Fumes extremely irritating to respiratory tract; pulmonary edema has resulted.	1 mg/m³	2000 mg/m³	…	White powder or colorless crystals that absorb moisture. The fume is white and has an acrid odor.
Zinc chromates (basic zinc chromate, ZnCrO₄; zinc potassium chromate, KZn₂(CrO₄)2(OH); zinc yellow): Found in a number of studies to cause lung cancer in workers. See pp 124 and 500.	0.01 mg/m³ (as Cr) A1	0.1 mg/m³ (C)	…	Basic zinc chromate is a yellow pigment; dichromates are orange.

(C) = ceiling air concentration (TLV-C); S = skin absorption can be significant; A1 = ACGIH-confirmed human carcinogen; A2 = ACGIH-suspected human carcinogen; NFPA Hazard Codes: H = health, F = fire, R = reactivity, OX = oxidizer, W = water-reactive, 0 (none) <—> 4 (severe). See expanded definitions on p 365.

continued

TABLE IV-12. HEALTH HAZARD SUMMARIES FOR INDUSTRIAL AND OCCUPATIONAL CHEMICALS (Continued)

Health Hazard Summaries	ACGIH TLV	PEL	IDLH	NFPA Codes H F R	Comments
Zinc oxide (CAS: 1314-13-2): Fumes irritating to the upper respiratory tract. Causes metal fume fever. Symptoms include headache, fever, chills, muscle aches, and vomiting. See p 201.	5 mg/m³ (fume) 10 mg/m³ (dusts)	5 mg/m³	…	…	A white or yellowish-white powder. Fumes of zinc oxide are formed when elemental zinc is heated.
Zirconium compounds (zirconium oxide, ZrO₂; zirconium oxychloride, ZrOCl; zirconium tetrachloride, ZrCL₄): Zirconium compounds are of generally low toxicity. Some compounds are irritating; zirconium tetrachloride releases HCl upon contact with moisture. Granulomata due to the use of deodorants containing zirconium have been observed. Dermal sensitization has not been reported.	5 mg/m³ (as Zr)	5 mg/m³	500 mg/m³	…	The elemental form is a bluish-black powder or a grayish-white, lustrous metal. The finely divided powder can be flammable.

(C) = ceiling air concentration (TLV-C); S = skin absorption can be significant; A1 = ACGIH-confirmed human carcinogen; A2 = ACGIH-suspected human carcinogen; NFPA Hazard Codes: H = health, F = fire, R = reactivity, OX = oxidizer, W = water-reactive, 0 (none) <—> 4 (severe). See expanded definitions on p 365.

KNOWN OR SUSPECTED HUMAN CARCINOGENS

Georganne M. Backman and Frank J. Mycroft, PhD

I. General considerations

A. Although exposure to low levels of industrial carcinogens is unlikely to be the major cause of cancer in the general population, environmental and occupational exposures to carcinogens are important health hazards.

B. Asbestos, β-naphthylamine, coal tar products, benzene, chromium, benzidine, and vinyl chloride are examples of industrial carcinogens that have been found to cause an increased incidence of cancer in exposed workers.

C. This chapter provides a quick means of identifying known or suspected human carcinogens as evaluated by a number of authoritative agencies. However, the limitations of carcinogenic risk assessment must be considered when using Tables IV–13 and IV–14.

II. Problems with assessing the risks of exposure to carcinogens

A. The magnitude of the risk associated with exposure to carcinogens is often difficult to determine. The risk is dependent on many factors: the potency of the agent, the level and duration of exposure, genetic susceptibility, and life-style factors that alter individual sensitivities (eg, smoking and the risk of lung cancer from asbestos exposure).

B. Because there is a strong correlation between the ability of a substance to cause cancer in humans and its ability to cause cancer in test animals, it is reasonable to regard agents that are shown to be carcinogens in animals as if they present a cancer risk to humans. However, there is as yet no reliable means of determining the potency of a carcinogen for humans from animal studies. A similar sensitivity is often assumed.

C. Information on the potency of carcinogens in humans is available only for the relatively small number of substances that have been identified by epidemiologic studies to cause cancer in humans. For the vast majority, the quantitative assessment of human risk is uncertain. It is therefore prudent to minimize as much as possible any exposure to known or suspected human carcinogens.

III. The table of human carcinogens

A. Table IV–13 is an extensive list of known or suspected human carcinogens as evaluated by several authoritative private, federal, and international agencies. The table is intended to provide a quick guide to identify known or suspected human carcinogens. The original documents prepared by each agency should be consulted for more complete information on the nature of the hazards.

B. It is prudent to regard animal carcinogens as potential human carcinogens. Table IV–13 includes all chemicals that have been judged by the agencies described below as having sufficient evidence of carcinogenicity in animals. For a comprehensive listing of the results of animal cancer bioassays, see the *Carcinogenic Potency Database* (Gold et al, 1984, 1986, 1987).

C. To interpret the table correctly, it is important to have an understanding of the agencies that have evaluated the substances and the meanings of the different classification systems used.

1. **IARC carcinogen evaluations**

   a. The International Agency for Research on Cancer (IARC) of the World Health Organization is the premier authority for the evaluation of carcinogenic potential. The IARC uses both human and animal data in its evaluations of the carcinogenic risk to humans.

   b. The **human evidence**, primarily of an epidemiologic nature, is judged to provide **sufficient (S)**, **limited (L)**, or **inadequate (I)** evidence of a causal relationship between exposure and cancer. A blank space indicates that data were not available to the IARC.

c. The **animal data** are derived primarily from laboratory studies on test animals and are similarly judged to provide S, L, or I evidence of carcinogenicity.

d. The **overall evaluations** are primarily based on both the human and animal data. **Group 1** substances have sufficient epidemiologic evidence to support a causal association between exposure and human cancer. In general, **group 2** compounds are considered to be probably carcinogenic for humans based on a combination of animal and human data. Group 2 is subdivided into 2 parts. **Group 2A** compounds are usually those for which there is limited evidence of carcinogenicity in humans; **group 2B** compounds are usually those for which there is inadequate evidence of carcinogenicity in humans and sufficient evidence in animals. The category **group 3** describes those compounds that could not be classified as to their carcinogenic potential for humans.

e. Table IV–13 includes all substances classified by the IARC as belonging to group 1, 2A, or 2B. Some compounds reviewed by the IARC have not yet been given an overall classification, although the human or animal evidence for these compounds has been evaluated. These substances, with the overall category left blank in the table, are included if the human evidence is sufficient (S) or limited (L) or if the animal evidence is sufficient (S).

f. In addition, Table IV–14 lists by known or suspected site of tumor development in humans all those substances recognized by the IARC as having sufficient or limited evidence of carcinogenicity in humans.

2. **ACGIH evaluations**

a. The **American Conference of Governmental Industrial Hygienists (ACGIH)** is a professional society that develops guidelines for controlling the exposure of workers to industrial chemicals, including carcinogens. Because the ACGIH has no regulatory authority, its guidelines are not legal standards. However, the ACGIH guidelines are updated more often than the federal standards and for that reason they are often used by occupational health professionals.

b. Table IV–13 lists those compounds designated by the ACGIH as being **confirmed (A1)** or **suspected (A2) human carcinogens**. The category A1 is further divided into 2 subcategories, A1a and A1b. Substances designated as A1a have an assigned threshold limit value (TLV; see p 000) that establishes the maximum 8-hour time-weighted average exposure. Substances with an A1b designation do not have an assigned TLV; for these substances, respiratory, skin, and oral exposures are not permitted.

3. **OSHA and NIOSH evaluations**

a. The **Occupational Safety and Health Administration (OSHA)** is the federal agency that sets and enforces occupational exposure standards. Table IV–13 lists all those substances that are OSHA "regulated carcinogens." They are designated with a "+."

b. The **National Institute for Occupational Safety and Health (NIOSH)** is the federal agency that investigates and assesses the health hazards of chemicals and recommends workplace standards to OSHA. Table IV–13 lists all those substances that NIOSH recommends be treated as potential human carcinogens. These compounds are also designated with a "+."

4. **NTP evaluations.** The **National Toxicology Program (NTP)** is charged with producing an annual report that contains a list of those sub-

stances that are either known or reasonably anticipated to be carcinogenic. Table IV-13 includes all those compounds classified as known (1a) or reasonably anticipated (1b) human carcinogens by the NTP.

IV. **Carcinogenic potency in animal tests**
  A. Standardized information on relative carcinogenic potencies has been included when available. The potency ranking (1-10) of a carcinogen is based on its most potent TD_{50} (see **B,** below, for definition) in a positive animal bioassay as calculated in the *Carcinogenic Potency Database of the Standardized Results of Animal Bioassays.* For half the compounds, a positive TD_{50} was not available.
  B. In simplified terms, the TD_{50} is the chronic daily dose of a carcinogen that will cause cancer in 50% of the test animals when administered over their lifetime. The most potent animal carcinogen in Table IV-13 is 2,3,7,8-tetrachlorodibenzo-p-dioxin (TD_{50} of 6.7 ng/kg/d). The least potent is di(2-ethylhexyl) phthalate (TD_{50} of 2.3 g/kg/d).
  C. The actual TD_{50}s are not presented in the table. Instead, the TD_{50} range of over 100 million has been divided into 10 summary ranks:

Rank	TD_{50} Range (mg/kg/d)
1	1-10 ng
2	10-100 ng
3	100 ng-1 μ g
4	1-10 μ g
5	10-100 μ g
6	100 μ g-1 mg
7	1-10 mg
8	10-100 mg
9	100 mg-1 g
10	1-10 g

Note: The extrapolation of animal potency data to estimate cancer risks for humans is controversial and uncertain. Despite the great range in potencies, simple ranking is not sufficient to assess the risk from exposure to a carcinogen. Consult the original sources of these evaluations for further information on the likely magnitude of the risks involved.

V. **Summary.** This section presents an extensive list of known or suspected human carcinogens. Its major purpose is to allow the rapid identification of chemical carcinogens, the first step in risk assessment. Whether exposure to one of these chemicals presents a significant risk of cancer depends on the degree of exposure and many other factors. To ascertain more fully the nature and magnitude of these risks, consult the original sources of these evaluations.

References

Code of Federal Regulations. 29 CFR Chapter XVII (7-1-85 ed.), 1910.1001-.1047. US Government Printing Office, 1985.

Fourth Annual Report on Carcinogens Summary. National Toxicology Program Publication No. NTP-85002. US Department of Health and Human Services, 1985.

Gold LS et al: A carcinogenic potency database of the standardized results of animal bioassays. *Environ Health Perspect* 1984;**58**:9.

Gold LS et al: Chronological supplement to the carcinogenic potency database: Standardized results of animal bioassays published through December 1982. *Environ Health Perspect* 1986;**67**:161.

Gold LS et al: Second chronological supplement to the carcinogenic potency database: Standardized results of animal bioassays published through December 1984 and by the National Toxicology Program through May 1986. *Environ Health Perspect* 1987;74:237.

IARC Monographs on the Evaluation of the Carcinogenic Risk of Chemicals to Humans. 42 vols. World Health Organization, 1972–1988.

NIOSH: Recommendations for occupational safety and health standards. *MMWR* 1986;35(Suppl 1S).

TABLE IV-13. KNOWN OR SUSPECTED HUMAN CARCINOGENS

Chemical or Process	IARC Evaluations[a] Overall	Human[b]	Animal	ACGIH[c]	NIOSH[d]	NTP[e]	potency[f]	Selected Uses or Occurrence
Acetaldehyde		I	S					Synthesis of acetic acid, plastics, rubber, resins, and dyes
Acetaldehyde methylformylhydrazone (gyromitrin)			S				7	Found in the false morel mushroom
2-Acetylaminofluorene				+	+	1b	6	Proposed pesticide before carcinogenicity discovered
Acrylamide			S	A2				Production of polyacrylamide resins
Acrylonitrile (AN)	2A	L	S	A2	+	1b	7	Manufacturing of synthetic fibers, fumigant, solvent
Actinomycin D	2B	I	L				3	Antineoplastic agent
Adriamycin	2B	I	S			1b		Antineoplastic agent
AF-2 (furylfuramide)		I	S				8	Former use as food preservative in Japan
Aflatoxins	2A	L	S			1b	3	Products of fungal metabolism, detected in certain foods
Aldrin	3	I	L		+		6	Insecticide
Aluminum production		L						Certain occupational exposures in aluminum foundries
Certain amino acid pyrolysis products			S					Certain pyrolysis products detected in some cooked foods

continued

TABLE IV-13. KNOWN OR SUSPECTED HUMAN CARCINOGENS (Continued)

Chemical or Process	IARC Evaluations[a] Overall	Human	Animal	Other Evaluations ACGIH[b]	OSHA[c]	NIH/HS[d]	NTP[e]	Potency[f]	Selected Uses or Occurrence
2-Aminoanthraquinone			L				1b	9	Synthesis of anthraquinone dyes
o-Aminoazotoluene			S					7	Dye
4-Aminodiphenyl	1		S	A1b	+	+	1a	6	Former use as rubber antioxidant, 2-aminobiphenyl contaminant
1-Amino-2-methylanthraquinone			L				1b	8	Intermediate in synthesis of anthraquinone dyes
2-Amino-5-(5-nitro-2-furyl)-1,3,4-thiadiazole			S					6	Former use as experimental agent
Amitrole	2B		I				1b		Herbicide, plant growth regulator
Analgesic mixtures containing phenacetin	1	S	L				1a		Analgesic drug
o-Anisidine (plus its HCl salt)			S	A2			1b	8	Synthesis of azo dyes
Antimony trioxide production			S	A2					Used to make flameproofing agents, pigments, and catalysts
Aramite			S				1b	8	Insecticide
Arsenic (certain compounds)[g]	1	S	L	A1		+	1a		Metallurgy, pesticide, wood preservative, pigments
Arsenic trioxide production			S	A2			1a		Preparation of arsenic trioxide
Arsine						+			Released by reaction of inorganic arsenic and nascent hydrogen

Agent							Uses/comments
Asbestos	1	S	S	A1a	+	1a	Electrical and heat insulation, filler for clays and cements
Asphalts (extracts of steam- and air-refined bitumens)		I	S				Used in paving materials, roof sealants, filler
Auramine (technical grade)	2B	L	L			8	Dye and dye intermediate
Auramine manufacturing	1	S					Auramine production
Azaserine			S			6	Experimental drug, antineoplastic agent
Azathioprine	1	S	L			1a	Immunosuppressive agent, antineoplastic agent
Benz(a)anthracene			S			1b	Product of incomplete combustion
Benzene	1	S	L	A2	+	8	Solvent, intermediate in the synthesis of many substances
Benzidine	1	S	S	A1b	+	7	Synthesis of dyes, hardener for rubber, analytic reagent
Benzidine-based dyes					+		See also direct blue 38, direct black 6, and direct brown 95
Benzo(b)fluoranthene			S			1b	Product of incomplete combustion
Benzo(j)fluoranthene			S				Product of incomplete combustion
Benzo(k)fluoranthene			S				Product of incomplete combustion
Benzo(a)pyrene	2A	I	S	A2		1b	Product of incomplete combustion
Benzotrichloride			S			1b	Used in production of synthetic dyes, organic synthesis
Benzyl violet 4B			S				Dye
Beryllium (certain compounds)[g]	2A	L	S	A2	+	1b	Alloys, ceramics, electronics, neutron reflector
Betel quid with tobacco		S	L				Chewing

continued

TABLE IV-13. KNOWN OR SUSPECTED HUMAN CARCINOGENS (Continued)

Chemical or Process	IARC Evaluations[a]			Other Evaluations					Selected Uses or Occurrence
	Overall	Human	Animal	ACGIH[b]	OSHA[c]	NIOSH[d]	EPA-P[e]	Potency-y[f]	
Bis-chloroethyl nitrosourea (BCNU)	2B	I	S				1b		Antineoplastic agent
Bis(chloromethyl) ether (BCME), or technical-grade chloromethyl methyl ether (CMME)	1	S	S	A1a	+	+	1a	4	Alkylating agent in synthesis of plastics, ion exchange resins
Boot and shoe manufacturing and repair	1	S							Certain occupations in boot and shoe manufacturing and repair
Bracken fern (*Pteridium aquilinium*)		I	S						Plant used for food
1,3-Butadiene		I	S	A2		+		8	Rocket fuel, monomer used in synthetic rubber manufacturing
1,4-Butanediol dimethanesulfonate (myleran)	1	S	L				1a		Antineoplastic agent
Butylated hydroxyanisole (BHA)			S					9	Antioxidant in foods and cosmetics, preservative
β-Butyrolactone			S					8	Solvent, chemical intermediate
Cadmium (plus certain compounds)[g]	2B	L	S			+	1b		Alloys, soldering, pigments, fungicides, stabilizers
Carbon blacks (solvent extracts)		I	S			+			Rubber and ink pigment, combustion product
Carbon tetrachloride	2B	I	S	A2		+	1b	6	Freon synthesis, solvent, degreasing agent, fire extinguisher
Carrageenan (degraded)			S					10	Stabilizer, emulsifier, thickener
Certain combined chemotherapy for lymphomas (including MOPP)	1		S				1a		Antineoplastic agents

Chlorambucil	1	S	S			1a	5	Antineoplastic agent, immunopressive agent
Chloramphenicol	2B	L	I					Antibiotic
Chlornaphazine (*N,N'*-bis[2-chloroethyl]-2-napthylamine)	1	S	L			1a		Antineoplastic agent
1-(2-Chloroethyl)-3-cyclohexyl-1-nitrosourea (CCNU)	2B	I	S			1b		Antineoplastic agent
Chloroform	2B	I	S	A2	+	1b	8	Solvent, manufacturing of fluorocarbons, dyes, drugs, pesticides
Chloromethyl methyl ether (CMME, technical grade with BCME)	1	S	S	A1a	+	1a	4	Alkylating agents in synthesis of plastics, ion exchange resins
Chlorophenols	2B	L						Occupational exposures to certain chlorophenols
4-Chloro-*o*-phenylenediamine		S				1b	9	Dye intermediate
Chloroprene	3	I	I		+		7	Used in synthetic rubber manufacturing
4-Chloro-*o*-toluidine		I	S				8	Chemical intermediate in the synthesis of dyes, pigments
Cholesterol, dietary		L	I					Consumption of cholesterol-containing foods
Chromite ore processing				A1a				Chromate production
Chromium (certain Cr[IV] compounds)[g]	1	S	S	A1a	+	1a		Alloys, electroplating, pigment, cements, antioxidant
Chrysene		L	L	A2	+			Reagent used in organic synthesis
Cisplatin	2B	I	L					Antineoplastic agent
Citrus red no. 2			S					Dye
Coal gasification		S	S					Occupational exposures involving gas production from coal
Coal tar pitches		S	S					Binder for aluminum smelting, roofing material

continued

TABLE IV-13. KNOWN OR SUSPECTED HUMAN CARCINOGENS (Continued)

Chemical or Process	IARC Evaluations[a]			Other Evaluations				Selected Uses or Occurrence
	Overall	Human[b]	Animal	ACGIH[c]	NIOSH[d]	NTP[e]	Potency[f]	
Coal tar pitch volatiles				A1a	+			Used in pitch-melting and roofing operations
Coal tars		S	S					Fuel, pharmaceutical, surface coating
Coke oven emissions				+	+	1a		Generated during coke oven operations
Coke production		S	S					Certain occupational exposures in foundries
Contraceptives, combined oral	2A	S						Contraceptive agents
Contraceptives, sequential oral	2B	L						Contraceptive agents
Creosotes		L	S		+			Wood preservative, fungicide
p-Cresidine			S			1b	8	Used in synthesis of azo dyes and pigments
Cupferron						1b	7	Analytic reagent
Cycasin			S			1b		Occurs in cycad plants
Cyclophosphamide	1	S				1a	7	Antineoplastic agent
Dacarbazine	2B	I	S			1b	6	Antineoplastic agent
Daunomycin			S					Antineoplastic agent

DDT	2B	I	S		+	1b	7	Insecticide
N,N'-Diacetylbenzidine			S					Dye intermediate
2,4-Diaminoanisole (plus its salts)			S		+	1b	9	Dye component and synthetic intermediate
4,4'-Diaminodiphenylether			S					Used in resin manufacturing
2,4-Diaminotoluene			S			1b	7	Dye and chemical synthetic intermediate
o-Dianisidine-based dyes					+			Dyes
Dibenz(*a,h*)acridine			S			1b		Product of incomplete combustion
Dibenz(*a,j*)acridine			S			1b		Product of incomplete combustion
Dibenz(*a,h*)anthracene			S			1b	7	Product of incomplete combustion
7-*H*-Dibenzo(*c,g*)carbazole			S			1b		Product of incomplete combustion
Dibenzo(*a,e*)pyrene			S					Product of incomplete combustion
Dibenzo(*a,h*)pyrene			S			1b		Product of incomplete combustion
Dibenzo(*a,l*)pyrene			S			1b		Product of incomplete combustion
Dibenzo(*a,i*)pyrene			S					Product of incomplete combustion
1,2-Dibromo-3-chloropropane (DBCP)			S		+	1b	6	Pesticide, nematocide, soil fumigant
3,3'-Dichlorobenzidine	2B	I	S	A2	+	1b	8	Synthesis of pigments, curing agent for isocyanate polymers
3,3'-Dichloro-4,4'-diaminodiphenyl ether			S					Industrial chemical; no commercial application
1,3-Dichloropropene (Telone II)		I	S				8	Fumigant

continued

TABLE IV-13. KNOWN OR SUSPECTED HUMAN CARCINOGENS (Continued)

Chemical or Process	IARC Evaluations[a] Overall	IARC Evaluations[a] Human[b]	IARC Evaluations[a] Animal	Other Evaluations ACGIH[c]	Other Evaluations OSHA[d]	Other Evaluations NIOSH[e]	Potency[f]	Selected Uses or Occurrence
Dieldrin	3	I	L			+	6	Insecticide
Dienestrol	2B	L	I					Synthetic nonsteroidal estrogen hormone, drug
Diepoxybutane			S			1b		Alkylating agent, drug synthesis
Di(2-ethylhexyl) phthalate			S	+		1b	10	Plasticizer
1,2-Diethylhydrazine			S					Chemical intermediate in organic synthesis
Diethylstilbestrol (DES)	1	S	S			1a	5	Synthetic nonsteroidal estrogen hormone, drug
Diethyl sulfate	2A	L	S			1b		Ethylating agent
Diglycidyl resorcinol ether			S					Component of liquid epoxy resin
Dihydrosafrole			S				8	Flavoring agent
3,3'-Dimethoxybenzidine (o-dianisidine)	2B	I	S			1b		Azo dye intermediate, analytic reagent
4-Dimethylaminoazobenzene			S	+	+	1b	7	Dye, analytic reagent; former use as food-coloring agent
trans-2[[Dimethylamino)methylimino]-5-(2-[5-nitro-2-furyl]vinyl)-1,3,4-oxydiazole			S				8	Nitrofuran compound; no commercial application

Dimethylcarbamoyl chloride	2B	I	S	A2		1b	7	Intermediate in synthesis of dyes, pesticides, drugs
1,1-Dimethylhydrazine			S	A2	+	1b	7	Jet rocket fuels, chemical intermediate
1,2-Dimethylhydrazine			S				6	Primarily used in research
Dimethyl sulfate	2A	I	S	A2		1b		Methylating agent in organic synthesis
2,4-Dinitrotoluene					+			Chemical intermediate for synthesis of dyes and explosives
1,4-Dioxane	2B	I	S		+	1b	9	Solvent, stabilizer
Direct black 38	2B	I	S			1b	6	Dye; see also benzidine-based dyes
Direct blue 6	2B	I	S			1b	7	Dye; see also benzidene-based dyes
Direct brown 95	2B	I	L				7	Dye; see also benzidene-based dyes
Epichlorohydrin	2B	I	S		+	1b		Raw material for epoxy and phenoxy resins, solvent, stabilizer
Erionite		S	S					Naturally occurring zeolite mineral
Estradiol, 17 β	2B		S			1b	6	Naturally occurring steroidal estrogen, drug
Estrogens (conjugated)	1	S	I			1a		Naturally occurring estrogens, drug
Estrone	2B		S			1b		Naturally occurring estrogen, drug
Ethinylestradiol	2B		S			1b		Drug, synthetic estrogen
Ethyl acrylate			S					Monomer, acrylic emulsion polymers
Ethylene dibromide (EDB, 1,2-dibromomethane)	2B	I	S	A2	+	1b	7	Gasoline additive, fumigant, synthesis of vinyl bromide
Ethylene dichloride (EDC, 1,2-dichloroethane)			S		+	1b	7	Antiknock agent for gasoline, solvent, pesticide

continued

TABLE IV-13. KNOWN OR SUSPECTED HUMAN CARCINOGENS (Continued)

Chemical or Process	IARC Evaluations[a]			Other Evaluations					Selected Uses or Occurrence
	Overall	Human[b]	Animal	ACGIH	OSHA[c]	NIOSH[d]	NTP[e]	Potency[f]	
Ethyleneimine (aziridine)					+	+		6	Chemical intermediate, flocculation aid, textile industry
Ethylene oxide	2B	L	S	A2	+	+	1b	7	Sterilant, fungicide, fumigant, common chemical intermediate
Ethylene thiourea	2B	I	S			+	1b	8	Rubber manufacturing, synthetic intermediate
Ethyl methanesulfonate			S						Mutagen used in experimental research
Formaldehyde (gas)	2B	I	S	A2	+	+	1b	6	Production of phenolic, urea, melamine, and acetyl resins, sterilant
2-(2-formylhydrazine)-4-(5-nitro-2-furyl)-thiazole			S					7	Primarily used in research
Furniture and cabinetmaking industry	1	S							Certain occupational exposures in furniture and cabinetmaking
Glycidaldehyde			S						Epoxide occurring in sunflower oil and rancid lard
Hematite underground mining	1	S					1a		Underground hematite mining (with exposure to radon)
Hexachlorobenzene			S				1b	7	Organic synthesis, fungicide, wood preservative
Hexachlorobutadiene				A2				8	Solvent, heat transfer liquid, transformer and hydraulic fluid
Hexachlorocyclohexane (certain isomers)[g]		I	S				1b	8	Insecticides

Agent								Uses
Hexachloroethane		L			+		9	Organic synthesis, insecticides, solvent, explosives
Hexamethylphosphoramide			S	A2		1b		Insect chemosterilant, solvent
Hydralazine		I	L					Antihypertensive drug
Hydrazine (plus its sulfate)	2B	I	S	A2	+		7	Rocket propellant, biocide, antioxidant, analytic reagent
Hydrazobenzene						1b	7	Dye intermediate
Indeno(1,2,3-cd)pyrene			S			1b		Product of incomplete combustion
Iron and steel production		L						Certain occupational exposures in iron and steel production
Iron dextran complex	3	I	S			1b		Drug for iron deficiency anemia
Isopropyl alcohol production	1		S		+	1a		Isopropyl alcohol manufacturing (strong acid process)
Isosafrole			S		+			Used in perfumes, flavoring agent, pesticide synergist
Kepone (chlordecone)			S		+	1b	6	Insecticide, fungicide, and larvacide
Lasiocarpine			S				6	Former uncommon use as drug
Lead (certain compounds)[g]	3	I	S			1b	9	Lead production, solder, batteries, pigment, insecticides
Lead chromate			S	A2				Pigment and analytic reagent
Magenta manufacturing	2A	L						Magenta production
Melphalan	1		S			1a	5	Antineoplastic agent, immunosuppressive agent
Merphalan			S					Antineoplastic agent, racemic form of melphalan
Mestranol	2B		S			1b		Estrogenlike drug

continued

TABLE IV-13. KNOWN OR SUSPECTED HUMAN CARCINOGENS (Continued)

Chemical or Process	IARC Evaluations[a] Overall	Human	Animal	Other Evaluations ACGIH[b]	OSHA[c]	NIOSH[d]	NTP[e]	potency[f]	Selected Uses or Occurrence
Methoxsalen with ultraviolet A therapy	1	S	S				1a		Therapy for psoriasis
Methylazoxymethanol acetate			S						Biologically active constituent of cycasin
Methyl bromide		I	L			+			Fumigant, solvent, methylating agent
Methyl chloride		I	I			+			Solvent, resin production, aerosol propellant, refrigerant
5-Methylchrysene			S						Combustion product
4,4'-methylenebis(2-chloroaniline) (MOCA)		I	S	A2		+	1b	7	Curing agent for polyurethanes and isocyanate resins
4,4'-Methylenebis (N,N-dimethyl) benzenamine			L				1b	8	Dye intermediate, analytic reagent for lead determinations
4,4'-Methylenebis(2-methyl aniline)			S					7	Curing agent for isocyanate-containing polymers
Methylene chloride (dichloromethane)		I	S		+	+		9	Solvent, paint remover, fire extinguisher, degreasing agent
4,4'-Methylenedianiline (plus its 2HCl salt)		I	S	A2		+	1b	8	Polymer and dye intermediate, epoxy- and resin-hardening agent
Methylhydrazine				A2		+		7	Missile propellant, intermediate, solvent
Methyl iodide			L	A2		+	1b		Used in pharmaceutical and other chemical synthesis
Methyl methanesulfonate			S					8	Experimental mutagen, alkylating reagent

Substance								Use
2-Methyl-1-nitroanthraquinone			S				7	Dye intermediate
4-(Methylnitrosamino)-1-(3-pyridyl)-1-butanone (NNK)			S					Formed during tobacco production and smoking
3-Methylnitrosaminopropionitrile			S					Derived from areca nut alkaloids
N-Methyl-N'-nitroso-N-nitroguanidine (MNNG)			S				6	N-Nitroso compound, research chemical
Methyl thiouracil			S				8	Antithyroid agent
Metronidazole	2B	I	S			1b	9	Antiprotozoal drug
Michler's ketone			S			1b	7	Synthetic intermediate for dyes and pigments
Mineral oils (untreated and mildly treated)[g]		S	S					Lubricants
Mirex			S			1b	7	Insecticide
Mitomycin C			S				3	Antineoplastic agent
Monocrotaline			S				6	Pyrrolizidine alkaloid found in some bush teas
5-(Morpholinomethyl)-3-[(5-nitrofurfurylidene)amino]-2-oxazolidinone			S				7	N-nitroso compound, research chemical
Mustard gas	1	S	L			1a		War gas, alkylating agent
Nafenopin			S					Antihyperlipoproteinemic drug
α-Naphthylamine	3	I	I	+	+		3	Intermediate in synthesizing dyes, insecticides, antioxidants
β-Naphthylamine	1	S	A1b	+	+	1a	7	Antioxidant, synthetic intermediate for dyes
Nickel (certain compounds)[g]	2A	L	S	+		1b		Metallurgy, electroplating, batteries, ceramics, catalysts

continued

TABLE IV–13. KNOWN OR SUSPECTED HUMAN CARCINOGENS (Continued)

Chemical or Process	IARC Evaluations[a]			Other Evaluations					Selected Uses or Occurrence
	Overall	Human	Animal	ACGIH[b]	OSHA[c]	NIOSH[d]	NTP[e]	Potency[f]	
Nickel refining	1	S		A1a			1a		Occupational exposures in the production of metallic nickel
Niridazole		S							Drug for treating schistosomiasis
Nitrilotriacetic acid							1b	9	Chelating agent for boiler feedwater, metal plating
5-Nitroacenaphthene			S					7	Dye intermediate in Japan
5-Nitro-o-anisidine			L				1b	8	Dye intermediate
4-Nitrodiphenyl			L	A1b	+	+			Chemical intermediate in synthesis of 4-aminobiphenyl
Nitrofen (technical grade)			S				1b	8	Herbicide
1-[(5-Nitrofurfurylidine]amino)-2-imidazolidinone			S					7	Primarily used in research
N-[4-[5-Nitro-2-furyl]-2-thiazolyl] acetamide			S					7	Primarily used in research
Nitrogen mustard	2A	I	S				1b	5	Antineoplastic agent
Nitrogen mustard n-oxide			S					6	Chemical intermediate in organic synthesis
2-Nitronaphthalene						+			By-product of dye production
2-Nitropropane		S		A2	+		1b		Solvent, chemical intermediate, rocket propellant

Compound							Uses
n-Nitrosodi-n-butylamine		S				1b	6	Chemical intermediate, produced by nitrosation of butylamines
n-Nitrosodiethanolamine		S				1b	7	Contaminant of some cutting fluids, pesticides, tobacco
n-Nitrosodiethylamine		S				1b	4	Antioxidant, contaminant, generated by nitrosation reactions
n-Nitrosodimethylamine		S	A2	+	+	1b	5	Other former uses as antioxidant, contaminant of cutting fluids
p-Nitrosodiphenylamine		I					9	Dye and drug synthesis, accelerator in rubber vulcanization
n-Nitrosodi-n-propylamine		S				1b	6	Contaminant of some cheese, brandy, liquors, pesticides
n-Nitroso-n-ethylurea		S				1b		Contaminant generated by nitrosation reactions
n-Nitroso-methylethylamine		S						Used in organic synthesis, microscopy
n-Nitroso-n-methylurea		S				1b	7	Contaminant generated by nitrosation reactions
n-Nitroso-n-methylurethane		S					6	Contaminant generated by nitrosation reactions
n-Nitrosomethylvinylamine		S				1b		Contaminant generated by nitrosation reactions
n-Nitrosomorpholine		S				1b	7	Contaminant generated by nitrosation reactions
n-Nitrosonornicotine		S				1b	8	Contaminant detected in cured tobacco
n-Nitrosopiperidine		S				1b	6	Epoxy resin and pacemaker manufacturing
n-Nitrosopyrrolidine		S				1b	7	Detected in some cured foods
n-Nitrososarcosine		S				1b		Detected in some foodstuffs
Norethisterone	2B	S				1b		Drug, progestational agent
Oil orange SS		S						Petroleum dye

continued

TABLE IV-13. KNOWN OR SUSPECTED HUMAN CARCINOGENS (Continued)

Chemical or Process	IARC Evaluations[a]			Other Evaluations					Selected Uses or Occurrence
	Overall	Human	Animal	ACGIH[b]	OSHA[c]	NIOSH[d]	NTP[e]	Potency[f]	
Oxymetholone	2A	L					1b		Anabolic, androgenic steroid, drug
Panfuran S (dihydroxymethylfuratrizine)			S						Former use in Japan as antibiotic
Phenacetin	2A	L	S				1b	10	Veterinary analgesic drug
Phenazopyridine (plus its HCl salt)	2B	I	S				1b	8	Analgesic drug
Phenoxyacetic acid herbicides		L							Occupational exposures to herbicides (2,4-D, 2,4,5-T, and MCPA)
Phenoxybenzamine (plus its HCl salt)			S					6	α-Adrenergic blocking agent, antihypertensive drug
Phenylhydrazine				A2		+		8	Reagent, intermediate
N-Phenyl-2-naphthylamine	3	I	I	A2		+			Rubber antioxidant, lubricant
Phenytoin (plus its Na salt)	2B	L	L				1b		Anticonvulsant drug
Polybrominated biphenyls		I	S				1b	6	Flame retardant
Polychlorinated biphenyls	2B	I	S			+	1b	7	Transformer, capacitors, heat transfer and hydraulic fluids
Ponceau MX			S						Dye
Ponceau SX			S						Dye

Compound							Use
Ponceau 3R		S					Dye
Potassium bromate		S				7	Maturing agent for flour, dough conditioner, malting of barley
Procarbazine (plus its HCl salt)	2A	I	S		1b	6	Antineoplastic agent
Progesterone	2B		S		1b		Drug, naturally occurring sex hormone
1,3-Propane sultone		S	A2		1b	7	Industrial chemical intermediate
β-Propiolactone		S	A2	+ +	1b	7	Acrylic acid and ester manufacturing, sterilant
Propylene imine (2-methylaziridine)		S	A2		1b		Industrial chemical intermediate
Propylene oxide		I	S			8	Synthesis of propylene glycol, fumigant, sterilant
Propylthiouracil	2B	I	S		1b	8	Antithyroid agent
Reserpine	3	I	L		1b	5	Antihypertensive drug
Rubber industry	1	S			1a		Certain occupations in rubber manufacturing
Saccharin (plus its sodium salt)	3	I	S		1b	10	Artificial sweetener
Safrole			S		1b	8	Flavoring agent
Selenium sulfide					1b	7	Antidandruff shampoos
Shale oils (certain compounds)g		S	S				Source of fuel
Silica, crystalline		L					Mineral used in sandblasting, filler in paints and ceramics
Soots, tars, and oils	1	S	S		1a		Combustion by-product, contaminant of some tars and oils
Sterigmatocystin		S				5	Product of fungal metabolism, detected in some food grains

continued

TABLE IV-13. KNOWN OR SUSPECTED HUMAN CARCINOGENS (Continued)

Chemical or Process	Overall	Human	Animal	IARC Group H[b]	OSHA A[c]	NIOSH H[d]	NTP P[e]	Potency[f]	Selected Uses or Occurrence
Streptozocin			S				1b	6	Antineoplastic agent
Styrene oxide	3	I	S					8	Epoxy resin manufacturing, chemical intermediate
Sulfallate (2-chloro-2-propenyl ester-diethylcarbamodithioic acid)			S				1b	8	Preemergence herbicide
Talc containing asbestiform fibers		S	I						Mineral and filler used in paints, ceramics, and plastics
Testosterone (plus its esters)			S						Drug, naturally occurring male sex hormone
2,3,7,8-Tetrachlorodibenzo-p-dioxin (TCDD)	2B	I	S			+	1b	1	Contaminant of 2,4,5-T, heating certain chlorinated aromatics
1,1,2,2-Tetrachloroethane			L			+		8	Solvent, artificial pearl industry
Tetrachloroethylene	3	I	L			+		8	Solvent, degreasing agent
Thioacetamide (TAA)			S				1b	7	Solvent, chemical intermediate, analytic reagent
4,4'-Thiodianiline			S					7	Dye intermediate
Thiourea			S				1b	8	Fire retardants, photographic chemicals, rust removers, glue
Thorium dioxide							1a		Nuclear reactors, x-ray medium, arc welding
Tobacco smoke		S	S						Inhalation of tobacco smoke from cigars, cigarettes, pipes

Agent								Use
Tobacco, smokeless products			S					Chewing tobacco
o-Tolidine (DMB, 3,3'-dimethyl-benzidine)			S	A2	+	1b		Dye and dye intermediate, analytic reagent
o-Tolidine-based dyes					+			Dyes
Toluene 2,4-diisocyanate		I	S			1b		Manufacturing of polyurethane foam and plastic products
o-Toluidine (plus its HCl salt)	2A	I	S	A2	+	1b	8	Dye intermediate
p-Toluidine				A2				8	Dye intermediate
Toxaphene			S			1b	7	Insecticide
Treosulfan	1	S						Antineoplastic agent
1,1,2-Trichloroethane					+		8	Chemical intermediate, solvent
Trichloroethylene		I	L		+		9	Solvent, dry cleaning and degreasing agent, chemical synthesis
2,4,6-Trichlorophenol	2B	I	S			1b	9	Wood and glue preservative, bactericide, herbicide
Tris(aziridinyl)-para-benzoquinone (triaziquone)	2B	I	L					Antineoplastic agent
Tris(1-aziridinyl)phosphine sulfide (thiotepa)	2B	I	S			1b	6	Antineoplastic agent
Tris(2,3-dibromopropyl) phosphate (TRIS)			S			1b	7	Former use as flame retardant for clothing
Trp-P-1(3-amino-1,4-dimethyl-5H-pyrido-[4,3,-b]indole) (plus its acetate)			S				8	Found in broiled fish and meat
Trp-P-2(3-amino-1-methyl-5H-pyrido-[4,3,-b]indole) (plus its acetate)			S				7	Found in broiled fish and meat
Trypan blue (commercial grade)			S					Dye

continued

TABLE IV-13. KNOWN OR SUSPECTED HUMAN CARCINOGENS (Continued)

Chemical or Process	IARC Evaluations[a]			Other Evaluations					Selected Uses or Occurrence
	Overall	Human	Animal	ACGIH[b]	OSHA[c]	NIOSH[d]	NTP[e]	Potency[f]	
Uracil mustard	2B								Antineoplastic agent
Urethane (ethyl carbamate)		S					1b	8	Antineoplastic agent, veterinary anesthetic
Vinyl bromide			S	A2		+		8	Intermediate in synthesis of fire retardants and some polymers
Vinyl chloride	1	S	S	A1a	+	+	1a	7	Vinyl chloride resin and methyl chloroform production
Vinylcyclohexane dioxide				A2					Chemical intermediate
Vinyl fluoride						+			Monomer
Vinylidine chloride (1,1-dichloroethylene)	3	I	L			+		8	Saran and adhesives production
Vinylidine fluoride (1,1-difluoroethylene)			I			+			Polymer, copolymer, chemical intermediate
Zinc chromate	3	S		A1a					See also chromium

[a] The International Agency for Research on Cancer (IARC) evaluations.

Overall heading:

Symbol	Meaning
1	IARC-recognized human carcinogen.
2A	Probable human carcinogen, with a higher degree of evidence (see text).
2B	Probable human carcinogen, with a lower degree of evidence (see text).
3	Could not be classified as to its carcinogenic potential for humans.

Human and Animal headings:

Symbol	Meaning
S	Sufficient human or animal evidence exists to show that an entry is a human or animal carcinogen.
L	Limited, but not conclusive, human or animal evidence exists to show that an entry is a human or animal carcinogen.
I	Inadequate human or animal evidence exists. The existing studies do not show a causal relationship.

[b]The American Council of Governmental Industrial Hygienists (ACGIH) evaluations.

Symbol	Meaning
A1a	Confirmed human carcinogen with an assigned TLV.
A1b	Confirmed human carcinogen without an assigned TLV.
A2	Suspected human carcinogen.

[c]The Occupational Safety and Health Administration (OSHA) evaluations. Under the OSHA heading, a "+" indicates that an entry is an OSHA-regulated carcinogen.

[d]The National Institute of Occupational Safety and Health (NIOSH) evaluation. A "+" indicates that they advise a substance be treated as a potential human carcinogen.

[e]The National Toxicology Program (NTP) evaluations. There are 2 possible entries under the NTP column:

Symbol	Meaning
1a	NTP known human carcinogen.
1b	Reasonably anticipated human carcinogen.

Note that blank entries under any of the headings indicate that the particular review was not available. Blank entries do not mean that an entry has been judged to be a noncarcinogen.

[f]The potency of a carcinogen is based on TD_{50} values derived from animal studies. The TD_{50} is the chronic daily dose that will cause cancer in 50% of the test animals when administered over their lifetime. The rankings found under the Potency heading range from 1 (the most potent carcinogens) to 10 (the least potent). The TD_{50} dose ranges assigned to each rank:

Rank	TD_{50} Range
1	1 ng–10 ng
2	10 ng–100 ng
3	100 ng–1 μg
4	1 μg–10 μg
5	10 μg–100 μg
6	100 μg–1 mg
7	1 mg–10 mg
8	10 mg–100 mg
9	100 mg–1 g
10	1 g–10 g

[g]See the original sources for the specific compounds included under this listing.

TABLE IV-14. KNOWN AND SUSPECTED HUMAN CARCINOGENS: TARGET ORGANS AND AGENTS

Organ or Disease	Sufficient Evidence	Limited Evidence
Bladder	4-Aminodiphenyl, auramine manufacturing, benzidine, chlornaphazine, cyclophosphamide, β-naphthylamine, rubber industry, soots, tobacco smoke	Aluminum production, auramine (technical grade), boot and shoe manufacturing and repair industry, coal gasification, coal tar pitches, magenta manufacturing
Brain	Vinyl chloride	Phenytoin (plus its sodium salt)
Breast	...	Cholesterol, dietary; oral contraceptives, combined
Colon and rectum	Asbestos	Cadmium (plus certain compounds); cholesterol, dietary; rubber industry; shale oils (certain compounds)
Esophagus	Soots, tobacco smoke	Coal tar pitches
Kidney	Analgesic mixtures containing phenacetin; tobacco smoke	Coke production, phenacetin
Larynx	Asbestos, tobacco smoke	Coal tar pitches, diethyl sulfate, isopropyl alcohol manufacturing, nickel (certain compounds), nickel refining
Leukemia	Benzene, boot and shoe manufacturing and repair, 1, 4-butanediol dimethanesulfonate (myleran), certain combined chemotherapy for lymphomas (including MOPP), chlorambucil, cyclophosphamide, melphalan, soots, treosulfan, vinyl chloride	Chloramphenicol, coal tar pitches, ethylene oxide, rubber industry
Liver	Azathioprine; oral contraceptives, combined; soots; vinyl chloride	Aflatoxins, oxymetholone
Lung	Arsenic trioxide production, asbestos, boot and shoe manufacturing and repair, bis(chloromethyl) ethyl or chloromethyl methyl ether or both, chromium (certain Cr[VI] compounds), coal gasification, coal tar pitches, coke production, erionite, hematite underground mining, mustard gas, nickel refining, rubber industry, soots, talc containing asbestiform fibers, tobacco smoke, vinyl chloride	Acrylonitrile; aluminum production; beryllium (certain compounds); cadmium (plus certain compounds); nickel (certain compounds); iron and steel production; silica, crystalline

Lymphoma	Azathioprine, vinyl chloride	Chlorophenols, phenoxyacetic acid herbicides, rubber industry
Nasal	Boot and shoe manufacturing and repair, furniture and cabinetmaking industry, isopropyl alcohol manufacture, nickel refining	Cadmium (plus certain compounds), nickel (certain compounds)
Oral cavity	Tobacco products, smokeless; betel quid with tobacco; tobacco smoke	Coal tars, coal tar pitches
Pancreas	Tobacco smoke	...
Pharynx	Betel quid with tobacco, tobacco smoke	Cadmium (plus certain compounds)
Prostate	...	Acrylonitrile, cadmium (plus certain compounds), rubber industry
Sarcoma	...	Chlorophenols, phenoxyacetic acid herbicides
Scrotum	Coal tar pitches, coal tars, shale oils (certain compounds), soots, tars, oils	Creosotes, rubber industry
Skin	Arsenic (certain compounds), azathioprine, coal tars, coal tar pitches, coke production, methoxsalen with ultraviolet A therapy, mineral oils (untreated and midly treated), shale oils (certain compounds), soots, tars, oils	Cresotes, rubber industry
Stomach	Rubber industry	Acrylonitrile, asbestos
Uterus	Estrogens, conjugated	Dienestrol; diethylstilbestrol (DES); oral contraceptives, combined and sequential
Vagina	Diethylstilbestrol (DES)	...

TABLE IV–15. REGIONAL OFFICES OF THE OCCUPATIONAL SAFETY AND HEALTH ADMINISTRATION (OSHA)

Region	Regional Office and Phone Number	States Served
I	Boston (617) 565-7164	Connecticut, Maine, Massachusetts, New Hampshire, Vermont
II	New York City (212) 337-2325	New York, New Jersey
III	Philadelphia (215) 596-1201	Delaware, District of Columbia, Maryland, Pennsylvania, Virginia, West Virginia
IV	Atlanta (404) 347-3573	Alabama, Florida, Georgia, Kentucky, Mississippi, North Carolina, South Carolina, Tennessee
V	Chicago (312) 353-2220	Illinois, Indiana, Michigan, Minnesota, Ohio, Wisconsin
VI	Dallas (214) 767-4731	Arkansas, Louisiana, New Mexico, Oklahoma, Texas
VII	Kansas City (816) 426-5861	Iowa, Kansas, Missouri, Nebraska
VIII	Denver (303) 844-3061	Colorado, Montana, North Dakota, South Dakota, Utah, Wyoming
IX	San Francisco (415) 995-5672	Arizona, California, Hawaii, Nevada, South Pacific Islands
X	Seattle (206) 442-5930	Alaska, Idaho, Oregon, Washington

CAS Chemical Numbers Index

NOTE: Page numbers in bold face type indicate a major discussion. A *t* following a page
number indicates tabular material and an *i* following a page number indicates an illustration.

Subject Index

NOTE: Page numbers in bold face type indicate a major discussion. A *t* following a page number indicates tabular material and an *i* following a page number indicates an illustration. Insofar as possible, drugs and chemical agents are listed under their generic or common names, and a cross reference is provided for the trade name. A separate index of chemicals by their CAS number is provided on pp. 505–515.

518

INDEX

Altered mental status (*cont.*)
seizures, 21–22
stupor, 17–18
α-Alumina, hazard summary for, 369*t*
Aluminum
carcinogenicity of, 481*t*
hazard summary for, 369*t*
Aluminum oxide (α-alumina)
hazard summary for, 369*t*
impure (emery), hazard summary for, 405*t*
Alveolitis, extrinsic, occupational causes of, 354*t*
Amanita mushrooms. *See also* Anticholinergics; Mushrooms, amatoxin-type
muscaria
tachycardia and, 12*t*
toxicity of, 211*t*
ocreata, toxicity of, 211*t*, 212–213
pantherina, toxicity of, 211*t*
phalloides
hepatic damage and, 34*t*
renal failure and, 33*t*
toxicity of, 211*t*, 212–213
toxicity of, 211*t*
verna, toxicity of, 211*t*, 212–213
virosa, toxicity of, 211*t*, 212–213
Amantadine
confusion and, 22*t*
delirium and, 22*t*
toxicity of, **59–60**
Amaryllis, 246*t*
Amatoxin-type mushrooms, **212–213**
hepatic damage and, 34*t*
hypotension and, 15*t*
renal failure and, 33*t*
rhabdomyolysis and, 24*t*
tachycardia and, 12*t*
toxicity of, 211*t*, **212–213**
American bittersweet, 246*t*
American Conference of Government Industrial Hygienists, exposure guidelines and, 478
American ivy, 246*t*
American mistletoe, 249*t*
American sea nettle envenomation, baking soda for, 184
Amikacin, 69*t*. *See also* Antibiotics
Amiloride, 145*t*. *See also* Diuretics
Amino acid pyrolysis products, carcinogenicity of, 481*t*
p-Aminoaniline (phenylenediamine), hazard summary for, 446*t*
2-Aminoanthraquinone, carcinogenicity of, 482*t*
o-Aminoazotoluene, carcinogenicity of, 482*t*
Aminobenzene (aniline)
hazard summary for, 370*t*
methemoglobinemia and, 204*t*
p-Aminobiphenyl (4-aminodiphenyl)
carcinogenicity of, 482*t*
hazard summary for, 369*t*
Aminocarb, 107*t*. *See also* Carbamate insecticides

Aminocyclohexane (cyclohexylamine), hazard summary for, 392*t*
4-Amino-6-(1,1-dimethylethyl)-3-(methylthio)-1,2,4-triazin-5(4H)-one (metribuzin), hazard summary for, 436*t*
4-Aminodiphenyl
carcinogenicity of, 482*t*
hazard summary for, 369*t*
2-Aminoethanol (ethanolamine), hazard summary for, 406*t*
Aminoglycosides. *See also* Antibiotics
renal failure and, 33*t*
toxicity of, 69*t*
1-Amino-2-methylanthraquinone, carcinogenicity of, 482*t*
2-Aminonaphthalene (β-naphthylamine)
carcinogenicity of, 493*t*
hazard summary for, 437*t*
2-Amino-5-(5-nitro-2-furyl)-1,3,4-thiadiazole, carcinogenicity of, 482*t*
Aminophenol, methemoglobinemia and, 204*t*
Aminophylline, for bronchospasm, 9. *See also* Theophylline
2-Aminopropane (isopropylamine), hazard summary for, 423*t*
Aminopterine, as teratogen, 53*t*
2-Aminopyridine, hazard summary for, 369*t*
4-Aminopyridine, for calcium antagonist overdose, 103
Aminoquinolines, toxicity of, **122–124**
3-Amino-1,2,4-triazole (amitrole)
carcinogenicity of, 482*t*
hazard summary for, 369*t*
4-Amino-3,5,6-trichloropicolinic acid (picloram), hazard summary for, 449*t*
Amiodarone. *See also* Antiarrhythmic drugs, newer
toxicity of, 66, 67*t*, 68
ventricular arrhythmias and, 13*t*
Amitriptyline. *See also* Cyclic antidepressants
elimination of, 49*t*
toxicity of, 137*t*
in toxicology screening, 35*t*
Amitrole
carcinogenicity of, 482*t*
hazard summary for, 369*t*
Ammonia. *See also* Gases, irritant
hazard summary for, 370*t*
toxicity of, **60–61**, 163*t*
Ammonium chloride, for radiation exposure, 260*t*
Ammonium chloroplatinate (platinum salt), hazard summary for, 450*t*
Amobarbital, 86*t*. *See also* Barbiturates
Amodiaquine, 122. *See also* Chloroquine
Amosite (asbestos)
carcinogenicity of, 483*t*
hazard summary for, 372*t*
toxicity of, **84–85**

Explosives manufacturing, occupational
exposures associated with, 351t
Extrapyramidal symptoms, drug-induced,
diphenhydramine for, 306
Extrinsic alveolitis, occupational causes
of, 354t
Eyes
decontamination of, 40, 41i
examination of in diagnosis of poisoning, 27
occupational exposures affecting, 354

False hellebore, 248t
Famphur, 226t. *See also* Organophos-
phates
Farm workers, occupational exposures as-
sociated with, 351t
Fasting, hypoglycemia and, 31t
Fava bean, 248t
Feldene. *See* Piroxicam
Felt making, occupational exposures as-
sociated with, 352t
Fenamiphos. *See also* Organophosphates
hazard summary for, 412t
toxicity of, 226t
Fenfluramine, 62t. *See also* Amphet-
amines
Fenitrothion, 226t. *See also* Organophos-
phates
Fenophosphon, 226t. *See also* Organo-
phosphates
Fenoprofen, 221t. *See also* Nonsteroidal
anti-inflammatory agents
Fenothrin, 254t. *See also* Pyrethrins
Fenpropanate, 254t. *See also* Pyrethrins
Fensulfothion. *See also* Organophos-
phates
hazard summary for, 412t
toxicity of, 226t
Fentanyl, 223t. *See also* Opiates/opioids
Fenthion. *See also* Organophosphates
hazard summary for, 412t
toxicity of, 226t
Fenvalerate, 254t. *See also* Pyrethrins
FEP test (free erythrocyte protoporphyrin
test), in lead poisoning, 186
Fer-de-lance envenomation, 269t. *See also*
Snakebite
Ferbam (ferric dimethyldithiocarbamate),
hazard summary for, 413t
Ferric ferrocyanide (ferric hexacyanofer-
rate, Prussian blue)
for radiation exposure, 260t
for thallium poisoning, 277
Ferrous gluconate, abdominal x-ray show-
ing, 39t. *See also* Iron
Ferrous sulfate, abdominal x-ray showing,
39t. *See also* Iron
Ferrovanadium dust, hazard summary for,
413t
Fibrous glass dust, hazard summary for,
413t
Ficus sap, 248t
Fire coral envenomation, 183–184

Fire fighters, occupational exposures associated with, 352t
Firethorn, 248t
Fish
anaphylactic/anaphylactoid reactions
and, 25t
food poisoning caused by, 158–159
Flecainide. *See also* Antiarrhythmic
drugs, newer
atrioventricular block and, 9t
bradycardia and, 9t
hypotension and, 15t
QRS interval prolongation and, 10t
toxicity of, 67, 67t
Flexeril. *See* Cyclobenzaprine
Fluid loss, hypotension and, 15t
Fluid therapy (intravenous fluids)
for anaphylactic/anaphylactoid reactions, 26
for circulatory maintenance, 9
for hypotension, 15
Flumazenil
for benzodiazepine overdose, 91, 313
for sedative-hypnotic overdose, 266
pharmacology/use of, 313–314
Flumethiazide, 145t. *See also* Diuretics
Fluoride, 154–155
calcium for poisoning with, 299
carbonyl, hazard summary for, 382t
chlorine (chlorine trifluoride), hazard
summary for, 383t
hazard summary for, 413t
hydrogen (hydrofluoric acid), 167–169
calcium for burns with, 299
hazard summary for, 419t
systemic effects of, 39t
topical treatment of burns with, 40t
toxicity of, 115t, 163t, 167–169
hyperkalemia and, 32
hypotension and, 15t
nitrogen (nitrogen trifluoride), hazard
summary for, 440t
oxygen (oxygen difluroide), hazard summary for, 443t
perchloryl, hazard summary for, 445t
seizures and, 21t
sulfuryl, hazard summary for, 461t
toxicity of, 154–155
ventricular arrhythmias and, 13t
vinyl, carcinogenicity of, 500t
vinylidine, carcinogenicity of, 500t
Fluorinated hydrocarbons. *See* Freons
Fluorine. *See also* Gases, irritant
hazard summary for, 413t
toxicity of, 163t
Fluorine monoxide (oxygen difluoride),
hazard summary for, 443t
Fluoroacetate
hazard summary for, 458t
toxicity of, 155–156
Fluorocarbon
12 (dichlorodifluoromethane), hazard
summary for, 396t
21 (dichlorofluoromethane), hazard
summary for, 398t

o-Isopropoxyphenyl N-methylcarbamate
(*cont*.)
hazard summary for, 452*t*
toxicity of, 107*t*
Isopropyl acetate, hazard summary for,
423*t*
Isopropyl alcohol (isopropanol), **181–183**
carcinogens in production of, 491*t*
elevated osmolar gap and, 29*t*
elimination of, 49*t*
estimation of level of from osmolar gap,
30*t*
hazard summary for, 423*t*
odor caused by, 29*t*
pupil size affected by, 28*t*
toxicity of, **181–183**
toxicologic blood tests affected by, 37*t*
in toxicology screening, 35*t*
Isopropylamine, hazard summary for, 423*t*
Isopropylbenzene (cumene), hazard summary for, 391*t*
Isopropyl cellosolve (2-isopropoxyetha-
nol), hazard summary for, 422*t*
Isopropyl ether, hazard summary for, 423*t*
Isopropyl glycidyl ether, hazard summary
for, 423*t*
Isoproterenol
for bradycardia and atrioventricular
block, 10, 318
pharmacology/use of, **318**
for torsades de pointes, 14, 318
Isoptin. *See* Verapamil
Isosafrole, carcinogenicity of, 491*t*
Isoxathion, 226*t*. *See also* Organophos-
phates
Isuprel. *See* Isoproterenol
Ivy
American, 246*t*
Boston, 246*t*
devils, 247*t*
English, 247*t*
glacier, 248*t*
heart, 247*t*
oakleaf, 250*t*
Ivy bush, 248*t*

Jack-in-the-pulpit, 248*t*
Jackhammer operators, occupational ex-
posures associated with, 352*t*
Jalap, 248*t*
Jasmolin I or II (pyrethrum), hazard sum-
mary for, 453*t*
Jatropha spp, 246*t*
Jaundice, occupational causes of, 356*t*
"Jaw thrust" maneuver, 1, 4*i*
Jellyfish envenomation, **183–184**
hair, baking soda for, 184
little mauve stinger, baking soda for,
184
Jequirity bean, 248*t*
Jerusalem cherry, unripe berries of, 248*t*
Jessamine, 248*t*
Carolina, 248*t*
day, 248*t*
night, 248*t*
yellow, 248*t*

Jetbead, 249*t*
Jetberry bush, 249*t*
Jimmyweed, 249*t*
Jimsonweed, 249*t*. *See also* Anticholin-
ergics
"Joints". *See* Marijuana
Juglans, 251*t*
Jumping spider envenomation, 272–274
Juniper (*Juniperus macropoda*), 249*t*

Kalmia spp, 248t, 249t
Kanamycin, 69*t*. *See also* Antibiotics
Karwinskia humboldtiana, 246*t*, 247*t*
Kava-kava, 249*t*
Kayexalate (sodium polystyrene sulfo-
nate)
for hyperkalemia, 32
for potassium toxicity, 46*t*
Kentucky coffee tree, 249*t*
Kepone (chlordecone). *See also* Chlorin-
ated hydrocarbon pesticides
carcinogenicity of, 491*t*
hazard summary for, 424*t*
repeat-dose activated charcoal for re-
moval of, 50*t*
toxicity of, 118*t*
Kerosene, 166*t*. *See also* Hydrocarbons
Ketamine, dyskinesias and, 23*t*
Ketene, hazard summary for, 424*t*
Ketone, Michler's, carcinogenicity of, 493*t*
Ketoprofen, 221*t*. *See also* Nonsteroidal
anti-inflammatory agents
Khat, 249*t*
Kidneys. *See also terms beginning with
Renal*
carcinogens affecting, 502*t*
occupational exposures affecting, 356,
357*t*
King snake envenomation, 269*t*. *See also*
Snakebite
Klonopin. *See* Clonazepam
KOH (potassium hydroxide), hazard sum-
mary for, 451*t*
Konakion. *See* Vitamin K₁
Krait envenomation, 269*t*. *See also* Snake-
bite
Kwell. *See* Lindane (gamma benzene hy-
drochloride)
KZn₂(CrO₄)₂(OH) (zinc potassium chro-
mate), hazard summary for, 475*t*

**L-Dopa, and monoamine oxidase inhibitor
interaction, 209t**
Labetalol. *See also* Beta-adrenergic
blockers
for hypertension, 17, 319
pharmacology/use of, **319**
toxicity of, 93*t*
Labrador tea, 249*t*
Laburnum anagyroides, 248*t*
Lampropeltis envenomation, 269*t*. *See
also* Snakebite
Lannate (methomyl). *See also* Carbamate
insecticides